29

DATE DUE

		PRINTED IN U.S.A.

ESSENTIALS OF KUMAR & CLARK'S CLINICAL MEDICINE

ESSENTIALS

SERIES EDITORS

PROFESSOR PARVEEN KUMAR
Professor of Medicine and Education,
Barts and the London School of Medicine and Dentistry,
Queen Mary University of London, and
Honorary Consultant Physician and Gastroenterologist,
Barts Health NHS Trust and Homerton University Hospital
NHS Foundation Trust, London, UK
and

DR MICHAEL CLARK
Honorary Senior Lecturer, Barts and the London School of
Medicine and Dentistry, Queen Mary University of London,
and Princess Grace Hospital, London, UK

Content Strategist: Pauline Graham
Content Development Specialist: Helen Leng
Project Manager: Andrew Riley
Designer: Christian Bilbow
Illustration Manager: Teresa McBryan

ESSENTIALS OF KUMAR & CLARK'S CLINICAL MEDICINE

SIXTH EDITION

EDITED BY

NICOLA ZAMMITT

MBCHB, BSC(MED SCI), MD, FRCP(EDIN)

Consultant Physician and Honorary Clinical Senior Lecturer,
Royal Infirmary of Edinburgh, Edinburgh, UK

ALASTAIR O'BRIEN

MBBS, BSC, PHD, FRCP

Reader in Experimental Hepatology, University College
London Consultant Hepatologist, UCLH &
The Royal Free Hospital NHS Trusts, London, UK

ELSEVIER

ELSEVIER

© 2018 Elsevier Ltd. All rights reserved.

First edition 1995
Second edition 2000
Third edition 2003
Fourth edition 2007
Fifth edition 2012
Sixth edition 2018

ISBN 9780702066030
Int'l ISBN 9780702066054

British Library Cataloguing in Publication Data
A catalogue record for this book is available from the British Library

Library of Congress Cataloging in Publication Data
A catalog record for this book is available from the Library of Congress

Notices

Knowledge and best practice in this field are constantly changing. As new research and experience broaden our understanding, changes in research methods, professional practices, or medical treatment may become necessary.

Practitioners and researchers must always rely on their own experience and knowledge in evaluating and using any information, methods, compounds, or experiments described herein. In using such information or methods they should be mindful of their own safety and the safety of others, including parties for whom they have a professional responsibility.

With respect to any drug or pharmaceutical products identified, readers are advised to check the most current information provided (i) on procedures featured or (ii) by the manufacturer of each product to be administered, to verify the recommended dose or formula, the method and duration of administration, and contraindications. It is the responsibility of practitioners, relying on their own experience and knowledge of their patients, to make diagnoses, to determine dosages and the best treatment for each individual patient, and to take all appropriate safety precautions.

To the fullest extent of the law, neither the publisher nor the authors, contributors, or editors, assume any liability for any injury and/or damage to persons or property as a matter of products liability, negligence or otherwise, or from any use or operation of any methods, products, instructions, or ideas contained in the material herein.

ELSEVIER   your source for books,
journals and multimedia
in the health sciences

www.elsevierhealth.com

Working together
to grow libraries in
developing countries

www.elsevier.com • www.bookaid.org

The
Publisher's
policy is to use
paper manufactured
from sustainable forests

Printed in China
Last digit is the print number: 9   8   7   6   5   4   3   2   1

Contents

Preface

This is the sixth edition of *Essentials of Kumar & Clark's Clinical Medicine* and we continue to strive to produce a small medical textbook with anatomy, physiology and pathophysiology as a key part to understanding clinical features and treatment for each disease process. The book is based on its parent textbook, *Kumar & Clark's Clinical Medicine*, from which we have taken these core principles. A key feature of the book is that it remains small and easy to carry around as a portable reference source.

The sixth edition has been extensively revised and updated, in line with changes in clinical medicine and with its parent text. Some updates reflect advances in medical science, including the increasing range of available biological therapies and the development of novel oral anticoagulants. Although it is beyond the scope of this book to provide an exhaustive drug list that covers prescribing in all patient groups, we have retained the section at the end of each chapter specifically dedicated to a description of common drugs relevant to that system. Some changes relate to the ethical approaches to medicine. The chapter on ethics and communication has been extensively revised in the light of the GMC's duty of candour and the recognition of the power and importance of apology and honesty when dealing with patients and families when things go wrong. The textbook has also been revised in the light of social changes, such as the increasing use of novel psychoactive substances and their medical consequences. Updated guidelines, such as those covering the treatment of malaria, are also included in this text. These represent just some of the advances in clinical medicine that have been incorporated into this edition.

The sixth edition of *Essentials of Clinical Medicine* has seen many changes from previous editions, including new editors. However, the current edition would never have evolved into its current state without the very significant work done in the past by Anne Ballinger, who edited the first five editions. It also goes without saying that the constant feature throughout every edition is the support and assistance of Mike Clark and Parveen Kumar, the editors of *Clinical Medicine* and this series of small textbooks.

Nicola Zammitt

Contributors

Jennifer C. Crane MRCP DTM&H
Consultant Acute Medicine and Infectious Diseases
Western General Hospital
Edinburgh, UK
2. Infectious diseases

Euan A. Sandilands MD FRCP(Edin) PGCert (MedEd)
Consultant Physician in Clinical Toxicology and Acute Medicine. National Poisons
Information Service (Edinburgh), Royal Infirmary of Edinburgh, UK
13. Clinical pharmacology and toxicology

Katharine F. Strachan MA, FRCP
Consultant Physician, Acute & General Medicine
Clinical Lead for Medical Ethics Education
Royal Infirmary of Edinburgh, UK
1. Ethics and communication

Medical emergencies

Abbreviations

AAT	α_1-antitrypsin
ABPM	ambulatory blood pressure monitoring
ABV	alcohol by volume
ABVD	chemotherapy involving doxorubicin, bleomycin, vinblastine, dacarbazine
ACBT	active cycle of breathing technique
ACE	angiotensin-converting enzyme
ACEI	angiotensin-converting enzyme inhibitor
ACR	urine albumin-to-creatinine ratio
ACSs	acute coronary syndromes
ACT	artemisinin combination therapy
ACTH	adrenocorticotrophic hormone
ADA	American Diabetes Association
ADC	AIDS–dementia complex
ADH	antidiuretic hormone
ADP	adenosine diphosphate
ADPKD	autosomal-dominant polycystic kidney disease
AED	automated external defibrillator
AEDs	antiepileptic drugs
AF	atrial fibrillation
AFP	α-fetoprotein
AIDS	acquired immunodeficiency syndrome
AIH	autoimmune hepatitis
AKI	acute kidney injury
AKIN	Acute Kidney Injury Network
ALL	acute lymphoblastic leukaemia
ALP	alkaline phosphatase
ALS	advanced life support
ALT	alanine aminotransferase
AMAs	antimitochondrial antibodies
AML	acute myeloid leukaemia
AMP	adenosine monophosphate
ANA	antinuclear antibodies
ANCA	antineutrophil cytoplasmic antibodies
ANF	antinuclear factor

ANP	atrial natriuretic peptide
anti-AChR antibodies	autoantibodies to acetylcholine receptors
anti-CCP	cyclic citrullinated peptide antibodies
anti-HBc	anti-hepatitis B core antibody
anti-HBe	anti-hepatitis e antibody
anti-HBs	anti-hepatitis B surface antibody
anti-MuSK antibodies	antibodies against a muscle-specific receptor tyrosine kinase
APACHE	acute physiology and chronic health evaluation
APML	acute promyelocytic leukaemia
APTT	activated partial thromboplastin time
ARA	angiotensin II receptor antagonist
ARD	autoimmune rheumatic disease
ARDS	adult respiratory distress syndrome
ARE	angiotensin II type 1 receptor antagonists
ARR	aldosterone:renin ratio
ART	antiretroviral therapy
ARVs	
5-ASA	aminosalicylic acid
AST	aspartate aminotransferase
AT	antithrombin
AT	angiotensin
AT$_1$ receptor	type 1 subtype of the angiotensin II receptor
ATN	acute tubular necrosis
ATRA	all-*trans*-retinoic acid
ATS	amfetamine-type stimulants
AV	atrioventricular
AVF	augmented vector foot (the name of an ECG lead)
AVL	augmented vector Left (the name of an ECG lead)
AVMs	arteriovenous malformations
AVNRT	atrioventricular nodal re-entry tachycardia
AVPU score	Alert, responds to Voice, responds to Pain, Unresponsive
AVR	augmented vector right (the name of an ECG lead)
AVRT	atrioventricular reciprocating tachycardia
AXR	abdominal X-ray
BCC	basal cell carcinoma
BCG	bacille Calmette–Guérin
β-hCG	β-human chorionic gonadotrophin
BHL	bilateral hilar lymphadenopathy
BiPAP	bilevel positive airway pressure

BLS	basic life support
BM	blood glucose monitoring
BMD	bone mineral density
BMI	body mass index
BMT	bone marrow transplantation
BNP	brain natriuretic peptide
BODE	**b**ody mass index, degree of airflow **o**bstruction — FEV_1, **d**yspnoea, **e**xercise capacity
BP	blood pressure
BPH	benign prostatic hypertrophy
BSE	bovine spongiform encephalopathy
CABG	coronary artery bypass grafting
CAD	coronary artery disease
cAMP	cyclic adenosine monophosphate
CAPD	continuous ambulatory peritoneal dialysis
CBD	common bile duct
CCF	congestive cardiac failure
CCU	coronary care unit
CD	cluster differentiation
CD	Crohn's disease
CDC	Centers for Disease Control and Prevention
CDI	cranial diabetes insipidus
CEA	carcinoembryonic antigen
CF	cystic fibrosis
CFTR	cystic fibrosis transmembrane conductance regulator
cGMP	cyclic guanosine monophosphate
CGRP	calcitonin gene-related peptide
CHADS$_2$ score	congestive heart failure, hypertension, age $\geq$75 years, diabetes mellitus and previous stroke or transient ischaemic attack
CHD	coronary heart disease
CHOP + R	chemo-immunotherapy involving cyclophosphamide, hydroxydaunorubicin, vincristine, prednisolone and rituximab
CJD	Creutzfeldt–Jakob disease
CK	creatine kinase, creatine phosphokinase
CKD	chronic kidney disease
CK-MB	the MB isoform of creatine kinase (CK)
CLL	chronic lymphatic leukaemia
CML	chronic myeloid leukaemia
CMR	cardiovascular magnetic resonance
CMV	cytomegalovirus

CNS	central nervous system
COHb	carboxyhaemoglobin
COPD	chronic obstructive pulmonary disease
COX	cyclo-oxygenase
CPAP	continuous positive airway pressure
CPR	cardiopulmonary resuscitation
Cr	creatinine
CRC	colorectal cancer
CREST syndrome	Calcinosis, Raynaud's phenomenon, Esophageal involvement, Sclerodactyly, Telangiectasia
CRGP	calcitonin gene-related peptide
CRH	corticotrophin-releasing hormone
CRP	C-reactive protein
CSII	continuous subcutaneous insulin infusion
CSF	cerebrospinal fluid
CT	computed tomography
CTH	corticotrophin-releasing hormone
CTPA	CT pulmonary angiogram
CTZ	chemoreceptor trigger zone
CVC	central venous catheter
CVP	central venous pressure
CVS	cardiovascular system
CXR	chest X-ray
DAEC	diffusely adhering *E. coli*
DAMPs	damage-associated molecular patterns
DaT	dopamine transporter
DBS	deep brain stimulation
DCM	dilated cardiomyopathy
DcSSc	diffuse cutaneous scleroderma
DCT	direct Coombs' test
δ-ALA	δ-aminolaevulinic acid
DHF	dengue haemorrhagic fever
DI	diabetes insipidus
DIC	disseminated intravascular coagulation
DIDMOAD syndrome	hereditary association of diabetes insipidus, diabetes mellitus, optic atrophy and deafness
DIPJs	distal interphalangeal joints
DKA	diabetic ketoacidosis
DM	dermatomyositis
DMARDs	disease-modifying antirheumatic drugs
DNA	deoxyribonucleic acid

DNACPR	do not attempt CPR
DOTS	directly observed therapy
DPLD	diffuse parenchymal lung diseases
DPTA	diethylenetriaminepentaacetic acid
ds	double-stranded
DSH	deliberate self-harm
DU	duodenal ulcer
DVLA	Driver and Vehicle Licensing Agency
DVT	deep venous thrombosis
DXA	dual-energy X-ray absorptiometry
EABV	effective arterial blood volume
EAggEC	enteroaggregative *E. coli*
EB	epidermolysis bullosa
EBNA	Epstein–Barr virus nuclear antigen
EBV	Epstein–Barr virus
ECG	electrocardiogram
EDR	extensively drug-resistant
EEG	electroencephalogram
eGFR	estimation of the glomerular filtration rate
EHEC	enterohaemorrhagic *E. coli*
EIA	enzyme-linked immunoassay
EIEC	enteroinvasive *E. coli*
ELISA	enzyme-linked immunosorbent assay
EM	erythema migrans
EM	erythema multiforme
EMA	endomysial antibodies
EMD	electromechanical dissociation
EMG	electromyography, electromyogram
EMR	endoscopic mucosal resection
ENT	ear, nose and throat
EPEC	enteropathogenic *E. coli*
EPR	electronic patient record
ERC	European Resuscitation Council
ERCP	endoscopic retrograde cholangiopancreatography
ESKD	end-stage kidney disease
ESR	erythrocyte sedimentation rate
ESWL	extracorporeal shock wave lithotripsy
ETEC	enterotoxigenic *E. coli*
EUS	endoscopic ultrasound
FAST	Face, Arm, Speech, Time
FAT	fluorescent antibody test

FBC	full blood count
FCU	first catch urine
FDG	fluorodeoxyglucose
FDPs	fibrin degradation products
FEV	forced expiratory volume
FEV$_1$	forced expiratory volume in 1 second
FFP	fresh frozen plasma
FNA	fine-needle aspiration
FSH	follicle-stimulating hormone
FVC	forced vital capacity
GABA	γ-aminobutyric acid
γ-GT	γ-glutamyl transpeptidase
GBM	glomerular basement membrane
GBS	Guillain–Barré syndrome
GCA	giant cell arteritis
GCS	Glasgow Coma Scale
G-CSF	granulocyte colony stimulating factor
GFR	glomerular filtration rate
GH	growth hormone
GHRH	growth hormone releasing hormone
GI	gastrointestinal
GIST	gastrointestinal stromal tumour
GLP-1	glucagon-like peptide-1
GMC	General Medical Council
GnRH	gonadotropin-releasing hormone
GORD	gastro-oesophageal reflux disease
Gp	glycoprotein
GPA	granulomatosis with polyangiitis (Wegener's granulomatosis)
G6PD	glucose-6-phosphate dehydrogenase
GPI	glycosylphosphatidylinositol
GRACE	Global Registry of Acute Coronary Events
GTN	glyceryl trinitrate
GTT	glucose tolerance test
GU	gastric ulcer
GVHD	graft-versus-host disease
H	haemagglutinin
HAV	hepatitis A virus
Hb	haemoglobin
HbA$_{1c}$	glycosylated haemoglobin
HBeAg	hepatitis B e antigen
HBPM	home blood pressure monitoring

HBsAg	hepatitis B surface antigen
HBV	hepatitis B virus
HCC	hepatocellular carcinoma
HCG	human chorionic gonadotrophin
HCM	hypertrophic cardiomyopathy
HCV	hepatitis C virus
HDLs	high-density lipoproteins
HDU	high-dependency unit
HGPRT	hypoxanthine-guanine phosphoribosyltransferase
HH	hereditary haemochromatosis
5-HIAA	5-hydroxyindoleacetic acid
HIV	human immunodeficiency virus
HLA	human leucocyte antigen
HMG-CoA	hydroxymethylglutaryl-coenzyme A
HNPCC	hereditary non-polyposis colorectal cancer
HPV	human papilloma virus
HRT	hormone replacement therapy
HSV	herpes simplex virus
5-HT	5-hydroxytryptamine
HTLV	human T-cell lymphotropic virus
IABCP	intra-aortic balloon counterpulsation
IBD	inflammatory bowel diseases
IBS	irritable bowel syndrome
ICAM-1	intercellular adhesion molecule-1
ICD	implantable cardioverter–defibrillator
ICD	International Classification of Diseases – the classification used to code and classify mortality data from death certificates
ICD-9-CM	ICD, Clinical Modification – used to code and classify morbidity data from the inpatient and outpatient records, general practices and Health Statistic surveys
ICP	intracranial pressure
ICU	intensive care unit
IDLs	intermediate-density lipoproteins
IFG	impaired fasting glucose
IFN	interferon
Ig	immunoglobulin (e.g. IgM = immunoglobulin M class)
IGF-1	insulin-like growth factor 1
IGT	impaired glucose tolerance
IHD	ischaemic heart disease
IL	interleukin

i.m.	intramuscular, intramuscularly
IMV	intermittent mandatory ventilation
INR	international normalized ratio
IPF	idiopathic pulmonary fibrosis
IPJs	interphalangeal joints
IPPV	intermittent positive-pressure ventilation
ITP	immune thrombocytopenic purpura
iu/IU	international unit
i.v.	intravenous
IVP	intravenous pyelogram, intravenous pyelography
IVU	intravenous urography
JVP	jugular venous pressure
KUB	kidney, ureters and bladder
LABA	long-acting selective inhaled β_2-adrenoceptor stimulants
LBBB	left bundle branch block
LcSSc	limited cutaneous scleroderma
LDH	lactate dehydrogenase
LDLs	low-density lipoproteins
L-dopa	levodopa
LEMS	Lambert–Eaton myasthenic syndrome
LFT	liver function test
LH	luteinizing hormone
LHRH	luteinizing hormone-releasing hormone
LMN	lower motor neurone
LMWH	low molecular weight heparin
LOS	lower oesophageal sphincter
LP	lumbar puncture
LTRA	leukotriene receptor antagonists
LVEF	left ventricular ejection fraction
LVF	left ventricular failure
LVSD	left ventricular systolic dysfunction
MAI	*Mycobacterium avium-intracellulare*
MALT	mucosa-associated lymphoid tissue
MALToma	mucosa-associated lymphoid tissue tumour
MCA	Mental Capacity Act
MCH	mean corpuscular haemoglobin
MCHC	mean corpuscular haemoglobin concentration
MCP	metacarpophalanges
MCV	mean corpuscular volume
MDIs	metered-dose inhalers

MDR	multidrug-resistant
MDRD	modification of diet in renal disease
MDS	myelodysplastic syndrome
MDT	multidisciplinary team
ME	myalgic encephalomyelitis
MEN	multiple endocrine neoplasia syndromes
MERS-CoV	Middle East respiratory syndrome coronavirus
MEWS	Modified Early Warning Score
MG	myasthenia gravis
MHRA	Medicines and Healthcare products Regulatory Agency
MI	myocardial infarction
mIBG	meta-[^{131}I]-iodobenzylguanidine
MMR	measles, mumps and rubella
MMSE	Mini Mental State Examination
MODS	multiple organ dysfunction syndrome
MPTP	methylphenyltetrahydropyridine
MR	magnetic resonance
MRCP	magnetic resonance cholangiopancreatography
MRI	magnetic resonance imaging
MRSA	meticillin-resistant *Staphylococcus aureus*
MS	multiple sclerosis
MSU	mid-stream urine
M–W tear	Mallory–Weiss tear
N	neuraminidase
Na$^+$	concentration of sodium ions
NAC	*N*-acetylcysteine
NAFLD	non-alcoholic fatty liver disease
NAPQI	*N*-acetyl-*p*-benzoquinoneimine
NBT-PABA	*N*-benzoyl-L-tryosyl-*p*-amino benzoic acid
nd	notifiable disease
NDI	nephrogenic diabetes insipidus
NERD	non-erosive reflux disease
NG	nasogastric
NHL	non-Hodgkin's lymphoma
NHS	National Health Service
NICE	National Institute for Health and Care Excellence
NIPPV	non-invasive positive-pressure ventilation
NK	natural killer (cell)
NMDA	N-methyl-D-aspartate
NOACs	novel oral anticoagulants

NPH	neutral protamine Hagedorn
NPS	novel psychoactive substances
NS1	non-structural protein 1
NSAIDs	non-steroidal anti-inflammatory drugs
NSTEMI	non-ST-segment elevation myocardial infarction
NTproBNP	N terminal fragment released from pro-BNP
NYHA	New York Heart Association
OA	osteoarthritis
OCP	oral contraceptive pill
OGD	oesophagogastroduodenoscopy
OPG	osteoprotegerin
ORS	oral rehydration solutions
OSA	obstructive sleep apnoea
OSCE	Objective Structured Clinical Examination
PA	postero-anterior, postero-anteriorly
$P_a\text{co}_2$	partial pressure of carbon dioxide in arterial blood
PAMPS	pathogen-associated molecular patterns
PAN	polyarteritis nodosa
pANCA	peripheral antineutrophilic cytoplasmic antibody
$P_a\text{o}_2$	partial pressure of oxygen in arterial blood
PAP	pulmonary artery pressure
PAS	periodic acid-Schiff
PBC	primary biliary cirrhosis
PCA	patient-controlled analgesia
PCI	percutaneous coronary intervention
PCOS	polycystic ovary syndrome
PCR	urine protein-to-creatinine ratio
PCR	polymerase chain reaction
PCT	porphyria cutanea tarda
PCV	packed cell volume
PD	Parkinson's disease
PD-1	programmed death receptor
PDE4	phosphodiesterase type 4
PDEI	phosphodiesterase inhibitor
PE	pulmonary embolism, pulmonary embolus
PE	phenytoin sodium equivalent
PEEP	positive end-expiratory pressure
PEFR	peak expiratory flow rate
PEG	percutaneous endoscopic gastrostomy
PET	positron emission tomography

Ph	Philadelphia
PHN	post-herpetic neuralgia
PIPJs	proximal interphalangeal joints
PM	polymyositis
PMF	progressive massive fibrosis
PML	progressive multi-focal leucoencephalopathy
PML-RARa	fusion protein involving promyelocytic leukaemia gene and retinoic acid receptor alpha
PMR	polymyalgia
POEM	per oral endoscopic myotomy
PPAR-γ	peroxisome proliferator-activated receptor-gamma
PPI	proton pump inhibitor
PPMS	primary progressive multiple sclerosis
PPS	phosphoribosyl-pyrophosphate synthetase
PR	per rectum (rectal instillation)
PSA	prostate-specific antigen
PSC	primary sclerosing cholangitis
PSE	portosystemic encephalopathy
PT	prothrombin time
PTC	percutaneous transhepatic cholangiography
PTCA	percutaneous transluminal coronary angioplasty
PTH	parathyroid hormone
PTTK	partial thromboplastin time with kaolin
PU	peptic ulcer, peptic ulceration
PUO	pyrexia (or fever) of unknown origin
PUVA	ultraviolet A radiation in conjunction with a photosensitizing agent, oral or topical psoralen
PVS	persistent vegetative state
PWP	pulmonary wedge pressure
RA	rheumatoid arthritis
RANK	receptor activator of nuclear factor-κB
RANKL	RANK ligand
RAPD	relative afferent pupillary defect
RAS	renal artery stenosis
RAST	radioallergosorbent test
RBBB	right bundle branch block
RCC	red cell count
RDW	red blood cell distribution width
RFA	radiofrequency ablation
Rh	rhesus
RhF	rheumatoid factor

RIA	radioimmunoassay
RIF	right iliac fossa
RIFLE criteria	Risk, Injury, Failure, Loss, End-stage renal disease
RNA	ribonucleic acid
RNP	ribonucleoprotein
r-PA	reteplase
RR	respiratory rate
RRMS	relapsing-remitting multiple sclerosis
RSR′	secondary R wave
RT-PCR	reverse transcriptase polymerase chain reaction
RUQ	right upper quadrant
RV	right ventricle
RV	residual volume
RVSD	right ventricular systolic dysfunction
SA node	sinus node
SAH	subarachnoid haemorrhage
SALT	Speech and Language Therapy
S_aO_2	arterial oxygen saturation
SARS	severe acute respiratory syndrome
SBAR	Situation-Background-Assessment-Recommendations
SBE	subacute (bacterial) endocarditis
SBFT	small bowel follow-through
SBP	spontaneous bacterial peritonitis
SBP	systolic blood pressure
s.c.	subcutaneous
SCC	squamous cell carcinoma
SCr	serum creatinine
$S_{cv}O_2$	central venous oxyhaemoglobin saturation
SDH	subdural haematoma
SDs	standard deviations
SERMs	selective oestrogen receptor modulators
SGLT2	sodium/glucose transporter 2
SIADH	syndrome of inappropriate ADH secretion
SIRS	systemic inflammatory response syndrome
SLE	systemic lupus erythematosus
SP	standardized patient
SPECT	single photon emission computed tomography
SR	slow-release
SRH	stigmata of recent haemorrhage
SS	Sjögren's syndrome

SSc	systemic scleroderma
STEMI	ST-elevation myocardial infarction
STI	sexually transmitted infection
SUNCT	short-lasting unilateral neuralgiform headache attacks with conjunctival injection and tearing
SVC	superior vena cava
SVR	sustained virological response
SVR	systemic vascular resistance
SVT	supraventricular tachycardia
T_3	triiodothyronine
T_4	thyroxine
TAVI	transcatheter aortic valve implantation
TB	tuberculosis
TBE	tick-borne encephalitis
TBG	thyroxine-binding globulin
TCAs	tricyclic antidepressants
TEN	toxic epidermal necrolyis
TF	tissue factor
TFPI	tissue factor pathway inhibitor
TFT	thyroid function test
Th	T helper
THC	tetrahydrocannabinol
TIA	transient ischaemic attack
TIBC	total iron-binding capacity
TIMI	Thrombolysis in Myocardial Infarction scoring system
TIN	tubulointerstitial nephritis
TIPS	transjugular intrahepatic portosystemic shunting
TLC	total lung capacity
TLESRs	transient lower oesophageal sphincter relaxations
TNF	tumour necrosis factor
TNK-PA	tenecteplase
TNM	tumour, node, metastasis classification
TOE	transoesophageal echocardiography
tPA	tissue plasminogen activator
TPN	total parenteral nutrition
TPMT	thiopurine methyltransferase
TRH	thyrotrophin-releasing hormone
TSH	thyroid-stimulating hormone
TT	thrombin time
TTE	transthoracic echocardiography
tTG	tissue transglutaminase

TTP	thrombotic thrombocytopenic purpura
UC	ulcerative colitis
U/E	urea and electrolytes
UMN	upper motor neurone
US	ultrasound
UTI	urinary tract infection
UVA	ultraviolet A radiation
VATS	video-assisted thoracoscopic (lung biopsy)
VCA	viral capsid antigen
VCAM	vascular cell adhesion molecule
VCAM-1	vascular cell adhesion molecule – 1
vCJD	variant Creutzfeldt–Jakob disease
VDRL	Venereal Disease Research Laboratory (test for syphilis)
VEGF	vascular endothelial growth factor
VF	ventricular fibrillation
VHF	viral haemorrhagic fever
VIP	vasoactive intestinal polypeptide
VLDLs	very-low-density lipoproteins
$\dot{V}/\dot{Q}$	ventilation–perfusion
VT	ventricular tachycardia
VTE	venous thromboembolism
vWF	von Willebrand factor
VZV	varicella-zoster virus
WBC	white blood (cell) count
WBI	whole bowel irrigation
WCC	white cell count
WE	Wernicke's encephalopathy
WHO	World Health Organization
WPW	Wolff–Parkinson–White
ZIG	zoster-immune immunoglobulin
ZN	Ziehl–Neelsen

Significant websites

General websites

Medical dictionaries

http://medical-dictionary.thefreedictionary.com/

http://www.online-medical-dictionary.org/

Guidelines and evidence-based medicine

http://www.nice.org.uk
UK National Institute for Health and Care Excellence

http://www.nih.gov/health
US National Institutes of Health

http://www.sign.ac.uk
Scottish Intercollegiate Guidelines Network

http://www.library.nhs.uk
NHS Evidence – evidence-based clinical and non-clinical information to help make decisions about treatment and use of resources

http://www.guideline.gov/
National Guideline Clearing House

http://www.dft.gov.uk/dvla/medical/ataglance.aspx
Driver and Vehicle Licensing Agency – guide to the current medical standards of fitness to drive and exclusions

http://www.cochrane.org/cochrane-reviews
Cochrane Reviews are part of the *Cochrane Library* and provide systematic reviews of primary research in human healthcare and health policy. They investigate the effects of interventions for prevention, treatment and rehabilitation. They also assess the accuracy of a diagnostic test for a given condition in a specific patient group and setting

http://www.medicine.ox.ac.uk/bandolier/index.html
Monthly journal on evidence-based healthcare

http://www.emedicine.com
eMedicine features up-to-date, searchable, peer-reviewed medical journals, on-line physician reference textbooks, a full-text article database and patient information leaflets

http://www.bma.org
British Medical Association. A library, excellent ethics section and healthcare information. More sections for members

Medical calculators

http://www.mdcalc.com/

http://medicineworld.org/online-medical-calculators.html
Clinical calculators and formulas for many conditions, e.g. sodium correction rate in hyponatraemia, APACHE II score and anion gap

Healthcare journals and magazines

www.bmj.com
BMJ (British Medical Journal)

Medical societies and organizations

http://www.gmc-uk.org/
UK General Medical Council

Others

http://www.medilexicon.com/icd9codes.php
Search for the definitions of ICD9/ICD-9-CM codes

http://www.ncbi.nlm.nih.gov/PubMed
PubMed: Medline on the Web

http://www.nhsdirect.nhs.uk

http://www.patient.co.uk
Information for patients on diseases, operations and investigations

http://www.medicalert.org.uk
Charity providing a life-saving identification system for individuals with hidden medical conditions and allergies

Chapter-specific websites

1 Ethics and communication

http://www.bma.org.uk/ethics
British Medical Association ethics site

http://www.ethics-network.org.uk
UK Clinical Ethics Network

http://www.gmc-uk.org/
General Medical Council

https://www.bioethics.nih.gov/home/index.shtml
  National Institutes of Health website – bioethics pages

www.each.eu
  European Association for Communication in Healthcare

https://www.wma.net/policy/
  World Medical Association policy

2 Infectious diseases

http://www.cdc.gov
  US Department of Health and Human Services, Centers for Disease Control and Prevention (CDC). The CDC has a major role in public health efforts to prevent and control infectious and chronic diseases, injuries, workplace hazards, disabilities and environmental health threats

https://www.gov.uk/government/groups/expert-advisory-group-on-aids#announcements-and-publications
  Department of Health Expert Advisory Group on AIDS: information about post-exposure prophylaxis, guidelines for pre-test discussion on HIV testing and risks of transmission

http://www.hivatis.org/
  Centers for Disease Control and Prevention: HIV/AIDS treatment/information service

http://ecdc.europa.eu/en/Pages/home.aspx
  European Centre for Disease Control

http://www.nfid.org
  National Foundation for Infectious Disease, USA

http://www.hpa.org.uk
  Health Protection Agency website. Provides up-to-date information for medical practitioners on some infectious diseases and their prevention, particularly those that are new or where an epidemic is expected

http://www.phls.co.uk/
  UK Public Health Laboratory Service: UK regional information on infections

http://www.who.int/en
  The World Health Organization is the United Nations specialized agency for health. The website provides information and fact sheets on many infectious diseases, and much more

3 Gastroenterology and nutrition

http://www.bsg.org.uk
  British Society of Gastroenterology. Regularly updated clinical practice guidelines for many common conditions

http://www.gastro.org/practice/medical-position-statements
American Gastroenterology Association medical position statements provide preferred approaches to specific medical problems or issues

Information for patients and relatives

http://www.coeliac.co.uk – Coeliac UK

http://www.corecharity.org.uk – Core

http://digestive.niddk.nih.gov/ddiseases/a-z.asp – National Digestive Diseases information clearing house

http://www.gastro.org/patient-care/patientinfo-center – American Gastroenterology Association Patient Centre

www.crohnsandcolitis.org.uk – National Association for Crohn's and Colitis

4 Liver, biliary tract and pancreatic disease

http://www.aasld.org/practiceguidelines/Pages/default.aspx
American Association for the Study of Liver Disease practice guidelines

http://www.easl.eu
European Association for the Study of the Liver

http://www.basl.org.uk/
British Association for the Study of the Liver

Information for patients and relatives

http://www.britishlivertrust.org.uk – British Liver Trust

http://www.liverfoundation.org – American Liver Foundation

http://pancreasfoundation.org – The National Pancreas Foundation

5 Haematological disease

http://www.bcshguidelines.com
The British Committee for Standards in Haematology. Guidelines for medical practitioners on diagnosis and treatment of haematological diseases

http://www.hematology.org
American Society of Haematology. Clinical guidelines, self-assessment programme, teaching cases and video library

Information for patients and relatives

http://www.blood.co.uk – UK National Blood Service

http://www.haemophilia.org.uk – The Haemophilia Society for patients affected by bleeding disorders http://www.leukaemia.org.au – Leukaemia Foundation

www.sicklecellsociety.org – Sickle Cell Society

6 Malignant disease

http://www.cancer.gov
US National Cancer Institute provides cancer statistics, patient information and clinical trials

http://www.endoflifecare-intelligence.org.uk/home
NHS National End of Life Care Programme

Information for patients and relatives

http://www.macmillan.org.uk – Macmillan Cancer Support

http://info.cancerresearchuk.org – Cancer Research UK

7 Rheumatology

http://www.rheumatology.org.uk
The British Society for Rheumatology. Clinical guidelines for medical practitioners

http://www.arthritisresearchuk.org
Arthritis Research UK. Publications on musculoskeletal conditions

http://www.nos.org.uk
National Osteoporosis Society. Guidance on investigation and management of osteoporosis

http://www.rheumatology.org/Practice-Quality/Clinical-Support/Clinical-Practice-Guidelines
American College of Rheumatology clinical practice guidelines

Information for patients and relatives

http://www.rheumatology.org.uk – British Society for Rheumatology

http://www.arthritisresearchuk.org – Arthritis Research UK

http://www.nos.org.uk – National Osteoporosis Society

http://www.nras.org.uk – National Rheumatoid Arthritis Society

8/9 Water, electrolytes and acid–base balance/Renal disease

http://www.arupconsult.com/Topics/ElectrolyteAbnormalities.html
ARUP Consult; the physician's guide to life-threatening electrolyte abnormalities

http://www.britishrenal.org
British Renal Society, guidance on clinical management

http://www.kidney.org/professionals/kdoqi/guidelines.cfm
National Kidney Foundation clinical practice guidelines

http://www.renal.org
The Renal Association guidelines

https://www.nice.org.uk/guidance/cg174/chapter/1-recommendations
NICE guideline (CG174): Intravenous fluid therapy in adults in hospital (published December 2013)

Information for patients and relatives

http://www.kidney.org – UK National Kidney Federation

10 Cardiovascular disease

http://www.erc.edu
European Resuscitation Council (ERC). Latest guidelines on resuscitation, as well as a full overview of the ERC educational tools such as manuals, posters and slides

http://www.resus.org.uk
Resuscitation Council (UK). Resuscitation guidelines

http://www.escardio.org
European Society of Cardiology clinical practice guidelines

http://www.cardiosource.org
American College of Cardiology

http://www.ecglibrary.com
ECG tracings library to help improve ECG skills

Information for patients and relatives

http://www.bhf.org.uk – British Heart Foundation

http://www.americanheart.org – American Heart Association

11 Respiratory disease

http://www.brit-thoracic.org.uk
British Thoracic Society. Clinical practice guidelines and clinical information

http://www.goldcopd.org
The WHO Global Initiative for Chronic Obstructive Lung Disease (GOLD). Clinical guidelines on diagnosis, treatment and prevention of COPD

http://www.thoracic.org
American Thoracic Society, clinical practice guidelines

Information for patients and relatives

http://www.brit-thoracic.org.uk – British Thoracic Society

http://www.asthma.org.uk – Asthma UK

http://www.goldcopd.org – The WHO Global Initiative for COPD

http://www.thoracic.org – American Thoracic Society

http://www.quitsmoking.com – The Quit Smoking Company

http://www.quitsmokinguk.com – NHS Quit Smoking Service

12 Intensive care medicine

http://www.esicm.org
European Society for Intensive Care guidelines and recommendations for medical practitioners

http://www.ics.ac.uk
UK Intensive Care Society standards and guidelines for medical practitioners

http://www.survivingsepsis.org
Surviving Sepsis Campaign clinical guidelines

Information for patients and relatives

http://www.ics.ac.uk – UK Intensive Care Society

http://www.survivingsepsis.org – Surviving Sepsis Campaign

13 Drug therapy, poisoning and alcohol misuse

http://www.mhra.gov.uk
Medicines and Healthcare Products Regulatory Agency includes http://yellowcard.mhra.gov.uk to report suspected side effects to any medication

http://www.toxbase.org
Toxbase. Database of UK National Poisons Information Service

http://www.toxnet.nlm.nih.gov
US National Library of Medicine Toxicology and Environmental Health Information Program. Toxicology, environmental health, chemical databases and other information resources

http://www.who.int/topics/poisons/en/
International Programme on Chemical Safety contact details of all poisons – centres world-wide.

https://www.gov.uk/government/collections/carbon-monoxide-co
Department of Health. Detailed information on carbon monoxide poisoning

Information for patients and relatives

www.patient.co.uk/dils.asp – Patient UK. Information leaflets on specific medicines and drugs

http://www.alcoholscreening.org helps people assess their drinking patterns. http://www.drinksafely.info – useful information about harmful effects of alcohol and guidelines for safe drinking

14 Endocrine disease

http://endocrine.niddk.nih.gov
US National Endocrine and Metabolic Diseases Information Service

http://www.endocrinology.org
Society for Endocrinology. Clinical updates, clinical cases and publications related to endocrinology

http://www.british-thyroid-association.org
British Thyroid Association

Information for patients and relatives

http://www.endocrineweb.com – website for diabetes, osteoporosis, thyroid, parathyroid and other endocrine disorders

http://www.btf-thyroid.org – The British Thyroid Foundation

http://tedct.org.uk – Thyroid Eye Disease Charitable Trust

http://www.pituitary.org.uk – The Pituitary Foundation (UK). Information and support for those living with pituitary disorders

15 Diabetes mellitus and other disorders of metabolism

http://www.idf.org
International Diabetes Federation

Information for patients, relatives and healthcare professionals

http://www.diabetes.org.uk – Diabetes UK

http://www.diabetes.org – American Diabetes Association.

http://www.jdrf.org.uk – Juvenile Diabetes Research Foundation (UK)

16 The special senses

http://www.nei.nih.gov
National Eye Institute with a professional section of statistics and pathology collection

http://www.eyeatlas.com/contents.htm
Online atlas of ophthalmology

http://www.entuk.org
British Association of Otorhinolaryngologists guidelines and position papers

Information for patients and relatives

https://www.actiononhearingloss.org.uk/ – Deafness Research UK

http://www.nei.nih.gov – National Eye Institute

http://www.entuk.org – British Association of Otorhinolaryngologists

17 Neurology

http://www.theabn.org
Documents relating to evidence-based neurology

Information for patients and relatives

http://www.epilepsy.org.uk – Epilepsy Action

http://www.gbs.org.uk – Guillain–Barré Syndrome Support Group

http://www.mssociety.org.uk – UK Multiple Sclerosis Society

http://www.parkinsons.org.uk – Parkinson's Disease Society

http://www.stroke.org.uk – The Stroke Association (UK)

18 Dermatology

http://www.dermatlas.net/
A collection of 11 750 images in dermatology and skin disease

http://www.bad.org.uk
British Association of Dermatologists clinical guidelines and other professional information.

Information for patients and relatives

http://www.eczema.org – UK National Eczema Society

http://www.paalliance.org – Psoriatic Arthropathy Alliance (psoriasis)

Therapeutics

http://bnf.org – *British National Formulary*. Authoritative and practical information on the selection and clinical use of drugs

http://www.dtb.org.uk/idtb – *Drug and Therapeutics Bulletin*. Independent reviews of medical treatment.
Registration is necessary for these websites.

1 Ethics and communication

Ethical and legal issues are integrally involved with patient care. A doctor with clinical responsibility for a patient has three corresponding duties of care:

- *Protect life and health.* Clinicians should practise medicine to a high standard and not cause unnecessary suffering or harm. Treatment should only be given when it is thought to be beneficial to that patient. Competent patients have the right to refuse treatment, including life-sustaining treatment. Such decisions should be informed by a clear explanation about the consequences of refusal.
- *Respect the right to autonomy.* Clinicians must protect the patient's right to respect for autonomy and self-determination, and support patients in reasoning, planning and making choices about their future. Wherever possible, patients should remain responsible for themselves. Informed consent gives meaning to autonomy and, alongside the duty to respect patient confidentiality and human dignity, represents a fundamental feature of good medical practice.
- *Protect life and health, and respect autonomy with fairness and justice.* All patients have the right to be treated equally and without prejudice or favouritism, regardless of race, fitness, gender, sexuality or social class.

Various regulatory bodies, common law and the Human Rights Act 1998 regulate medical practice and ensure that doctors take their duties of care seriously. The ethical standards expected of healthcare professionals by their regulatory bodies (for example in the UK, the General Medical Council (GMC), the Royal College of Physicians and British Medical Association) may at times be higher than the minimum required by law.

LEGALLY VALID CONSENT

It is a general legal and ethical principle that valid consent must be obtained before starting a treatment or physical investigation, or providing personal care for a patient. This principle gives meaning to respect for autonomy and reflects the right of patients to determine what happens to their own bodies. For instance, common law has established that touching a patient without valid consent may constitute the offence of battery. Furthermore, failure to obtain valid consent may be a factor in a claim of negligence against the health professional involved, particularly if the patient suffers harm as a result of treatment.

In order for consent to be valid it must be:

- Given by a patient who has capacity to make decisions about his/her care
- Voluntarily given, i.e. free from coercion

- Sufficiently informed
- Continuing, i.e. patients can change their mind at any time.

Capacity

Patients must have capacity in order to make choices about their health or treatment. Patients over the age of 16 are presumed to have capacity to consent to treatment unless it can be shown otherwise, and judgements about capacity must not be assumed by specific diagnoses or impairments. Capacity to consent to treatment requires that the patient must be able to comprehend and retain information given about the proposed treatment, use this information in the decision-making process and be able to communicate their decision. Capacity is not an 'all-or-nothing' concept; patients may have the capacity for some choices but not others, and capacity can fluctuate. Hence, assessments of capacity are decision specific and should be reviewed regularly. Doctors should be aware of factors which can enhance or diminish a patient's capacity. A competent patient's decision about their care or treatment must be respected regardless of whether doctors agree with it or not.

Information disclosure

The amount of information doctors provide to each patient will vary according to factors such as the nature and severity of the condition, the complexity of the treatment, the risks associated with the treatment or procedure and the patient's own wishes.

In the consent process, enough information must be provided to inform the patient's decisions. Any discussion with the patient should be supplemented by written information where relevant. The amount of information that doctors share with patients will vary depending upon what the individual patient will want or need to know. For a patient who does not speak the native language this must be done with the aid of a health advocate. The type of information provided should include:

- Details and uncertainties of the diagnosis
- The purpose of the investigation or treatment
- Options for treatment including the option not to treat
- The likely benefits and probabilities of success for each option
- Known possible side effects or risks of treatment: decide what information about risks a 'reasonable person' in the position of the patient would want to know before agreeing to treatment. Doctors should be alert to the particular concerns or priorities of the individual patient and risks which may be significant for that patient must be discussed, even if the likelihood of occurrence is small.
- The name of the doctor who will have overall responsibility
- A reminder that the patient can change his or her mind at any time.

Obtaining consent

The clinician providing the treatment or investigation is responsible for ensuring that the patient has given valid consent before treatment begins. Consent may be verbal (e.g. for venepuncture) or written (e.g. always for a surgical procedure). However, it should be remembered that a signed consent form is not legal or professional proof that proper informed consent has been obtained. The person obtaining consent should be the surgeon/physician who is doing the procedure or an assistant who is fully competent to carry out the procedure and therefore understands the potential complications. It is not acceptable for a junior doctor who does not perform and fully understand the procedure to obtain consent.

Special circumstances

Adults who lack capacity to consent

In an emergency situation, doctors treating an adult patient who lacks capacity to consent to treatment can legally give treatment if it is necessary to save their life, or to prevent them from incurring serious and permanent injury.

The treatment of adults who lack capacity is governed by the Mental Capacity Act (MCA) 2005 in England and Wales and the Adults with Incapacity (Scotland) Act 2000 in Scotland. Doctors treating patients who lack capacity to consent to treatment must decide if the proposed treatment is in the overall best interests of the patient. This assessment goes beyond the patient's medical interests and should take account of their wishes or preferences if these can be ascertained. The proposed treatment should be discussed with the relatives (if appropriate) in order to obtain an indication of what the patient's wishes or preferences would be, but family should not be asked to provide consent. However, patients may appoint a proxy decision maker (e.g. lasting power of attorney) with the legal authority to express consent or refuse treatment on their behalf in the event of incapacity. Any treatment(s) provided in the patient's best interests should be proportionate i.e offer a reasonable chance of benefit without being overly burdensome and should be the least restrictive option available.

Advance decisions

Competent adults acting free from pressure and who understand the implications of their choice(s) can make an advance decision (sometimes known as a living will) about how they wish to be treated should they lose capacity. The advance decision should be a clear oral or written instruction refusing one or more medical procedures, or a statement that specifies a degree of irreversible deterioration after which no life-sustaining treatment should be given (advance decisions to refuse life-sustaining treatment must be written and witnessed). An advance decision cannot be used to demand treatment or refuse basic care. Advance statements are binding provided that the patient criteria outlined above are fulfilled, the statement is specific and clearly applicable to the current circumstances and there is no reason to believe that the patient has changed their mind. Where ambiguity exists about the validity of an advance decision, the presumption should be to save life. Advance decisions have different legal force within the UK and doctors should familiarize themselves with the relevant legislation in the jurisdiction in which they work.

Children

In the UK, the legal age of presumed competence to consent to treatment is 16 years. Below this age, those with parental responsibility are the legal proxies for their children and usually consent to treatment on their behalf. In the absence of someone with parental responsibility, e.g. in an emergency where urgent treatment is required, doctors can proceed on the basis of the child's best interests. Some children under 16 years may be able to legally give effective consent to medical treatment provided they have sufficient understanding and intelligence (so called Gillick competence). At any age, an attempt should be made to explain fully the procedures and potential outcomes to the child, even if the child is too young to be fully legally competent.

Teaching

It is necessary to obtain a patient's consent for a student or observer to sit in during a consultation. The patient has the right to refuse without affecting the subsequent consultation. Consent must also be obtained if any additional procedure or examination is to be carried out on an anaesthetized patient solely for the purposes of teaching. Consent must also be obtained if a video or audio recording is to be made of a procedure or consultation and subsequently used for teaching purposes.

Human immunodeficiency virus testing

Doctors must obtain verbal consent from patients before testing for human immunodeficiency virus (HIV), however lengthy pre-test counselling is no longer necessary. The offer of HIV testing should be within the competence of any qualified health care professional. In rare circumstances such as in unconscious patients, HIV testing can be carried out without consent where testing would be in the patient's immediate clinical interests, e.g. to help make a diagnosis and direct treatment.

End-of-life decisions including assisted dying

Competent patients can refuse life-sustaining treatment. Similarly, a patient who lacks capacity may have a valid advance decision or proxy decision maker who is authorized to refuse treatment on their behalf. For patients who lack capacity without an advance decision or proxy decision maker, decisions at the end of life are made as per other treatment decisions on the basis of best interests. Treatments may be lawfully withheld or withdrawn towards the end of life if they are deemed to be physiologically futile (e.g. will not confer significant benefit) or burdensome. Such decisions should be made in consultation with the multidisciplinary team and those closest to the patient. The team is acting in the patient's best interests where the intention is to reduce suffering, rather than to deliberately end life, which would constitute murder. In ethical terms, it is the nature of the doctor's good intention and the moral status of withholding/withdrawing treatment (which are classified as omissions) that differentiates these practices from acts of assisted dying (where the intention is to end life) which are unlawful in the UK.

Cardiopulmonary resuscitation

Decisions about cardiopulmonary resuscitation (CPR) should be made in consultation with the patient (or their representatives if they lack capacity), unless discussing this would cause significant harm. Harm must constitute more than the patient getting upset. A 'do not attempt CPR' (DNACPR) order is appropriate when a patient refuses CPR or when it offers no realistic chance of success. If CPR might be successful it may still be inappropriate due to the likelihood of adverse outcomes based on the patient's current circumstances. If it is not practical to discuss CPR with the patient or their representative and a decision is needed, the decision should be discussed at the earliest, practicable opportunity. Discussions about CPR should form part of a wider discussion about goals of care and the type of treatment(s) patients wish to receive in the event of deteriorating health.

CONFIDENTIALITY

Confidentiality is an essential prerequisite for a therapeutic relationship. Medical information belongs to the patient and should not be disclosed to other parties, including relatives, without the informed consent of the patient. Doctors who breach confidentiality may face legal and professional sanctions. However, the duty of confidence may be breached if disclosure is required by law or is justified in the public interest. In the UK, guidance on such circumstances is available from the GMC. In this event, doctors should seek patient consent for disclosure. Where a breach of confidence is justified, patients should be informed (where appropriate) about the doctor's intention to breach and disclosure should be proportionate and limited to those who need to know. Doctors should be able to justify their decision to breach confidentiality.

COMMUNICATION

Patient-centred communication improves health outcomes and symptom resolution, increases patient adherence to therapies, increases patient and clinician satisfaction, reduces litigation and enhances patient safety. A relationship based on trust and mutual respect allows information to be exchanged to reach a shared understanding between the patient and his/her doctor about the illness and/or its treatment. Most complaints against doctors are not based on failures of biomedical practice but on poor communication. Patients identify the following features of a good consultation:

- Explanation of the process to the patient
- Asking the patient relevant questions to formulate a diagnosis
- Asking patients to express their opinion
- Use of active listening and avoidance of inappropriate interruptions
- Tailored explanations followed by a check of the patient's understanding
- Sufficient time allowed for the interview.

The medical interview

There are seven essential steps in the medical interview (the following applies to a first consultation):

1. Building a relationship

Good first impressions are vital. This will be helped by well-organized arrangements. The doctor should come out of the room to greet the patient, establish eye contact and shake hands if appropriate. Clinicians should tell patients their name, status and responsibility to the patient. The clinician should sit beside the patient and not on the far side of a desk to convey interest and engagement.

2. Opening the discussion

The aim is to address all the patient's concerns (usually they have more than one). Start by asking a question such as: 'What problems have brought you to see me today?'. Listen to the answer without interrupting, then ask 'Is there anything else?' to screen for problems before exploring the history in detail.

3. Gathering information

The components of a complete medical interview are: the nature of the key problems, timing of symptom onset, development over time, precipitating factors, help given to date, impact on the patient's life and availability of support. The clinician should use non-verbal cues to encourage the patient to tell the whole story in their own words. Start with open questions ('Tell me about the pain you have been having' rather than 'Where is your chest pain?'). Then move on to screening ('Is there anything else?'). Leading questions ('You have given up drinking alcohol, haven't you?') should be avoided.

4. Understanding the patient

Empathy is a key skill in building the patient–clinician relationship and involves the patient's experiences being recognized and accepted with some feedback to demonstrate this. Some patients may need encouragement, e.g. 'What were you worried this might be?'. Be alert to non-verbal cues, for instance, 'You look worried, what are you concerned might be causing this pain?'. Doing so demonstrates the patient's concerns have been recognized.

5. Sharing information

Patients generally want to know whether their problem is serious, how will it affect them, what is causing it and what can be done. Verbal information can be supported by leaflets, patient support groups and reputable websites. Verbal information is best provided in assimilable chunks in a logical sequence, using simple language and avoiding medical terminology. It is helpful to check that the patient has understood what has been said before moving on to the next section of the information.

6. Reaching agreement on management

The clinician and patient need to agree on the plan for investigations and treatment. Some patients will want to be more involved than others. The clinician's opinion and the patient's views on management options should be discussed to negotiate a plan together. Summarizing at the end will allow any misunderstandings to be corrected.

7. Providing closing

Closing the interview may start with a brief summary of the patient's agenda and then that of the clinician. The patient should be told the arrangements for follow-up and the commitment to informing other healthcare professionals involved with the patient's care. It is important to record what the patient has been told in their notes. It can be helpful if the patient knows how to contact an appropriate team member as a safety net before the next interview. The interview is closed with an appropriate farewell.

Breaking bad news

Breaking bad news can be difficult, and the way that it is broken has a major psychological and physical effect on patients. Patients often know more than the doctor thinks they do. They welcome clear information and do not want to be drawn into a charade of deception that prevents discussion of their illness and the future. The S-P-I-K-E-S strategy sets a framework for breaking bad news:

S – Setting. The patient should be seen as soon as information is available in a quiet place with everyone seated. Ask not to be disturbed and hand pagers/phones to a colleague. If possible the patient should have someone with them and be introduced to everyone who is with you. Indicate your status and the extent of your responsibility towards the patient.

P – Perception. Begin by finding out how much the patient knows and if anything new has developed since the last encounter.

I – Invitation. Indicate to the patient that you have the results, and ask if they would like you to explain them. A few patients will want to know very little information, and they will indicate that they would prefer for you to talk to a relative or friend.

K – Knowledge. The clinician should give the patient a warning if the news is bad ('I am afraid it looks more serious than we had hoped') before giving the details. At this point, pause to allow the patient to think this over and only continue when the patient gives some lead to follow. The clinician should give small chunks of information and ensure that the patient understands before moving on. Pauses allow the patient to think and ask questions. The patient should be provided with some positive information and hope tempered with realism, for instance, emphasize which problems are reversible and which are not. The importance of maintaining a good quality of life should be stressed. It is often impossible to give an accurate time frame for a terminal disease, but survival rates should be discussed if the patient wants to know these.

E – Empathy. The clinician will need to respond appropriately to a range of emotions that the patient may express (denial, despair, anger, bargaining, depression and acceptance). These must be acknowledged and where necessary, the clinician should wait for them to settle before moving on. Sometimes the interview will need to be stopped and resumed later.

S – Strategy and summary. The clinician must ensure that the patient has understood what has been discussed. Written information may be helpful. The interview should close with a further interview date set (preferably soon) and the patient provided with a contact name before the next interview and details regarding further sources of information. The clinician should offer the patient the opportunity to meet their relatives if they could not be there at this time. A written summary should be recorded in the patient's notes detailing accurately what was said and to whom.

Communication in difficult circumstances

When things go wrong

The professional duty of candour requires doctors to be open and honest when something goes wrong in the care of a patient that causes, or has the potential to cause, harm or distress. In such circumstances, the doctor should offer the patient (or those close to the patient if the patient lacks capacity) a full apology, an explanation of the consequences of the harm and a remedy to put matters right. An apology is an expression of regret, not an admission of liability, and may reduce the likelihood of a formal complaint. Any clinician faced with legal action must seek specialist advice. The professional duty of candour also involves being open and honest with colleagues, employers or other relevant organizations in disclosing adverse events or near misses to encourage a culture of learning which fosters patient safety. Doctors should always follow their organization's clinical governance procedures for reporting and investigating incidents and should not stop someone from raising concerns.

Complaints

Many complaints result from poor communication or miscommunication. The majority of complaints stem from the exasperation felt by patients who:

- Have not been able to get clear information
- Feel that they are owed an apology
- Are concerned that other patients will go through what they have experienced.

Complaints should be dealt with as soon as possible. Be honest and never alter the medical records.

Culture and communication

Patients from minority cultures tend to get poorer healthcare than others of the same socioeconomic status, even when they speak the same language. Consultations tend to be shorter and with less engagement of the patient by the clinician. Cultural issues may affect a patient's behaviour, e.g. when to seek medical care or willingness to discuss sensitive topics. If an interpreter is required this should not be a family member. Advocates (interpreters from the patient's culture who can do more than translate by putting explanations in culturally relevant terms) should be used wherever possible. The clinician should still speak directly to the patient rather than the interpreter.

Patients with impaired faculties for communication

Patients with impaired hearing may require help from a signer. If they can lip read, this can be facilitated by the use of good lighting, plain language and by checking patient understanding. Conversation aids (microphones and amplifier, adapted textphones) can help. Patients with impaired vision will be helped by large print or Braille information sheets. Clinicians should remember these patients can miss non-verbal cues, so sudden touch during the interview should be avoided. For patients with dysphasia, closed questioning is often helpful with a few key headings written down. Speech and language therapists can be very useful for patients with dysphasia.

Medical record keeping

Clinical notes should contain a complete record of every encounter with the patient (including results, information given to the patient obtaining consent, treatment prescribed, follow-up and referrals) and a summary of any discussions with relatives (after obtaining patient consent). If clinicians communicate with patients via e-mail or text, confidentiality must be respected, consideration given to who else might read the information and copies of e-mails or texts kept in the notes. Emails should not be sent from non-NHS email accounts.

A patient has a legal right to see their records, and these are an essential part of the investigation into any complaint or claim for negligence. Criteria for good records are:

- Clear, accurate and legible
- Every entry should be signed, dated and time of consultation recorded. The healthcare worker should also print their name and record where they have seen the patient, e.g. emergency department, ward name.
- Entries should be written in pen and not retrospectively
- Records should never be altered. An additional note should be made, signed and dated alongside any mistake
- Records should always be kept secure. Any patient details kept electronically requires the computer to be encrypted.

Computer records (electronic patient records, EPRs) are increasingly replacing written records; EPRs are more legible, contain more information and reduce prescribing errors.

Team communication

Patients are frequently looked after by multiple healthcare professionals across different teams. Good handover between teams is vital for patient safety and can be facilitated by everyone adopting a clear system. Frameworks such as the SBAR (Situation-Background-Assessment-Recommendations) use standardized prompts to ensure relevant information is shared concisely (Table 1.1).

Table 1.1 SBAR: a structure for team communication

S – Situation	My name is … I am the junior doctor on ward … I am calling about Mr …, under consultant … The reason I am calling is …
B – Background	The patient was admitted on … for … Brief summary background: history, medications, laboratory results, diagnostic tests, procedures
A – Assessment	Summarize relevant information gathered on examination of patient, charts and results Vital signs and early warning or similar score What has changed? Interpretation of this
R – Recommendation (examples)	I need your advice on how to proceed … I think the patient needs urgent review in the next … (time frame)

2 Infectious diseases

Infection remains the main cause of morbidity and mortality in humans, particularly in developing areas where it is associated with poverty and overcrowding. Although the prevalence of infectious disease has reduced in the developing world as a result of increasing prosperity, immunization and antibiotic availability, antibiotic-resistant strains of microorganisms and diseases such as human immunodeficiency virus (HIV) infection have emerged. Increasing global mobility and climate change have aided the spread of infectious disease world-wide. In the elderly and immunocompromised, the presentation of infectious disease may be atypical, with few localizing signs, and the normal physiological responses to infection (fever and sometimes neutrophilia) may be diminished or absent. A high index of suspicion is required in these populations.

Notification of specific infectious diseases is a legal requirement in the UK (Table 2.1) and reporting of certain infections is international practice. These are indicated in the text by the superscripted abbreviation [nd] where appropriate. Scotland and Northern Ireland have slightly different reporting practices. Notification includes reporting of the patient's demographic details along with the disease that is being reported. This allows analyses of local and national trends, tracing of the source and the prevention of spread to others. Registered medical practitioners should notify the local health protection team of a patient attending who is suspected to have a notifiable disease.

Common investigations in infectious disease

- *Blood tests.* Full blood count, erythrocyte sedimentation rate (ESR) and C-reactive protein (CRP), biochemical profile, urea and electrolytes and liver function testing.
- *Imaging.* X-ray, ultrasound, echocardiography, computed tomography (CT) and magnetic resonance imaging (MRI) are used to identify and localize infections. Positron emission tomography (PET) (p. 73) and single photon emission computed tomography (SPECT) have proved useful in localizing infection, especially when combined with CT. Biopsy or aspiration of tissue for microbiological examination may also be facilitated by ultrasound or CT guidance.
- *Radionuclide scanning* after injection of indium- or technetium-labelled white cells (previously harvested from the patient) may occasionally help to localize infection. It is most effective when the peripheral white cell count (WCC) is raised, and is of particular value in localizing occult abscesses.

Table 2.1 Diseases notifiable to local authority proper officers under the Health Protection (Notification) Regulations 2010

Acute encephalitis	Measles
Acute infective hepatitis	Meningococcal septicaemia
Acute meningitis	MERS*
Acute poliomyelitis	Mumps
Anthrax	Plague
Botulinism	Rabies
Brucellosis	Rubella
Cholera	Scarlet fever
Diphtheria	Severe acute respiratory syndrome (SARS)
Ebola	
Enteric fever – paratyphoid/typhoid	Smallpox
Food poisoning	Tetanus
Haemolytic uraemic syndrome (HUS)	Tuberculosis
Infectious bloody diarrhoea	Typhus fever
Invasive group A streptococcal disease	Viral haemorrhagic fever
	Viral hepatitis
Legionnaires' disease	Whooping cough
Leprosy	Yellow fever
Malaria	Zika

*MERS, Middle East respiratory syndrome.

- *Microbiological investigations*
  - *Microscopy and culture* of blood, urine, cerebrospinal fluid (CSF) and faeces should be performed as clinically indicated.
  - *Immunodiagnostic tests*. These detect either a viral/bacterial antigen using a polyvalent antiserum, a monoclonal antibody or the serological response to infection.
  - *Nucleic acid detection*. Nucleic acid probes can be used to detect pathogen-specific nucleic acids in body fluids or tissue. The utility of this approach has been enhanced by amplification techniques such as the polymerase chain reaction (PCR), which increases the amount of target DNA/RNA in the sample to be tested.

Pyrexia of unknown origin

Pyrexia (or fever) of unknown origin (PUO) is defined as 'a documented fever persisting for >2 weeks, with no clear diagnosis despite intelligent

Table 2.2 Causes of pyrexia of unknown origin

Infection (20–40%)	Pyogenic abscess, e.g. liver, pelvic, subphrenic, epidural
	Tuberculosis
	Infective endocarditis
	Toxoplasmosis
	Viruses: Epstein–Barr, cytomegalovirus
	Primary HIV infection
	Brucellosis
	Lyme disease Whipple's disease
Malignant disease (10–30%)	Lymphoma
	Leukaemia
	Renal cell carcinoma
	Hepatocellular carcinoma
Vasculitides (15–20%)	Adult Still's disease
	Rheumatoid arthritis
	Systemic lupus erythematosus
	Granulomatosis with polyangiitis
	Giant cell arteritis
	Polymyalgia rheumatica
Miscellaneous (10–25%)	Drug fevers
	Thyrotoxicosis
	Inflammatory bowel disease
	Sarcoidosis
	Granulomatous hepatitis, e.g. tuberculosis, sarcoidosis
	Factitious fever (switching thermometers, injection of pyogenic material)
	Familial Mediterranean fever
Undiagnosed (5–25%)	

and intensive investigation'. Occult infection remains the most common cause in adults (Table 2.2).

Investigations

A detailed history and examination is essential, and the examination should be repeated on a regular basis in case new signs appear. First-line investigations are usually repeated as the results may have changed since the tests were first performed:

- Full blood count, including a differential WCC and blood film
- ESR and CRP
- Serum urea and electrolytes, liver biochemistry and blood glucose
- Blood cultures – several sets from different sites at different times
- Microscopy and culture of urine, sputum and faeces
- HIV testing
- Chest X-ray
- Serum rheumatoid factor and antinuclear antibody.

Second-line investigations are performed in conditions that remain undiagnosed and when repeat physical examination is unhelpful:

- Abdominal imaging with ultrasound, CT or MRI to detect occult abscesses and malignancy
- Echocardiography for infective endocarditis
- Biopsy of liver and bone marrow occasionally; temporal artery biopsy (p. 311) should be considered in the elderly.

Management

The treatment is of the underlying cause. Blind antibiotic therapy should not be given unless the patient is very unwell. In a few patients, no diagnosis is reached after thorough investigation and in most of these the fever will resolve on follow-up.

Septicaemia

- *Bacteraemia* refers to the transient presence of organisms in the blood (generally without causing symptoms) as a result of local infection or penetrating injury.
- *Septicaemia* is reserved for the clinical picture that results from the systemic inflammatory response to infection.

Inflammation is normally intended to be a local and contained response to infection. Activated polymorphonuclear leucocytes, macrophages and lymphocytes release inflammatory mediators, including tumour necrosis factor, interleukin-1 (IL-1), platelet-activating factor, IL-6, IL-8, interferon and eicosanoids. In some cases, mediator release exceeds the boundaries of the local environment leading to a generalized response that affects normal tissues. Clinical features include fever, tachycardia, an increase in respiratory rate and hypotension. Septicaemia has a high mortality without treatment, and demands immediate attention. The pathogenesis and management of septic shock is discussed on pages 578 and 579.

Aetiology

Overall, about 40% of cases are the result of Gram-positive organisms and 60% of Gram-negative organisms. Fungi are much less common but can occur, particularly in the immunocompromised. In the previously healthy adult, septicaemia may occur from a source of infection in the chest (e.g. with pneumonia), urinary tract (often Gram-negative rods) or biliary tree (commonly *Enterococcus faecalis, Escherichia coli*). Intravenous drug users develop septicaemia often from skin flora or environmental organisms. Commonly, there is endovascular involvement. Hospitalized patients are susceptible to infection from wounds, indwelling urinary catheters and intravenous cannulae.

Clinical features

Fever, rigors and hypotension are the cardinal features of severe septicaemia. Lethargy, headache and a minor change in conscious level may be preceding features. In elderly and immunocompromised patients the clinical features may be quite subtle and a high index of suspicion is needed. Certain bacteria are associated with a particularly fulminating course:

- Staphylococci that produce an exotoxin called toxic shock syndrome toxin-1. Toxic shock syndrome is characterized by an abrupt onset of fever, rash, diarrhoea and shock. It is associated with infected tampons in women but may occur in anyone, including children.
- The Waterhouse–Friderichsen syndrome is most commonly caused by *Neisseria meningitidis*. This is a rapidly fatal illness (without treatment) with a purpuric skin rash and shock. Adrenal haemorrhage (and hypoadrenalism) may be present.

Investigations

In addition to blood count, serum electrolytes, liver biochemistry and lactate measurement:

- Blood cultures
- Cultures from possible source: urine, abscess aspirate, sputum
- Chest radiography and if necessary abdominal ultrasonography and CT.

Management

The Surviving Sepsis Campaign advocates the use of the care bundle 'Sepsis six', which is associated with decreased mortality, decreased length of stay in hospital and fewer intensive care bed days. The following three diagnostic and three therapeutic steps in the bundle should be instituted within 1 hour of the initial recognition of sepsis.

- Deliver high-flow oxygen
- Take blood cultures
- Administer empiric intravenous antibiotics

- Measure serum lactate and send full blood count
- Start intravenous fluids
- Commence accurate urine output measurement.

Antibiotic therapy should be appropriate for the probable site of origin of sepsis in accordance with local antibiotic policies. In some cases the source of sepsis will not be immediately apparent and empirical broad spectrum antibiotic cover will be required. Therapy should subsequently be rationalized on the basis of culture and sensitivity results. In severe sepsis and septic shock, significant attention should be paid to fluid resuscitation and often the patient will be best managed in a critical care environment.

COMMON VIRAL INFECTIONS

Viral infections that are confined to a single organ (or system) are discussed in the relevant chapter, e.g. the common cold caused by one of the rhinoviruses is discussed in Chapter 11 on respiratory diseases.

Measles[nd]

Measles is caused by infection with an RNA paramyxovirus. With the introduction of aggressive immunization policies, the incidence fell in the West (when immunization schedules were adhered to), but it remains common in developing countries, where it is associated with a high morbidity and mortality. One attack confers lifelong immunity. It is spread by droplet infection and the period of infectivity is from 4 days before and up to 4 days after the onset of the rash (after which the infected person can return to work or school).

Clinical features

The incubation period is 7–18 days. Two distinct phases of the disease can be recognized.

The pre-eruptive and catarrhal stage is characterized by fever, cough, rhinorrhoea, conjunctivitis and pathognomonic Koplik's spots in the mouth (small, grey, irregular lesions on an erythematous base, commonly on the inside of the cheek).

The eruptive or exanthematous stage is characterized by the presence of a maculopapular rash, which starts on the face and spreads to involve the whole body. The rash becomes confluent and blotchy. It fades in about a week.

Complications

These are uncommon in the healthy child but carry a high mortality in the malnourished or those with other diseases. Complications include gastroenteritis, pneumonia, otitis media, encephalitis and myocarditis. Rarely, persistence of the virus with reactivation pre-puberty results in subacute sclerosing panencephalitis with progressive mental deterioration and death.

Management

The diagnosis is usually clinical but acute infection can be confirmed by saliva or serum testing for measles-specific immunoglobulin (Ig)M. Treatment is symptomatic. Measles vaccine is given to children of 13 months (9 months in developing countries) to prevent infection. In some countries, including the UK, it is given in combination with mumps and rubella vaccines (MMR). For some patient groups who have been exposed to the virus, human normal immunoglobulin or the MMR vaccine can be used as post-exposure prophylaxis.

Mumps

Mumps is also caused by infection with a paramyxovirus, spread by droplets. The incubation period averages 18 days.

Clinical features

It is primarily an infection of school-aged children and young adults. There is fever, headache and malaise, followed by painful parotid gland swelling. Less common features are orchitis, meningitis, pancreatitis, oophoritis, myocarditis and hepatitis. Sensorineural deafness is a recognized complication.

Management

Diagnosis is usually clinical. Acute infection can be confirmed by PCR analysis of buccal mucosa or demonstration of specific IgM. Treatment is symptomatic. The disease is prevented by administration of a live attenuated mumps virus vaccine (as MMR, see above). Children can return to school 5 days after the onset of the swelling.

Rubella

Rubella ('German measles') is caused by an RNA virus and has a peak age of incidence of 15 years. The incubation period is 14–21 days. During the prodrome the patient complains of malaise, fever and lymphadenopathy (suboccipital, post-auricular, posterior cervical nodes). A pinkish macular rash appears on the face and trunk after about 7 days and lasts for up to 3 days. Maternal infection during pregnancy may affect the fetus, particularly if infection is acquired in the first trimester.

Diagnosis

The diagnosis may be suspected clinically and a definitive diagnosis is made by demonstrating a rising serum IgG titre in paired samples taken 2 weeks apart, or by the detection of rubella-specific IgM.

Management

Treatment is symptomatic. Complications are uncommon but include arthralgia, encephalitis and thrombocytopenia. Prevention is with a live vaccine (see Measles). Children can return to school 4 days after the onset of the rash.

Herpes viruses

Herpes simplex virus (HSV)

HSV-1 causes:

- Herpetic stomatitis with buccal ulceration, fever and local lymphadenopathy
- Herpetic whitlow: damage to the skin over a finger allows access of the virus, with the development of irritating vesicles
- Keratoconjunctivitis
- Acute encephalitis
- Disseminated infection in immunocompromised patients.

HSV-2 is transmitted sexually and causes genital herpes, with painful genital ulceration, fever and lymphadenopathy. Anorectal infection may occur in male homosexuals. There may be systemic infection in the immunocompromised host, and in severe cases death may result from hepatitis and encephalitis. These divisions are not rigid, because HSV-1 can also give rise to genital herpes.

Recurrent HSV infection occurs when the virus lies dormant in ganglion cells and is reactivated by trauma, febrile illnesses and ultraviolet irradiation. This leads to recurrent labialis ('cold sores') or recurrent genital herpes. HSV-2 is also associated with recurrent 'aseptic' meningitis.

Investigations

The diagnosis is often clinical. A firm diagnosis is made by detection of virus from the lesions usually by HSV DNA detection by PCR. Herpes simplex encephalitis is discussed on page 775.

Management

Oral aciclovir, famciclovir and valaciclovir for 5 days are useful if started while lesions are still forming; after this time there is little clinical benefit. Long-term suppressive therapy for 6–12 months reduces the frequency of attacks in recurrent genital herpes. Topical antiviral preparations are available but are less effective in the treatment of anogenital lesions.

Varicella zoster virus

Varicella (chickenpox)

Primary infection with this virus causes chickenpox, which may produce a mild childhood illness, although this can be severe in adults and immunocompromised patients.

Clinical features After an incubation period of 14–21 days there is a brief prodromal period of fever, headache and malaise. The rash, predominantly on the face, scalp and trunk, begins as macules and develops into papules and vesicles, which heal with crusting. Complications include pneumonia and central nervous system involvement, presenting as acute truncal cerebellar ataxia. Individuals are considered infective for 2 days before the appearance of the vesicles until the lesions crust over.

Investigations The diagnosis is usually clinical but is confirmed by detection of viral DNA in vesicular fluid by PCR, electron microscopy or immunofluorescence.

Management Healthy children require no treatment. Anyone over the age of 16 years should be considered for antiviral therapy with aciclovir (if they present within 48 hours) because they are more at risk of severe disease. Because of the risk to both mother and fetus during pregnancy, susceptible pregnant women exposed to the varicella zoster virus should receive prophylaxis with zoster-immune immunoglobulin (ZIG), and treatment with aciclovir if they develop chickenpox. The risk to the fetus depends on the stage of pregnancy. Immunocompromised patients are treated in a similar manner. A live vaccine is available for non-immune health workers and some other specific patient groups.

Herpes zoster (shingles)

After the primary infection, the varicella virus remains dormant in dorsal root ganglia and/or cranial nerve ganglia, and reactivation causes herpes zoster or shingles. A person with shingles (particularly if the rash is weeping) could cause chickenpox in a non-immune person after close contact and touch.

Clinical features Pain and tingling in a dermatomal distribution precede the rash by a few days. The rash consists of papules and vesicles in the same dermatome. The most common sites are the lower thoracic dermatomes and the ophthalmic division of the trigeminal nerve.

Management Treatment is with oral acyclovir, valaciclovir or famciclovir given as early as possible. The main complication is post-herpetic neuralgia (PHN), which can be severe and last for years. Treatment is with amitriptyline, gabapentin or topical agents such as capsaicin cream. The development of PHN is reduced by prompt treatment with aciclovir or similar. The national shingles immunization programme recommends vaccination to be offered to all individuals over the age of 70 years to reduce PHN.

Epstein–Barr virus infection

Acute Epstein–Barr virus (EBV), also referred to as infectious mononucleosis or glandular fever, predominantly affects young adults. EBV is transmitted in saliva and by aerosol. EBV is also the major aetiological agent responsible for Burkitt's lymphoma, nasopharyngeal carcinoma and post-transplant lymphoproliferative disorders. In HIV patients it is associated with non-Hodgkin lymphoma and oral hairy leukoplakia.

Clinical features

Many cases of acute EBV infection are subclinical. If clinical symptoms are present they include fever, headache, sore throat and a transient macular rash (more common following administration of amoxicillin given inappropriately for a sore throat). There may be palatal petechiae, cervical lymphadenopathy, splenomegaly and hepatitis. Rare complications include splenic rupture, myocarditis and meningitis. Cytomegalovirus (CMV), toxoplasmosis and acute HIV infection produce a similar illness.

Investigations

Atypical lymphocytes (activated CD8-positive T lymphocytes) on a peripheral blood film strongly suggest EBV infection. In association with a compatible clinical syndrome, detection of heterophile antibodies to sheep red cells (the Paul-Bunnell reaction) or horse red blood cells (the Monospot test) is diagnostic. However, false negatives may occur in the early stages of infection. False-positive results can occur in leukaemias, lymphoma, systemic lupus erythematosus (SLE) and HIV infection. If the diagnosis is in question, then measurement of EBV-specific antibodies may be necessary. IgM and IgG antibodies against the viral capsid antigen (VCA) are present in acute illness because of the long incubation period. IgG to EBV nuclear antigen (EBNA) appears 6–12 weeks post infection; therefore, a positive EBV VCA IgM and negative EBNA IgG is indicative of acute infection. PCR can be used for EBV DNA quantification in peripheral blood but is most useful in the assessment of lymphoproliferative disease in the post-transplant setting.

Management

Most cases require only symptomatic treatment. Corticosteroids are considered if there is neurological involvement (encephalitis, meningitis), when tonsillar enlargement causes airway obstruction or if there is severe aplastic anaemia.

BACTERIAL INFECTIONS

Most of the bacterial infections are discussed under the relevant system, e.g. meningitis in Chapter 17, cellulitis in Chapter 18 and pneumonia in Chapter 11.

Lyme disease

Lyme disease is a multisystem inflammatory disease caused by the spirochaete *Borrelia burgdorferi* and occasionally other *Borrelia* species. Infection is spread from deer and other wild mammals by *Ixodes* ticks. It is widespread in Europe and North America and present in some parts of Asia. It is most likely to occur in rural wooded areas in the spring and summer months.

Clinical features

- *Early localized infection.* The first stage, usually within 1 month of infection, is characterized by erythema migrans (EM) at the site of the tick bite and, in some cases, constitutional symptoms. EM is pathognomic of Lyme disease and characterized by an erythematous rash expanding over several days with central clearing ('bull's eye' appearance).
- *Early disseminated infection.* The second stage follows weeks to months later and there may be no history of previous EM. Neurological manifestations include meningoencephalitis and cranial or polyneuropathies. Cardiac manifestations include myocarditis or conduction defects.
- *Late Lyme.* This stage often presents months to years after primary infection. Most commonly there is arthritis affecting the large joints – often the knee. There may also be a subtle encephalopathy or polyneuropathy.
  Acrodermatitis chronica atrophicans is a skin manifestation seen particularly in Europe.

Patients may develop persistent non-specific symptoms following treatment but there is no objective evidence that this is due to persistent infection with *Borrelia*.

Investigations

In endemic areas, EM is pathognomonic and no further investigation is required prior to treatment.

Serology is used to confirm early disseminated or late disease. If there is a history of tick bite this should be sent after 6–8 weeks to reduce false-negative results. PCR testing can be carried out on CSF, joint fluid or skin biopsies.

Management

Doxycycline 100 mg twice daily given for 14 days is the treatment of choice for early-stage disease with amoxicillin as an alternative. In arthritis, doxycycline treatment is extended to 1 month. Intravenous ceftriaxone is used for neurological or cardiac involvement. To prevent infection in tick-infested areas, repellents and protective clothing should be worn and ticks removed promptly from the site of a bite.

Leptospirosis[nd]

This zoonosis is caused by a Gram-negative organism, *Leptospira interrogans,* which is excreted in animal urine and enters the host through a skin abrasion or intact mucous membranes. Individuals who work with animals, take part in water sports or have occupational exposure which bring them into close contact with rodents (e.g. freshwater swimming, sewage workers) are most at risk.

Clinical features

Most cases are mild, however some are severe and life threatening. Following an incubation period of about 10 days the initial leptospiraemic phase is characterized by fever, headache, malaise and myalgia and conjunctival suffusion. The 'immune phase' follows, which is most commonly manifest by meningism. A small proportion of cases go on to develop hepatic and renal failure, haemolytic anaemia and circulatory collapse (Weil's disease). Rhabdomyolysis, myocarditis, acute respiratory distress syndrome (ARDS) and pulmonary haemorrhage are also seen.

Investigations

Serology is most often used to confirm the diagnosis but in patients with appropriate environmental exposure, empirical treatment should not be delayed. Blood or CSF culture can identify the organisms in the first week of the disease, but this is insensitive and requires prolonged culture. The organism may be detected in the urine during the second week. Molecular diagnostics are not widely available.

Management

Oral doxycycline is given for mild disease and intravenous penicillin or ceftriaxone for more severe disease. The complications of the disease may require renal replacement therapy or ventilatory support.

Rickettsia

A variety of Rickettsial species with wide geographical distribution can cause travel-related infection, but most commonly *Rickettsia africae* (African tick-bite fever) or *Rickettsia conorii* (Mediterranean spotted or tick bite fever) is identified. Incubation is 5–7 days. *R. africae* is endemic in cattle ticks and infection is seen in those returning from game parks in southern Africa. Fever, malaise, lymphadenitis, rash and particularly eschar all suggest infection. Diagnosis is by serology. Treatment with doxycycline 100 mg BD should not be delayed in patients with a suggestive clinical picture and appropriate travel history.

FEVER IN THE RETURNED TRAVELLER

Fever is the most common symptom in people returning from tropical travel. Malaria is the most common cause of febrile illness in recent travellers and is potentially fatal; therefore, prompt assessment of these patients is necessary. Most patients in this group present within 1 month of travel. Table 2.3 lists the causes of fever in travellers from the tropics; however, in some patients no specific cause is found. The most common causes are discussed in greater detail below.

Table 2.3 Common causes of fever after travel to the tropics

Malaria	
Enteric fever (typhoid and paratyphoid fevers)	
Arbovirus infection (Dengue/Chikungunya)	
Rickettsia	Consider early in the
HIV seroconversion	assessment
Amoebic liver abscess	
Acute schistosomiasis – Katayama fever	
Viral hepatitis	
Viral respiratory tract infection – influenza, avian influenza, MERS-CoV, SARS	
Gastroenteritis	
Leptospirosis	
Tuberculosis	
Febrile illness unrelated to foreign travel – includes respiratory and urinary tract infection	

Viral haemorrhagic fever (VHF)[nd] is caused by a heterogeneous number of zoonotic viruses. The Ebola outbreak in West Africa has brought them to global attention. VHF is a rare cause of fever in returning travellers, but due to the transmissibility and significant mortality associated with a number of these viruses, potential cases require strict isolation and infection control practices. VHF should be considered when assessing patients with fever who have returned from high-risk countries, particularly countries in sub-Saharan or West Africa (Lassa, Marberg and Ebola viruses). Crimean-Congo haemorrhagic fever is found in southern Africa and parts of Asia. Suspected cases should be discussed immediately with the local Infectious Diseases team and Health Protection unit as per local policy. Within the UK, risk assessment information can be found on http://www.gov.uk.

Approach to diagnosis

In addition to a full medical history, a detailed travel history and physical examination will help to formulate an appropriate differential diagnosis:

- *Dates of travel and illness onset:* this will allow assessment of the incubation period; Table 2.4
- *Destination:* all countries visited should be noted on a timeline, including airport stopovers. Details of travel in rural and urban areas including types of accommodation used should also be recorded.
- *Exposure:* to vectors (mosquitos, flies, ticks, snails), animals, fresh water, healthcare facilities (needle and blood exposure, surgery) and sexual exposure

Table 2.4 Typical incubation periods for tropical infections

Incubation period	Infection
Short (<10 days)	Arboviral infections, gastroenteritis, melioidosis, meningitis, respiratory infection (bacterial and viral), rickettsial infection
Medium (10–21 days)	Malaria, enteric fever, brucellosis, leptospirosis, African trypanosomiasis, EBV, CMV, HIV, viral haemorrhagic fevers
Long (>21 days)	Viral hepatitis (A–E), tuberculosis, HIV, schistosomiasis, amoebic liver abscess, visceral leishmaniasis, filariasis, brucellosis, tuberculosis, malaria

- *Activities:* such as working in hospitals or refugee camps, caving, visiting game parks
- *Pre-travel vaccination and prophylaxis used:* no vaccination is 100% effective, however some confer extremely effective protection such as vaccination against yellow fever and hepatitis A and B. Malaria prophylaxis has to be appropriate for the area visited and taken reliably without premature cessation. Appropriate prophylaxis with full adherence does not exclude malaria within the differential.

Investigations

The initial work-up of a febrile patient who has recently travelled is listed below. Additional studies depend on exposure and other factors:

- Full blood count with differential WCC, urea and electrolytes, liver function testing, blood glucose
- Malaria rapid antigen test followed by thick and thin blood malaria films; repeat after 12–24 hours if initial films negative. At least three in total
- Blood cultures
- Urine microscopy and culture and stool culture
- Chest X-ray ± liver and spleen ultrasound scan
- HIV test
- Serology for specific antibody detection as necessary
- Pregnancy test for women with childbearing potential.

Malaria[nd]

Malaria is a protozoan parasite widespread in the tropics and subtropics (Fig. 2.1). Approximately half of the world's population is at risk of malaria; however, sub-Saharan Africa is disproportionally affected, with the region

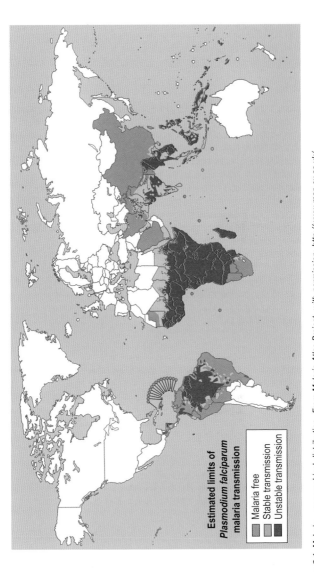

Fig. 2.1 Malaria – geographical distribution. *From Malaria Atlas Project, with permission; http://www.map.ox.ac.uk/.*

seeing 89% of malaria cases globally in 2015. Increasing prevention and control strategies have seen the global mortality rates for malaria drop by 60% since 2000. In endemic areas, mortality is principally in infants, and those who survive to adulthood acquire significant immunity. In hyperendemic areas, an exaggerated immune response to repeated malarial infections leads to massive splenomegaly, anaemia and elevated IgM levels.

Aetiology

Malaria is transmitted by the bite of infected female *Anopheles* mosquitoes. Occasionally it is transmitted in contaminated blood (transfusions, contaminated equipment, injecting drug users sharing needles). Rarely the parasite is transmitted by importation of infected mosquitoes by air (airport malaria).

Five malaria parasites infect humans. *Plasmodium falciparum* is responsible for most malaria-related deaths, and infection can rapidly progress from an acute fever with rigors to severe multiorgan failure, coma and death. Once successfully treated this form does not relapse. Of the other malaria parasites, *P. vivax* is the most dominant malaria parasite outside sub-Saharan Africa. Along with *P. ovale, P. malariae* and *P. knowlesi, P. vivax* causes a more benign illness. However, *P. ovale* and *P. vivax* may relapse and *P. malariae* may run a chronic course over months or years.

In the UK, between 1300 and 1800 cases of malaria are reported each year. Most often this occurs in people of African or South Asian origin and 50% of cases occur in patients who have visited friends and family in endemic areas.

Specific country information for malaria can be found at http://travelhealthpro.org.uk.

Pathogenesis

The infective form of the parasite (sporozoites) passes through the skin and, via the bloodstream, enters the liver. Here they multiply inside hepatocytes as merozoites. After a few days the infected hepatocytes rupture, releasing merozoites into the blood where they are taken up by erythrocytes and pass through further stages of development, which terminate with the rupture of the red cell. Rupture of red blood cells contributes to anaemia and releases pyrogens, causing fever. Red blood cells infected with *P. falciparum* adhere to the endothelium of small vessels and the consequent vascular occlusion causes severe organ damage, chiefly in the gut, kidney, liver and brain. *P. ovale* and *P. vivax* remain latent in the liver as hypnozoites, and this is responsible for the relapses that may occur.

Clinical features

The incubation period varies:
- 10–14 days in *P. vivax, P. ovale* and *P. falciparum* infection
- 18 days to 6 weeks in *P. malariae* infection.

The onset of symptoms may be delayed (up to 3 months, 1 year in vivax malaria) in the partially immune or after prophylaxis. There is an abrupt onset of fever, tachycardia and rigors, followed by profuse sweating some hours later. This may be accompanied by anaemia and hepatosplenomegaly. Atypical presentations without fever.

P. falciparum infection is a medical emergency because patients may deteriorate rapidly. These patients must be discussed with local infection experts and should be managed in a high-dependency or intensive care setting. *P. falciparum* infection can also be complicated by Gram-negative septicaemia and consideration should be made for the addition of empirical antibiotic cover.

Investigations

The conventional method for diagnosing malaria is examination of a thick and thin blood film. Thick smears detect malaria parasites and thin smears are used for parasite identification and for quantification of the percentage of parasitized red cells (in *P. falciparum* infection). Rapid diagnostic tests detect parasite antigens and are used in many UK laboratories in addition to blood films and are useful as an immediate screen when the expertise for reading blood films is not readily available. If clinical suspicion for malaria remains but initial blood films are negative, these should be repeated in 12–24 hours and again at 24 hours. Pregnancy testing should be undertaken in all women of childbearing potential, as falciparum malaria in pregnancy is more likely to be complicated, diagnosis can be difficult, treatment strategies are different and expert opinion should be sought.

Assessment should include careful evaluation for the features of severe malaria in Table 2.5 and would routinely include full blood count, urea, creatinine and electrolytes, liver function tests and blood glucose. Blood gases,

Table 2.5 Major features of severe or complicated falciparum malaria in adults

Impaired consciousness or seizures
Renal impairment
Oliguria
Haemoglobinuria
Acidosis
Hypoglycaemia
Pulmonary oedema or acute respiratory distress syndrome (ARDS)
Haemoglobin ≤80 g/L
Disseminated intervascular coagulation or spontaneous bleeding
Shock (blood pressure <90/60)
Parasitaemia >10%

serum lactate, clotting studies and blood cultures should be taken in patients who are unwell. Thrombocytopenia is common and in isolation does not reflect severe or complicated disease.

Management

Treatment of uncomplicated falciparum malaria

Patients should be admitted to hospital at least for the first 24 hours as there can be rapid deterioration. Careful evaluation for the features of severe disease must be made. Although a parasitaemia of >10% is considered to represent severe disease, with a parasitaemia of >2% there is increased risk of developing severe disease and these patients should receive parenteral therapy – see below.

Most cases of uncomplicated falciparum malaria are now treated with artemisinin combination therapy (ACT), but other therapeutic options are available (Table 2.6). Symptomatic treatment with antipyretics and intravenous fluid is often necessary. **Severe falciparum malaria** (indicated by the presence of any of the features listed in Table 2.5) is a medical emergency, and patients should be cared for in an appropriate high-dependency or intensive care environment. Expert advice should be sought. Parenteral therapy should be given to patients who have a >2% parasitaemia, are pregnant (following specialist advice) or in which the oral route is unavailable.

Intravenous artesunate is unlicensed in the EU but is available in most centres. Parenteral quinine should be commenced immediately if artesunate is unavailable.

- *Parenteral artesunate:* 2.4 mg/kg body weight i.v. given at 0, 12 and 24 hours and then daily. After completing at least 24 hours of therapy and once oral medication can be tolerated, a full course of ACT should be given (Table 2.6).
- *Parenteral quinine:* Quinine dihydrochloride 20 mg/kg loading dose in 5% dextrose or dextrose saline over 4 hours, then 10 mg/kg every 8 hours for the first 48 hours. Parenteral quinine should be continued until the patient can take oral therapy. At this point, quinine sulphate 600 mg three times daily should be given to complete a 5–7 day course. Quinine must always be accompanied by a second agent, most often doxycycline 200 mg orally for 7 days from when the patient can swallow. Clindamycin should be used for pregnant women.

Careful monitoring of blood sugar, renal function, fluid balance, clotting studies and for respiratory distress is required so that supportive measures can be instituted early. Development of shock may be secondary to Gram-negative septicaemia and broad spectrum antibiotics should be considered.

Non-falciparum malaria

Treatment is twofold for *P. vivax* and *P. ovale* – ACT or chloroquine is used to treat the acute erythrocytic stages and primaquine is used for elimination of liver hypnozoites (Table 2.6). Primaquine may cause haemolysis in patients

Table 2.6 Treatment of acute uncomplicated malaria in adults

Type of malaria	Oral drug treatment
Acute treatment of Non-falciparum malaria	Chloroquine: 620 mg followed by 310 mg at 6, 24 and 48 hours
	or
	Artemether-lumefantrine: four tablets at 0, 8, 24, 36, 48 and 60 hours Or DHA-piperaquine: 36–60 kg three tablets daily for 3 days, >60 kg four tablets daily for 3 days
In p. vivax and p. ovale after treatment of acute infection to eradicate liver cysts	
	Oral primaquine* (15 mg base/day for p. ovale, 30 mg/day for p. vivax) for 14 days. In mild to moderate G6PD deficiency primaquine 0.75 mg/kg as a single weekly dose for 8 weeks
P. falciparum	Artemether-lumefantrine: four tablets at 0, 8, 24, 36, 48 and 60 hours
	or
	DHA-piperaquine: 36–60 kg three tablets daily for 3 days, >60 kg four tablets daily for 3 days
	or
	Atovaquone-proguanil: four 'standard' tablets daily for 3 days Or Oral quinine sulphate 600 mg 8 hourly for 5–7 days **plus** doxycycline 200 mg daily (clindamycin 450 mg 8 hourly for pregnant women) for 7 days.

*Check for glucose-6-phosphate dehydrogenase deficiency first.
DHA, dihydroartemisinin.
(Adapted from UK Malaria Treatment Guidelines.)

with glucose-6-phosphate dehydrogenase (G6PD) deficiency; therefore, all patients must be screened before treatment is commenced. ACT or chloroquine can be used for *P. malariae* and *P. knowlesi*.

Prevention and control

Effective prevention of malaria includes the following elements (ABC):

- Awareness of risk
- Bite avoidance – using mosquito repellents, covering up with permethrin-impregnated clothing, sleeping under impregnated bednets
- Chemoprophylaxis.

As a result of changing patterns of resistance, advice about chemoprophylaxis should be sought from an appropriate travel advice centre before leaving for a malaria-endemic area. Prophylaxis does not afford full protection.

Enteric fever[nd]

Typhoid fever and paratyphoid fever are caused by *Salmonella typhi* and *S. paratyphi* (types A, B and C), respectively. Humans are the only reservoir of infection and spread is faecal–oral. The incubation period is 10–14 days. Typhoid fever is most prevalent in overcrowded areas with poor sanitation.

Clinical features

The incubation period is 5–21 days after organism ingestion. There is an insidious onset of intermittent fever, headache and dry cough and relative bradycardia. In the second week of the illness there is an erythematous maculopapular rash ('rose spots') on the upper abdomen and thorax, splenomegaly, cervical lymphadenopathy and hepatomegaly. Diarrhoea may develop. Complications, usually occurring in the third week, are pneumonia, meningitis, acute cholecystitis, osteomyelitis, intestinal perforation and haemorrhage.

Investigations

Diagnosis requires the culture of *S. typhi* or *S. paratyphi* from the patient. Organisms can be cultured from the blood, faeces and urine, depending on the stage in the illness that individuals present for medical attention. Where the diagnosis is in doubt, bone marrow cultures may be positive even after starting antibiotics. A blood count shows non-specific leukopenia. The Widal test has limited clinical use.

Management and prevention

Due to the increasing resistance of *S. typhi* and *S. paratyphi* to fluroquinolones, intravenous ceftriaxone is considered first-line treatment until fluroquinolone sensitivity is assessed. Azithromycin is an alternative in uncomplicated disease. To reduce relapse rates and persistent carriage, treatment should be continued for 14 days. Some patients become chronic carriers, with the focus of infection in the gall bladder, and prolonged antibiotic treatment is indicated. Vaccination with injectable inactivated or oral live attenuated vaccines gives partial protection.

Enterocolitis

Other *Salmonella* species (*S. choleraesuis* and *S. enteritidis*) cause a self-limiting infection presenting with diarrhoea and vomiting (Table 2.7) and are a cause of travellers' diarrhoea – see below and Table 2.8.

Table 2.7 Pathogenic mechanisms of bacterial gastroenteritis where established

Pathogenesis	Mode of action	Clinical presentation	Examples
Mucosal adherence	Effacement of intestinal mucosa	Moderate watery diarrhoea	Enteropathogenic *E. coli* (EPEC)
			Enteroaggregative *E. coli* (EAggEC)
			Diffusely adhering *E. coli* (DAEC)
Mucosal invasion	Penetration + destruction of mucosa	Bloody diarrhoea	*Shigella* spp.
			Campylobacter spp.
			Enteroinvasive *E. coli* (EIEC)
Toxin production			
Enterotoxin	Fluid secretion without mucosal damage	Profuse watery diarrhoea	*Vibrio cholera*
			Salmonella spp.
			Campylobacter spp.
			Enterotoxigenic *E. coli* (ETEC)
			Bacillus cereus
			Staph. aureus producing enterotoxin B
			Clostridium perfringens type A
Cytotoxin	Damage to mucosa	Bloody diarrhoea	*Salmonella* spp.
			Campylobacter spp.
			Enterohaemorrhagic *E. coli* (EHEC)

Dengue fever

Dengue viruses (a member of the *Flaviviridae* family) are transmitted to humans through bites of infected female *Aedes aegypti* mosquitoes. These are found mainly in Asia, Africa, Central America and South America, where it is a common cause of fever and may be fatal. After an incubation period of 4–7 days, there is an abrupt onset of fever, headache, retro-orbital pain and severe

Table 2.8 Causes of travellers' diarrhoea

Bacteria: 70–90% of cases	E. coli (enterotoxigenic)
	E. coli (enteroaggregative)
	Shigella spp.
	Salmonella spp.
	Campylobacter jejuni
	Aeromonas and Plesimonas spp.
	Vibrio cholera
Viruses: 10%	Rotavirus
	Noroviruses*
Protozoa: <5%	Giardia intestinalis
	Entamoeba histolytica
	Cryptosporidium parvum
	Cyclospora cayetanensis

Note: Co-infection with multiple pathogens occurs in approximately 10% of cases.
*Often associated with outbreaks of diarrhoea or cruise ships and in holiday resorts.

myalgia, often with a skin rash. Dengue haemorrhagic fever (DHF) is a severe form with thrombocytopenia, increased vascular permeability (indicated by a rising haematocrit), ongoing fever and spontaneous bleeding. Additional signs of circulatory failure indicate dengue shock syndrome. Initial diagnosis is mainly clinical and it should be considered in all travellers returning from endemic regions. Laboratory diagnosis usually relies on serology, which should be taken 5 days after the onset of illness. PCR detection of the virus or its components (non-structural protein, NS1) in the blood is also available for earlier confirmation. Treatment is supportive as no specific therapy is available. Early recognition of deterioration to DHF should identify patients who require more aggressive supportive approaches.

Schistosomiasis

Schistosomiasis is a parasitic infection caused by five schistosome species. These parasites live in freshwater snails and the infectious forms of the parasite – cercariae – penetrate skin when it comes in contact with contaminated water. Prevalence is highest in sub-Saharan Africa, but schistosomiasis is also found in other areas of Africa, South America, South East Asia, China and the Middle East. Acute symptoms are more common in non-immune individuals such as travellers. Parasite penetration through the skin may cause a localized pruritic papular rash ('swimmer's itch'). Parasite migration through the lungs and hepatic circulation 3–4 weeks after infection may cause fever, arthralgia and dry cough (Katayama fever). Chronic complications of

Schistosoma infection usually occur only in endemic areas where there is a high parasite load; there may be intestinal, hepatosplenic, pulmonary, genito-urinary or neurological manifestations, but it is often asymptomatic (Table 2.9).

Diagnostic approaches differ between returning travellers and those in endemic settings. In returning travellers, serology taken at least 6 weeks after exposure is the most useful diagnostic tool, as parasite load is usually low and ova may not be detected in stool or urine by microscopy.

Swimmer's itch is treated symptomatically. Acute schistosomiasis syndrome is initially treated with corticosteroids to reduce the hypersensitivity reaction to schistosome antigens and then praziquantel is administered after acute symptoms have resolved and at least 4–6 weeks following exposure. Chronic infection is treated with praziquantel.

MISCELLANEOUS VIRAL INFECTIONS

Zika

Zika virus is a mosquito-borne arbovirus first isolated in the 1940s in Uganda. The first major outbreak was in 2007. More recently there has been a rapidly expanding epidemic in Latin America. Although the illness is mild and self-limiting, causing fever, rash, headache and myalgia/arthralgia, recent evidence confirms that congenital infection is associated with microcephaly and other abnormalities. Given the now world-wide distribution of other arboviruses, there is significant concern that Zika virus could spread globally. Diagnosis is by serology and treatment is supportive. Pregnant women are monitored through pregnancy with fetal ultrasound. Following clinical illness compatible with Zika or confirmed diagnosis, men are advised to use barrier contraception for 6 months to avoid sexual transmission through infected semen.

MERS Co-V

Middle East respiratory syndrome coronavirus (MERS-CoV) was first isolated in 2012 in Saudi Arabia. Since then it has been reported in many countries on the Arabian Peninsula. Camels appear to be the primary animal host. Case clusters in imported infection strongly suggests that human-to-human transmission occurs and therefore rigorous infection control practices must be adhered to if there is epidemiological and clinical risk for infection. Suspected cases should be discussed immediately with the local Infectious Diseases team and Health Protection unit as per local policy. The incubation period is not certain, but up to 14 days is widely used in the risk assessment of cases. Most patients have presented with severe pneumonia, ARDS and some with acute kidney injury but mild and asymptomatic infection has been reported. Diagnosis is by PCR of upper or lower respiratory tract specimens. There is no antiviral treatment available, and full supportive measures, particularly mechanical ventilation, are often required.

Table 2.9 Summary of intestinal diseases caused by helminths (parasitic worms)

Helminth		Clinical manifestations	Diagnosis	Treatment of choice
Nematodes (roundworms)				
Small intestine	*Strongyloides stercoralis*	Local dermatitis at site of skin penetration, diarrhoea, malabsorption, disseminated disease. Symptoms may continue for years as a result of autoinfection	Larvae in fresh stool, serology	Ivermectin/albendazole
	Hookworm: *Ancylostoma duodenale, Necator americanus*	Local dermatitis at the site of skin penetration, nausea, epigastric pain, iron deficiency anaemia	Detection of eggs in faeces	Albendazole/mebendazole
	Roundworm: *Ascaris lumbricoides*	Often asymptomatic. Vomiting, abdominal discomfort, anorexia, intestinal obstruction. Pulmonary eosinophilia after migration to the lungs	Detection of eggs in faeces	Albendazole/mebendazole
	Trichinella spiralis	Abdominal pain and diarrhoea. Larvae penetrate the bowel wall and invade striated muscle causing pain. Periorbital oedema may be present	Serology, muscle biopsy	Albendazole/mebendazole
	Toxocara canis	Penetration of small intestine to lungs (bronchospasm), liver (hepatomegaly), heart, brain and eye	Serology	Albendazole

Continued

Large intestine	Whipworm: *Trichuris trichiura*	Often asymptomatic. Mucosal damage may result in bloody diarrhoea	Detection of eggs in faeces	Albendazole/mebendazole
	Threadworm: *Enterobius vermicularis*	Pruritus ani	Apply adhesive paddle to perineum and identify eggs	Albendazole/mebendazole
	Trematodes (flukes)			
Water-borne	*Schistosoma* species	Parasite eggs, released in urine or faeces, hatch on contact with water before infecting freshwater snails. Snail vectors release cercariae which penetrate human skin (causing swimmer's itch). Worms migrate to pelvic veins and bladder (*S. haematobium*) causing haematuria, hydronephrosis, renal failure. *S. mansoni* and *S. japonicum* migrate to mesenteric veins and bowel causing bloody diarrhoea, intestinal strictures, hepatic fibrosis and portal hypertension	Detection of eggs in urine, stool or rectal biopsy. Serology	Praziquantel
Food-borne	Liver flukes (*Clonorchis sinensis*, *Opisthorchis felineus*, *O. viverrin*)	Cholangitis, biliary carcinoma	Eggs on stool microscopy	Praziquantel
	Fasciola hepatica	Fever/right upper quadrant pain (RUQ pain)/ hepatomegaly	+ serology	Triclabendazole

Table 2.9 Summary of intestinal diseases caused by helminths (parasitic worms)—cont'd

Helminth		Clinical manifestations	Diagnosis	Treatment of choice
	Lung fluke (*Paragonimus*)	Chest pain, dyspnoea, fever, cough, haemoptysis	Ova on sputum or in stool/serology	Praziquantel/triclabendazole
Cestodes (tapeworms)				
	Taenia saginata	Beef tapeworm acquired by eating insufficiently cooked beef. Causes abdominal pain and malabsorption	Detection of eggs or proglottids on stool microscopy	Praziquantel
	Taenia solium	Pork tapeworm from undercooked pork. Larvae penetrate the intestinal wall and cause disseminated disease involving skin, skeletal muscle and brain (neurocysticercosis) often presenting with seizure	Serology, imaging of cysts in muscle and brain by X-ray, CT or MRI	Albendazole ± praziquantel (neurological parenchymal disease requires additional corticosteroids and antiepileptics)
	Echinococcus granulosus	Hydatid disease acquired by eating meat (from sheep, cattle) contaminated with ova excreted by dogs. Large cysts develop in liver, lung and brain. Anaphylactic reactions if cyst contents escape	Ultrasound, CT and MRI show the cysts and daughter cysts. Diagnosis by serology	Surgical excision and albendazole

GASTROENTERITIS AND FOOD POISONING[nd]

Most causes of acute diarrhoea (lasting less than 14 days) with or without vomiting are due to a gastrointestinal infection with bacteria, virus or protozoa. Not all cases of gastroenteritis are food poisoning, as the pathogens are not always food- or water-borne, e.g. *C. difficile* as a complication of antibiotic use (see below). Individuals at increased risk of infection include infants and young children, the elderly, travellers (principally to developing countries), the immunocompromised and those with reduced gastric acid secretion (e.g. individuals using proton pump inhibitors or with pernicious anaemia). Viral gastroenteritis is a common cause of diarrhoea and vomiting in young children. Helminthic gut infections are rare in the West but relatively common in developing countries.

Bacteria can cause diarrhoea in three different ways resulting in two broad clinical syndromes: watery diarrhoea and bloody diarrhoea, i.e. dysentery (Table 2.7).

The clinical features based on the principal presenting symptom associated with the causative organisms of food poisoning are summarized in Table 2.10. Listeriosis (infection with *Listeria monocytogenes*) is associated with contaminated coleslaw, non-pasteurized soft cheeses and other packaged chilled foods. The most serious complication of listerial infection is meningitis, occurring perinatally and in immunocompromised adults. Hepatitis A (p. 150) and *Toxoplasma gondii* (p. 58) are also acquired from infected foods and their major effects are extraintestinal.

Most infectious causes of diarrhoea are self-limiting. Routine stool examination for culture, microscopy for ova and parasites (three samples, since excretion is intermittent) and stool testing for *C. difficile* toxin are not usually necessary other than in the following groups of patients: immunosuppressed, patients with inflammatory bowel disease (to distinguish a flare from infection), certain employees such as food handlers, bloody diarrhoea, persistent diarrhoea (>7 days, possible *Giardia, Cryptosporidium, Cyclospora*), severe symptoms (fever, volume depletion) or recent antibiotic treatment or hospitalization. The management of patients with acute diarrhoea includes adequate hydration. Antibiotic therapy is not given in most cases since the illness is usually self-limited. Antibiotics are avoided in patients with suspected or proven enterohaemorrhagic *E. coli* infection as they may increase the risk of haemolytic uraemic syndrome. As a result, the use of empirical antibiotic therapy (e.g. ciprofloxacin and metronidazole for severely unwell patients) should be discussed with an infection specialist first.

Clostridium difficile

C. difficile is responsible for some cases of antibiotic-related diarrhoea and nearly all cases of pseudomembranous colitis. Some patients have recurring episodes following initial infection.

Table 2.10 Major food-borne microbes by the principal presenting gastrointestinal symptom in immunocompetent adults[nd]

Clinical presentation	Organism	Source/vehicles	Incubation period	Diagnosis	Recovery
Vomiting	Staph. aureus	Prepared food (e.g. sandwiches)	2–4 h	Diagnosis usually clinical for all organisms – PCR for norovirus available in outbreak situations	<24 h
	Bacillus cereus	Rice, meat	1–6 h		2–3 days
	Norovirus	Shellfish, prepared food	24–48 h		2–3 days
Watery diarrhoea	Clostridium perfringens	All by contaminated food and water	8–22 h	Stool culture	2–3 days
	Enterotoxigenic E. coli (ETEC)		24 h		1–4 days
	Enteric viruses		Variable		Variable
	Cryptosporidium parvum and C. hominis		5–28 days		7–14 days
	Cyclospora cayetanensis		7 days		Weeks to months
	Yersinia enterocolitica		2–14 h		1–22 days
	Vibrio cholera		Hours to 6 days		2–3 days

Diarrhoea with blood (dysentery)	*Campylobacter jejuni*	Cattle and poultry – meat and milk	48–96 h	Stool culture	3–5 days
	Non-typhoidal salmonella	Cattle and poultry – eggs, meat	12–48 h		3–6 days, may be up to 2 weeks
	Enterohaemorrhagic *E. coli* (usually serotype O157:H7)*	Cattle – meat, milk	12–48 h		10–12 days
	Shigella spp.	Contaminated food and water	24–48 h		7–10 days
	Vibrio parahaemolyticus	Contaminated seafood	2–48 h		1–12 days
Non-gastrointestinal manifestations	*Clostridium botulinum* Paralysis due to neuromuscular blockade	Environment – bottled or canned food	18–24 h	Toxin in food or faeces	10–14 days
	Listeria monocytogenes Meningitis	Contaminated packaged chilled foods	Up to 6 weeks	CSF culture	Variable

*It is vital that there is a low threshold for suspecting E. coli O157 infection in gastroenteritis because it can cause serious complications. Between 1% and 15% of cases progress to haemolytic uraemic syndrome (acute kidney injury, haemolytic anaemia, thrombocytopenia). Antibiotics are contraindicated in E. coli O157 infection.

Pathology and clinical features

C. difficile can be cultured from the stool of 3% of healthy adults and about one-third of hospital inpatients. Most colonized patients remain asymptomatic. Clinical disease develops when the normal colonic microbiota is altered, usually by antibiotics, and creates an environment which favours the proliferation of *C. difficile*. Infection with toxigenic strains of *C. difficile* causes colonic inflammation and diarrhoea by secretion of toxins A and B. There is focal epithelial ulceration and an inflammatory exudate that appears as a pseudomembrane on endoscopic examination. The clinical picture varies from mild diarrhoea to life-threatening severe disease with profuse diarrhoea, abdominal pain and toxic megacolon.

Diagnosis is a two-test process used to differentiate those with *C. difficile*-associated diarrhoea from those who are potential *C. difficile* excretors in the absence of clinical symptoms. Initial screening is with a glutamate dehydrogenase enzyme-linked immunoassay (EIA) or toxin gene NAAT. If this is positive then a toxin EIA is undertaken. Characteristic pseudomembranes may be seen at colonoscopy. In potential outbreak situations, ribotyping is undertaken to determine the strain involved as some are associated with increased severity, i.e. ribotype 027.

Management

Patients with *C. difficile*-associated diarrhoea should have specific multidisciplinary assessment and input at least weekly. Patients require isolation with barrier precautions and daily review of severity markers, fluid resuscitation, electrolyte replacement and nutritional status. If at all possible, ongoing antibiotic treatment should be discontinued, and if the patient is receiving acid-suppressing medications such as proton-pump inhibitors, these should be reviewed and if possible stopped. Evidence is increasing that these may be a risk factor for *C. difficile* infection.

Antimicrobial approaches depend on the severity of the infection and whether this is a first episode or recurrence. Certain patient groups, particularly the elderly and those with multiple comorbidities, are more likely to have severe disease and recurrent episodes.

Any one of the following is considered a severity marker:

- WCC >15 10^9/L
- Acutely rising blood creatinine
- Temperature >38.5°C
- Evidence of severe colitis (abdominal examination/radiology/colonoscopy)

Mild/moderate disease is treated with oral metronidazole 500 mg 8 hourly for 10–14 days.

Severe disease is treated with oral vancomycin 125 mg 6 hourly. Some centres now use fidaxomicin in this patient group. If there is no response to initial treatment the vancomycin dose can be increased up to 500 mg 6 hourly and delivered via nasogastric (NG) tube or per rectally if necessary with the addition of intravenous (i.v.) metronidazole 500 mg 8 hourly. Surgical assessment for intervention is required. Severe *C. difficile*-associated diarrhoea is included as an appropriate use for i.v. immunoglobulin.

Recurrent disease is treated with fidaxomicin or vancomycin. Tapering doses of vancomycin over a number of weeks may be used. Donor faecal transplant has shown to be effective in achieving resolution of persistently recurrent *C. difficile*.

Prevention of *C. difficile* infection is achieved by preventing cross infection (see above) and by reducing overprescribing and inappropriate antibiotic use (avoid broad spectrum agents, use the shortest treatment course likely to be effective, avoid intravenous antibiotics and use single antibiotic doses for surgical prophylaxis).

Travellers' diarrhoea

This is one of the most common illnesses in people who travel internationally and affects 20–50% of travellers depending on destination. The risk is highest in people travelling to areas with poor food and water hygiene.

Clinical features

The clinical features of travellers' diarrhoea consist of diarrhoea (with or without blood), abdominal cramps, fever, nausea and vomiting, which usually resolve without treatment over several days. A prolonged illness lasting weeks is more likely to be caused by protozoan parasites (Table 2.10).

Treatment and prevention

To reduce the risk of infection, travellers are advised to drink bottled water, peel fruit before eating it and avoid salads because the ingredients may have been washed in contaminated water. Antibiotic prophylaxis with ciprofloxacin is not indicated for most travellers but is given when an underlying medical illness would be compromised by diarrhoea, e.g. patients with an ileostomy, immunosuppression and chronic kidney disease.

Treatment of travellers' diarrhoea is for the most part symptomatic. Fever and significant bloody diarrhoea is concerning for amoebic dysentery or invasive bacterial infection and empirical treatment should be considered with fluoroquinolones or cephalosporins. Campylobacter isolates are becoming increasingly fluoroquinolone resistant, especially in Asia, and in this case azithromycin should be used.

Colonoscopy and biopsy are occasionally necessary in patients with persistent diarrhoea, when an alternative diagnosis to travellers' diarrhoea, such as inflammatory bowel disease, seems likely. Irritable bowel syndrome (p. 119) can occur after travellers' diarrhoea.

Amoebiasis[nd]

Amoebiasis is caused by the protozoal organism *Entamoeba histolytica*. Infection occurs world-wide, although much higher incidence rates are found in the tropics and subtropics. Transmission of infection is by ingestion of cysts in contaminated food and water or spread directly by person-to-person contact.

Clinical features

Intestinal amoebiasis (amoebic dysentery) *E. histolytica* invades the colonic epithelium, leading to tissue necrosis and ulceration. Ulceration may deepen and progress under the mucosa to form typical flask-like ulcers. The presentation varies from mild bloody diarrhoea to fulminating colitis, with the risk of toxic dilatation, perforation and peritonitis. An amoeboma (inflammatory fibrotic mass) may develop, commonly in the caecum or rectosigmoid region, which may bleed, cause obstruction or intussusception, or be mistaken for a carcinoma.

Amoebic liver abscess An amoebic liver abscess (often single and in right lobe of liver) develops when organisms invade through the bowel serosa, enter the portal vein and pass into the liver. The incubation period is 8–20 weeks. There is tender hepatomegaly, a high swinging fever and profound malaise. There may not be a history of colitis.

Investigations

Serology Amoebic fluorescent antibody test (FAT) is positive in 90% of patients with liver abscess and in 60–70% of patients with active colitis.

Colonic disease Microscopic examination of fresh stool or colonic exudate obtained at sigmoidoscopy shows the motile trophozoites, which contain red blood cells. *E. histolytica* must be distinguished by molecular techniques from the non-pathogenic *E. dispar,* which appears identical but has no clinical relevance.

Liver disease Liver abscesses should be considered when liver function testing is abnormal. There may be a raised right hemidiaphragm on chest X-ray. Liver ultrasonography or CT scan will confirm the presence of an abscess.

Differential diagnosis

Amoebic colitis must be differentiated from the other causes of bloody diarrhoea: inflammatory bowel disease, bacillary dysentery, *E. coli*, *Campylobacter* sp., salmonellae and, rarely, pseudomembranous colitis. An amoebic liver abscess must be differentiated from a pyogenic abscess and/or a hydatid cyst. In patients with exposure in the Middle East, Central Asia and some parts of Africa, hydatid disease should be excluded by serological testing (Table 2.9).

Management

- *Colitis* – oral metronidazole or tinidazole, followed by a luminal amoebicide such as diloxanide furoate or paromomycin to clear the bowel of parasites.
- *Liver abscess* – metronidazole 500 mg three times daily for 7–10 days. A large tense abscess may require percutaneous drainage under ultrasound guidance. As a pyogenic abscess may be difficult to distinguish from, broad spectrum antibiotic therapy is often used until the diagnosis is confirmed.

Shigellosis (bacillary dysentery)[nd]

Shigellosis is an acute self-limiting intestinal infection which occurs world-wide but is more common in tropical countries and in areas of poor hygiene. Transmission is by the faecal–oral route. The four *Shigella* species (*S. dysenteriae*, *S. flexneri*, *S. boydii* and *S. sonnei*) invade and damage the intestinal mucosa (Table 2.10). Some strains of *S. dysenteriae* secrete a cytotoxin which results in diarrhoea. Differential diagnosis is from other causes of bloody diarrhoea (see above). Sigmoidoscopic appearances may be the same as those in inflammatory bowel disease. Some infections settle spontaneously but Ciprofloxacin 500 mg orally twice daily is the treatment of choice; however, there is increasing world-wide resistance.

Cholera[nd]

Cholera is caused by the Gram-negative bacillus, *Vibrio cholerae* (Tables 2.7 and 2.10). Infection is common in tropical and subtropical countries in areas of poor hygiene. Infection is by the faecal–oral route, and spread is predominantly by ingestion of water contaminated with the faeces of infected humans.

Pathophysiology and clinical features

Following attachment to and colonization of the small intestinal epithelium, *V. cholerae* produces its major virulence factor, cholera toxin. The toxin binds to its enterocyte surface receptor (monosialoganglioside G_1), which in turn activates cyclic adenosine monophosphate (cAMP). The increase in cAMP activates intermediates (e.g. protein kinase and Ca^{2+}), which then act on the apical membrane causing chloride ion secretion (with water) and inhibition of sodium and chloride absorption. This produces massive secretion of isotonic fluid into the intestinal lumen. Cholera toxin also increases serotonin release from enterochromaffin cells in the gut, which contributes to the secretory activity and diarrhoea. Additional enterotoxins have been described in *V. cholerae* which may contribute to its pathogenic effect. Profuse watery diarrhoea ('rice-water stools') may result in dehydration, hypotension and death.

Management

Management is aimed at aggressive volume replacement which is mainly oral. Intravenous fluids are given in severe cases. The mechanism of action of oral rehydration solutions (ORS) depends on the fact that there is a glucose-dependent sodium absorption mechanism not related to cAMP and thus unaffected by cholera toxin. The World Health Organization ORS contains sodium (75 mmol/L) and glucose (75 mmol/L), along with potassium, chloride and citrate. Cereal-based regimens also contain cooked rice. Single-dose azithromycin or doxycycline helps to eradicate the infection, decrease stool output, shorten the duration of the illness and reduce bacterial shedding.

Prevention and control

Good hygiene and sanitation are the most effective measures for the reduction of infection. Oral live attenuated and killed vaccine are recommended in potential or actual outbreak situations.

Giardiasis

Giardia intestinalis is a flagellated protozoan that is found world-wide but is more common in developing countries. It is a cause of travellers' diarrhoea and may cause prolonged symptoms.

Clinical features

The clinical features are the result of damage to the small intestine, with subtotal villous atrophy in severe cases, and consist of diarrhoea, nausea, abdominal pain and distension, with malabsorption and steatorrhoea in some cases. Repeated infections can result in growth retardation in children.

Investigations

Treatment is often given based on clinical suspicion. If necessary, the diagnosis is made by finding cysts on stool examination (but negative stool does not exclude the diagnosis) or parasites in duodenal aspirates or biopsies.

Management

Metronidazole 2 g as a single dose daily for 3 days will cure most infections; some patients need two or three courses. Alternative drugs include tinidazole and mepacrine.

HELMINTHIC INFECTIONS

The helminths or worms that infect humans are of three classes (Table 2.9). In the UK, only three species are commonly encountered: *Enterobius vermicularis*, *Ascaris lumbricoides* and *Taenia saginata*. Other species occur in tropical and subtropical countries and may be imported into the UK. A raised blood eosinophil count (eosinophilia) occurs at some stage in nearly all helminth infections.

SEXUALLY TRANSMITTED INFECTIONS

Sexually transmitted infections (STIs) remain endemic in all societies, and the range of diseases spread by sexual activity continues to increase. The three common presenting symptoms are:

- Urethral discharge (see below)
- Genital ulcers (see below)
- Vaginal discharge – this is caused by *Candida albicans*, *Trichomonas vaginalis*, *Neisseria gonorrhoeae*, *Chlamydia trachomatis* and herpes simplex. Bacterial vaginosis is also characterized by a vaginal discharge but is not regarded as an STI. It occurs when the normal lactobacilli of the vagina are replaced by a mixed flora of *Gardnerella vaginalis* and anaerobes, resulting in an offensive discharge. Other causes of vaginal discharge are retained tampon, chemical irritants, cervical polyps and neoplasia.

The STIs predominantly seen in the tropics are chancroid (caused by *Haemophilus ducreyi*), donovanosis (*Klebsiella granulomatis*) and lymphogranuloma venereum (*Chlamydia trachomatis* types LGV 1, 2 and 3). They present with genital ulceration and inguinal lymphadenopathy.

The aspects of management of all the STIs are:

- Accurate diagnosis and effective treatment
- Screening for other STIs including HIV, hepatitis viruses and syphilis
- Patient education
- Contact tracing: the patient's sexual partners must be traced so that they can be treated, thereby preventing the disease from spreading further
- Follow-up to ensure that infection is adequately treated.

Urethritis

Urethritis in men presents with urethral discharge and dysuria. It is often asymptomatic in women. The causes are infection with *N. gonorrhoeae*, *C. trachomatis*, *Ureaplasma urealyticum*, *Bacteroides* sp. and *Mycoplasma* sp.

Gonorrhoea

The causative organism, *N. gonorrhoeae* (gonococcus), is a Gram-negative intracellular diplococcus which infects epithelium, particularly of the urogenital tract, rectum, pharynx and conjunctivae. Infection is via mucous membranes by direct contact.

Clinical features

The incubation period ranges from 2 to 14 days. In men the symptoms are purulent urethral discharge and dysuria. In men who have sex with men (MSM), proctitis may produce anal pain, discharge and itch. Women may be asymptomatic or complain of vaginal discharge, dysuria, lower abdominal pain and intermenstrual bleeding. Pharyngeal infection is asymptomatic in >90%. Complications include epididymo-orchitis and prostatitis in men. In women, complications include salpingitis, Bartholin's abscess, pelvic inflammatory disease and perihepatitis. Haematogenous spread causes disseminated infection with rash and arthritis (p. 286). Infants born to infected mothers may develop ocular infections (ophthalmia neonatorum).

Diagnosis

Testing is carried out for symptomatic patients, contacts of those infected and in those with risk factors. In men a first catch urine (FCU) and in women vaginal or endocervical swabs are taken for nucleic acid amplification tests (NAAT). This technique is highly sensitive but can give false-positive results. Rectal and pharyngeal swabs should be sent for culture and sensitivity testing. A positive NAAT must be followed up by samples for culture to allow sensitivity testing to be carried out. In disseminated disease blood/synovial fluid cultures should be taken.

Management

Uncomplicated anogenital infection in adults is treated with ceftriaxone 500 mg intramuscularly (i.m.) and azithromycin 1 g orally, both as single doses. Dual therapy is used to prevent the resistance to β-lactam antibiotics. Gonococcal epididymo-orchitis and PID is treated with i.m. ceftriaxone and 10–14 days of doxycycline, with the addition of metronidazole for PID. Disseminated disease is usually treated with higher doses of intravenous ceftriaxone.

Test of cure is recommended in all cases at 3 days if symptoms remain or 2 weeks if asymptomatic. Recent outbreaks of high level azithromycin resistant gonorrhoea in parts of England have the potential to render gonococcal infection untreatable.

Chlamydia urethritis

Urogenital *C. trachomatis* is the most common curable STI in the UK. The majority of infections are asymptomatic. Men present with urethral discharge and dysuria. Women present with vaginal discharge, intermenstrual bleeding and dysuria. In MSM, rectal infection distinct from lymphogranuloma venereum is seen. The diagnosis is made by NAAT from vulvo-vaginal swabs in women and FCU or rectal swabs in men. Treatment for uncomplicated urogenital infection is with doxycycline for 7 days or single-dose azithromycin 1 g. Test of cure is not usually necessary.

Genital ulcers

The infective causes of genital ulceration in the UK include syphilis, herpes simplex and herpes zoster. Non-infective causes are Behçet's disease (p. 312), toxic epidermal necrolysis (p. 817), Stevens–Johnson syndrome (p. 817), carcinoma and trauma.

Syphilis

Syphilis is a multisystem and multistage disease. The causative organism, *Treponema pallidum,* is a motile spirochaete which enters the new host through breaches in squamous or columnar epithelium either by direct contact or vertical transmission.

Early stages

Primary infection After an incubation period of 10–90 days a papule (usually anogenital) develops at the site of inoculation often with regional lymphadenopathy. This ulcerates to become a painless, firm chancre, which heals spontaneously within 2–3 weeks.

Secondary infection In 25% of patients, 4–10 weeks after the appearance of the primary lesion, constitutional symptoms appear with fever, sore throat and arthralgia. There may be generalized lymphadenopathy, widespread skin rash (except the face, but may affect palms and soles), superficial ulcers in the mouth and on the genitalia (snail-track ulcers) and condylomata lata (warty perianal lesions). Many systems may be affected (hepatitis, glomerulonephritis, arthritis, meningitis, uveitis). In most patients, symptoms subside within 3–12 weeks and the disease enters an asymptomatic, latent phase.

Late stages

Tertiary syphilis This occurs after a latent period of 2 years or more. The characteristic lesion is a gumma (granulomatous, sometimes ulcerating lesion) occurring in the skin, bones, liver and testes. Cardiac syphilis and neurosyphilis are discussed on page 773.

Congenital syphilis Two-thirds of cases are asymptomatic at birth, but 2–6 weeks after birth there is nasal discharge, skin and mucous membrane lesions and failure to thrive. Signs of late syphilis (see above) appear after 2 years of age, when there are also characteristic bone ('sabre tibia') and teeth abnormalities (Hutchinson's teeth) as a result of earlier damage. Screening programmes are undertaken in pregnant women in the UK.

Diagnosis

A full sexual history including all partners over many weeks to decades is necessary depending on the stage of infection at presentation.

- *Dark ground microscopy of fluid* taken from lesions shows organisms in primary and secondary disease. Serological tests may be negative early in primary disease.
- *PCR* can be performed from swabs of oral and other lesions and samples such as CSF.
- *Serology*. Treponemal antibody tests cannot differentiate *T. pallidum* from endemic treponemal infections (yaws/bejel/pinta); therefore, consideration must be made for travel history etc.

Primary screening is most commonly with the *T. pallidum* EIA, *Treponema pallidum* particle agglutination assay (TPPA) or *T. pallidum* haemagglutination assay (TPHA). Positive results should be confirmed with a different screening method and a second specimen should be tested to confirm positive results. These may be negative in early disease.

Serological activity of syphilis is carried out by quantitative methods; RPR or Venereal Disease Research Laboratory (VDRL). A titre of >16 usually indicates active disease. False negatives may occur in late disease. Other diseases, e.g. autoimmune disease and malignancy, may give false-positive results.

Monitoring serological effect of treatment is carried out by quantitative RPR/VDRL.

Management

- *Primary, secondary and early latent syphilis* – intramuscular benzathine penicillin G 2.4 MU as a single dose. Porcaine penicillin G, doxycycline, ceftriaxone and azithromycin are alternatives.
- *Late latent, cardiovascular and gummatous disease* – extend early-stage treatment weekly for 3 weeks.
- *Neurosyphilis* – procaine penicillin 1.8–2.4 MU intramuscularly once daily plus probenecid 500 mg QDS for 14 days.

The Jarisch–Herxheimer reaction, characterized by malaise, fever and headache, occurs most commonly in early syphilis and resolves within 24 hours.

HUMAN IMMUNODEFICIENCY VIRUS

HIV is a retrovirus and since the 1980s has become a major global public health problem. Without viral suppression the infection eventually leads to acquired immune deficiency syndrome (AIDS) and death. Estimates for 2014 suggested 37 million people were living with HIV world-wide but only 54% of people with HIV knew their status. Between 2000 and 2015, HIV infection rates have fallen but sub-Saharan Africa remains the most seriously affected and 70% of new HIV diagnoses occur here. Highly active antiretroviral therapy (ART) has transformed the outcome for individuals with HIV infection, but there is still variable access in developing countries. The challenge in developed countries is to diagnose HIV infection at an earlier stage and thus reduce transmission and avoid late diagnosis. In the UK, approximately 17% of those with HIV are unaware of their diagnosis. Forty per cent of newly diagnosed adults in the UK are diagnosed late, which is associated with an impaired response to ART and increased morbidity and mortality.

Routes of acquisition

Transmission is by:

- *Sexual intercourse (vaginal and anal)*. World-wide, heterosexual intercourse accounts for the vast majority of infections. In the UK, diagnoses in MSM still account for over half of the infections per annum, with black African heterosexuals the next most commonly diagnosed group. Coexistent STIs, especially those causing genital ulceration, enhance transmission.
- *Mother to child.* Transmission can occur in utero, although the majority of infections take place perinatally or via breast milk.
- *Contaminated blood, blood products and organ donations*. The risk is now minimal in developed countries since the introduction of screening blood products in 1985.
- *Contaminated needles.* This is a major route of transmission of HIV among intravenous drug addicts who share needles and syringes. Healthcare workers have a risk of approximately 0.3% following a single needle-stick injury with known HIV-infected blood but post-exposure prophylaxis is available.

HIV infection is not spread by ordinary social or household contact.

Pathogenesis of HIV infection

There are two types, HIV-1 and HIV-2. HIV-2 is mainly confined to West Africa, runs a more indolent course than HIV-1 and may not respond to many of the drugs used in HIV-1. The virus consists of an outer envelope and an inner core. The core contains RNA and the enzyme reverse transcriptase, which allows viral RNA to be transcribed into DNA and then incorporated into the host cell genome (i.e. a retrovirus). The rapid emergence of viral quasi-species (closely related but genetically distinct variants) is due to the high mutation rate of reverse transcriptase and the high rate of viral turnover. This genetic diversification has implications for the evolution of viral variants with resistance to antiviral drugs.

HIV surface glycoprotein gp120 binds to the CD4 molecule on host lymphocytes and other cells bearing the CD4 receptor. The interaction between CD4 and HIV surface glycoprotein together with host chemokine co-receptors CCR5 and CXCR4 is responsible for HIV entry into cells and release of viral RNA. There is a progressive and severe depletion of infected CD4 helper lymphocytes, which results in host susceptibility to infections with intracellular bacteria and mycobacteria. The coexisting antibody abnormalities predispose to infections with capsulated bacteria, e.g. *Streptococcus pneumoniae* and *Haemophilus influenzae*. The clinical illness associated with HIV infection is due to this immune dysfunction, and also to a direct effect of HIV on certain tissues.

Natural history of HIV infection

The typical pattern of HIV infection is shown in Fig. 2.2. Throughout the course of HIV infection, viral load and immunodeficiency progress steadily, despite the absence of observed disease during the latency period.

HIV infection is divided into the following stages:

- *Primary HIV infection or seroconversion.* Illness occurs in most individuals 2–4 weeks after infection. Symptoms are non-specific and include fever, maculopapular rash, myalgia, headache/aseptic meningitis. The illness lasts up to 3 weeks and recovery is usually complete.

- *Clinical latency.* Most are asymptomatic. A subgroup of patients have *persistent generalized lymphadenopathy* defined as lymphadenopathy (>1 cm) at two or more extra inguinal sites for more than 3 months in the absence of causes other than HIV infection. There may be splenomegaly.

- *Early symptomatic HIV infection* is associated with a rise in viral load, a fall in CD4 count and development of symptoms and signs due to direct HIV effects and immunosuppression. Non-HIV-related malignancies are more common.

- *Significant immunosuppression* sees the patient develop opportunistic infections and specific malignancies. AIDS is a term used to describe these potentially life-threatening infections and cancers. In most patients the CD4 count will be below 200 and often much lower (Table 2.11).

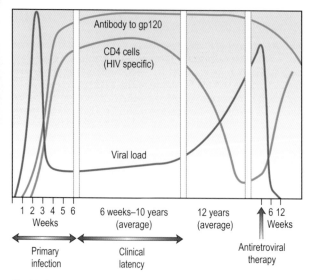

Fig. 2.2 Schematic representation of the course of human immunodeficiency virus (HIV) infection. The effect of antiretroviral therapy is also shown.

Table 2.11 AIDS-defining conditions*

Candidiasis of bronchi, trachea or lungs
Candidiasis, oesophageal
Cervical carcinoma, invasive
Coccidioidomycosis, disseminated or extrapulmonary
Cryptococcosis, extrapulmonary
Cryptosporidiosis, chronic intestinal (1 month duration)
CMV disease (other than liver, spleen or nodes)
CMV retinitis (with loss of vision)
Encephalopathy (HIV-related)
Herpes simplex, chronic ulcers (1 month duration); or bronchitis, pneumonitis or oesophagitis
Histoplasmosis, disseminated or extrapulmonary
Isosporiasis; chronic intestinal (1 month duration)
Kaposi's sarcoma
Lymphoma, Burkitt's
Lymphoma, immunoblastic (or equivalent term)
Lymphoma (primary) of brain
Mycobacterium avium-intracellulare complex or *M. kansasii,* disseminated or extrapulmonary
Mycobacterium tuberculosis, any site
Mycobacterium, other species or unidentified species, disseminated or extrapulmonary
Pneumocystis jiroveci (formerly P. carinii) pneumonia
Pneumonia, recurrent
Progressive multifocal leucoencephalopathy
Salmonella septicaemia, recurrent
Toxoplasmosis of brain
Wasting syndrome, due to HIV

*USA definition also includes those with a CD4 count <200 cells/mm^3.

Clinical features

The spectrum of illnesses associated with HIV infection is broad and is the result of direct HIV infection (Table 2.12), infections associated with immunodeficiency (p. 48), co-infections (e.g. hepatitis B and C) (pp. 153–160) and side effects of the drugs used to treat the condition.

Diagnosis

Informed consent and testing for HIV infection is within the competence of any doctor, nurse, midwife or trained healthcare worker. UK national guidelines for HIV testing are intended to facilitate an increase in testing and prevent late diagnosis (Table 2.13). Testing should be offered to those with signs and symptoms

Table 2.12 Direct HIV infection effects

Neurological disease	AIDS dementia complex
	Sensory polyneuropathy
	Autonomic neuropathy causing diarrhoea and postural hypotension
	Aseptic meningitis
Eye	Retinal cotton wool spots – rarely troublesome
Mucocutaneous	Dry, itchy, flaky skin
	Pruritic papular eruption
	Aphthous ulceration in the mouth
Haematological	Anaemia of chronic disease
	Neutropenia
	Autoimmune thrombocytopenia
Gastrointestinal	Anorexia leading to weight loss in advanced disease
	HIV enteropathy leading to diarrhoea and malabsorption
Renal	Renal impairment
	Nephrotic syndrome (due to focal glomerulosclerosis)
Respiratory	Chronic sinusitis and otitis media
	Lymphoid interstitial pneumonitis – lymphocytic infiltration of the lung, causing dyspnoea and a dry cough
Endocrine	Reduced adrenal function – infection may precipitate clear adrenal insufficiency
Cardiac	Myocarditis and cardiomyopathy

of acute or chronic infection and those with risk exposure (i.e. MSM, intravenous drug users), but it should also be incorporated into the routine care of healthy individuals. Some centres in the UK have adopted a universal screening policy for new admissions/A&E attendances. HIV testing should be considered in any demographic of patient. All pregnant women are offered testing to prevent vertical transmission in the UK.

- Combination immunoassays detecting HIV-1 and HIV-2 antibodies and the HIV P24 antigen are used for initial screening and, when positive, confirmatory testing is undertaken. These assays have improved identification of early infection by reducing the 'window period' where antibody may not be detected, but this is still an important consideration and repeat testing may be required.
- Plasma HIV RNA levels are very high in early infection and may be used when the above approach is indeterminate to confirm early infection.

Table 2.13 Clinical indicator diseases for adult HIV infection and testing

Respiratory	Bacterial pneumonia
	Aspergillosis
Neurology	Aseptic meningitis/encephalitis
	Cerebral abscess
	Space occupying lesion of unknown cause
	Guillain-Barré syndrome
	Transverse myelitis
	Peripheral neuropathy
	Dementia
	Leucoencephalopathy
Dermatology	Severe or recalcitrant seborrheic dermatitis
	Severe or recalcitrant psoriasis
	Multidermatomal or recurrent herpes zoster
Gastroenterology	Oral candidiasis
	Oral hairy leukoplakia
	Chronic diarrhoea of unknown cause
	Weight loss of unknown cause
	Salmonella, shigella or campylobacter
	Hepatitis B
	Hepatitis C
Oncology	Anal cancer or anal intraepithelial dysplasia
	Lung cancer
	Seminoma
	Head and neck cancer
	Hodgkin's lymphoma
	Castleman's disease
Gynaecology	Vaginal intraepithelial neoplasia
	Cervical intraepithelial neoplasia grade 2 or above
Haematology	Any unexplained blood dyscrasia
	- thrombocytopenia
	- neutropenia
	- lymphopenia
Ophthalmology	Infective retinal disease including toxoplasmosis and herpesvirus
	Any unexplained retinopathy

Continued

Table 2.13 Clinical indicator diseases for adult HIV infection and testing—cont'd

ENT	Lymphadenopathy of unknown cause
	Chronic parotitis
	Lymphoepithelial parotid cysts
Other	Mononucleosis-like syndrome
	Pyrexia of unknown origin
	Lymphadenopathy of unknown cause
	Any sexually transmitted infection

- Rapid point-of-care and home testing kits are now available but positive results need to be confirmed in a laboratory setting.
- Viral genotype analysis is undertaken for all newly diagnosed patients with HIV along with resistance testing.
- All newly diagnosed patients should also have routine bloods, testing for co-infection with hepatitis B and C, syphilis serology and sexual health screen, screening for antibody detection for a variety of vaccine-preventable infections and, if aged over 50 years, estimation of cardiovascular risk and fracture risk.

Monitoring

Patients are monitored to assess the progression of the infection and ongoing treatment. As patient survival has dramatically improved since the availability of ART, so has the recognition of non-AIDS-defining HIV comorbidities, particularly cardiovascular, renal, metabolic, and bone disease and non-HIV-related malignancy, all of which require monitoring.

- CD4 lymphocyte count is measured at least biannually but often more regularly in ART naïve patients or following the initiation of ART. Patients with counts below 200 cells are at greatest risk of HIV-related pathology, particularly opportunistic infection.
- Plasma levels of HIV RNA ('viral load', measured in copies of RNA per mL) are a measure of viral replication. The viral load is the best indicator of long-term prognosis but more immediately reflects the effectiveness of a chosen ART regimen. A rising viral load in a patient receiving ART suggests drug failure as a result of poor compliance or emerging resistance.

Management

Management involves treatment with antiretroviral drugs, social and psychological care, prevention of opportunistic infections and prevention of transmission of HIV. Although HIV infection cannot be cured, the advent of highly active ART in the 1990s has transformed HIV into a chronic controllable condition. The aims of treatment are to maintain physical and mental health and to avoid transmission of the virus. It is paramount that the patient is actively involved in treatment decision-making. General health promotion advice on smoking cessation, alcohol, diet, drug misuse and exercise should be given, particularly in light of the cardiovascular, metabolic and hepatotoxic risks associated with ART. Antiretroviral drugs available in the UK are listed in Table 2.14. Some ART combinations now come in a combined pill offering the patient the freedom of once-daily dosing and improved adherence.

Treatment regimens for HIV infection are complicated and require a long-term commitment to high levels of adherence. A combination of clinical assessment and laboratory marker data, including viral load and CD4 counts, together with individual circumstances, should guide therapeutic decision-making.

Table 2.14 Antiretroviral drugs*

Class of drug	Mechanism of action
Reverse transcriptase inhibitors	
1. Nucleoside/nucleotide* reverse transcriptase inhibitors	
Abacavir Didanosine Emtricitabine Lamivudine Stavudine Tenofovir* Zidovudine NRTI Fixed dose combinations Kivexa – abacavir/lamivudine Trizivir – abacavir/lamivudine/ zidovudine Truvada – emtricitabine/tenofovir (disoproxil) Descovy – Emtricitabine/Tenofovir (alafenamide) Combivir – lamivudine/zidovudine	Inhibit synthesis of DNA by reverse transcription and also act as DNA chain terminators
2. Non-nucleoside reverse transcriptase inhibitors	
Efavirenz Etravirine Nevirapine Rilpivirine	Bind directly to and inhibit reverse transcriptase

Continued

Table 2.14 Antiretroviral drugs—cont'd

Class of drug	Mechanism of action
Protease inhibitors	
Atazanavir Darunavir Fosamprenavir Indinavir Lopinavir Ritonavir* Saquinavir Tipranavir *Ritonavir is often used as a low-dose booster to increase the effect of other protease inhibitors	Act competitively on HIV aspartyl protease enzyme, which is involved in production of functional viral proteins and enzymes
Pharmacokinetic enhancers	
Cobicistat used to increase the effect of atazanavir or darunavir	
Fusion inhibitors	
Enfuvirtide	Inhibits fusion of HIV with target cell
Co-receptor blockers	
Maraviroc	Blocks the CCR5 chemokine co-receptor
Integrase inhibitors	
Raltegravir Dolutegravir	Prevents insertion of HIV DNA into the human genome
Single tablet regimens:	
Atripla – efavirenz/emtricitabine/tenofovir (disoproxil) Eviplera – rilpivirine/emtricitabine/tenofovir (disoproxil) Genvoya – Elvitegravir/cobicistat/emtricitabine/tenofovir (alafenamide) Stribild – Elvitegravir/cobicistat/emtricitabine/tenofovir (disoproxil) Triumeq – Dolutegravir/abacavir/lamivudine All ARVs are given orally as capsules tablets or liquid formulation except enfuvirtide (s.c. injection)	

ARVs have significant side effects, the extent of which is beyond the scope of this text. Specialist advice should be sought on the use of ARVs.

Within the last decade the CD4 count threshold at which patients are first offered ART treatment has risen such that recent guidelines published by the British HIV Association recommend that all patients are offered treatment regardless of their CD4 count.

Treatment is initiated with a combination of drugs started simultaneously; initial resistance data should be considered. The preferred starting regimen is two nucleoside/nucleotide reverse transcriptase inhibitors plus one of a ritonavir-boosted protease inhibitor, a non-nucleoside transcriptase inhibitor or an integrase inhibitor. The goal is to suppress the viral load to an undetectable level (<50 copies/mL) within 3–6 months of starting therapy. Patients may need to change therapy because of drug resistance or intolerance/adverse drug reactions. Adverse drug reactions are relatively common; product literature and specialist advice should be sought. Many antiretroviral drugs have significant interactions with other classes of compounds and when commencing any new medication in a patient receiving ART it is highly recommended that these be considered. Comprehensive interaction data are available at http://www.hiv-druginteractions.org.

Conditions due to immunodeficiency

Immunodeficiency allows the development of opportunistic infections. These are diseases caused by organisms that are not usually considered pathogenic, or are unusual presentations of known pathogens, or the occurrence of tumours that have an oncogenic viral aetiology. Susceptibility increases as the patient becomes more immunosuppressed. When patients are profoundly immunocompromised (CD4 count <100 cells/mm^3), disseminated infections with organisms of very low virulence such as *M. avium-intracellulare* and *Cryptosporidium* are able to establish themselves. The mortality and morbidity associated with HIV infection have declined dramatically since the introduction of highly active ART. Similarly, long-term secondary chemoprophylaxis for previously life-threatening infections may not be necessary when ART maintains the CD4 count above 200 cells/mm^3 and the viral load is low.

Fungi

Pneumocystis jiroveci (formerly *P. carinii*) causes pneumonia in
   immunocompromised patients, usually when CD4 count <200. There is
   an insidious onset of breathlessness, specifically exertional dyspnoea, a
   non-productive cough, fever and malaise. The chest X-ray may be normal
   or show bilateral perihilar interstitial infiltrates, which can progress to
   more diffuse shadowing. Pneumothorax may complicate *P. jiroveci*
   pneumonia (PCP). High-resolution CT scans of the chest are abnormal
   even if there is little on the chest X-ray. *Histoplasmosis* can produce a
   similar appearance. Definitive diagnosis is made by PCR amplification of
   the fungal DNA from induced sputum or bronchoalveolar lavage.
   Treatment depends on severity assessment and is usually with co-
   trimoxazole, either orally or intravenously. Treatment should not be
   delayed if clinical suspicion is high. High-dose corticosteroids reduce
   mortality in severe cases ($P_aO_2 < 9.3$ kPa). Long-term prophylaxis, usually
   with oral co-trimoxazole, is required in patients whose CD4 count
   remains below 200 cells/mm^3 despite ART.

Cryptococcus neoformans most commonly causes meningitis in HIV patients. There is an insidious onset of fever and headache. Nausea, vomiting and impaired consciousness may suggest raised intracranial pressures. Diagnosis is made by demonstration of cryptococcal antigen in serum. CSF microscopy with Indian ink staining shows the organisms directly, and culture of the organism from CSF and/or blood is possible. CT scan is performed before lumbar puncture to exclude a space-occupying lesion. Treatment is with intravenous amphotericin B $\pm$ flucytosine or fluconazole. Serial lumbar punctures may be necessary to reduce intracranial pressure. *Candida* infection (usually *Candida albicans*) presents as creamy plaques in the mouth, vulvovaginal region and oesophagus (producing odynophagia and dysphagia). Treatment is with fluconazole (preferred if *Candida* is disseminated) or other azoles. Disseminated infection with *Aspergillus fumigatus* occurs in advanced HIV infection. Treatment is with voriconazole or liposomal amphotericin B.

Protozoal infections

Toxoplasma gondii most commonly causes cerebral abscess in immunocompromised HIV-infected patients. Clinical features include focal neurological signs, fits, fever, headache and confusion. Toxoplasma infection in the immunocompromised is usually caused by reactivation of previous infection and diagnosis is made on the basis of positive *Toxoplasma* serology. Multiple ring-enhancing lesions on contrast-enhanced CT or MRI of the brain are characteristic. Treatment is with anticonvulsants and combination pyrimethamine, sulfadiazine and folinic acid for at least 6 weeks. Lifelong maintenance is required to prevent relapse unless the CD4 count can be restored by ART. The differential diagnosis of multiple ring-enhancing central nervous system (CNS) lesions in these patients includes lymphoma, mycobacterial (e.g. tuberculoma), progressive multifocal leucoencephalopathy or focal cryptococcal infection.

Cryptosporidium species (*parvum* and *hominis*) cause self-limiting watery diarrhoea and abdominal cramps in immunocompetent individuals and a severe chronic watery diarrhoea in HIV patients, in whom it also causes sclerosing cholangitis. Diagnosis is made by demonstrating cysts on stool microscopy or on small bowel biopsy specimens obtained at endoscopy. ART and immune restoration is associated with resolution of symptoms. Treatment is otherwise symptomatic. Paromomycin and nitazoxanide have a limited effect on diarrhoea.

Microsporidia infection (*Enterocytozoon bieneusi* and *Septata intestinalis*) cause diarrhoea. Diagnosis is made by demonstrating spores in the stools. Treatment is with ART and albendazole.

Leishmaniasis in HIV-infected patients occurs as in any immunocompetent host with either visceral (weight loss, fever, hepatosplenomegaly), mucocutaneous or cutaneous disease. In Europe most cases are cutaneous. Diagnosis is by parasitological or histological confirmation and may require splenic, bone marrow or skin biopsy. Visceral disease is treated with liposomal amphotericin B.

Viruses

Cytomegalovirus causes retinitis, colitis, oesophageal ulceration, encephalitis, pneumonitis, polyradiculopathy and adrenalitis. Retinitis presents with floaters, loss of visual acuity and orbital pain, usually in a patient with CD4 count <100. The diagnosis is made on fundoscopy, which shows a characteristic appearance of the retina with haemorrhages and exudate. Colitis presents with bloody diarrhoea and abdominal pain. Diagnosis is made by demonstrating characteristic 'cytomegalic cells' (large cells containing an intranuclear inclusion and sometimes intracytoplasmic inclusions) on pathology examination of mucosal biopsy specimens. CMV DNA via PCR can be detected in peripheral blood but high titres do not always correlate with clinical infection and it is best used to monitor treatment response. Treatment of CMV infection is with intravenous ganciclovir, foscarnet or oral valganciclovir. Reactivation occurs in CMV retinitis and oral or topical ganciclovir is given long term, unless immune competence can be restored with ART.

Herpes virus Primary infection with herpes simplex virus causes genital and oral ulceration, and systemic infection. Varicella zoster occurs at any stage of HIV infection, but may be more aggressive and longer lasting than in immunocompetent patients. Treatment is with aciclovir. Human herpesvirus 8 is associated with Kaposi's sarcoma (see below). EBV causes oral hairy leucoplakia, presenting as a pale, ridged lesion on the side of the tongue. EBV is also associated with primary cerebral lymphoma and non-Hodgkin's lymphoma (see below).

Human papilloma virus (HPV) produces genital and plantar warts. HPV infection is associated with the more rapid development of squamous cell cancer of the cervix and anal cancer.

Polyomavirus (JC virus) causes progressive multifocal leucoencephalopathy, which presents with intellectual impairment and often hemiparesis and aphasia.

Hepatitis virus B and C Because of the comparable routes of transmission of hepatitis viruses and HIV, co-infection is common, particularly in drug users and those infected by blood products. Hepatitis B does not seem to influence the natural history of HIV, though there is a reduced rate of clearance of the hepatitis B e antigen in co-infected patients and thus the risk of developing chronic infection is increased. Hepatitis C, however, is associated with a more rapid progression of HIV infection, and the progression of hepatitis C is more likely and more rapid.

Bacterial infection

This may present early in HIV infection, is often disseminated and frequently recurs. *Mycobacterium tuberculosis* can cause disease at all stages of HIV infection, but extrapulmonary tuberculosis (TB) is more common with advanced disease. *M. tuberculosis* infection usually responds well to standard treatment regimens, although the duration of therapy may be extended, especially in extrapulmonary infection. Treatment of TB in HIV co-infected patients presents specific challenges, particularly with regard to drug interactions and multidrug resistance (p. 540), and requires input from a specialist physician.

Mycobacterium avium-intracellulare (MAI) occurs only in the later stages of HIV infection when patients are profoundly immunosuppressed (CD4 cell count <50/mm^3). Clinical features include fever, anorexia, weight loss, diarrhoea and anaemia with bone marrow involvement. MAI is typically resistant to standard anti-tuberculous therapies. A combination of ethambutol, rifabutin and clarithromycin reduces the burden of organisms and provides symptomatic benefit. Other infections include *Strep. pneumoniae, H. influenzae,* staphylococcal skin infection and salmonella.

Neoplasia

The most common tumours are Kaposi's sarcoma and non-Hodgkin's lymphoma. The incidence of all HIV-related malignancies has fallen dramatically since the introduction of ART.

- Kaposi's sarcoma is a vascular tumour that appears as red-purple, raised, well-circumscribed lesions on the skin, hard palate and conjunctivae, and in the gastrointestinal tract. The lungs and lymph nodes may also be involved. Human herpesvirus 8 is implicated in the pathogenesis. Localized disease is treated with radiotherapy; systemic disease is treated with chemotherapy. Initiation of ART may cause regression of lesions and prevent new ones emerging.
- Non-Hodgkin's lymphoma occurs in the brain, gut and lung.
- Squamous cell carcinoma of the cervix and anus is associated with HIV. Infection with oncogenic strains of HPV has a causal association with invasive cancer.
- Non-HIV-related malignancy is more common in people living with HIV.

Prevention and control

- The risk of HIV transmission following a needle-stick injury involving contaminated blood is reduced by using combination ART. Occupational Health and local HIV specialists must be involved. Prophylaxis should be started as soon as possible after exposure following risk assessment.
- Pregnant HIV-positive women should receive antiviral therapy to reduce the risk of vertical transmission. For patients not adequately treated with ART, delivery by caesarean section dramatically reduces perinatal infection but access to these interventions is limited in resource-poor countries. In the UK, guidance suggests that infants with mothers known to be HIV positive should be exclusively formula fed.

- The use of condoms reduces sexual transmission of HIV. Male circumcision protects those individuals against infection with HIV and also other sexually transmitted diseases, such as syphilis and gonorrhoea.
- People who inject recreational drugs should not share needles; some areas provide free sterile needles as part of needle exchange programmes.

Prognosis

The rate of progression among patients infected with HIV varies greatly. The average life expectancy for an HIV-infected patient in the absence of treatment is approximately 10 years. The introduction of ART has resulted in a dramatic decrease in mortality and opportunistic infections in patients with HIV who now lead long and productive lives while managing a chronic health condition.

THERAPEUTICS

Antimicrobial agents are natural or synthetic chemical substances that suppress the growth of, or destroy, microorganisms including bacteria, fungi and viruses. Antimicrobial treatment must be started immediately in patients with life-threatening infection using 'blind therapy' based on the likely causative organisms and system involved. Treatment must then be adjusted later based on antimicrobial susceptibility data from specimens (e.g. pus, blood, foreign bodies) sent before or coinciding with start of treatment. Treatment should be prescribed for the shortest course likely to be effective and agents selected to minimize collateral damage and side effects. Antimicrobials should always be prescribed in accordance with local policies, formularies and guidelines. Such antimicrobial stewardship is of paramount importance in reducing the use of broad-spectrum antibiotics, particularly those associated with *C. difficile* infection, and minimizing the ongoing emergence of resistant organisms to allow infection to be treated successfully for future generations.

Antibacterials

β-Lactam antibacterials

Mechanism of action

The β-lactam antibacterials inhibit synthesis of the peptidoglycan layer of the cell wall, which surrounds certain bacteria and is essential for their survival.

Indications

Benzylpenicillin (penicillin G) is effective for many streptococcal and meningococcal infections, leptospirosis and treatment of Lyme disease. *Phenoxymethylpenicillin* (penicillin V) has a similar antibacterial spectrum to benzyl-penicillin but it should not be used for serious infections because gut absorption is unpredictable. *Flucloxacillin* is effective for infections due to β-lactamase-producing staphylococci (most staphylococci are resistant to benzyl-penicillin because they produce penicillinases). *Ampicillin* is principally indicated for the treatment of exacerbations of chronic bronchitis and middle ear infections. *Amoxicillin* is derived of ampicillin and has a similar antibacterial spectrum. It is better absorbed than ampicillin when given by mouth. *Co-amoxiclav* consists of amoxicillin with the β-lactamase inhibitor clavulanic acid, which extends the spectrum of activity of amoxicillin. *Piperacillin* is an extended spectrum β-lactam antibiotic. It is usually used together with a β-lactamase inhibitor such as tazobactam. The combination has activity against many Gram-positive and Gram-negative pathogens and anaerobes including *Pseudomonas aeruginosa*.

Preparations and dose

Benzylpenicillin Injection: 600 mg vial.

IM/IV (slow injection or infusion): 2.4–4.8 g daily in four divided doses. Higher doses may be needed in serious infections.

Flucloxacillin Capsules: 250 mg, 500 mg; Solution: 125 mg/5 mL, 250 mg/5 mL; Injection: 250 mg vial.

Oral 250–500 mg every 6 hours, at least 30 minutes before food.

IM 250–500 mg every 6 hours.

IV (slow injection or infusion): 0.25–2 g every 6 hours.

Amoxicillin Capsules: 250 mg, 500 mg; Suspension: 125 mg/5 mL, 250 mg/5 mL; Injection: 250 mg vial.

Oral 250–500 mg depending on infection.

IM/IV (slow injection or infusion): 500 mg every 8 hours increased to 1 g every 6 hours in severe infections.

Piperacillin + tazobactam Injection 2.25 g (2 g/250 mg) or 4.5 g (4 g/ 500 mg) vial.

IV (slow injection or infusion): 4.5 g every 8 hours increased to every 6 hours with an aminoglycoside in neutropenia.

Side effects

Hypersensitivity reactions include urticaria, fever, rashes and anaphylaxis. Individuals with a history of anaphylaxis, urticaria or rash immediately after penicillin administration are at risk of immediate hypersensitivity to a penicillin and should not receive a penicillin or cephalosporin (10% of penicillin-allergic patients are also allergic to cephalosporins). Encephalopathy with fits results from excessively high doses or in patients with severe renal failure. Diarrhoea and *C. difficile* infection (p. 34) can occur as a result of disturbance of the normal colonic flora. Other effects are interstitial nephritis, hepatitis, cholestatic jaundice, reversible neutropenia and eosinophilia. Aminopenicillins (e.g. amoxicillin) frequently produce a non-allergic maculopapular rash in patients with glandular fever.

Cautions/contraindications

Contraindicated in penicillin hypersensitivity (see above); macrolides are an alternative in these patients.

Cephalosporins

Mechanism of action

Cephalosporins inhibit bacterial wall synthesis in a manner similar to the penicillins.

Indications

Broad-spectrum antibiotics – used for treatment of septicaemia, pneumonia, meningitis, biliary tract infections, peritonitis and urinary tract infections.

Preparations and dose

Cephalosporins are often classified by 'generations'. The members within each generation share similar antibacterial activity. Succeeding generations tend to have increased activity against Gram-negative bacilli, usually at the expense of Gram-positive activity, and increased ability to cross the blood–brain barrier.

First generation

E.g. Cefalexin Capsules: 250 mg, 500 mg; Suspension: 125 mg/5 mL, 250 mg/5 mL.

Oral 250 mg every 8 hours, doubled for severe infections; maximum 4 g daily.

Second generation

E.g. Cefuroxime Tablets: 125 mg, 250 mg; Suspension: 125 mg/mL; Injection: 250 mg, 750 mg, 1.5 g vial.

Oral 250 mg twice daily in most infections; double dose for pneumonia. Gonorrhoea: 1 g as a single dose; Lyme disease: 500 mg twice daily for 20 days.

IM/IV 750 mg every 6–8 hours; 1.5 g every 6–8 hours in severe infections. Single injected doses over 750 mg by intravenous route only.

Third generation

E.g. Cefotaxime Injection: 500 mg, 1 g, 2 g.

IM/IV (injection or infusion): 1 g every 12 hours, increased in severe infections (e.g. meningitis) to 8 g daily in four divided doses.

Side effects

Skin rashes, nausea and vomiting, diarrhoea (including *C. difficile* colitis), hypersensitivity reactions (see penicillin).

Cautions/contraindications

Penicillin hypersensitivity other than with a minor rash only.

Aminoglycosides

Mechanism of action

Aminoglycosides inhibit protein synthesis in bacteria by binding irreversibly to the 30S ribosomal unit. This inhibits translation from mRNA to protein. Aminoglycosides are bactericidal.

Indications

Aminoglycosides are active against many Gram-negative bacteria (including *Pseudomonas* species) and some Gram-positive bacteria but are inactive against anaerobes. Aminoglycosides are often used for serious Gram-negative infections when they have a complementary and synergistic action with agents that disrupt cell wall synthesis (e.g. penicillins).

Preparations and dose

Examples: gentamicin (the most widely used), amikacin, neomycin, netilmicin, streptomycin, tobramycin.

Gentamicin Injection: 40 mg/mL

IM/IV (slow injection over 3 min or infusion): 3–5 mg/kg in divided doses every 8 hours or once daily by intravenous infusion, 5–7 mg/kg, then adjust according to serum gentamicin concentration.

Side effects

Most unwanted effects are dose related and are probably related to high trough concentrations of the drug. Ototoxicity can lead to both vestibular and auditory dysfunction, which result in often irreversible disturbances of balance or deafness. Other side effects are renal toxicity, acute neuromuscular blockade, nausea, vomiting, rash and antibiotic-associated colitis.

Cautions/contraindications

Aminoglycosides are contraindicated in myasthenia gravis. Monitor serum concentrations in all patients and reduce the dose in renal impairment. In patients with normal renal function, serum aminoglycoside concentrations should be measured after three to four doses (earlier and more frequent measurements in patients with renal failure), 1 hour after i.m. or i.v. administration ('peak' concentration to ensure bactericidal efficacy) and also just before the next dose ('trough' concentration to minimize the risk of toxic effects). For once-daily dose regimen, consult local guidelines on monitoring.

Macrolides

Mechanism of action

Macrolides interfere with bacterial protein synthesis by binding reversibly to the 50S subunit of the bacterial ribosome. The action is primarily bacteriostatic unless at high concentrations.

Indications

Erythromycin has an antibacterial spectrum that is similar to that of penicillin; it is thus an alternative in penicillin-allergic patients. Indications for erythromycin include respiratory infections, whooping cough, Legionnaires' disease, *Chlamydia* infections and *Campylobacter* enteritis. Erythromycin has poor activity against *H. influenzae*. Clarithromycin is a derivative of erythromycin with slightly greater activity. Azithromycin has slightly less activity than erythromycin against Gram-positive bacteria but enhanced activity against Gram-negative bacteria.

Preparations and dose

Clarithromycin Tablets: 250 mg, 500 mg; Injection: 500 mg vial.

Oral 250 mg every 12 hours; increased in severe infections to 500 mg every 12 hours.

IV infusion into larger proximal vein: 500 mg twice daily.

Side effects

Gastrointestinal upsets (epigastric discomfort, nausea, vomiting and diarrhoea) are common with the oral preparation of erythromycin; azithromycin and clarithromycin are better tolerated. Skin rashes, cholestatic jaundice (with erythromycin), prolongation of the QT interval on the electrocardiogram (ECG), with a predisposition to ventricular arrhythmias. Erythromycin and clarithromycin inhibit P450 drug-metabolizing enzymes and can elevate levels of drugs (e.g. carbamazepine and ciclosporin) requiring these enzymes for metabolism (see national formulary for list).

Metronidazole

Mechanism of action

A toxic metabolite inhibits bacterial DNA synthesis and breaks down existing DNA. Only some anaerobes and some protozoa contain the enzyme (nitroreductase) that converts metronidazole to its toxic metabolite. It is bactericidal.

Indications

Anaerobic infections, protozoal infections, *Helicobacter pylori* eradication, *C. difficile* colitis. Metronidazole is more commonly used than tinidazole.

Preparations and dose

Metronidazole Tablets: 200 mg, 400 mg; Suspension: 200 mg/5 mL; Intravenous infusion: 5 g/5 mL; Flagyl® suppositories.

Oral 400 mg every 8 hours; for surgical prophylaxis, 400 mg before surgery and three further doses of 400 mg every 8 hours for high-risk procedures.

IV infusion over 20 minutes: 500 mg every 8 hours; for surgical prophylaxis, 500 mg at induction and up to three further doses of 500 mg every 8 hours for high-risk procedures.

By rectum 500 mg every 8 hours; for surgical prophylaxis, 1 g 2 hours before surgery and up to three further doses of 1 g every 8 hours for high-risk procedures.

Side effects

Nausea, vomiting, metallic taste, disulfiram-like reaction (unpleasant hangover symptoms) with alcohol, skin rashes, and abnormal liver biochemistry. With prolonged therapy, peripheral neuropathy, transient epileptiform seizures and leucopenia can occur.

Cautions/contraindications

Caution with alcohol ingestion; reduce dose in severe liver disease and avoid in porphyria.

Quinolones

Mechanism of action

Quinolones inhibit replication of bacterial DNA. The effect is bactericidal.

Indications

Ciprofloxacin has a broad spectrum of activity and is particularly active against Gram-negative bacteria. It has only weak activity against streptococci, staphylococci and anaerobes.

Preparations and dose

Examples: ciprofloxacin, norfloxacin, levofloxacin.

Ciprofloxacin Tablets: 100 mg, 250 mg, 500 mg, 750 mg; Suspension: 250 mg/5 mL; Intravenous infusion: 2 mg/mL.

Oral 250–750 mg twice daily depending on infection.

IV infusion (over 30–60 minutes): 200–400 mg twice daily.

Side effects

Gastrointestinal upset (nausea, vomiting, diarrhoea), CNS effects (dizziness, headache, tremors, rarely convulsions), photosensitive skin rashes, tendon damage (pain, inflammation, rupture).

Cautions/contraindications

Contraindicated in patients with a history of tendon disorders related to quinolone use; risk of tendon rupture is increased by corticosteroids. If tendonitis is suspected, stop quinolone immediately.

3 Gastroenterology and nutrition

GASTROENTEROLOGY

Gastrointestinal symptoms are a common reason for attendance in primary care and hospital clinics. In developed countries they are often a manifestation of functional bowel diseases, but the clinician needs to consider that 20% of all cancers occur in the gastrointestinal tract. In developing countries infection is a more common diagnosis.

SYMPTOMS OF GASTROINTESTINAL DISEASE

Dyspepsia and indigestion

Dyspepsia is common and describes a range of upper gastrointestinal tract symptoms, e.g. epigastric pain or burning, nausea, heartburn, fullness and belching. Patients are likely to use the term 'indigestion' for these symptoms. Dyspeptic symptoms are caused by disorders of the oesophagus, stomach, pancreas or hepatobiliary system, but the most common cause is functional dyspepsia. Other causes include peptic ulceration, gastro-oesophageal reflux disease or rarely a gastro-oesophageal cancer. Investigation and management of dyspepsia is discussed on page 86.

Dysphagia

Dysphagia is difficulty in swallowing and suggests an abnormality in the passage of liquids or solids from the oral cavity through the oesophagus and into the stomach. The causes are listed in Table 3.1 and investigation discussed on page 75.

Vomiting

Vomiting occurs as a result of stimulation of the vomiting centres in the medulla. This may result from stimulation of the chemoreceptor trigger zones or from gut vagal afferents. Vomiting is associated with many gastrointestinal conditions, but nausea and vomiting without abdominal pain are frequently non-gastrointestinal in origin, e.g. due to central nervous system (CNS) disease (e.g. raised intracranial pressure, migraine), excess alcohol, drugs (especially chemotherapeutic agents), metabolic conditions (e.g. uraemia, diabetic keto-acidosis) and pregnancy. Persistent nausea and vomiting without any other symptoms may also be functional in origin (p. 118).

Table 3.1 Causes of dysphagia

Disorders of the mouth and tongue	Extrinsic pressure
E.g. tonsillitis	Mediastinal glands
Neuromuscular disorders	Goitre
Pharyngeal disorders	Enlarged left atrium
Bulbar palsy	
Myasthenia gravis	**Intrinsic lesion**
	Benign stricture
Oesophageal motility disorders	Malignant stricture
Primary oesophageal disease	Oesophageal web or ring
Achalasia	Foreign body
Other oesophageal dysmotility	Pharyngeal pouch
Eosinophilic oesophagitis*	
Systemic disease	
Diabetes mellitus	
Chagas' disease	
Scleroderma	

*Increasingly apparent cause of dysphagia (? due to discoordination of longitudinal muscle of the oesophagus), characterized by eosinophil infiltration of the oesophagus and diagnosed on mucosal biopsies.

Flatulence

Flatulence describes excessive wind, presenting as belching, abdominal distension and the passage of flatus per rectum. It is rarely indicative of serious underlying disease.

Diarrhoea and constipation

These are common complaints and not usually due to serious disease. Diarrhoea implies the passage of increased amounts of loose stool (stool weight >250 g/24 h) (p. 115). This must be differentiated from the frequent passage of small amounts of stool (that patients often refer to as diarrhoea), which is commonly seen in functional bowel disorders. Investigation and management are discussed on page 117. Constipation is difficult to define because there is considerable individual variation, but it is usually taken to mean infrequent passage of stool (< three times per week) or the difficult passage of hard stools.

Steatorrhoea

Steatorrhoea is the passage of pale bulky stools that contain fat (>17 mmol or 6 g per day) and indicates fat malabsorption as a result of small bowel, pancreatic disease (resulting in lipase deficiency), or cholestatic liver/biliary disease (resulting in intestinal bile salt deficiency). The stools are offensive, often float because of increased air content and are difficult to flush away.

Abdominal pain

Table 3.2 lists the common causes of abdominal pain based on the usual site of pain. Abdominal pain presenting as an acute abdomen is also discussed on page 119.

INVESTIGATION OF GASTROINTESTINAL DISEASE

Other than blood tests, which will often include coeliac serology, endoscopy and radiological imaging are the common investigations in patients with gastrointestinal complaints. Faecal markers of intestinal inflammation and tissue damage, e.g. faecal calprotectin, are used in some centres. They are able to distinguish organic from non-inflammatory functional disease with high diagnostic accuracy.

Table 3.2 Causes of abdominal pain by location

Epigastric	Lower abdomen
Peptic ulceration	Functional pain
Functional dyspepsia	Diverticulitis
Gastric cancer	Appendicitis
Pancreatitis	Gynaecological: salpingitis, ovarian cyst/cancer
Pancreatic cancer	Ectopic pregnancy
	Renal or urinary tract
Upper abdomen	Inflammatory bowel disease
Hepatitis	
Hepatic congestion	**Diffuse or varied site**
Pancreatitis	Gastroenteritis
Biliary pain	Mesenteric ischaemia
Subdiaphragmatic abscess	Bowel obstruction
Functional pain	Peritonitis
Splenic abscess or infarct	Ruptured aortic aneurysm
Cardiac (myocarditis, ischaemia)	Metabolic (DKA, porphyria)
Pneumonia	Familial Mediterranean fever
	Herpes zoster (pain precedes the rash)

DKA, diabetic ketoacidosis.

Endoscopy

Video endoscopes relay colour images to a high definition television monitor. The tip of the endoscope can be angulated in all directions and channels in the instrument are used for air insufflation, water injection, suction, and for the passage of accessories such as biopsy forceps or brushes for obtaining tissue, snares for polypectomy and needles for injection therapies. Permanent photographic or video records of the procedure are obtained. Mucosal biopsy is often an integral part of the examination; multiple biopsies (8–10) are taken in suspected cancer to reduce sampling error and a false-negative result.

Oesophagogastroduodenoscopy (OGD, 'gastroscopy')

A flexible endoscope is passed through the mouth into the oesophagus, stomach and duodenum following the administration of local anaesthetic spray to the pharynx and/or light sedation with intravenous midazolam. Patients fast for 6 hours prior to the procedure and must not drive for 24 hours after intravenous sedation. OGD is used in the investigation of dyspepsia, dysphagia, weight loss and iron deficiency anaemia. Duodenal biopsies can be obtained to establish a diagnosis of coeliac disease, and therapeutic options include arresting upper gastrointestinal bleeding, dilatation of oesophageal strictures and stent insertion for palliation of oesophageal malignancy. The mortality for diagnostic endoscopy is 0.001% with significant complications in 1:10 000, usually when performed as an emergency (e.g. GI haemorrhage).

Sigmoidoscopy

This is performed with a rigid instrument to examine the rectum and distal sigmoid, or with a flexible instrument to examine the whole of the left colon. Bowel preparation is achieved with one or two phosphate enemas, and sedation is rarely required.

Colonoscopy

This allows visualization of the entire colon and terminal ileum. Bowel cleansing solutions (p. 133) are given in advance of the procedure to clear the bowel of solid contents. Intravenous analgesia (with fentanyl) and sedation (with midazolam) may be required. Colonoscopy is useful for the investigation of patients with altered bowel habit, rectal bleeding or as a screening tool for colorectal cancer. Cancer, polyps and diverticular disease are the most common significant findings. The success rate for reaching the caecum should be at least 90% after training. Therapeutic options include removal of polyps (polypectomy) or diathermy of bleeding lesions such as angiodysplasia. Perforation occurs in 1:1000 examinations, but this is higher (up to 2%) after polypectomy and endoscopic mucosal resection. Complications of colonoscopy (± polypectomy) are bowel perforation and bleeding, and respiratory depression and hypotension as a result of the sedation.

Endoscopic retrograde cannulation of biliary and pancreatic duct (ERCP) combines endoscopy and fluoroscopy to visualize the pancreatico biliary tree. It is not used diagnostically but used for intervention such as gallstone extraction and stenting benign and malignant strictures in the common bile duct. Complications include perforation, pancreatitis and sepsis.

Endoscopic ultrasound (EUS) is performed with a gastroscope incorporating an ultrasound probe at the tip. It is used diagnostically for lesions in the oesophageal or gastric wall, including the detailed TNM staging (see Table 3.16) of oesophageal/gastric cancer and for the detection and biopsy of pancreatic tumours and cysts.

Endoanal and endorectal ultrasonography are performed to define the anatomy of the anal sphincters to detect perianal disease and to stage superficial rectal tumours.

Balloon enteroscopy, either double or single balloon, can examine the small bowel from the duodenum to the ileum, from both the cranial and caudal approach using specialized enteroscopes in expert centres.

Capsule endoscopy is used for the evaluation of obscure GI bleeding (after negative gastroscopy and colonoscopy) and for the detection of small bowel tumours and occult inflammatory bowel disease. It should be avoided if strictures are suspected.

Imaging

Plain X-rays of the chest and abdomen are used in the investigation of the acute abdomen. They may show free gas with a perforated viscus, dilated loops of bowel with intestinal obstruction and colonic dilatation in a patient with severe ulcerative colitis (UC). Calcification in the pancreas (just to the left of L1) indicates chronic pancreatitis, and faecal loading is seen with constipation.

Ultrasound

Transabdominal ultrasound is useful for visualization of the liver, gall bladder and biliary tree, and kidneys. It is commonly used for investigation of abnormal liver blood tests, hepatomegaly and for characterization of abdominal masses. It is also used for the detection of bowel wall thickening and for determining the extent of involved segments in Crohn's disease, but is not disease specific. It is used to guide needle placement for biopsies of the liver and solid mass lesions and for drainage of ascites and inflammatory collections.

Computed tomography (CT) scan

CT scanning (p. 822) is frequently used in the investigation of gastrointestinal disease, particularly in the staging of intra-abdominal malignancy and in the investigation and assessment of the acute abdomen (demonstrating perforated viscus, inflammation, e.g. appendicitis, the site and cause of intestinal obstruction and renal calculi). CT colonography/CT pneumocolon (virtual colonoscopy) provides a computer-simulated intraluminal view of the air-filled colon. Like conventional colonoscopy it requires full bowel preparation (p. 133) and air distension of the colon. The images obtained can visualize colonic polyps (Fig. 3.1) and cancer, but biopsies cannot be taken or polyps removed. It is mainly used where conventional colonoscopy cannot be performed because of patient intolerance or technical difficulties. Unprepared abdominal and pelvic CT scanning is a good test for colon cancer in the frail or elderly patient who may not tolerate the necessary bowel preparation for conventional or CT colonography.

Risks associated with CT scanning are allergy to intravenous contrast and exposure to radiation. The effective radiation dose from abdominal and pelvic CT scan or CT colonography is 10 mSv and equivalent to about 3 years' natural background radiation. Multiple CT scans in an individual may increase cancer risk as a result of radiation exposure.

Magnetic resonance imaging (MRI)

MRI uses no radiation and is particularly useful in the evaluation of rectal cancers and abscesses and fistulae in the perianal region. It is also useful in small bowel disease (MR enteroclysis) and in hepatobiliary and pancreatic disease.

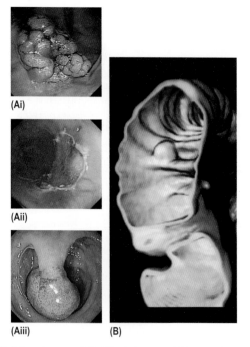

(Ai)

(Aii)

(Aiii)   **(B)**

Fig. 3.1 Colon polyps seen at (Ai–Aiii) colonoscopy and (B) computed tomography (CT) colonography. Aii is after endoscopic resection of the polyps in Ai.

Positron emission tomography (PET) relies on detection of the metabolism of fluorodeoxyglucose. It is used for staging oesophageal, gastric and colorectal cancer and in the detection of metastatic and recurrent disease. PET/CT adds additional anatomical information.

Contrast studies

Ingestion of barium followed by X-rays allows examination of the oesophagus (barium swallow), stomach and duodenum (barium meal) and small intestine (barium follow-through). These techniques are less sensitive than endoscopy particularly for small mucosal lesions. However, unlike endoscopy, barium swallow will demonstrate motility problems in the investigation of dysphagia. MRI of the small bowel is being used more frequently as it does not involve radiation.

Oesophageal physiology testing

Insertion of probes into the lower oesophagus via the nose allows continual measurement over 24 hours of acid (pH monitoring) and volume (by impedance testing) reflux of gastric contents. Data are captured on a small device worn on a belt and transferred to a computer at the end of the 24-hour period. These methods record the frequency and duration of reflux episodes and correlation with symptoms. They are performed prior to surgical treatment of reflux or in difficult diagnostic cases.

Oesophageal manometry involves the passage of a small tube containing several pressure transducers into the oesophagus via the nose. Oesophageal peristalsis and pressure are assessed on swallowing. Manometry is used in the investigation of suspected oesophageal motility disorders in patients with dysphagia.

THE MOUTH

Problems in the mouth are common and although often trivial, they can cause severe symptoms.

Mouth ulcers

Non-infective

- Recurrent aphthous ulceration is common and affects at least 20% of the population; in most cases the aetiology is unknown. There are recurrent self-limiting episodes of painful oral ulcers (rarely on the palate). Topical corticosteroids are used for symptomatic relief, but they have no effect on the natural history. In a few cases ulcers are associated with trauma or gastrointestinal and systemic diseases, e.g. anaemia, inflammatory bowel disease, coeliac disease, Behçet's disease, Reiter's disease, systemic lupus erythematosus, pemphigus, pemphigoid and fixed drug reactions.

- Squamous cell carcinoma presents as an indolent ulcer, usually on the lateral borders of the tongue or floor of the mouth. Aetiological factors include tobacco (smoking and chewing) and alcohol. Treatment is with surgery, radiotherapy or a combination of both.

Infective

Many infections can affect the mouth, though the most common are viral and include Herpes simplex virus type 1, Coxsackie A virus and Herpes zoster virus.

Oral white patches

Transient white patches are either due to *Candida* infection or very occasionally systemic lupus erythematosus. Local causes include mechanical, irritative or chemical trauma from drugs (e.g. ill fitting dentures or aspirin). Oral candidiasis in adults is seen following therapy with broad-spectrum antibiotics or inhaled steroids and in people with diabetes, patients who are seriously ill or immunocompromised.

Persistent white patches can be due to *leucoplakia*, which is associated with alcohol and (particularly) smoking, and is pre-malignant. A biopsy should always be taken; histology shows alteration in the keratinization and dysplasia of the epithelium. Treatment is unsatisfactory. Isotretinoin possibly reduces disease progression. *Oral lichen planus* presents as white striae, which can rarely extend into the oesophagus.

The tongue

The tongue may be affected by inflammatory or malignant processes with similar lesions to those described above.

- **Glossitis** is a red, smooth, sore tongue associated with B_{12}, folate, iron, riboflavin and nicotinic acid deficiency. It is also seen in infections due to *Candida*.
- **A black hairy tongue** is due to a proliferation of chromogenic microorganisms causing brown staining of elongated filiform papillae. The causes are unknown, but heavy smoking and the use of antiseptic mouthwashes have been implicated.
- **A geographic tongue** is an idiopathic condition occurring in 1–2% of the population and may be familial. There are erythematous areas surrounded by well-defined, slightly raised irregular margins. The lesions are usually painless and the patient should be reassured.

Periodontal disorders

Gum bleeding is most commonly caused by gingivitis, an inflammatory condition of the gums associated with dental plaque. Bleeding may also be associated with generalized conditions such as bleeding disorders and leukaemia. Acute ulcerative gingivitis (Vincent's infection) is characterized by the development of crater-like ulcers, with bleeding, involving the interdental papillae, followed by lateral spread along the gingival margins. It is thought to be the result of spirochaetal infection occurring in the malnourished and immunocompromised. Treatment is with oral metronidazole and good oral hygiene.

Salivary gland disorders

Xerostomia (mouth dryness) may be caused by anxiety, drugs such as tricyclic antidepressants, Sjögren's syndrome and dehydration. Infection (parotitis) may be viral, e.g. mumps virus, or bacterial (staphylococci or streptococci). Calculus formation usually occurs in the duct of the submandibular gland, and causes painful swelling of the gland before or during mastication. Among the salivary glands, tumours most commonly develop in the parotid gland and are usually benign, e.g. pleomorphic adenoma. Treatment is with surgical resection. Involvement of the VIIth cranial nerve raises the suspicion of malignancy.

THE OESOPHAGUS

Symptoms of oesophageal disorders

- Dysphagia (difficulty in swallowing) has mechanical and neuromuscular causes (Table 3.1). A short history of progressive dysphagia initially for solids and then liquids is suggestive of a mechanical stricture. Investigation is with urgent OGD particularly to look for a malignant oesophageal stricture. A barium swallow is more appropriate as the first-line investigation when the history (slow onset of dysphagia for both solids and liquids) suggests a motility disorder such as achalasia. Oesophageal manometry may subsequently be necessary.
- Heartburn is a retrosternal or epigastric burning sensation produced by the reflux of gastric acid into the oesophagus. The pain may radiate up to the throat and be confused with chest pain of cardiac origin. It is often aggravated by bending or lying down and relieved by antacids.
- Regurgitation is the effortless reflux of oesophageal contents into the mouth and pharynx. It occurs in reflux disease and oesophageal strictures.
- Odynophagia is pain during swallowing particularly with alcohol and hot liquids. It suggests oesophageal inflammation (oesophagitis) due to gastro-oesophageal reflux disease, infections of the oesophagus (herpes simplex virus, *Candida*) or drugs such as slow release potassium or bisphosphonates.

Gastro-oesophageal reflux disease (GORD)

Pathophysiology

The reflux of gastric acid, pepsin, bile and duodenal contents back in to the oesophagus can be influenced by many factors which overcome the innate defence mechanisms, primarily the lower oesophageal sphincter. Between swallows, the muscles of the oesophagus are relaxed except for those of the two sphincters. The lower oesophageal sphincter (LOS) in the distal oesophagus remains closed due to the unique property of the muscle and relaxes when swallowing is initiated. *Transient Lower Oesophageal Sphincter Relaxations* (TLESRs) are part of normal physiology, but occur more frequently in patients with GORD, allowing gastric acid to flow back in to the oesophagus. Increased abdominal pressure (pregnancy) and low LOS pressure also predispose to GORD. Delayed gastric emptying and prolonged post-prandial and nocturnal reflux also contribute. Mechanical or functional aberrations associated with a hiatus hernia may contribute to GORD, but reflux disease can occur in the absence of a hiatus hernia. Other predisposing factors in GORD include obesity, systemic sclerosis and certain drugs (e.g. nitrates, tricyclics).

Clinical features

Heartburn is the major symptom. There may also be regurgitation and odynophagia. Cough and nocturnal asthma can occur from aspiration of gastric contents into the lungs. The correlation between heartburn and severity of oesophagitis is poor.

Investigations

The diagnosis is clinical and most patients are treated without investigation. OGD is indicated in patients with new-onset heartburn over 55 years of age or patients with alarm symptoms (weight loss, dysphagia, haematemesis, anaemia) suspicious for upper gastrointestinal malignancy. It is also performed to document complications of reflux (e.g., Barrett's oesophagus) and in patients who do not respond well to treatment.

OGD may show oesophagitis (mucosal erythema, erosions and ulceration), a hiatus hernia, e.g., Barrett's oesophagus (p. 78) or may be normal.

24-Hour intraluminal pH monitoring or impedance (pp. 72–73) is usually reserved for the confirmation of GORD prior to surgery or where there is an inadequate response to standard doses of proton pump inhibitors (PPIs) (p. 130).

Management

Conservative measures with lifestyle changes (weight loss, avoidance of excess alcohol or aggravating foods, smoking cessation) and simple antacids are often sufficient for mild symptoms in the absence of oesophagitis. Patients with severe symptoms or with proven pathology (oesophagitis or complications) require PPIs.

- *Alginate-containing antacids* (10 mL three times daily) are the most frequently used 'over the counter' agents for GORD. They form a gel or 'foam raft' with gastric contents to reduce reflux. Magnesium-containing antacids tend to cause diarrhoea while aluminium-containing compounds may cause constipation.

- *The dopamine antagonist prokinetic agents* metoclopramide and domperidone are occasionally helpful as they enhance peristalsis and speed gastric emptying, but there is little data to substantiate this. The role of domperidone has been limited still further following reports of serious cardiac side effects.

- *H_2-receptor antagonists* (e.g. cimetidine, ranitidine, famotidine and nizatidine) are frequently used for acid suppression if antacids fail as they can easily be obtained.

- *Proton pump inhibitors* (PPIs: omeprazole, rabeprazole, lansoprazole, pantoprazole, esomeprazole) inhibit gastric hydrogen/potassium-ATPase. PPIs reduce gastric acid secretion by up to 90% and are the drugs of choice for all but mild cases. Most patients with GORD will respond well, with approximately 60% symptom free after 4 weeks of a once-daily PPI. Patients with severe symptoms may need twice-daily PPIs and prolonged treatment, often for years. Once oesophageal sensitivity has normalized, a lower dose, e.g. omeprazole 10 mg, may be sufficient for maintenance. Long-term PPI prescription is not uncommon and although there has been some recent data to suggest side effects, such as osteoporosis and increase gastrointestinal infections such as *Clostridium difficile;* these are uncommon and tend to occur in at risk patients. Patients who do not respond to a PPI and have continuing symptoms with a normal endoscopy are described as having *non-erosive reflux disease (NERD)*. These patients are usually female and often the symptoms are functional, although a small group have a 'hypersensitive' oesophagus, giving discomfort with only slight changes in pH.

- *Surgery* may be necessary. Via a laparoscopic approach the fundus of the stomach is sutured around the lower oesophagus to produce an antireflux valve (Nissen fundoplication, 'lap wrap'). *Indications for operation* are not clear cut but include intolerance to medication, the desire for freedom from medication, the expense of therapy and the concern of long-term side-effects. The most common cause of mechanical fundoplication failure is recurrent hiatus hernia.

- The *Linx Reflux Management System* is a device with a row of magnets which increase LOS closure pressure, allowing food passage during swallowing. Patients with oesophageal dysmotility unrelated to acid reflux, patients with no response to PPIs and those with underlying functional bowel disease should rarely have surgery.

Complications

Peptic stricture

Since the advent of PPIs peptic strictures have become far less common. They usually occur in patients over the age of 60 and present with intermittent dysphagia for solids which worsens gradually over a long period. Mild cases may respond to PPI alone. More severe cases need endoscopic dilatation and long-term PPI therapy. Surgery is required if medical treatment fails.

Barrett's oesophagus

Barrett's oesophagus is diagnosed at endoscopy showing proximal displacement of the squamocolumnar mucosal junction and biopsies demonstrating columnar lining above the proximal gastric folds; intestinal metaplasia is no longer a requirement of the British Society of Gastroenterology definition, but is central to the American College of Gastroenterology guidelines.

Central obesity increases the risk of Barrett's by 4.3 times. Long segment (>3 cm) and short segment (<3 cm) Barrett's is found respectively in 5% and 15% of patients undergoing endoscopy for reflux symptoms. Barrett's is also often found incidentally in endoscoped patients without reflux symptoms. The major concern is that approximately 0.12–0.5% of Barrett's patients develop oesophageal adenocarcinoma per year, the majority, probably, through a gradual transformation from intestinal metaplasia to low-grade then high-grade dysplasia, before invasive adenocarcinoma. A Barrett's typical patient has a 1% lifetime risk.

Although there is an absence of high quality evidence, endoscopic surveillance is recommended by some. This involves use of a high definition gastroscope and targeted biopsies taken of any focally abnormal tissue in addition to random biopsies. Chromo-endoscopy (topical application of stains or pigments via the endoscope), narrow band, and autofluorescence imaging may aid the diagnosis of dysplasia and carcinoma. Endoscopic technology has improved the detection of pre-malignant lesions, enabling removal with either endoscopic mucosal resection (EMR) or endoscopic submucosal dissection, therefore preventing surgical oesophagectomy.

If *low-grade* dysplasia is found on endoscopic surveillance, a repeat endoscopy with quadrantic biopsies every 1 cm is usually performed within 6 months, while on high-dose proton pump inhibition. Long-term surveillance is controversial.

If *high-grade* dysplasia is found, it is usually in the context of an endoscopically visible lesion which, if nodular, is removed by endoscopic mucosal resection for more accurate histological staging. If high-grade dysplasia is detected in the absence of any endoscopically visible lesion high-dose proton pump inhibition is started and repeat biopsies taken within 3 months. Endoscopic ultrasound is frequently used to more accurately stage this patient group to exclude cancer and associated significant lymphadenopathy.

Radiofrequency ablation (RFA) has superseded photodynamic therapy as the technique of choice for endoscopic treatment of dysplasia within Barrett's segments following removal of any nodular lesions, returning the oesophagus to squamous lining. The benefit of RFA in low-grade dysplasia is currently under evaluation.

Achalasia

Achalasia is a condition of unknown aetiology characterized by oesophageal aperistalsis and impaired relaxation of the lower oesophageal sphincter. The lower oesophageal pressure is elevated in more than half of patients.

Clinical features

The incidence of achalasia is 1:100 000 and is equal in males and females. It occurs at all ages but is rare in childhood. There is usually a long history of dysphagia for both liquids and solids, which may be associated with regurgitation. Retrosternal chest pain may occur and be misdiagnosed as cardiac pain.

Investigations

- *Chest X-ray* shows a dilated oesophagus, sometimes with a fluid level seen behind the heart. The fundal gas shadow is absent.
- *Barium swallow* shows lack of peristalsis and often synchronous contractions in the body of the oesophagus, sometimes with dilatation. The lower end shows a 'bird's beak' due to failure of the sphincter to relax.
- *Oesophagoscopy* is performed to exclude a carcinoma at the lower end of the oesophagus, as this can produce a similar X-ray appearance. When there is marked dilatation, a 24-hour liquid-only diet and a washout, prior to endoscopy, is useful to remove food debris.
- *CT scan* excludes distal oesophageal cancer.
- *Manometry* shows aperistalsis of the oesophagus and failure of relaxation of the lower oesophageal sphincter.

Management

All current forms of treatment for achalasia are for symptom relief. Drug therapy rarely produces satisfactory or durable relief; nifedipine (20 mg sublingually), nitrates or sildenafil can be tried.

Endoscopic balloon dilatation (2% risk of oesophageal perforation) or surgical division of the LOS (Heller's cardiomyotomy) are the most effective treatments. Per oral endoscopic myotomy (POEM) is a novel technique, which is a division of the LOS using a gastroscope. The early results show great promise.

Reflux oesophagitis complicates all procedures and the aperistalsis of the oesophagus remains.

Complications

There is a slight increase in the incidence of squamous carcinoma of the oesophagus in both treated and untreated patients.

Systemic sclerosis

There is oesophageal involvement in most patients with systemic sclerosis. The smooth muscle layer is replaced by fibrous tissue and LOS pressure is reduced, thereby permitting gastro-oesophageal reflux. Symptoms are the result of reflux (leading to oesophagitis and strictures) and oesophageal hypomotility. Treatment is as for reflux and stricture formation.

Other oesophageal dysmotility disorders

Three types are characterized on oesophageal manometry: diffuse oesophageal spasm (simultaneous contractions in the distal oesophagus), nutcracker oesophagus (high-amplitude peristaltic waves) and hypertensive lower oesophageal sphincter (raised resting pressure). They present with dysphagia and chest pain and abnormalities may be seen on barium swallow ('corkscrew' appearance in diffuse oesophageal spasm) and manometry. Nitrates and calcium-channel blockers, e.g. oral nifedipine, sometimes help symptoms. Treatment of GORD may help.

Hiatus hernia

Part of the stomach herniates through the oesophageal hiatus of the diaphragm:

- *Sliding* accounts for more than 95% of cases. The gastro-oesophageal junction slides through the hiatus and lies above the diaphragm. A sliding hiatus hernia does not cause any symptoms unless there is associated reflux.
- *Para-oesophageal hernias* are uncommon. The gastric fundus rolls up through the hiatus alongside the oesophagus, the gastro-oesophageal junction remaining below the diaphragm. These pose a serious risk of complications including gastric volvulus (rotation and strangulation of the stomach), bleeding and respiratory complications and should be treated surgically.

Benign oesophageal strictures

The causes vary geographically; benign peptic stricture secondary to long-standing GORD is the commonest cause in developed countries. Other causes are ingestion of corrosives, after radiotherapy or endoscopic treatment of oesophageal varices, and following prolonged nasogastric tube placement. Dysphagia is the main symptom and treatment is with endoscopic dilatation, PPIs and sometimes surgery.

Oesophageal perforation

Iatrogenic perforation occurs after endoscopic dilatation of oesophageal strictures (usually malignant) or achalasia, or rarely after passage of a nasogastric tube. Management involves placement of an expanding covered oesophageal stent, which usually seals the hole. A water-soluble contrast X-ray is performed after 2–3 days to check the perforation has sealed.

Traumatic or spontaneous oesophageal rupture occurs after blunt chest trauma or forceful vomiting (Boerhaave's syndrome). There is severe chest pain, fever, hypotension and surgical emphysema (crepitation). Chest X-ray may be normal or show air in the mediastinum and neck, and a pleural effusion. Diagnosis is made with CT scan or water soluble contrast swallow. The best outcomes are associated with early diagnosis and definitive surgical management within 12 hours of rupture.

Malignant oesophageal tumours

Pathology

This is the sixth most common cancer world-wide. Squamous cancers occurring in the middle third account for 40% of tumours, and in the upper third, 15%. Adenocarcinomas occur in the lower third of the oesophagus and at the cardia and represent approximately 45%. Primary small cell cancer of the oesophagus is extremely rare.

Epidemiology and aetiological factors

Squamous carcinoma The incidence is 5–10 per 100 000 in the UK, but there is great world-wide variation, being particularly high in China and parts of Africa and Iran. It is most common in the 60–70-year age group. Major risk factors are smoking and excess alcohol consumption. Other risk factors are important in specific regions with a high incidence (high intake of salted fish and pickled vegetables and ingestion of very hot food and beverages). Pre-existing oesophageal disease (achalasia and caustic strictures) and coeliac disease increase the risk.

Adenocarcinoma arises from Barrett's metaplasia (p. 78). Smoking and obesity are also risk factors.

Clinical features

There is progressive dysphagia (initially for solids and later for liquids) and weight loss. Bolus food impaction or local infiltration may cause chest pain. Physical signs are usually absent.

Investigations

These are to confirm the diagnosis and stage the tumour (TNM system, p. 829).

- Diagnosis is by OGD and tumour biopsy. *Barium swallow* can be useful where the differential diagnosis of dysphagia includes a motility disorder such as achalasia.

- Staging is initially by CT scan of the chest and abdomen to look for distant metastases. Patients without evidence of metastatic disease and who are potentially curable, then undergo EUS (p. 71) to locally stage the tumour (depth of wall invasion and local lymph node involvement), PET scanning (more sensitive than CT to detect distant metastases) and sometimes laparoscopy to detect occult peritoneal disease.

Management

Surgical resection provides the best chance of cure and is performed when the tumour has not infiltrated outside of the oesophageal wall. It is combined with pre-operative chemotherapy with or without radiotherapy (neo-adjuvant treatment). However, over half of patients present with incurable locally advanced or metastatic disease. Systemic chemotherapy may temporarily improve symptoms in patients with metastatic disease although local treatments may be necessary for relief of dysphagia. These include endoscopic insertion of an expanding metal stent across the tumour or laser and alcohol injections to cause tumour necrosis. For patients with non-metastatic but locally unresectable disease, combined radiotherapy and chemotherapy may limit disease progression and increase survival.

Prognosis

The prognosis overall is poor with 10% 5-year survival.

Benign oesophageal tumours

See page 89 (gastrointestinal stromal tumour, GIST).

THE STOMACH AND DUODENUM

Acid secretion is central to the functionality of the stomach. Acid is not essential for digestion but does prevent some food-borne infections. It is under neural and hormonal control and both stimulate acid secretion through the direct action of histamine on the parietal cell. Acetylcholine and gastrin also release histamine via the enterochromaffin cells. Somatostatin inhibits both histamine and gastrin release and therefore acid secretion.

Other major functions are:

- Reservoir for food
- Emulsification of fat and mixing of gastric contents
- Secretion of intrinsic factor
- Absorption (minimal importance).

Helicobacter pylori infection

H. pylori is a Gram-negative urease-producing spiral-shaped bacterium found predominantly in the gastric antrum and in areas of gastric metaplasia in the duodenum. It is closely associated with chronic active gastritis, peptic ulcer disease (gastric and duodenal ulcers), gastric cancer and gastric B cell lymphoma. However, most patients are asymptomatic.

Epidemiology

Infection is acquired in childhood and persists for life unless treated. Infection is associated with lower socioeconomic status and is commoner in developing countries. Transmission is most likely via the oral–oral or faecal–oral routes.

Clinicopathological features

H. pylori infection produces gastritis mainly in the antrum of the stomach. In some individuals gastritis can involve the body of the stomach, leading to atrophic gastritis and in some cases intestinal metaplasia, which is a premalignant condition.

Diagnosis of infection

This is by non-invasive (serology, breath test or stool antigen) or invasive (antral biopsy for patients undergoing an endoscopy) tests (Table 3.3).

Management

Eradication of *H. pylori* is indicated for all patients with peptic ulcer disease, atrophic gastritis, gastric B cell lymphoma, after gastric cancer resection and in patients with dyspepsia ('test and treat' strategy). It is also indicated for individuals who have a first-degree relative with gastric cancer. Recurrence is rare after successful eradication. Several treatment regimens are available, although PPI-based triple therapy regimens for 14 days are favoured. Examples include:

- Omeprazole 20 mg + metronidazole 400 mg + clarithromycin 500 mg – all twice daily
- Omeprazole 20 mg + amoxicillin 1 g + clarithromycin 500 mg – all twice daily.
- Quadruple therapy using bismuth chelate with above is increasingly used

Peptic ulcer disease

A peptic ulcer (PU) is an ulcer of the mucosa in or adjacent to an acid-bearing area. Most occur in the stomach or proximal duodenum.

Epidemiology

Duodenal ulcers (DUs) are two to three times more common than gastric ulcers (GUs) and occur in 15% of the population at some time. They are more common in the elderly, and there is a significant geographical variation.

Table 3.3 Diagnosis of *Helicobacter pylori* infection

	Method	Main use	Comments
Non-invasive tests			
^{13}C-Urea breath test	Hydrolysis of ingested ^{13}C-Urea by *H. pylori* to produce ^{13}C in expired air	Diagnosis of infection Monitoring of infection after eradication	Highly sensitive and specific False-negative results after recent use of PPIs or antibiotics
Stool antigen test	Immunoassay using monoclonal antibodies		
Serology	Serum antibody detection	Diagnosis of infection Epidemiological studies	Inaccuracy limits use Antibodies remain positive after infection cleared
Invasive tests (endoscopic gastric mucosal biopsy)			
Rapid urease (CLO) test	Urease from *H. pylori* breaks down urea to produce ammonia causing a pH-dependent colour change in the indicator present	Diagnosis of infection in patients already undergoing endoscopy	Highly sensitive and specific False-negative results after recent upper gastrointestinal bleeding and recent use of PPIs or antibiotics
Histology	Direct visualization of the organism		Subject to sampling error and observer variability

PPI, proton pump inhibitors.

Aetiology

H. pylori and non-steroidal anti-inflammatory drugs (NSAIDs)/aspirin are the cause of most PUs. Co-administration of corticosteroids and NSAIDs further increases the risk of an ulcer. Potential pathogenic mechanisms for *H. pylori*-induced ulcers are listed in Table 3.4; reduction of gastric mucosal resistance is thought to be the main factor in causation of GUs as, in contrast to DUs, gastric acid secretion is reduced. Aspirin and NSAIDs cause ulcers, at least in part, by reduced production of prostaglandins (through inhibition of cyclooxygenase-1) which provide mucosal protection in the upper gastrointestinal tract. Less common causes of PUs are hyperparathyroidism,

Table 3.4 Proposed pathogenic mechanisms of *H. pylori*

Increased gastric acid secretion due to:
    Increased gastrin secretion
    Increased parietal cell mass
    Decreased somatostatin production due to antral gastritis
Disruption of mucous protective layer
Reduced duodenal bicarbonate production
Production of virulence factors:
    Vacuolating toxin (Vac A)
    Cytotoxic associated protein (CagA)
    Urease
    Adherence factors

Zollinger–Ellison syndrome, vascular insufficiency, sarcoidosis and Crohn's disease.

Clinical features

Burning epigastric pain is the most common presenting symptom, typically relieved by antacids and a variable relationship to food. DU pain often occurs when the patient is hungry and classically occurs at night. Other symptoms, such as nausea, heartburn and flatulence, may occur. Occasionally ulcers may present with the complications of perforation or painless haemorrhage.

Investigations

Patients less than 55 years with ulcer-type symptoms should undergo non-invasive testing for *H. pylori* infection (Table 3.3); upper gastrointestinal endoscopy is not usually necessary (see management of dyspepsia). In patients who undergo endoscopy and are found to have a GU, multiple biopsies from the centre and edge of the ulcer are taken because it is often impossible to distinguish by naked eye a benign from malignant ulcer. A barium meal is useful if gastric outlet obstruction is suspected.

Management

Ulcers associated with *H. pylori* Treatment regimens (p. 83) that successfully eradicate *H. pylori* result in ulcer healing rates of over 90% and prevent ulcer recurrence. There is usually no need to continue antisecretory treatment (with a PPI or H_2-receptor antagonist) unless the ulcer is complicated by haemorrhage or perforation. This approach to treatment is indicated in all patients with *H. pylori*-associated peptic disease. Eradication is confirmed by either a urea breath test or faecal antigen testing in patients who remain symptomatic or who have had an ulcer complication.

H. pylori-negative peptic ulcers are usually associated with aspirin or NSAID ingestion. Treatment is with PPIs (p. 130) and stopping aspirin/NSAID if at all possible. After ulcer healing, NSAIDs can only be continued with PPI prophylaxis, or NSAID therapy is switched to a selective cyclo-oxygenase-2 inhibitor.

Follow-up endoscopy plus biopsy is performed for all GUs to demonstrate healing and exclude malignancy (initial biopsies may be false negatives).

Surgery is now rarely necessary for PU but is reserved for the treatment of complications.

Complications

Perforation is uncommon. DUs perforate more commonly than GUs, usually into the peritoneal cavity. Treatment is surgical closure of the perforation and drainage of the abdomen. *H. pylori* should subsequently be eradicated. Conservative treatment with intravenous fluids and antibiotics may be indicated in elderly or very ill patients.

Gastric outlet obstruction Ulcer disease causing obstruction is now rare and carcinoma is the commonest cause. Outflow obstruction occurs because of surrounding oedema or scarring following healing. Copious projectile vomiting is the main symptom, and a succussion splash may be detectable clinically. Metabolic alkalosis may develop as a result of loss of acid. In patients with PU disease the oedema will usually settle with conservative management with nasogastric suction, replacement of fluids and electrolytes and PPIs. Surgery is rarely required.

Haemorrhage See page 89.

Management of dyspepsia

Significant gastrointestinal pathology is uncommon in most young people with dyspepsia (p. 65). Furthermore, the close association of *H. pylori* with peptic ulcer disease and the ability to detect *H. pylori* by non-invasive methods means that investigation with endoscopy is unnecessary in most patients. An approach to the management of dyspepsia is outlined in Fig. 3.2.

Gastropathy

The commonest cause of gastropathy is mucosal damage associated with the use of aspirin or other NSAIDs. These drugs deplete mucosal prostaglandins, by inhibiting the cyclo-oxygenase pathway, which leads to mucosal damage. Other causes include infections, e.g. cytomegalovirus and herpes simplex virus, and alcohol in high concentrations. Gastric erosions can also be seen after severe stress (stress ulcer), burns (Curling's ulcer), and in renal and liver disease. Symptoms include indigestion, vomiting and haemorrhage, although these correlate poorly with endoscopic and pathological findings. Erosions (superficial breaks in the mucosa <3 mm) and subepithelial haemorrhage are most commonly seen at endoscopy. Treatment is with a PPI with removal of the offending cause if possible. Prophylaxis is also given to prevent future damage in patients who continue to take aspirin or NSAIDs.

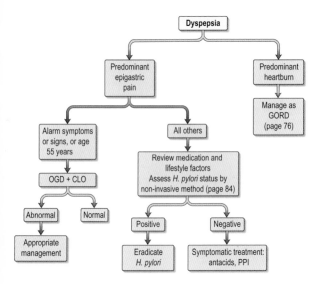

Notes:
- Alarm symptoms or signs: dysphagia, weight loss, vomiting, gastrointestinal bleeding, epigastric mass.
- Think if pain could be originating from biliary tract (page 141) or pancreas (page 189) and patient needs US or CT scan.

Fig. 3.2 Approach to the investigation of patients with dyspepsia. CLO, rapid urease test; CT, computed tomography; GORD, gastro-oesophageal reflux disease; OGD, oesophagogastroduodenoscopy; PPI, proton pump inhibitor; US, ultrasound.

Gastritis

The commonest cause of gastritis is *H. pylori* infection. Other causes are autoimmune gastritis (the cause of pernicious anaemia associated with antibodies to gastric parietal cells and intrinsic factor), viruses and duodeno-gastric reflux. Gastritis is a histological diagnosis and is usually discovered incidentally when a gastric mucosal biopsy is taken for histology at endoscopy. It is classified as acute or chronic. Acute inflammation is associated with neutrophilic infiltration, while chronic inflammation is characterized by mononuclear cells, chiefly lymphocytes, plasma cells and macrophages. Gastritis is usually asymptomatic; whether *H. pylori* gastritis itself produces functional dyspepsia is controversial. At endoscopy the mucosa may appear reddened or normal. No specific treatment is required although eradication treatment for *H. pylori* is often given.

Gastric cancer

Epidemiology

Gastric cancer is the fourth most common cancer world-wide and the second leading cause of cancer-related mortality. Incidence increases with age and is more common in men. The frequency varies throughout the world, being more common in Japan and Chile, and relatively less common in the USA. Although the incidence overall is decreasing world-wide, proximal gastric cancers are increasing in frequency in the West.

Aetiology

This is unknown; *H. pylori* infection is implicated, causing chronic gastritis which in some individuals leads to atrophic gastritis and pre-malignant intestinal metaplasia. Other risk factors are lifestyle (tobacco smoking, diets low in fruits and vegetables or high in salted, smoked or preserved foods), pernicious anaemia, family history of gastric cancer and after partial gastrectomy.

Pathology

Tumours most commonly occur in the antrum and are almost always adenocarcinomas. They are localized ulcerated lesions with rolled edges (intestinal, type 1), or diffuse with extensive submucosal spread, giving the picture of linitis plastica (diffuse, type 2).

Clinical features

Pain similar to peptic ulcer pain is the most common symptom. With more advanced disease, nausea, anorexia and weight loss are common. Tumours near the pylorus cause outflow obstruction and vomiting and dysphagia occurs with lesions in the cardia. Almost 50% have a palpable epigastric mass, and a lymph node is sometimes felt in the supraclavicular fossa (Virchow's node). Metastases in the peritoneum and liver cause ascites and hepatomegaly. Skin manifestations of malignancy, such as dermatomyositis (p. 308) and acanthosis nigricans, are occasionally associated.

Investigations

Gastroscopy and biopsy is the initial investigation of choice. CT, EUS and laparoscopy are then used to stage the tumour in a similar manner to oesophageal cancer.

Management

Surgery is the most effective form of treatment if the tumour is operable. Adjuvant (post-operative) chemoradiotherapy is given for more advanced tumours. Palliative chemotherapy is sometimes used for unresectable lesions, with a modest improvement in survival.

Prognosis

The overall survival is poor (10% 5-year survival). Five-year survival after 'curative' surgery is 50%. In Japan there is an active endoscopic screening programme, and earlier diagnosis and an aggressive surgical approach have resulted in a 5-year survival of 90%.

Other gastric tumours

Gastrointestinal stromal tumours (GISTs) are the most common type of stromal or mesenchymal tumour of the gastrointestinal tract and occur most commonly in the stomach and proximal small intestine. They were previously considered to be benign but on prolonged follow-up, most have malignant potential. They are usually asymptomatic and discovered incidentally when an upper gastrointestinal endoscopy is performed for dyspepsia. They can ulcerate and bleed. Treatment is surgical as far as possible. Imatinib, a tyrosine kinase inhibitor, is used for unresectable or metastatic disease, and is now used as adjunctive therapy after surgical removal of the primary in the absence of metastatic disease.

Gastric lymphoma arises from mucosal areas and is called mucosa-associated lymphoid tissue tumour (MALToma). Gastric lymphoma presents similarly to gastric carcinoma. Most are associated with *H. pylori* infection and some can be treated by eradication of *H. pylori* only. Other patients are treated with surgery or chemotherapy with or without radiotherapy.

Gastric polyps are uncommon and usually regenerative. Adenomatous polyps are rare.

GASTROINTESTINAL BLEEDING

Acute upper gastrointestinal bleeding

This is a common emergency admission with an overall mortality rate of 5–12%. Haematemesis is the vomiting of blood. Melaena is the passage of black tarry stools (the result of altered blood) and usually indicates bleeding from a site proximal to the jejunum. Acute massive upper gastrointestinal bleeding may present with fresh rectal bleeding, almost always in association with shock.

Aetiology

PU is the most common cause often associated with aspirin or NSAID ingestion (Fig. 3.3). Relative incidences vary according to patient population. Anticoagulants do not cause bleeding *per se* but bleeding from any cause is greater if the patient is anticoagulated.

Management

This is summarized in Emergency Box 3.1.

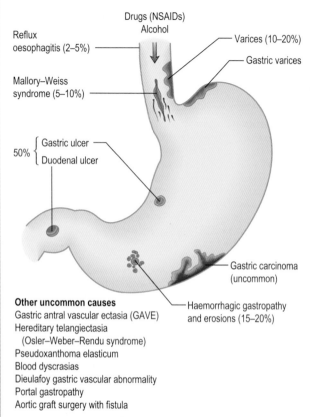

Drugs (NSAIDs)
Alcohol

Reflux oesophagitis (2–5%)

Varices (10–20%)

Gastric varices

Mallory–Weiss syndrome (5–10%)

50% { Gastric ulcer / Duodenal ulcer

Gastric carcinoma (uncommon)

Other uncommon causes
Gastric antral vascular ectasia (GAVE)
Hereditary telangiectasia
  (Osler–Weber–Rendu syndrome)
Pseudoxanthoma elasticum
Blood dyscrasias
Dieulafoy gastric vascular abnormality
Portal gastropathy
Aortic graft surgery with fistula

Haemorrhagic gastropathy and erosions (15–20%)

Fig. 3.3 Causes of upper gastrointestinal haemorrhage. The approximate frequency is also given.

Immediate management   Two large-bore (16-gauge) intravenous cannulas should be placed in a peripheral vein and blood taken for full blood count, liver biochemistry, urea and electrolytes, clotting screen and 'group and save'; cross-match at least 4 units of blood if there is evidence of a large bleed (blood pressure <100 mmHg, pulse >100 beats per min, cool or cold extremities with slow capillary refill, Hb <100 g/L). Intravenous fluids (0.9% saline) are started while the patient is assessed further, including a history and physical examination.

Risk assessment is made using a scoring system such as the 'Rockall' Score (Table 3.5). It helps to identify those at high risk of recurrent or life-threatening haemorrhage and those at low risk who may be suitable for early hospital discharge (pre-endoscopy score 0, post-endoscopy ≤1).

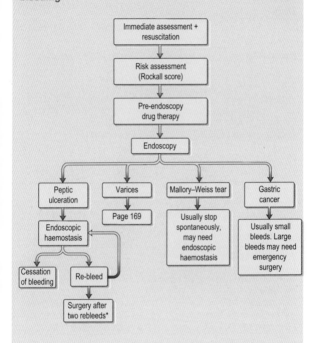

✛ Emergency Box 3.1

Approach to the management of upper gastrointestinal bleeding

*NB: less common causes of upper gastrointestinal bleeding are not indicated on this figure.
Consider angiography with transcatheter embolization of bleeding lesions if high-risk surgical patient.*

In many patients no specific treatment is required, bleeding stops spontaneously and the patient remains well compensated. In patients with large bleeds (see above) or clinical signs of shock urgent blood transfusion is required. Monitoring pulse rate and central venous pressure will guide transfusion requirements.

Pre-endoscopy drug therapy

- *Aspirin, NSAIDs and warfarin* are stopped and the INR reversed if necessary. Cardiology advice should be sought before stopping aspirin and clopidogrel in patients with low-risk bleeds.

Table 3.5 Rockall score for upper gastrointestinal haemorrhage

	Score 0	Score 1	Score 2	Score 3
Age (years)	<60	60–79	>80	
Shock	None	Pulse >100	Pulse >100	
		Systolic BP >100	Systolic BP <100	
Comorbidity	None		Cardiac failure, IHD, co-morbidity	Renal/liver failure, any other disseminated malignancy
Endoscopic stigmata	None or dark spot seen		Blood in upper gastrointestinal tract Adherent clot Visible or spurting vessel	
Diagnosis	M–W tear: no lesion seen and no SRH	All other diagnoses	Malignancy of upper gastrointestinal tract	

*Parameters indicated in bold calculate a pre-endoscopy Rockall score – maximum 7.
Final Rockall score – maximum 11.
M–W tear, Mallory–Weiss tear; SRH, stigmata of recent haemorrhage; IHD, ischaemic
heart disease.
Low-risk patients (post-endoscopy score ≤1) 5% risk of re-bleeding, 0% risk of death.
High-risk patients (post-endoscopy score 5–11), 11–41% risk of death.
Death and re-bleeding are particularly common in inpatients and patients with varices.*

- *PPIs* (omeprazole 80 mg bolus i.v. followed by infusion of 8 mg/h) are given to high-risk patients (Rockall score ≥4) in whom endoscopy cannot be performed immediately.
- *Antibiotics* are given to patients with suspected variceal haemorrhage. Consider also terlipressin in these patients.

Determine site of bleeding This may be evident from the history, e.g. bleeding from a PU is suggested by recent aspirin or NSAID ingestion or previous PU. A history of vomiting preceding the haematemesis suggests a Mallory–Weiss tear (linear mucosal tear at the oesophagogastric junction). Suspect variceal bleeding in patients with liver disease or known varices. After resuscitation, upper gastrointestinal endoscopy should be performed as soon as possible and preferably within 24 hours. More urgent endoscopy is indicated in patients with shock, continued bleeding or suspected varices (e.g. signs of chronic liver disease).

Specific management Varices are treated with banding or glue sclerotherapy. Ulcers with high-risk stigmata for continued or re-bleeding (active bleeding, visible vessel, overlying clot) should undergo endoscopic haemostasis by injection of dilute adrenaline (epinephrine) together with coagulation of the vessel with thermal therapy (heater or bipolar probe), or application of mechanical clips (endoclips) to the vessel. Intravenous PPIs are given for 72 hours following endoscopic therapy in PU bleeding; they reduce re-bleeding rates and transfusion requirements. Surgery is required for persistent or recurrent bleeding from ulcers.

Post-endoscopy

In general, young patients with PU bleeding who are otherwise fit and haemodynamically stable and who have no stigmata of recent bleeding can be discharged from hospital within 24 hours (post-endoscopy Rockall Score ≤1). *H. pylori* eradication treatment is given and eradication confirmed by urea breath test or faecal antigen testing. Assessment of ongoing need for antiplatelet therapy is made and essential treatment is co-prescribed with a PPI.

Lower gastrointestinal bleeding

Bright red or altered blood per rectum suggests bleeding from the colon or small intestine. Massive bleeding is rare and usually from diverticular disease or ischaemic colitis (Table 3.6). Minor bleeds from haemorrhoids and anal fissure are common.

Table 3.6 Causes of lower gastrointestinal bleeding

Colonic
Haemorrhoids
Anal fissure
Neoplasms: benign and malignant
Colitis: ulcerative colitis, Crohn's, infective, ischaemic
Angiodysplasia (abnormal collections of blood vessels)
Diverticular disease
Small intestine
Neoplasms
Ulcerative disease: Crohn's disease, vasculitis, NSAIDs
Angiodysplasia
Meckel's diverticulum

NB: acute massive upper gastrointestinal bleeding may present with fresh rectal bleeding usually with haemodynamic instability.
NSAIDs, non-steroidal anti-inflammatory drugs.

Management

Resuscitation with intravenous fluids or blood is necessary with large bleeds. The site of bleeding is determined from the history and physical examination including a rectal examination and the following investigations as appropriate:

- Proctoscopy to look for anorectal disease, e.g. haemorrhoids.
- Sigmoidoscopy or colonoscopy for inflammatory bowel disease, polyps, colon cancer, diverticular disease, ischaemic colitis, vascular lesions.
- Angiography for vascular abnormality, e.g. angiodysplasia.

In the non-emergency setting, bright red fresh rectal bleeding is likely to originate from a source distal to the splenic flexure and can be investigated with a flexible sigmoidoscopy rather than full colonoscopy.

Specific management Lesions are treated as appropriate.

Chronic gastrointestinal bleeding

Chronic gastrointestinal bleeding presents with iron deficiency anaemia. All such patients require investigation of the gastrointestinal tract particularly to exclude a malignancy. The exception is menstruating women less than 50 years of age without gastrointestinal symptoms, in whom anaemia is assumed to be due to menstrual blood loss. Causes of chronic blood loss are those that cause acute bleeding (see Fig. 3.3, p. 89 and Table 3.6). However, oesophageal varices, duodenal ulcers and diverticular disease rarely bleed chronically. Malabsorption (most frequently from coeliac disease), previous gastrectomy and, rarely, poor dietary intake are causes of iron deficiency and will also present with anaemia.

Investigations

Iron deficiency anaemia is investigated with OGD and colonoscopy ('top and tail') performed at the same endoscopic session; a distal duodenal biopsy is taken to look for coeliac disease. Further investigations, usually in the order listed, are only warranted in anaemia not responding to iron treatment or if there is abdominal pain or visible blood loss:

- Small bowel barium follow-through or MRI (usually only helpful if there are symptoms to suggest Crohn's disease)
- Video capsule endoscopy
- Enteroscopy (push and/or balloon-assisted) is particularly useful for endoscopic therapy of vascular lesions seen at capsule endoscopy
- Coeliac axis and mesenteric angiography
- Technetium-labelled red cell scan.

Management

The cause of the bleeding is treated and oral iron is given to treat the anaemia.

Table 3.7 Disorders of the small intestine causing malabsorption

Coeliac disease
Crohn's disease
Dermatitis herpetiformis
Tropical sprue
Bacterial overgrowth
Intestinal resection
Whipple's disease
Radiation enteritis
Parasite infection, e.g. *Giardia intestinalis*

THE SMALL INTESTINE

The principal role of the small intestine is the digestion and absorption of nutrients. Vitamin B_{12} and bile salts have specific receptors in the terminal ileum but other nutrients are absorbed throughout the small intestine.

Presenting symptoms of small bowel disease are diarrhoea, steatorrhoea, abdominal pain or discomfort, and anorexia causing weight loss. Small bowel disease may also be found after investigation for specific deficiencies such as vitamin B_{12}. The two most common causes of small bowel disease in developed countries are coeliac disease and Crohn's disease. Disorders of the small intestine causing malabsorption are shown in Table 3.7. Investigation of suspected small bowel disease (e.g. in a symptomatic patient and/or folate/B_{12} deficiency) is initially with coeliac serology, small bowel barium follow or MRI and endoscopic small bowel biopsy.

Coeliac disease (gluten-sensitive enteropathy)

This is an autoimmune condition characterized by an abnormal jejunal mucosa that improves when gluten (contained in wheat, rye and barley) is withdrawn from the diet and relapses when gluten is reintroduced. About 1 in 100 individuals in European-derived populations have coeliac disease, most of whom are undiagnosed.

Aetiopathogenesis

A strong association exists between coeliac disease and two human leucocyte antigen (HLA) class II molecules, HLA DQ2 and DQ8. The peptide α-gliadin is the toxic portion of gluten. Gliadin is resistant to proteases in the small intestinal lumen and passes through a damaged (as a result of an infection or possibly gliadin itself) epithelial barrier of the small intestine where it is deaminated by tissue transglutaminase so increasing its immunogenicity. Gliadin then interacts with antigen-presenting cells in the lamina propria via HLA DQ2 and DQ8 and activates gluten-sensitive T cells. The resultant inflammatory cascade and release of mediators contribute to the villous atrophy and crypt hyperplasia that are typical histological features of coeliac disease. There is an increase in intraepithelial lymphocytes but the pathogenic role of these lymphocytes, compared with lamina propria lymphocytes, is controversial.

Clinical features

Presentation is at any age but there are two peaks in incidence: infancy (after weaning on to gluten-containing foods) and in adults in the fifth decade. There may be non-specific symptoms of tiredness and malaise, or symptoms of small intestinal disease (see above). Physical signs are usually few and non-specific, and related to anaemia and nutritional deficiency. There is an increased incidence of atopy and autoimmune diseases (Table 3.8).

Investigations

Serum antibodies IgA tissue transglutaminase (tTG) antibodies have a very high sensitivity and specificity for coeliac disease. False negatives occur in IgA deficiency (2% of coeliacs) when IgG based tests should be used. IgA endomysial (EMA) antibodies are less sensitive. Serological testing is offered to patients with signs or symptoms or in conditions where there is an increased risk of disease (Table 3.8). Patients with positive serology or if serology is negative but coeliac disease is strongly suspected are referred for intestinal biopsy.

Distal duodenal biopsies (obtained endoscopically) are required for a definitive diagnosis. Histological changes are of variable severity and show an increase in the number of intraepithelial lymphocytes, crypt hyperplasia with chronic inflammatory cells in the lamina propria and villous atrophy. The latter is seen in other conditions (e.g. tropical sprue, Whipple's disease), but coeliac disease is the commonest cause of subtotal villous atrophy.

Blood count A mild anaemia is present in 50% of cases. There is almost always folate deficiency, commonly iron deficiency and, rarely, vitamin B_{12} deficiency.

Table 3.8 Individuals who should be offered serological testing for coeliac disease

Autoimmune disease
    Type 1 diabetes mellitus
    Thyroid disease
    Autoimmune liver disease
    Addison's disease
Irritable bowel syndrome with diarrhoea (symptoms may be similar to coeliac disease)
Unexplained osteoporosis
Those with a first degree relative (10-fold increase compared to general population)
Down's syndrome (20-fold increase)
Turner's syndrome
Infertility and recurrent miscarriage

Small bowel radiology or capsule endoscopy is usually only performed when a complication is suspected such as lymphoma.

Bone densitometry (dual energy X-ray absorptiometry [DXA] scan) is performed at diagnosis because of the increased risk of osteoporosis.

Management

Treatment is with a lifelong gluten-free diet and correction of any vitamin deficiencies. Pneumococcal vaccine is given as coeliac disease is associated with hyposplenism. Symptoms and serologic testing (undetectable antibodies indicate a response) are used to monitor recovery and compliance with the diet; re-biopsy is reserved for patients who do not respond or in whom there is diagnostic uncertainty.

Complications

There is an increased incidence of malignancy, particularly intestinal T cell lymphoma, small bowel and oesophageal cancer. The incidence may be reduced by a gluten-free diet.

Dermatitis herpetiformis

Dermatitis herpetiformis is an itchy, symmetrical eruption of vesicles and crusts over the extensor surfaces of the body, with deposition of granular immunoglobulin (Ig) A at the dermoepidermal junction of the skin including areas not involved with the rash. Patients also have a gluten-sensitive enteropathy, which is usually asymptomatic. The skin condition responds to dapsone, but both the gut and the skin will improve on a gluten-free diet.

Tropical sprue

This is a progressive small intestinal disorder presenting with diarrhoea, steatorrhoea and megaloblastic anaemia. It occurs in residents or visitors to endemic areas in the tropics (Asia, some Caribbean islands, Puerto Rico, parts of South America). The aetiology is unknown but likely to be infective. Diagnosis is based on demonstrating evidence of malabsorption (particularly of fat and vitamin B_{12}) together with a small bowel mucosal biopsy showing features similar, but not identical, to those in untreated coeliac disease. Infective causes of diarrhoea, particularly *Giardia intestinalis,* should be excluded. Treatment is with folic acid and tetracycline for 3–6 months and correction of nutritional deficiencies.

Bacterial overgrowth

The upper small intestine is almost sterile. Bacterial overgrowth occurs when there is stasis of intestinal contents as a result of abnormal motility, e.g. systemic sclerosis, or a structural abnormality, e.g. previous small bowel surgery or a diverticulum.

Clinical features

The bacteria deconjugate bile salts causing diarrhoea and/or steatorrhoea and metabolize vitamin B_{12}, which may result in deficiency.

Diagnosis

A therapeutic trial of antibiotics is given when clinical suspicion is high. Otherwise, diagnosis is usually by a hydrogen breath test in which hydrogen is measured in exhaled air after oral lactulose. With bacterial overgrowth an early peak is seen in the breath hydrogen followed by the later colonic peak (normally present due to metabolism of lactulose by colonic bacteria).

Management

The underlying cause should be corrected if possible. Otherwise, rotating courses of antibiotics, e.g. tetracycline and metronidazole, are given.

Intestinal resection

The effects of small intestinal resection depend on the extent and the area involved. Resection of the terminal ileum leads to malabsorption of:

- Vitamin B_{12}, leading to megaloblastic anaemia
- Bile salts, which overflow into the colon. This causes secretion of water and electrolytes and diarrhoea, and increased oxalate absorption, which may result in renal oxalate stones (p. 377).

More extensive resection leaving less than 1 m of small bowel is followed by the *short bowel syndrome*. The majority of cases occur after resection due to Crohn's disease, mesenteric ischaemia, trauma, volvulus or surgical complications. Parenteral nutrition is the mainstay of treatment for patients in whom absorptive function has failed. Intestinal transplantation is used in a few centres.

The ability of patients to cope without supplemental intravenous fluids or nutrition depends on:

- *Amount* of resected bowel – most patients with <100 cm of jejunum and no colon will require supplements.
- *Location* of resected bowel (jejunal resection is better tolerated than ileal).
- *Colon* intact which absorbs water and electrolytes.
- *Health* of the residual intestine, i.e. there are fewer problems after resection following trauma than in patients with Crohn's disease.

Whipple's disease

This is a rare disease caused by the bacterium *Tropheryma whipplei*. Steatorrhoea, abdominal pain, fever, lymphadenopathy, arthritis and neurological involvement occur. Small bowel biopsy shows periodic acid-Schiff

(PAS)-positive macrophages which on electron microscopy are seen to contain the causative bacteria. Treatment is with co-trimoxazole for 1 year.

MISCELLANEOUS SMALL INTESTINAL CONDITIONS

Tuberculosis

This results from reactivation of the primary disease caused by *Mycobacterium tuberculosis*. In developed countries it is most commonly seen in ethnic minority groups or patients who are immunocompromised due to human immunodeficiency virus (HIV) infection or drugs. The ileocaecal valve is the most common site affected.

Clinical features

There is abdominal pain, diarrhoea, anorexia, weight loss and fever. A mass may be palpable. Presentation can be similar to Crohn's disease.

Diagnosis

Imaging Chest X-ray shows evidence of pulmonary tuberculosis in 50% of cases. The small bowel follow-through may show features similar to those of Crohn's disease (p. 101). US or CT shows mesenteric thickening and lymphadenopathy.

Histology and culture of tissue is desirable but not always possible, and treatment is started if there is a high degree of suspicion. Specimens can be obtained at laparoscopy; laparotomy is rarely required.

Management

Treatment is similar to that for pulmonary tuberculosis but given for 1 year.

Protein-losing enteropathy

Increased protein loss across an abnormal intestinal mucosa occasionally leads to hypoalbuminaemia and oedema. Causes include Crohn's disease, Ménétrier's disease (thickening and enlargement of gastric folds), coeliac disease and lymphatic disorders, e.g. lymphangiectasia.

Meckel's diverticulum

A diverticulum projects from the wall of the ileum approximately 60 cm from the ileocaecal valve. About 50% contain gastric mucosa which secretes acid, and peptic ulceration may occur. Presentation is with lower gastrointestinal bleeding, perforation, inflammation (presents similarly to appendicitis) or with obstruction (due to an associated band). Treatment is surgical removal.

Intestinal ischaemia

Ischaemia is usually due to reduced arterial inflow as a result of atheroma, embolism (e.g. in atrial fibrillation), vasculitis or profound and prolonged shock. It presents acutely with severe abdominal pain but often little to find on abdominal examination. Surgery is necessary to resect the gangrenous bowel and the mortality is high. It may also present chronically with post-prandial abdominal pain and weight loss. Diagnosis is made by angiography.

Tumours of the small intestine

These are rare and present with abdominal pain, diarrhoea, anorexia and anaemia. Carcinoid tumours have additional clinical features, described below.

Malignant tumours

Adenocarcinoma accounts for 50% of malignant small bowel tumours; there is an increased incidence in coeliac disease and Crohn's disease. Non-Hodgkin's lymphoma constitutes 15% of malignant small bowel tumours and may be B cell or T cell in origin. The latter occur with increased frequency in coeliac disease. Treatment is surgical excision with or without chemotherapy and radiotherapy.

Benign small bowel tumours

- Peutz–Jeghers syndrome is an autosomal dominant condition with mucocutaneous pigmentation (circumoral, hands and feet) and hamartomatous gastrointestinal polyps. Polyps may occur anywhere in the gastrointestinal tract, but are most common in the small bowel. They may bleed or cause intussusception, and may undergo malignant change.
- Adenomas, leiomyomas and lipomas are rare. They are usually asymptomatic and discovered incidentally.
- Familial adenomatous polyposis (p. 111).

Carcinoid tumours

Pathology

These originate from enterochromaffin cells (serotonin producing) of the intestine. *Carcinoid syndrome* is the term applied to the symptoms that arise as a result of serotonin (5-hydroxytryptamine, 5-HT), kinins, histamine and prostaglandins, released into the circulation from secondaries in the liver.

Clinical features

Patients with gastrointestinal carcinoid tumours have the carcinoid syndrome only if they have liver metastases. Tumour products are then able to drain directly into the hepatic vein (without being metabolized by the liver) and into the systemic circulation, where they cause flushing, wheezing, diarrhoea, abdominal pain, and right-sided cardiac valvular fibrosis causing stenosis and regurgitation.

Investigations

A high level of 5-hydroxyindoleacetic acid (5-HIAA), the breakdown product of serotonin, is found in the urine in the carcinoid syndrome. A liver ultrasound confirms the presence of metastases.

Management

Treatment of the carcinoid syndrome is symptomatic and aimed at:

- Inhibition of tumour products with the somatostatin analogue, octreotide, or with 5-HT antagonists, e.g. cyproheptadine
- Reducing tumour mass through surgical resection, hepatic artery embolization, radiofrequency ablation or chemotherapy.

INFLAMMATORY BOWEL DISEASE

Inflammatory bowel diseases (IBD) are a group of chronic systemic diseases involving inflammation of the intestine and include: ulcerative colitis (UC), which only affects the colon; Crohn's disease (CD), which can affect the entire gastrointestinal tract; and indeterminate colitis, which shows features of both CD and UC.

Epidemiology

IBD occurs world-wide but is most common in Northern Europe, the UK and North America. Presentation is usually in the teens and twenties. In the UK, there are about 400 IBD patients per 100 000 population.

Aetiology

IBD represents the outcome of three essential interacting co-factors: genetic susceptibility, the environment and host immune response.

Genetic susceptibility

- Genetic association is stronger for CD than UC.
- There is familial aggregation of disease.
- Concordance rates are higher in monozygotic (58% for CD) than dizygotic twins (4%).
- Disease susceptibility genes, e.g. mutations in the *CARD15 (NOD2)* gene on chromosome 16, confer susceptibility to stricturing small bowel CD.
- Increased incidence of HLA-B27 in IBD with ankylosing spondylitis.

Environment

- Smoking is associated with a twofold increased risk for CD. In contrast, current smoking is associated with a reduced risk for developing UC compared with non-smokers.
- Stress and depression may precipitate relapses in IBD.
- Enteric microflora is altered and the intestinal wall is contaminated by adherent and invading bacteria.

Host immune response IBD results from a defective mucosal immune system producing an abnormal response to luminal antigens such as bacteria which enter the intestine via a leaky epithelium. In the genetically predisposed individual, there is an exaggerated immune response with effector T cells (T helper (Th)1, Th2 and Th17) predominating over regulatory T cells. Pro-inflammatory cytokines (interleukin (IL)-12, interferon (IFN)-γ, IL-5, IL-17) released by these activated T cells stimulate macrophages to produce tumour necrosis factor (TNF)-α, IL-1 and IL-6. There is also activation of other cells (neutrophils, mast cells and eosinophils) that together lead to increased production of a wide variety of inflammatory mediators, all of which can lead to cell damage.

Pathology

CD and UC have some overlapping clinical and pathological features but also key differences at macroscopic and microscopic levels (Table 3.9).

Table 3.9 Differences between Crohn's disease and ulcerative colitis

	Crohn's disease	Ulcerative colitis
Macroscopic	Affects any part of gastrointestinal tract	Affects only the colon
	Oral and perianal disease	Begins in rectum and extends proximally in varying degrees
	Discontinuous involvement ('skip lesions')	Continuous involvement
	Deep ulcers and fissures in mucosa: 'cobblestone appearance'	Red mucosa, bleeds easily
		Ulcers and pseudopolyps (regenerating mucosa) in severe disease
Microscopic	Transmural inflammation	Mucosal inflammation
	Granulomas present in 50%	No granulomata
		Goblet cell depletion
		Crypt abscesses

Clinical features

Crohn's disease Symptoms depend on the region(s) of involved bowel; the commonest site is ileocaecal in 40% of patients. Small bowel disease causes abdominal pain, usually with weight loss. Less commonly, terminal ileal disease presents as an acute abdomen with right iliac fossa pain mimicking appendicitis. Colonic disease presents with diarrhoea, bleeding and pain related to defecation. In perianal disease there are anal tags, fissures, fistulae and abscess formation.

Ulcerative colitis presents with diarrhoea, often containing blood and mucus. The clinical course may be one of persistent diarrhoea, relapses and remissions or severe fulminant colitis (Table 3.10). Patients with IBD may also have one or more extraintestinal manifestations (Table 3.11).

Table 3.10 Ulcerative colitis severity index

	Mild	Severe
Bloody diarrhoea	<4 per day	>6 per day
Fever	Absent	>37.5°C
Tachycardia	Absent	>90/min
Erythrocyte sedimentation rate	<20 mm/h	>30 mm/h
Anaemia	Absent	Hb <100 g/L
Serum albumin	Normal	<30 g/L

Severe colitis requires bloody diarrhoea plus any one of the systemic features. Moderate colitis lies between these two definitions.

Table 3.11 Extragastrointestinal manifestations of inflammatory bowel disease

Eyes	Uveitis, episcleritis, conjunctivitis
Joints	Arthralgia*, small joint arthritis, monoarticular arthritis (knees and ankles), ankylosing spondylitis, inflammatory back pain
Skin	Erythema nodosum, pyoderma gangrenosum (necrotizing ulceration of the skin, commonly on lower legs)
Hepatobiliary	Fatty liver*, sclerosing cholangitis, chronic hepatitis, cirrhosis, gallstones*
Renal calculi	Oxalate stones in patients with small bowel disease or after resection
Venous thrombosis	

All uncommon, occur in less than 10% of patients other than those marked.*

Investigations

The purpose of investigations is to establish the diagnosis of IBD with differentiation between CD and UC, to define the extent and severity of bowel involvement, identify any extraintestinal manifestations and exclude other diseases that may present similarly.

Blood tests Anaemia is common and may be normochromic, normocytic anaemia of chronic disease or due to deficiency of iron, B_{12} or folate. The platelet count, erythrocyte sedimentation rate (ESR) and C-reactive protein are often raised in acute CD, and the serum albumin is low in severe disease. Liver biochemistry may be abnormal related to associated liver disease.

Radiology and imaging

Rigid or flexible sigmoidoscopy will establish the diagnosis of UC and CD (if the rectum and/or sigmoid colon is involved). A rectal biopsy is taken for histological examination to determine the nature of the inflammation.

Colonoscopy allows the exact extent and severity of colonic and terminal ileal inflammation to be determined and biopsies to be taken.

Small bowel imaging is performed to determine the extent of small bowel involvement with CD. Specific imaging type depends on local expertise and includes small bowel barium follow-through or MR enteroclysis with oral contrast. Affected bowel shows an asymmetrical alteration in the mucosal pattern, with deep ulceration and areas of narrowing ('string sign') commonly confined to the ileum. Skip lesions may be seen. Video capsule endoscopy is increasingly used to detect small bowel disease and is more sensitive than a barium follow-through. It is contraindicated in stricturing disease.

Perianal CD is usually assessed by MRI and sometimes by endoanal ultrasound.

Ultrasonography is particularly helpful in delineating abdominal and pelvic abscesses and will show thickened bowel in involved areas. Abdominal CT scanning is also used in patients with suspected abscesses.

Plain abdominal X-ray should be performed in all patients admitted to hospital with acute severe colitis. It helps to assess extent of colonic involvement and identifies toxic dilatation of the colon.

Radiolabelled white cell scanning is a safe, non-invasive investigation. It helps to identify small bowel and colonic disease but lacks specificity.

Differential diagnosis

CD must be differentiated from other causes of chronic diarrhoea, malabsorption and malnutrition. In children it is a cause of short stature. Other causes of terminal ileitis are tuberculosis and *Yersinia enterocolitica* infection (causing an acute illness). IBD affecting the colon must be differentiated from other causes of colitis: infection, ischaemia, radiation and microscopic colitis.

Management

Medical The aim of treatment is to induce and maintain a remission. Patients with CD who smoke should be advised to stop with help offered to achieve this. Therapy for IBD is a rapidly evolving field and new drugs are likely to appear in the next decade. In general the treatments used have many anti-inflammatory and immunosuppressive properties combined with an antibacterial action in some cases (e.g. metronidazole).

Treatment of CD depends on the site and severity of disease and also if the disease is stricturing or fistulating:

- *Oral 5-ASA* is less efficacious than in UC and is used in mild disease only. It is generally well tolerated. Rare potentially serious side effects are bloody diarrhoea (resembling acute colitis), Stevens–Johnson syndrome, acute pancreatitis and renal impairment.

- *Steroids:* Oral prednisolone (40 mg/day) is used for moderate/severe disease. It is reduced gradually according to severity and patient response, generally over 8 weeks. A few patients with severe disease require inpatient admission and intravenous hydrocortisone. Budesonide is a poorly absorbed oral corticosteroid with limited bioavailability and extensive first-pass metabolism that has therapeutic benefit with reduced systemic toxicity in ileocaecal CD.

- *Liquid enteral nutrition* with an elemental (liquid preparation of amino acids, glucose and fatty acids) or polymeric diet induces a remission in active CD. The exact mode of action is not known. These diets are unpalatable and may have to be given via a nasogastric tube.

- *The thiopurine drugs*, azathioprine (2.5 mg/kg/day) or its metabolite 6-mercaptopurine 1.5 mg/kg/day), are used to maintain a remission and are given to patients who require two or more corticosteroid courses per year. Major side effects are bone marrow suppression (neutropenia, thrombocytopenia and anaemia), acute pancreatitis and allergic reactions. The enzyme, thiopurine methyltransferase (TPMT), is essential in metabolism of thiopurines and activity should be measured on a blood sample before treatment is given. Approximately 1 in 300 patients have absent TPMT activity and will not metabolize the drug. These patients are at high risk for pancytopenia and treatment is contraindicated. About 10% of patients have reduced TMPT activity and a lower drug dose is indicated (a half to one-third of normal dosing).

- *Metronidazole* is useful in severe perianal CD as a result of both its antibacterial and immunosuppressive action.

- *Methotrexate* (intramuscular) is used in a minority of patients with active CD that is resistant to conventional treatment with steroids. It is also used to maintain a remission in those refractory or intolerant to azathioprine/6-mercaptopurine.

- *Anti-TNF antibodies* (infliximab, adalimumab, certolizumab) are used to induce a remission in patients resistant to corticosteroids/ immunosuppressives. Scheduled treatment at 8-weekly intervals is then given to maintain a remission.

Treatment of UC depends on severity (Table 3.10) and distribution of disease (Table 3.12). The management of acute, severe UC is summarized in Emergency Box 3.2.

Surgery In CD and UC, surgery is indicated for:

- Failure of medical therapy with acute or chronic symptoms producing ill health
- Complications (Table 3.13)
- Failure to grow in children despite medical treatment.

Resections are kept to a minimum in CD as recurrence is almost inevitable in the remaining bowel. In some patients with small bowel disease, strictures can be widened (stricturoplasty) without resection.

The surgical options in UC are:

- Colectomy with ileoanal anastomosis: the terminal ileum is used to form a reservoir (a 'pouch'), and the patient is continent with a few bowel motions per day. The pouch may become inflamed ('pouchitis'), leading to bloody diarrhoea which is treated initially with metronidazole. Probiotics (live

Table 3.12 Summary of treatments used in ulcerative colitis

Disease severity	Medication	Indications
Mild/moderate	Oral 5-ASA	First line for left sided/extensive
	Rectal 5-ASA/ steroids	For proctitis or proctosigmoiditis
	Oral prednisolone	Second line, if inadequate response to 5-ASA
Severe	Oral prednisolone	
Severe with systemic features	Hydrocortisone	See Emergency Box 3.2
	Ciclosporin	
	Infliximab	
Maintain remission	5-ASA	Most patients require maintenance treatment
	Azathioprine/6-mercaptopurine	For patients who relapse frequently despite ASA or are ASA-intolerant

5-ASA, aminosalicylic acid; left sided disease, up to splenic flexure; proctitis, rectal inflammation.

✚ Emergency Box 3.2

Management of acute severe colitis

Admit to hospital

- Joint inpatient management between gastroenterologist and colorectal surgeon

Investigations

- FBC, CRP, liver biochemistry, serum albumin and electrolytes
- Blood cultures (Gram-negative sepsis occurs)
- Plain abdominal X-ray looking for colonic dilatation (transverse colon diameter >5 cm), and mucosal islands
- Stool cultures (×3) and *C. difficile* toxin to exclude coincidental infection (do not delay steroids while awaiting result)

Treatment

- Stop drugs that may precipitate colonic dilatation (anticholinergics, antidiarrhoeals, non-steroidal anti-inflammatory drugs, opioids)
- i.v. hydrocortisone 100 mg 6-hourly
- Correct electrolyte and fluid imbalance
- Low molecular weight heparin to reduce the risk of venous thrombosis
- Consider i.v. ciclosporin (2 mg/kg over 24 hours) or infliximab if no response after 4 days of i.v. hydrocortisone. Colectomy may be necessary.

Monitor

- Stool chart: frequency, type and presence of blood
- Vital signs at least four times daily
- Daily bloods and abdominal X-ray if admitting film abnormal

---

Table 3.13 Complications of inflammatory bowel disease

Toxic dilatation of the colon + perforation
Stricture formation*
Abscess formation (Crohn's disease)
Fistulae and fissures (Crohn's)*
Colon cancer

*Surgical intervention only necessary if symptomatic and not responding to medical treatment.

---

microorganisms that modify composition of enteric bacteria) are sometimes used to prevent and treat pouchitis.

- Panproctocolectomy with ileostomy: the whole colon and rectum are removed and the ileum brought out on to the abdominal wall as a stoma.

Cancer in inflammatory bowel disease

Extensive UC and Crohn's colitis of more than 10 years' duration is associated with an increased risk of colorectal cancer (CRC, cumulative risk 12% after 25 years). Patients with colitis should undergo colonoscopy at 10 years from diagnosis and an assessment of cancer risk is made. High risk patients (extensive colitis with moderate/severe activity, primary sclerosing cholangitis or family history of CRC in first degree relative <50 years) are offered a further colonoscopy and multiple colonic biopsies (to look for dysplasia) 1 year later. Lower risk patients undergo colonoscopy 3–5 years later. Colectomy is recommended if high grade dysplasia is discovered and increased surveillance (6–12 monthly) with low-grade dysplasia.

Prognosis

Both diseases are characterized by relapses and remissions. Almost all patients with CD have a significant relapse over a 20-year period. The prognosis of UC is variable. Only 10% of patients with proctitis develop more extensive disease, but with severe fulminant disease there is a risk of colonic perforation and death.

Microscopic colitis

The colonic mucosa looks normal at endoscopy but histological examination of mucosal biopsies shows lamina propria inflammation and increased intra-epithelial lymphocytes in *lymphocytic colitis* and thickening of the subepithelial collagen layer in *collagenous colitis*. Presentation is most commonly with chronic, watery diarrhoea in a middle-aged or elderly person. Microscopic colitis can be drug induced, e.g. NSAIDs, and occurs with increased frequency in coeliac disease. Treatment is symptomatic initially with antidiarrhoeal drugs such as loperamide. Budesonide is the first-line therapy for both induction and maintenance of response in patients not controlled with symptomatic treatment. Aminosalicylates, bismuth subsalicylate, colestyramine and systemic steroids are used in resistant cases. Microscopic colitis does not progress to overt inflammatory bowel disease.

THE COLON AND RECTUM

The main role of the colon is absorption of water and electrolytes and propulsion of contents from the caecum to the anorectal region. About 9000 mL of water containing electrolytes enters the gastrointestinal tract each day; the majority from gastrointestinal secretions (stomach, pancreas, bile, intestinal secretion) and only a small amount from the diet. Most is absorbed in the small intestine and only about 1500 mL passes through the ileocaecal valve into the colon, of which about 1350 mL is normally absorbed.

Constipation

This is a common problem in the general population, particularly in the elderly (associated with immobility and poor diet), and in young women (associated with slow colonic transit or post-partum pelvic floor abnormalities). Constipation is a consistent difficulty in defecation. Specific definitions are infrequent passage of stools (<3/week), straining, passage of hard stools, incomplete evacuation and sensation of anorectal blockage. There is a long list of possible causes (Table 3.14), but in many patients it is their perception that there is an abnormality and requires no more than dietary advice and reassurance. In many patients it is part of the irritable bowel syndrome.

Investigation

Initial evaluation is with a history and physical examination, including a rectal examination during which the patient is asked to strain. A patient with a defecatory disorder has paradoxical contraction rather than the normal relaxation of the puborectalis and external anal sphincter during straining, which may prevent defecation.

Table 3.14 Causes of constipation

General
Pregnancy, inadequate fibre intake, immobility
Metabolic/endocrine
Diabetes mellitus, hypothyroidism, hypercalcaemia, porphyria
Functional
Irritable bowel syndrome, idiopathic slow transit
Drugs
Opiates, antimuscarinics, calcium channel blockers, e.g. verapamil
Antidepressants, e.g. tricyclics, iron
Neurological
Spinal cord lesions, Parkinson's disease
Psychological
Depression, anorexia nervosa, depressed urge to defecate
Gastrointestinal disease
Intestinal obstruction (e.g. by colon cancer) and pseudo-obstruction
Painful anal conditions, Hirschsprung's disease
Defecatory disorders
Rectal prolapse, pelvic floor dyssynergia
Megarectum, large rectocele

Routine blood tests, radiography and endoscopy are not usually indicated in the evaluation of patients with constipation without alarm symptoms; the latter includes rectal bleeding, anaemia or recent onset of constipation in the middle aged or elderly (>50 years) particularly if associated with a sense of incomplete evacuation.

A few patients with no obvious underlying cause (idiopathic constipation) may require studies of colonic transit (measured using radiopaque markers taken orally) and anorectal physiology to determine if they have normal colonic transit, slow transit or a defecatory disorder.

Management

Any underlying cause should be corrected. Patients with normal and slow transit constipation are treated with a high-fibre diet together with plenty of liquids. Long-term laxatives are only used in severe and unresponsive cases (p. 131). A wide variety of laxatives are available but many patients are not satisfied with their treatments. Prucalopride is a high affinity $5HT_4$ agonist which increases colonic transit and is an effective therapy for refractory constipation. Linaclotide, a minimally absorbed peptide agonist of guanylate cyclase-C receptor increases gastrointestinal fluid secretion. Lubiprostone is an orally active agonist for type-2 chloride channels and therefore also increases GI fluid secretion. Patients with defecatory disorders may require referral to a specialist centre.

Faecal incontinence

This is recurrent uncontrolled passage of flatus and/or stool. Continence depends on a number of factors including mental function, stool volume and consistency, structural and functional integrity of the anal sphincters, puborectalis muscle, pudendal nerve function, rectal distensibility and anorectal sensation. Faecal impaction is a common cause of faecal incontinence in the elderly (overflow diarrhoea). Anal sphincter tears or trauma to the pudendal nerve can occur after childbirth or anal surgery (e.g. for haemorrhoids). Impaired rectal sensation occurs with diabetes mellitus, multiple sclerosis, dementia and spinal cord injuries. A detailed history and examination with digital rectal examination will help diagnose and exclude most common causes. Specific investigations include sigmoidoscopy to exclude mucosal disease, imaging of the anal sphincters (by anal endosonography, or MRI), anorectal manometry (to assess anal sphincter pressures), and sensory testing by rectal balloon distension to assess rectal sensation and compliance. Treatment depends on the cause.

Diverticular disease

Pouches of mucosa extrude through the colonic muscular wall via weakened areas near blood vessels to form diverticula. The term *diverticulosis* means the presence of diverticula. *Diverticulitis* implies inflammation, which occurs when faeces obstruct the neck of the diverticulum. Diverticula are common, affecting 50% of the population over 50 years of age.

Aetiology

The precise cause of diverticular disease is unknown, although it appears to be related to the low-fibre diet eaten in Western populations; insufficient dietary fibre leads to increased intracolonic pressure, which causes herniation of the mucosa at sites of weakness.

Clinical features

It is asymptomatic in 95% and usually discovered incidentally when a barium enema or colonoscopy is performed for other reasons. Symptoms are the result of luminal narrowing (causing pain and constipation), bleeding which may be massive, or diverticulitis. The latter present with left iliac fossa pain, fever and nausea and may result in perforation (leading to abscess formation or peritonitis), fistula formation into the bladder or vagina, or intestinal obstruction. Acute diverticulitis is diagnosed by CT scan or in some cases by ultrasound.

Management

Acute attacks are treated with antibiotics (cephalosporin and metronidazole). Surgery is indicated rarely for complications and for frequent attacks of diverticulitis.

Miscellaneous conditions

Megacolon

This term describes a number of conditions in which the colon is dilated. The most common cause is chronic constipation. Other causes are Chagas' disease and Hirschsprung's disease (congenital aganglionic segment in the rectum). Treatment is with laxatives, although Hirschsprung's disease responds to surgical resection.

Ischaemic colitis

Blood supply to the colon is from the superior and inferior mesenteric arteries. Watershed areas in the splenic flexure and caecum are most susceptible to ischaemia. Ischaemic colitis is most common in the elderly and related to underlying atherosclerosis and vessel occlusion. It also occurs in a younger population associated with use of contraceptives, thrombophilia and vasculitis. Presentation is with abdominal pain and rectal bleeding, and occasionally shock. Sigmoidoscopy is often normal apart from blood. Treatment is symptomatic, although surgery may be required for gangrene, perforation or stricture formation.

Colon polyps and the polyposis syndromes

A polyp is an abnormal growth of tissue projecting into the intestinal lumen from the normally flat mucosal surface. Polyps may be single or multiple and are usually asymptomatic. Most polyps in the colon are adenomas, which are the precursor lesions of most colorectal cancer (CRC). Other types are hyperplastic, inflammatory (in patients with IBD) and hamartomatous, of which only the latter carry a malignant potential.

Adenomatous polyps These are tumours of benign neoplastic epithelium and are more common with increasing age. The aetiology is unknown, although genetic and environmental factors are implicated. They rarely produce symptoms, although large polyps can bleed and cause anaemia, and large villous adenomas can occasionally present with diarrhoea and hypokalaemia. Although most adenomas do not become malignant during the patient's lifetime they are removed at endoscopy to reduce the risk of developing CRC. The risk of malignant change in a polyp increases with:

- Size >1 cm
- Sessile polyps (base attached to colon wall) > pedunculated polyps (mucosal stalk is interposed between polyp and colon wall)
- Severe dysplasia > mild dysplasia
- Villous histology > tubular
- Polyp number: multiple > single.

About 5% of CRCs occur on a background of a genetic syndrome associated with colonic polyps and an increased risk of colon cancer (Table 3.15). A family history suggestive of one of these syndromes may lower the threshold for investigation in a patient presenting with gastrointestinal symptoms. In addition, referral for genetic testing may be appropriate in a patient with colon polyps or cancer when one of these syndromes is suspected (e.g. young age at diagnosis <50 years, affected family members, other associated cancers).

Colorectal cancer

Most colorectal cancers occur sporadically. Family colon cancer syndromes (Table 3.15) or cancers occurring on a background of longstanding colitis account for a small percentage.

Epidemiology

CRC is the third most common cancer world-wide and the second most common cause of cancer deaths in the UK. Increasing age is the greatest risk factor and the average age at diagnosis is 60–65 years. Family history, next to age, is the most significant risk factor. In the West, the lifetime risk of CRC is 1 in 50, increasing to 1 in 17 in those with one affected first-degree relative and greatly increased in the family cancer syndromes (Table 3.15). Colon cancer is rare in Africa and Asia, largely because of environmental differences. A diet high in meat and animal fat and low in fibre is thought to be one aetiological factor.

Table 3.15 The family colon cancer syndromes

Name	Mutated gene (s)	Description	Cancer risk
HNPCC (Lynch's syndrome)	DNA mismatch repair genes	Accelerated progression from adenoma to CRC. Increased risk several extracolonic malignancies; endometrial is commonest.	Over half develop CRC, onset in fourth decade
Familial adenomatous polyposis (FAP)	*APC* gene	Numerous colorectal polyps (>100) develop in teenage years Increased risk of extracolonic malignancies. FAP variants are Turcot's (with brain tumours), Gardner's (with desmoid tumours, skull osteomas) and attenuated FAP (fewer polyps at a later age).	100% lifetime risk of CRC, onset in young adults
MYH-associated polyposis	Base-excision repair gene	Multiple polyps (>15) at a young age (<50 years)	Increased risk of CRC, onset in fourth decade
Peutz–Jeghers syndrome	*STK-11*	Numerous pigmented spots on lips and buccal mucosa. Multiple hamartomas, polyps. Small intestinal polyps may bleed, obstruct or cause intussusception.	Increased risk of non-gastrointestinal and gastrointestinal cancer (through adenomatous change in polyps)

All are autosomal dominant inheritance, other than MYH-associated polyposis.
CRC, colorectal cancer; HNPCC, hereditary non-polyposis colorectal cancer.

Inheritance

In sporadic CRC, a stepwise accumulation of abnormalities in a number of critical growth regulating genes drives the progression from normal mucosa to adenoma to invasive cancer. These include the activation of tumour-promoting genes or oncogenes, e.g. K-*ras* and the inactivation of tumour suppressor genes.

Table 3.16 TNM staging of colon cancer

TNM stage	Description	5-Year survival (%)
Stage 0	Tumour confined to the mucosa	>95
Stage 1	Tumour invades submucosa (T1) or muscularis propria (T2). No involved nodes (N0) or distant metastases (M0)	80–95
Stage II	Tumour invades into subserosa (T3) or directly into other organs (T4). No involved nodes (N0) or distant metastases (M0)	65–85
Stage IIIa	T1/T2 and 1–3 regional lymph nodes involved (N1).	55–65
Stage IIIb	T3, N1 or T4, N1	35–42
Stage IIIc	Any T, ≥4 regional lymph nodes (N2)	25–27
Stage 4	Any T, any N + distant metastases	5–7

Pathology

Spread is by direct invasion through the bowel wall, with later invasion of blood vessels and lymphatics and spread to the liver and lung. Mortality of CRC is related to the TNM stage at presentation (Table 3.16). Synchronous (i.e. more than one) tumours are present in 2% of cases.

Clinical features

Most tumours are in the left side of the colon. They cause rectal bleeding and stenosis, with symptoms of increasing intestinal obstruction such as an alteration in bowel habit and colicky abdominal pain. Carcinoma of the caecum and ascending colon often present with iron deficiency anaemia or a right iliac fossa mass. Clinical examination is usually unhelpful, although a mass may be palpable transabdominally or in the rectum. Hepatomegaly may be present with liver metastases.

Investigation

The purpose of investigation is to confirm the diagnosis and stage the tumour.

Colonic examination with colonoscopy, CT colonography or barium enema are all used to examine the colon in suspected CRC but colonoscopy and biopsy of lesions remains the gold standard.

Blood tests A full blood count may show anaemia, and abnormal serum liver biochemistry suggests the presence of liver secondaries. Serum levels of the tumour marker carcinoembryonic antigen (CEA) are often raised in CRC but are used in follow-up (rising levels suggest recurrence) rather than diagnosis.

Radiology CT scan of the chest, abdomen and pelvis is the initial staging investigation to look for local spread and metastatic disease. PET scanning is often used for evaluation of suspicious lesions found on CT. MRI and endoanal ultrasound are used to locally stage rectal cancer.

Faecal occult blood tests are used in population screening studies (see below) but are not of value diagnostically.

Management

Treatment is surgical, with tumour resection and end-to-end anastomosis of bowel if possible. In very low rectal cancers abdominoperineal resection with permanent end colostomy is necessary. Post-operative (adjuvant) chemotherapy increases survival in stage III and selected stage II tumours. Pre-operative radiotherapy improves survival in some patients with rectal cancer, and radiotherapy can also offer effective palliation in patients with locally advanced disease. Patients with up to two or three liver metastases confined to one lobe of the liver may be offered hepatic resection. Patients with unresectable metastatic disease are commonly offered palliative chemotherapy, which increases median survival and improves quality of life.

Prognosis

This is related to tumour stage at presentation (Table 3.16).

Screening

High-risk individuals, e.g. from family colon cancer syndromes or with a first-degree relative developing colon cancer aged <45 years, are offered screening colonoscopy. Many countries now have population screening programmes to detect early-stage cancer and hence improve outcome. In the UK, screening with biannual faecal occult blood tests (with colonoscopy when positive) for individuals 60–69 years is predicted to reduce CRC mortality by 16%.

DIARRHOEA

Diarrhoea is a common complaint in clinical practice.

Acute diarrhoea is usually due to infection or dietary indiscretion. Stool cultures ($\times 3$ for ova, parasites and cysts) are sent and a flexible sigmoidoscopy with colonic biopsy is then performed if symptoms persist and no diagnosis has been made. Treatment is symptomatic to maintain hydration, with antidiarrhoeal agents (p. 134) for short-term relief and antibiotics for specific indications.

Chronic diarrhoea is defined as diarrhoea persisting for more than 14 days. Organic causes (resulting in stool weights >250 g) have to be distinguished from functional causes (frequent passage of small volume stools with stool weights <250 g) which can usually be done from the history. Sometimes faecal markers of intestinal inflammation are used to differentiate functional disorders from organic disease.

Mechanisms of diarrhoea

Osmotic diarrhoea

Large quantities of non-absorbed hypertonic substances in the bowel lumen draw fluid into the intestine. The diarrhoea stops when the patient stops eating or the malabsorptive substance is discontinued. The causes of osmotic diarrhoea are as follows:

- Ingestion of non-absorbable substance, e.g. a laxative such as magnesium sulphate
- Generalized malabsorption so that high concentrations of solute (e.g. glucose) remain in the lumen
- Specific malabsorptive defect, e.g. disaccharidase deficiency.

Secretory diarrhoea

There is active intestinal secretion of fluid and electrolytes as well as decreased absorption. Secretory diarrhoea continues when the patient fasts. The causes are:

- Enterotoxins, e.g. from *Escherichia coli*, cholera toxin
- Hormone-secreting tumours, e.g. VIPoma
- Bile salts (in the colon) following ileal disease, resection or idiopathic bile acid malabsorption
- Fatty acids (in the colon) following ileal resection
- Some laxatives.

Inflammatory diarrhoea (mucosal destruction)

Damage to the intestinal mucosal cell leads to loss of fluid and blood and defective absorption of fluid and electrolytes. Common causes are infective (e.g. *Shigella*, salmonella) and inflammatory conditions (e.g. UC and CD).

Motility related

Abnormal motility often produces frequency rather than true diarrhoea. Causes are thyrotoxicosis, diabetic autonomic neuropathy and post-vagotomy.

Approach to the patient with diarrhoea

An assessment of the likely cause of diarrhoea is initially made on the history:

Step 1: Determine if the diarrhoea is likely to have an organic or functional basis. Frequent passage of small-volume stools (often formed) points to a functional cause; the exceptions are distal colon cancer and proctitis – organic causes that present with stool frequency and normal stool volumes. Symptoms suggestive of an organic cause include large-volume watery stools, nocturnal diarrhoea, bloody stools, weight loss or a stool description suggesting steatorrhoea.

Step 2: Distinguish malabsorptive from colonic/inflammatory forms of diarrhoea. Colonic, inflammatory and secretory (see below) causes of diarrhoea typically present with loose liquid or watery stools. Inflammatory diarrhoea is associated with blood or mucous discharge. Malabsorption is often accompanied by steatorrhoea.

Step 3: Rarely, measurement of stool weight by a 3-day stool collection as a hospital inpatient may be necessary where differentiation between organic and functional bowel disease is difficult. Occasionally diarrhoea is factitious due to surreptitious laxative ingestion, or the patient deliberately dilutes the faeces by adding water or urine.

Investigation

Chronic diarrhoea of likely organic origin always requires investigation. Fig. 3.4 outlines an approach to investigation. Laxative abuse, usually seen in young females, must be excluded as a cause. Patients taking anthraquinone purgatives, e.g. senna, develop pigmentation of the colonic mucosa

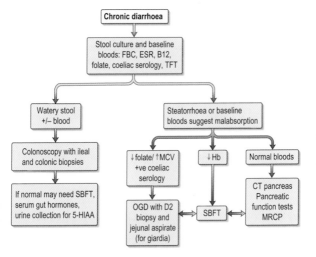

- Patients with presumed functional diarrhoea, based on history, age and normal baseline investigations (FBC, ESR coeliac serology) are excluded from this algorithm.
- High-risk patients (immunosuppressed, recent travel or antibiotics) should have multiple stool cultures including a search for unusual organisms.

Fig. 3.4 Approach to the investigation of chronic diarrhoea. SR, erythrocyte sedimentation rate; FBC, full blood count; HIAA, hydroxyindoleacetic acid; MCV, mean corpuscular volume; MRCP, magnetic resonance cholangiopancreatography; OGD, oesophagogastroduodenoscopy; SBFT, small bowel follow-through; TFT, thyroid function test.

(melanosis coli) which may be seen at sigmoidoscopy. Other laxatives may be detected in the stool or urine. Treatment of chronic diarrhoea depends on the cause.

FUNCTIONAL BOWEL DISORDERS

This is a large group of gastrointestinal disorders that are termed 'functional' because symptoms occur in the absence of any demonstrable abnormalities in the digestion and absorption of nutrients, fluid and electrolytes, and no structural abnormality can be identified in the gastrointestinal tract. Functional bowel disorders are extremely common world-wide, accounting for up to 80% of patients seen in the gastroenterology clinic. Rather than a diagnosis of exclusion after normal investigations (as the definition would suggest), this is frequently a positive diagnosis made in a patient with symptoms suggestive of a functional gastrointestinal disorder (Table 3.17). It is estimated that only 25% of persons with this condition seek medical care for it, and studies suggest that those who seek care are more likely to have behavioural and psychiatric problems than those who do not seek care.

Altered bowel motility, visceral hypersensitivity (they have a lower pain threshold when tested with balloon distension of the rectum), psychosocial factors, an imbalance in neurotransmitters and gastrointestinal infection have all been proposed as playing a part in the development of functional bowel disorders. Low-dose antidepressant treatment, e.g. amitriptyline 10 mg daily, is frequently used for these disorders if initial symptom-based treatments do not prove beneficial. Common functional gastrointestinal disorders are listed below.

- *Functional oesophageal disorders* occur in the absence of dysphagia, pathological gastrooesophageal reflux disease or other oesophageal disorder. They include globus (a sensation of a lump in the throat persisting between meals), regurgitation and midline chest pain. Sometimes these symptoms will respond to high-dose acid suppression or antidepressants, e.g. amitriptyline or citalopram.

Table 3.17 Chronic gastrointestinal symptoms suggestive of a functional gastrointestinal disorder

Nausea alone
Vomiting alone
Belching
Chest pain unrelated to exercise
Post-prandial fullness
Abdominal bloating
Abdominal discomfort/pain (right or left iliac fossa)
Passage of mucus per rectum
Frequent bowel actions with urgency first thing in the morning

- *Functional dyspepsia*. Common symptoms include epigastric pain or discomfort, early satiety, bloating and nausea. Symptoms are sometimes similar to peptic ulceration. Investigation is frequently unnecessary in younger people (<55 years) but endoscopy is usually required in older people or in those with 'alarm symptoms' (for management of dyspepsia, see p. 86). Management is mainly by reassurance and lifestyle changes (reducing intake of fat, coffee, alcohol and cigarette smoking). PPIs help some patients with epigastric pain. Prokinetic agents, e.g. metoclopramide and domperidone (p. 136), are sometimes helpful, particularly in those with fullness and bloating. Eradication of *H. pylori* is helpful in some patients.

- *Irritable bowel syndrome (IBS)*. Crampy abdominal pain relieved by defecation or the passage of wind, altered bowel habit, a sensation of incomplete evacuation, abdominal bloating and distension are common symptoms. Subtypes of IBS can be identified according to the predominant stool pattern: IBS with constipation, IBS with diarrhoea and mixed IBS with alternating diarrhoea and constipation. In other patients with IBS, diarrhoea without pain (formed stools followed by loose mushy stools mainly in the morning) or abdominal pain without alteration in bowel habit are the major symptoms.

Symptoms are more common in women than men, and the history is usually prolonged. Characteristically the patient looks healthy. Examination is usually normal, although sigmoidoscopy and air insufflation may reproduce the pain. If frequency of defecation is a feature, a rectal biopsy should be performed to exclude IBD. Investigation depends on the individual patient. Young patients with classic symptoms need only simple blood tests (full blood count, C-reactive protein and coeliac serology) to look for evidence of other gastrointestinal diseases that present similarly, e.g. IBD and coeliac disease. Onset of symptoms in an older patient (>50 years) should be investigated further, e.g. colonoscopy, to exclude other pathology. The approach to investigating a patient presenting with constipation or diarrhoea is discussed elsewhere, respectively. Management is reassurance, with a discussion of lifestyle and diet. Initial treatment is symptom based with soluble fibre supplements for constipation, e.g. ispaghula husk (p. 130), and antidiarrhoeal drugs, e.g. loperamide (p. 134), for bowel frequency. Smooth muscle relaxants, such as peppermint oil and mebeverine, are useful in some patients with abdominal pain. Second-line treatment is with low-dose amitriptyline or citalopram. Psychological interventions (hypnotherapy, cognitive behavioural therapy and psychotherapy) are used for patients with resistant symptoms.

THE ACUTE ABDOMEN

Most are admitted under the care of the surgical team, and some will need a laparotomy. Medical conditions that present as an acute abdomen include diabetic ketoacidosis, myocardial infarction and pneumonia. IBS occasionally presents with acute severe abdominal pain. A leaking abdominal aortic aneurysm may present similarly to renal colic and should be considered in the over 50s presenting with apparent colic. Mesenteric ischaemia is easily missed and should be considered in a patient presenting with abdominal pain and prior weight loss. A plain abdominal X-ray and erect chest X-ray is usually performed in the acute abdomen but the most useful imaging investigations are ultrasound (for cholangitis, cholecystitis, appendicitis, gynaecological conditions) and CT (site and cause of intestinal obstruction, renal colic, acute pancreatitis).

History

The history, including gynaecological (vaginal discharge, last menstrual period) and urinary symptoms, will often point to the cause of the pain.

- *Onset* of pain may be sudden or gradual. Sudden onset suggests perforation of a viscus (e.g. duodenal ulcer), rupture of an organ (e.g. aortic aneurysm) or torsion (e.g. ovarian cyst). The pain of acute pancreatitis often begins suddenly. Ruptured ectopic pregnancy, rupture or torsion of ovarian cysts and acute salpingitis cause lower abdominal pain in women.
- *Site* of pain and radiation must be noted. In general, upper abdominal pain is produced by pathology of either the upper abdominal viscera – e.g. acute cholecystitis, acute pancreatitis – or the stomach and duodenum. The pain of small bowel obstruction is often in the centre of the abdomen. A common cause of acute right iliac fossa pain is acute appendicitis. Pain from acute pancreatitis, rupture of an aortic aneurysm or renal tract disease often radiates to the back.
- *Pain may be intermittent or continuous.* Intermittent (colicky) pain describes pain that occurs for a short period (usually a few minutes) and is interspersed with pain-free periods lasting a few minutes or up to half an hour. This is characteristic of mechanical obstruction of a hollow viscus, e.g. ureteric calculus or bowel obstruction (Table 3.18). Additional symptoms of bowel obstruction, which may or may not be present, are abdominal distension,

Table 3.18 Some causes of mechanical intestinal obstruction

Small intestinal obstruction
Adhesions (80% in adults)
Hernias
Crohn's disease
Intussusception
Obstruction due to extrinsic involvement by cancer

Colonic obstruction
Carcinoma of the colon
Sigmoid volvulus
Diverticular disease

vomiting and absolute constipation (i.e. failure to pass flatus or stool). Biliary pain (previously called biliary colic) resulting from obstruction of the gall bladder or bile duct is not colicky but usually a constant upper abdominal pain.

- *Continuous pain* is relentless with no periods of complete relief. It occurs in many abdominal conditions.

Examination

- The presence of shock (pale, cool peripheries, tachycardia, hypotension) suggests rupture of an organ, e.g. aortic aneurysm, ruptured ectopic pregnancy. It also occurs in the later stages of generalized peritonitis resulting from bowel perforation (see below).
- Fever is common in acute inflammatory conditions.
- The signs of peritonitis are tenderness, guarding (involuntary contraction of the abdominal muscles when the abdomen is palpated) and rigidity on palpation. Bowel sounds are absent with generalized peritonitis.
- Mechanical bowel obstruction produces distension and active 'tinkling' bowel sounds. A strangulated hernia may produce obstruction, and the hernial orifices must always be examined.

A rectal and pelvic examination should be performed in most patients with an acute abdomen.

Investigations

- Blood tests. The white cell count is raised in inflammatory conditions. The serum amylase is raised in any acute abdomen, but levels greater than five times normal indicate acute pancreatitis.
- Urinalysis may show evidence of infection or blood in renal colic. Women of childbearing age should have a pregnancy test.
- Imaging. An erect chest X-ray may show air under the diaphragm with a perforated viscus, but its absence does not exclude perforation. Plain abdominal X-ray shows dilated loops of bowel and fluid levels in obstruction. Ultrasound examination is useful in the diagnosis of acute cholecystitis, cholangitis, appendicitis and gynaecological conditions such as ruptured ovarian cyst and ectopic pregnancy. Spiral CT scan is the most accurate modality in the investigation of the acute abdomen but is usually reserved for patients with inconclusive or negative ultrasound results.
- Surgery. Laparoscopy or laparotomy may be necessary depending on the diagnosis.

Acute appendicitis

Acute appendicitis occurs when the lumen of the appendix becomes obstructed by a faecolith.

Epidemiology

It affects all age groups but is rare in the very young and very old.

Clinical features

The typical clinical presentation is the onset of central abdominal pain which then becomes localized to the right iliac fossa (RIF), accompanied by anorexia and sometimes vomiting and diarrhoea. The patient is pyrexial, with tenderness and guarding in the RIF due to localized peritonitis. There may be a tender mass in the presence of an appendix abscess.

Investigations

The white cell count, C-reactive protein and ESR are raised, but these are not specific. Ultrasonography may show an inflamed appendix and can also show an appendix mass. CT is highly sensitive and specific, and has reduced removal of histologically normal appendices by 90%.

Differential diagnosis

Non-specific mesenteric lymphadenitis, terminal ileitis due to Crohn's disease or *Yersinia* infection, acute salpingitis in women, inflamed Meckel's diverticulum and functional bowel disease can all mimic acute appendicitis.

Management

The treatment is surgical, with removal of the appendix either by open surgery or laparoscopically. An appendix mass is treated conservatively initially with intravenous fluids and antibiotics and later appendicectomy.

Complications

These arise from gangrene and perforation, leading to localized abscess formation or generalized peritonitis.

Acute peritonitis

Localized peritonitis occurs with all acute inflammatory conditions of the gastrointestinal tract, and management depends on the underlying condition, e.g. acute appendicitis, acute cholecystitis.

Generalized peritonitis occurs as a result of rupture of an abdominal viscus, e.g. perforated duodenal ulcer, perforated appendix. There is a sudden onset of abdominal pain which rapidly becomes generalized. The patient is shocked and lies still, as movement exacerbates the pain. A plain abdominal X-ray may show air under the diaphragm; serum amylase must be checked to exclude acute pancreatitis.

Intestinal obstruction

Intestinal obstruction is either mechanical or functional.

Mechanical (Table 3.18) The bowel above the level of the obstruction is dilated, with increased secretion of fluid into the lumen. The patient complains of colicky abdominal pain, associated with vomiting (occurs earlier with small bowel than large bowel obstruction) and absolute constipation (occurs earlier with large bowel than small bowel obstruction). On examination there is distension and 'tinkling' bowel sounds. Small bowel obstruction may settle with conservative management (i.e. nasogastric suction and intravenous fluids to maintain hydration). Large bowel obstruction is treated surgically.

Functional This occurs with a paralytic ileus, which is often seen in the post-operative stage of peritonitis or of major abdominal surgery, or in association with opiate treatment (acute colonic pseudo-obstruction, Ogilvie's syndrome). It also occurs when the nerves or muscles of the intestine are damaged, causing intestinal pseudo-obstruction. Unlike mechanical obstruction, pain is often not present and bowel sounds may be decreased. Gas is seen throughout the bowel on a plain abdominal X-ray. Management is conservative.

THE PERITONEUM

The peritoneal cavity is a closed sac lined by mesothelium. It contains a little fluid to allow the abdominal contents to move freely. Conditions which affect the peritoneum are:

- Infective (peritonitis)
  - Secondary to gut disease, e.g. appendicitis, perforation
  - Chronic peritoneal dialysis
  - Spontaneous (associated with cirrhotic ascites)
  - Tuberculous
- Neoplasia
  - Secondary deposits, e.g. from ovary
  - Primary mesothelioma
- Vasculitis: connective tissue disease.

NUTRITION

Dietary requirements

Food is necessary to provide the body with energy. The average daily requirement (Table 3.19) of a 55 year old female in the UK is 8100 kJ (1940 kcal), and a 55 year old man is 10 600 kJ (2550 kcal). This is at present made up of about 50% carbohydrate, 35% fat, 15% protein ± 5% alcohol. In developing countries, however, carbohydrate may be >75% of the total energy input, and fat <15% of

Table 3.19 Protein, energy and water requirement of normal and hypercatabolic adults

Metabolic state	Nutritional requirements Normal	Hypercatabolic
Protein (g/kg)	1	2–3
Nitrogen (g/kg)	0.17	0.3–0.45
Energy (kcal/kg)	25–30	35–50
Water (mL/kg)	30–35	30–35

the total energy input. Energy requirements increase during periods of rapid growth, such as adolescence, pregnancy and lactation and with sepsis.

Bodyweight is maintained at a 'set point' by a precise balance of energy intake and total energy expenditure (the sum of the resting or basal metabolic rate, physical activity, and the thermic effect of food eaten). Weight gain is almost always due solely to an increase in energy intake which exceeds total energy expenditure. Occasionally weight gain is due to a decrease in energy expenditure, e.g. hypothyroidism, or fluid retention, e.g. heart failure or ascites. On the other hand, weight loss associated with cancer and chronic diseases is due to a reduction in energy intake secondary to a loss of appetite (anorexia). In a few conditions, such as sepsis and severe trauma, there is an increase in energy requirements (hypercatabolic or hypermetabolic) which will result in a negative energy balance if there is no compensatory increase in energy intake.

A balanced diet also requires sufficient amounts of minerals and vitamins. In the developed world vitamin deficiency is rare except in specific groups, e.g. alcohol dependent and patients with small bowel disease, and patients with liver and biliary tract disease, who are susceptible to deficiency of the fat-soluble vitamins (A, D, E, K). Deficiencies of the B vitamins, riboflavin and biotin are rare in all patient groups. Dietary deficiency of vitamin B_6 (pyridoxine, pyridoxal and pyridoxamine) is also extremely rare, but drugs (e.g. isoniazid and penicillamine) that interact with pyridoxal phosphate may cause deficiency and a polyneuropathy.

NUTRITIONAL SUPPORT

Patients should be screened for nutritional status on admission to hospital and during their stay. Current recommendations suggest:

- Patients should be asked about recent weight loss, their usual weight and whether they have been eating less than usual.
- Their weight and height should be recorded and body mass index (BMI) calculated (weight [kg]/height [m]^2). The acceptable range of BMI is 20–25 kg/m^2 for men and 19–24 kg/m^2 for women.

Nutritional supplementation is required in those patients who cannot eat, should not eat, will not eat or cannot eat enough. It is necessary to provide nutritional support for:

- All severely malnourished patients (indicated by a BMI less than 15 kg/m^2) on admission to hospital
- Moderately malnourished patients (BMI 15–19 kg/m^2) who, because of their physical illness, are not expected to eat for 3–5 days
- Normally nourished patients not expected to eat for 7–10 days.

Enteral nutrition is cheaper, more physiological and has fewer complications than parenteral (intravenous) nutrition, and should be used if the gastrointestinal tract is functioning normally. With both enteral and parenteral nutrition a complete feeding regimen consisting of fat, carbohydrates, protein, vitamins, minerals and trace elements can provide the nutritional requirements of the individual (Table 3.17). Ideally a multidisciplinary nutrition support team should supervise the provision of artificial nutritional support.

Enteral nutrition

Foods can be given by:

- Mouth
- Fine-bore nasogastric tube for short-term enteral nutrition
- Percutaneous endoscopic gastrostomy (PEG): this is useful for patients who need feeding for longer than 2 weeks
- Percutaneous jejunostomy where a tube is inserted directly into the jejunum either endoscopically or at laparotomy.

A polymeric diet with whole protein, carbohydrate and fat is usually used; an elemental diet composed of amino acids, glucose and fatty acids may be used for patients with CD.

Total parenteral nutrition (TPN)

Parenteral nutrition may be given via a feeding catheter placed in a peripheral vein or a silicone catheter placed in the subclavian vein. Central catheters must only be placed by experienced clinicians under strict aseptic conditions in a sterile environment. These catheters should only be used for feeding purposes, and not the administration of drugs or blood to reduce the risk of introducing infection. Complications of TPN are given in Table 3.20.

Table 3.20 Complications of total parenteral nutrition

Catheter related: sepsis, thrombosis, embolism and pneumothorax
Metabolic, e.g. hyperglycaemia, hypercalcaemia
Electrolyte disturbances
Liver dysfunction

Monitoring of artificial nutrition

Patients receiving nutritional support should be weighed twice weekly: they require regular clinical examination to check for fluid overload or depletion. Patients receiving nutritional support in hospital initially require daily measurements of urea and electrolytes and blood glucose. More frequent measurement of blood glucose with BM sticks is indicated in patients beginning TPN. Liver biochemistry, calcium and phosphate are measured twice weekly. Serum magnesium, zinc and nitrogen balance (see below) are measured weekly. The frequency of biochemical monitoring is adjusted according to the patient's clinical and metabolic status.

It is necessary to give 40–50 g of protein per 24 hours to maintain nitrogen balance, which represents the balance between protein breakdown and synthesis. The aim of any regimen is to achieve a positive nitrogen balance, which can usually be obtained by giving 3–5 g of nitrogen in excess of output. The amount of protein required to maintain nitrogen balance in a particular individual can be calculated from the amount of urinary nitrogen loss, using the formula:

$$N_2 \text{loss (g/24 h)} = \text{Urinary urea (mmol/24 h)} \times 0.028 + 2$$

$$\text{Urinary nitrogen} \times 6.25 = \text{grams of protein required (most proteins contain about 16\% nitrogen)}$$

Most patients require about 12 g of nitrogen per 24 hours, but hypercatabolic patients require about 15 g/day.

Refeeding syndrome

The refeeding syndrome occurs within the first few days of refeeding by the oral, enteral or parenteral route. It is underrecognized and can be fatal. It involves a shift from the use of fat as an energy source during starvation to the use of carbohydrate as an energy source during refeeding. With the introduction of artificial nutrition and carbohydrate by any source, insulin release is augmented and there is rapid intracellular passage of phosphate, magnesium and potassium resulting in hypophosphataemia, hypomagnesaemia, and hypokalaemia. Phosphate is an integral part of cellular machinery. Deficiency results in widespread organ dysfunction (muscle weakness, rhabdomyolysis, cardiac failure, immune suppression, haemolytic anaemia, thrombocytopenia, coma, hallucinations, fits). Thiamine deficiency can be precipitated. Patients at risk of refeeding are underweight (e.g. anorexia nervosa, alcohol dependent syndrome) or those with recent rapid weight loss (5% within preceding month), including patients after treatment for morbid obesity. These at-risk patients should receive high-dose vitamin B and C vitamins, e.g. Pabrinex® 1 pair twice daily, for 5–7 days beginning before feeding, and begin feeding at 25–50% of estimated calorie requirements, increasing by 100 calories per day. Serum phosphate, magnesium, calcium, potassium, urea and creatinine, bodyweight and evidence of fluid overload should be checked daily for the first week, and electrolyte deficiencies corrected as necessary.

DISORDERS OF BODYWEIGHT

Obesity

Obesity, defined as an excess of body fat contributing to comorbidity, is an increasingly common problem in developed and developing countries. It is defined as a BMI of 30 kg/m^2 or greater. Overweight is defined as a BMI of 25–30 kg/m^2 and may be associated with a mildly increased risk of complications that have been identified in obese patients (see below). In almost all obese individuals weight gain is a result of increased energy intake and energy expenditure is normal or indeed increased. In a few conditions, e.g. hypothyroidism, weight gain is due at least in part to reduced energy expenditure. Obese patients are at risk of a premature death, mainly from diabetes, ischaemic heart disease and cerebrovascular disease. Obesity is also associated with an increased risk of hypertension, hyperlipidaemia, obstructive sleep apnoea, osteoarthritis of the knees and hips, fatty liver disease, gallstones and an increased cancer risk. Weight reduction can be achieved with a reduction in calorie intake and an increase in physical activity, although this is often difficult to achieve. The most common diets allow a daily energy intake of 4200 kJ (1000 kcal) which in a middle-aged woman would result in a daily energy deficit (expenditure vs intake) of about 4200 kJ. A week of dieting would result in a total energy deficit of 25–29 MJ (6000–7000 kcal) and weight loss of about 1 kg. A 10% loss of body weight (i.e. 10 kg in a 100 kg person) is associated with a fall in blood pressure and a reduced risk of diabetes and overall mortality. Drug treatment such as orlistat, an inhibitor of pancreatic lipase and hence fat digestion, may be used in the severely obese patient for a 3 month trial period. Bariatric surgery is increasingly performed in patients with morbid obesity (BMI >40 kg/m^2) or patients with a BMI >35 kg/m^2 and obesity-related complications, after conventional medical treatment has failed. The techniques used are restrictive, such as gastric banding (which restricts the ability to eat) or intestinal bypass (which reduces the ability to absorb nutrients) or a combination Roux-en-Y.

Anorexia nervosa

Anorexia nervosa is a psychological illness, predominantly affecting young females and characterized by marked weight loss (BMI <17.5 kg/m^2), intense fear of gaining weight, a distorted body image and amenorrhoea. Patients with anorexia nervosa control their body weight by a process of semi-starvation and/ or self-induced vomiting (bulimia) and may develop consequences of undernutrition. Treatment is difficult and should be undertaken in a specialist eating disorders unit.

THERAPEUTICS

Drugs for dyspepsia and peptic ulceration

Antacids

Mechanism of action

Main effect is to neutralize gastric acid. Alginate-containing antacids form a 'raft' that floats on the surface of the stomach contents to reduce reflux and protect the gastro-oesophageal mucosa.

Indications

Symptomatic relief in dyspepsia, gastro-oesophageal reflux and peptic ulceration. Healing of peptic ulcers is much less than with antisecretory drugs (see below) and antacids should not be used for this indication.

Preparations and dose

Aluminium hydroxide   Tablets: 500 mg; Capsules (Alu-Cap®) 475 mg.

1–2 tablets chewed or 1 capsule four times daily and at bedtime, or as required.

Magnesium trisilicate mixture   Oral suspension, 5% each of magnesium trisilicate, light magnesium carbonate, and sodium bicarbonate.

10–20 mL in water three times daily or as required.

Co-magaldrox (Mucogel®)   *Suspension.* Mixture of aluminium hydroxide 220 mg, and magnesium hydroxide 195 mg/5 mL.

10–20 mL 20–60 minutes after meals and at bedtime, or as required.

Alginate-containing antacid   *Tablets, suspension.* Gaviscon® Advance contains potassium bicarbonate, sodium alginate.

1–2 tablets chewed or 10–20 mL four times daily after meals and at bedtime.

Side effects

Magnesium-containing antacids tend to be laxative, whereas aluminium-containing antacids may be constipating; antacids containing both aluminium and magnesium may reduce these colonic side effects.

Cautions/contraindications

Antacids may interfere with the absorption of other drugs and in general other drugs should be given at least 1 hour before or after each dose of antacid. The sodium content of preparations with a high sodium content, e.g. magnesium trisilicate mixture (6.3 mmol/10 mL) and Gaviscon® Advance (4.6 mmol/ 10 mL; 2.25 mmol/tablet) should be taken into account in patients on a 'no added' salt diet (cardiac, renal or hepatic disease). Aluminium hydroxide is contraindicated in hypophosphataemia. Constipating antacids (i.e. those containing aluminium) should be avoided in liver disease.

H$_2$-receptor antagonists

Mechanism of action

Reduce gastric acid secretion as a result of histamine H$_2$-receptor blockade.

Indications

GORD, healing of benign gastric and duodenal ulcers, prevention of gastroduodenal damage in patients requiring intensive care, prevention of NSAID-induced DUs, and in high doses prevention of GUs. However, for all indications, PPIs are more effective and more commonly used in clinical practice.

Preparations and dose

Ranitidine Tablets: 150 mg, 300 mg; Syrup 75 mg/5 mL; Injection (Zantac®) 25 mg/mL.

Oral

- Gastric and duodenal ulceration 150 mg twice daily or 300 mg at night for 4–8 weeks.
- GORD: 150 mg twice daily or 300 mg at night, 150 mg four times daily in severe cases for up to 12 weeks. Reduce to lowest dose possible to relieve symptoms in maintenance treatment.
- NSAID-associated ulceration: 150 mg twice daily or 300 mg at night, 300 mg twice daily can be given for higher healing rate.
- Prophylaxis of NSAID-induced peptic ulceration, 300 mg twice daily.
  IV 50 mg diluted to 20 mL and given over at least 2 minutes every 6–8 hours *or* infusion 25 mg/h for 2 hours repeated every 6–8 hours.

Cimetidine Tablets: 200 mg, 400 mg, 800 mg; Syrup 200 mg/5 mL.

Oral

- GORD: 400 mg four times daily for 4–8 weeks; reduce down to lowest dose possible for maintenance treatment.
- Peptic ulceration: 400 mg twice daily or 800 mg at night for at least 4 weeks, 8 weeks in NSAID-associated ulceration.

Side effects

Diarrhoea, altered liver biochemistry, headache, dizziness, rash. Rarely, other side effects (see national formulary).

Cautions/contraindications

Cimetidine retards oxidative hepatic drug metabolism by binding to microsomal cytochrome P450. It should be avoided in patients stabilized on warfarin, phenytoin, and theophylline (or aminophylline) but other interactions (see national formulary) may be of less clinical relevance.

Proton pump inhibitors

Mechanism of action

Inhibit gastric acid secretion by blocking the hydrogen/potassium-adenosine triphosphate enzyme system (the 'proton pump') of the gastric parietal cell.

Indications

GORD; healing of peptic ulcers; prevention of NSAID-induced peptic ulcers; in combination with antibacterials for eradication of *H. pylori*; intravenously and after endoscopic therapy to reduce re-bleeding rates in patients with bleeding peptic ulcers; inhibition of gastric acid in pathological hypersecretory conditions, e.g. gastrinoma; prevention of peptic ulcers in critically ill patients; prophylaxis of acid aspiration during general anaesthesia; dyspepsia.

Preparations and dose

Omeprazole Capsules and tablets: 10 mg, 20 mg, 40 mg; Dispersible tablets: 10 mg, 20 mg, 40 mg; Intravenous infusion: 40 mg vial.

- GORD: 20–40 mg once daily for 4–8 weeks, maintenance 10–20 mg once daily.
- Healing of peptic ulcers (not *H. pylori* associated): 20 mg daily for 4 weeks.
- Prevention of NSAID-induced ulcers: 20 mg daily.
- Eradication of *H. pylori* (in combination with antibacterials): 20 mg twice daily for 1 week.
- By i.v. injection in bleeding peptic ulcers: 80 mg over 5 minutes and then 8 mg/h (1 vial diluted in 100 mL 0.9% sodium chloride or 5% dextrose).
- Gastrinoma: 60 mg once daily, usual range 20–120 mg daily.
- Gastric acid reduction during general anaesthesia: 40 mg on preceding evening then 40 mg 2–6 hours before surgery.
  Lansoprazole Capsules: 15 mg, 30 mg; Orodispersible tablet: 15 mg, 30 mg.
- GORD: 30 mg once daily for 4–8 weeks, maintenance 15–30 mg once daily.
- Healing of peptic ulcers (not *H. pylori* related): 30 mg daily for 4 weeks.
- Prevention of NSAID-induced ulcers: 15–30 mg daily.
- Eradication of *H. pylori* (in combination with antibacterials): 20 mg twice daily for 1 week.
- Gastrinoma: 60 mg once daily, usual range 30–120 mg daily.

Side effects

Gastrointestinal disturbance (diarrhoea, nausea, vomiting), liver dysfunction, hypersensitivity reactions, headache, skin reactions, increased risk of gastrointestinal infections (due to reduced gastric acidity). Rarely, acute kidney injury, deficiency of vitamin B_{12}, calcium (leading to hip fracture) and magnesium due to reduced intestinal absorption.

Cautions/contraindications

Omeprazole and esomeprazole competitively inhibit the CYP2C19 isoenzyme (which metabolises clopidogrel to its active metabolite) and may reduce the ability of clopidogrel to inhibit platelet aggregation. Omeprazole may decrease the effect of warfarin, phenytoin and diazepam. Lansoprazole may increase the effect of warfarin, phenytoin and theophylline. Reduce dose in severe liver disease.

Constipation

Treatment of constipation is initially with lifestyle changes and drugs are reserved for use as second-line treatment. It may be necessary to use a combination of two different types of laxative, e.g. stimulant plus faecal softener. All laxatives are contraindicated in intestinal obstruction or perforation, paralytic ileus, and severe inflammatory conditions of the gut such as CD and UC.

Bulk-forming laxatives

Mechanism of action

Absorb water and increase faecal mass, which stimulates peristalsis.

Indications

Treatment of slow-transit constipation and bulking of stool in patients with a colostomy, diverticular disease and irritable bowel syndrome.

Preparations and dose

Unprocessed wheat bran is one of the most effective fibre laxatives, and patients can add it to meals, e.g. cereal (2–6 tablespoons per day).

> **Ispaghula husk** Granules: 3.5 g sachet.
> 1 sachet or 2 level 5 mL spoonfuls in water twice daily after meals.
> **Methycellulose** Tablets: 500 mg.
> 3–6 tablets twice daily with at least 300 mL of liquid.
> **Sterculia** Granules: 7 g sachets.
> 1–2 sachets or 1–2 heaped 5 mL spoonfuls washed down with plenty of liquid once or twice daily after meals.

Side effects

Flatulence, abdominal distension.

Cautions/contraindications

Maintain adequate fluid intake to prevent faecal impaction; contraindications (see above).

Stimulant laxatives

Mechanism of action

Increase colonic motor activity.

Indications

Short-term treatment of constipation.

Preparations and dose

Bisacodyl Tablets: 5 mg; Suppositories: 10 mg.
> *Oral* 5–10 mg at night, occasionally increase to 15–20 mg.
> *By rectum* in suppositories, 10 mg in the morning.

Docusate sodium Capsules: 100 mg; Solution: 50 mg/5 mL; Micro-enema: 120 mg in 10 g single-dose pack.

Oral 500 mg daily in two to three divided doses.

By rectum 10 g unit daily.

Glycerol (glycerin)

Suppositories: glycerol 700 mg.

1 suppository moistened with water before use.

Senna Tablets: 7.5 mg; Syrup: 7.5 mg/5 mL.

2–4 tablets, 10–20 mL of syrup at night.

Side effects

Abdominal cramps, diarrhoea and hypokalaemia.

Cautions/contraindications

Contraindications (see above).

Osmotic laxatives

Mechanism of action

Attract or retain water in the intestinal lumen, leading to softer stools and improved propulsion.

Indications

Treatment of constipation. Lactulose is used in the treatment of hepatic encephalopathy. Phosphate enemas are used to evacuate the bowel before radiological procedures, flexible sigmoidoscopy and surgery.

Preparations and dose

Lactulose Solution: 3.1–3.7 g/5 mL.

Initially 15 mL twice daily; hepatic encephalopathy: 30–50 mL three times daily adjusted to produce two to three soft stools daily.

Macrogols (polyethylene glycol) Movicol® (polyethylene glycol '3350' with electrolytes).

1–3 sachets daily in divided doses; each sachet dissolved in 125 mL of water. For smaller dosing, Movicol-Half® is also available.

Magnesium salts Magnesium hydroxide mixture; Magnesium sulphate (Epsom salts).

30–45 mL when required of magnesium hydroxide. 5–10 g of magnesium sulphate in a glass of warm water before breakfast.

Phosphates (rectal) Fleet® Ready-to-use Enema: 133 mL pack.

One enema inserted 30 minutes before evacuation required.

Sodium citrate (rectal) Micralax Micro-enema®: 5 mL.

One enema as required.

Side effects

Abdominal distension, colic, nausea, local irritation after phosphate enema.

Cautions/contraindications

Contraindications (see above). May also cause electrolyte disturbance. Use with caution in hepatic and renal impairment. Although magnesium ions are absorbed poorly, similar to all osmotic ions some absorption does occur, which can cause problems in patients with abnormal renal function.

Bowel-cleansing solutions

Indications

Used before colonic surgery, colonoscopy or radiological examination to ensure the bowel is free of solid contents. They are not treatments for constipation. Bowel-cleansing agents are coupled with a low residue diet for at least 3 days before the procedure, copious intake of water or other clear fluids and cessation of all solid foods on the day before the procedure. All are contraindicated in bowel obstruction, perforated bowel or severe colitis and Moviprep® is contraindicated in glucose-6-phosphate dehydrogenase deficiency.

Mechanism of action

This is variable depending on the drug.

Preparations and dose

Citramag® Magnesium carbonate 11.57 g and citric acid 17.79 g/sachet.

1 sachet at 8.00 a.m. and 1 sachet between 2 and 4 p.m. on day before procedure.

Fleet Phospho-soda® Sodium dihydrogen phosphate dehydrate 24.4 g, disodium phosphate dodecahydrate 10.8 g/45 mL.

45 mL diluted with 120 mL of water (half glass), followed by one full glass of water. For morning procedures, the first dose should be taken at 7 a.m. and the second dose at 7 p.m. the day before the procedure. For afternoon procedures, the first dose should be taken at 7 p.m. on the day before and the second dose at 7 a.m. on the day of the procedure.

Klean-prep® Macrogol '3350' (polyethylene glycol '3350') with electrolytes.

2 sachets diluted with water to 2 L, and 250 mL drunk rapidly every 10–15 minutes. 2 sachets on evening before examination, and 2 sachets on morning of examination.

Moviprep® Sachet A containing macrogol '3350' (polyethylene glycol '3350') with electrolytes and Sachet B containing ascorbic acid 4.7 g and sodium ascorbate 5.9 g.

Dilute sachet A and B in 1 L of water. Drink 2 L of reconstituted solution on the evening before the procedure or 1 L on the evening before and 1 L early on the morning of the procedure.

Picolax® Sodium picosulfate 10 mg/sachet with magnesium citrate.

Dosing as for Citramag®.

Side effects

Nausea, vomiting, abdominal cramps. Occasionally dehydration and hypotension, electrolyte disturbance.

Diarrhoea

Most cases of acute diarrhoea are infective and will settle without treatment. Oral rehydration salts (Dioralyte®), 1 sachet after every loose motion, are often used especially in the elderly and children. Antidiarrhoeal agents relieve symptoms of acute diarrhoea but are not recommended routinely. Antidiarrhoeal agents, e.g. loperamide, are sometimes used in the management of chronic diarrhoea.

Loperamide hydrochloride

Capsules or tablets: 2 mg.

Mechanism of action

Antimotility agent.

Indications

Symptomatic treatment of acute diarrhoea; chronic diarrhoea in adults.

Side effects

Constipation, abdominal cramps, dizziness.

Cautions/contraindications

Active ulcerative colitis or infective diarrhoea associated with bloody stools.

Nausea and vomiting

Antiemetics should be prescribed only when the cause of vomiting is known (e.g. drugs particularly cytotoxic chemotherapy, post-operative, motion sickness, pregnancy and migraine) because otherwise they may delay diagnosis. If antiemetic drug treatment is indicated, the drug is chosen according to the aetiology of vomiting. Dexamethasone has antiemetic effects and is used in vomiting associated with cancer chemotherapy. It has additive effects when given with high-dose metoclopramide or with a $5-HT_3$-receptor antagonist such as ondansetron. The mechanism of action of dexamethasone as an antiemetic is unknown but may involve reduction of prostaglandin synthesis.

Antihistamines

Indications

Motion sickness, drug-induced vomiting, vestibular disorders, such as vertigo and tinnitus.

Mechanism of action

Competitive antagonist at the histamine H_1 receptor.

Preparations and dose

Cyclizine Valoid® tablets: 50 mg; Injection 50 mg/mL.

Oral 50 mg up to three times daily.

IM/IV injection 50 mg three times daily.

Promethazine Phenergan® tablets: 10 mg, 25 mg; Elixir: 5 mg/mL; Injection: 25 mg/mL.

Oral for motion sickness prevention, 20–25 mg (at bedtime the night before travel).

IM/IV 25–50 mg.

Side effects

Drowsiness, antimuscarinic effects (urinary retention, dry mouth, blurred vision), palpitations, arrhythmias and rashes.

Cautions/contraindications

Caution in prostatic hypertrophy, urinary retention, glaucoma and pyloroduodenal obstruction (due to antimuscarinic effects). Drug interactions – see national formulary.

Phenothiazines

Mechanism of action

Dopamine antagonists. Act centrally by blocking the chemoreceptor trigger zone (CTZ) in the fourth ventricle. Many drugs produce vomiting by an action on the CTZ.

Indications

Phenothiazines are used for the prophylaxis and treatment of nausea and vomiting associated with diffuse neoplastic disease, radiation sickness and vomiting caused by drugs such as general anaesthetics, opioids and cytotoxics. Chlorpromazine is associated with more sedation and is usually reserved for nausea and vomiting of terminal illness.

Preparations and dose

Chlorpromazine hydrochloride Tablets: 25 mg, 50 mg, 100 mg; Solution: 25 mg/5 mL, 100 mg/5 mL; Injection: 25 mg/mL; Suppositories: 25 mg and 100 mg.

Oral 10–25 mg every 4–6 hours.

IM 25 mg then 25–50 mg every 3–4 hours.

By rectum In suppositories: 100 mg every 6–8 hours.

Prochlorperazine Tablets 5 mg; Stemetil® tablets and suppositories: 5 mg; Syrup: 5 mg/mL; Injection: 12.5 mg/mL.

Oral 20 mg initially, then 10 mg after 2 hours; prevention: 5–10 mg two to three times daily.

IM 12.5 mg followed if necessary after 6 hours by an oral dose.

Side effects
As for other antipsychotic agents.

Cautions/contraindications
As for other antipsychotic agents.

Domperidone and metoclopramide

Mechanism of action
Block dopamine receptors and inhibit dopaminergic stimulation of the CTZ.

Indications
Domperidone is used particularly in post-operative nausea and vomiting and also gastro-oesophageal reflux disease and dyspepsia. Metoclopramide is particularly used in nausea and vomiting associated with cytotoxics or radiotherapy.

Preparations and dose
Metoclopramide Tablets: 10 mg; Syrup: 5 mg/mL; Injection: 5 mg/mL.
 Oral/IM/IV (over 1–2 minutes): 10 mg three times daily.
 Domperidone Tablets: 10 mg; Motilium® tablets: 10 mg; Suspension: 5 mg/mL; Suppositories: 30 mg.
 Oral 10–20 mg three to four times daily; maximum 80 mg.
 By rectum 60 mg twice daily.

Side effects
Central nervous system effects are produced by metoclopramide and to a lesser extent by domperidone (due to limited passage across the blood–brain barrier). Extrapyramidal effects include acute dystonias (treated by drug cessation and procyclidine 5–10 mg i.m./i.v.), akathisia and a parkinsonism-like syndrome. Drowsiness with high doses of metoclopramide. Galactorrhoea is caused by hyperprolactinaemia as a result of dopamine receptor blockade.

Cautions/contraindications
Contraindicated in gastrointestinal obstruction, 3–4 days after gastrointestinal surgery where increased motility may be harmful, and phaeochromocytoma.

5-HT$_3$-receptor antagonists

Mechanism of action
Block the 5-HT$_3$-receptors in the CTZ (see phenothiazines, p. 135) and in the gut.

Indications

Particularly effective against vomiting induced by highly emetogenic chemotherapeutic agents and radiotherapy used for treating malignancy and postoperative vomiting that is resistant to other agents.

Preparations and dose

Examples: dolasetron, granisetron, ondansetron, palonosetron.

Ondansetron Tablets: 4 mg; Injection: 2 mg/mL; Zofran$^®$ syrup: 4 mg/5 mL; Suppositories: 16 mg.

- Chemotherapy: 8 mg by mouth, or 16 mg by rectum 1–2 hours before treatment; or by i.m./i.v. injection, 8 mg immediately before treatment, then by mouth, 8 mg every 12 hours; or by rectum, 16 mg daily. With severely emetogenic chemotherapy, treatment is given i.m./i.v. and continued by infusion 1 mg/h for up to 24 hours.
- Prevention of post-operative nausea and vomiting: by mouth, 16 mg 1 hour before anaesthesia; or by i.m./i.v. injection, 4 mg at induction of anaesthesia.

Side effects

Headache, constipation, hypersensitivity reactions. Following i.v. administration: seizures, chest pain, arrhythmias, hypotension and bradycardia.

Cautions/contraindications

Caution with prolonged QT interval and cardiac conduction disorders.

4 Liver, biliary tract and pancreatic disease

Liver disease is common throughout the world. In the developed world, it is most often due to non-alcoholic fatty liver disease (NAFLD) and alcohol excess. In the developing world, chronic viral hepatitis B or hepatitis C are the leading causes of liver mortality. Cirrhosis represents the final common pathway for liver diseases and is characterized by progressive fibrosis of the liver parenchyma leading to portal hypertension and deterioration of liver function. In decompensated cirrhosis, the median overall survival is 2 years, which is a far worse prognosis than for many cancers.

The liver is the main site for metabolism of most drugs and alcohol; other major functions include:

- *Control of synthesis and metabolism of protein.* All circulating proteins except γ-globulins (made by lymphocytes) are synthesized in the liver. These include albumin (maintains intravascular oncotic pressure and transports water-insoluble substances, e.g. bilirubin and some drugs in the plasma), transport and carrier proteins (e.g. transferrin), components of the complement system and all factors involved in coagulation. The liver eliminates nitrogenous waste by degradation of amino acids and conversion to urea for renal excretion.

- *Maintenance of blood sugar.* The liver releases glucose into the blood stream in the fasting state, either by breakdown of stored glycogen or by synthesizing glucose from amino acids (from muscle) or glycerol (from adipose tissue).

- *Lipid metabolism.* Most of the body's cholesterol is manufactured in the liver but the remainder comes from food. Cholesterol is used to make bile salts and certain hormones, including oestrogen, testosterone and the adrenal hormones. The liver also synthesizes lipoproteins and triglycerides (most are of dietary origin).

- *Metabolism and excretion of bilirubin and bile acids.* Bile acids are formed from cholesterol, excreted into bile and pass into the duodenum via the common bile duct (CBD), where they solubilize lipid for digestion and absorption. Bilirubin is formed from the breakdown of mature red cells and eventually excreted in urine and faeces.

LIVER BIOCHEMISTRY AND LIVER FUNCTION TESTS

A routine blood sample for liver biochemistry will be processed by an automated multichannel analyser to produce serum levels of bilirubin, aminotransferases, alkaline phosphatase, γ-glutamyl transpeptidase (γ-GT) and total proteins.

These tests are often referred to as 'liver function tests' (LFTs) which is misleading as they do not accurately reflect the liver's function. They are best referred to as 'liver blood tests' or 'liver biochemistry'. Liver synthetic function is determined by measuring the prothrombin time (clotting factors are synthesized in the liver) and serum albumin, which are increased and reduced, respectively, with impaired function. Hypoalbuminaemia is also found in hypercatabolic states (e.g. chronic inflammatory disease and sepsis) and where there is excessive renal (nephrotic syndrome) or intestinal (protein-losing enteropathy) albumin loss. A prolonged prothrombin time may also occur as a result of vitamin K deficiency in biliary obstruction (low concentration of intestinal bile salts results in poor absorption of vitamin K); however, unlike in liver disease, clotting will be corrected by administering 10 mg vitamin K intravenously (i.v.) for 2–3 days.

- *Bilirubin* (normal range <17 μmol/L, 1.00 mg/dL) is the breakdown product of haemoglobin (see p. 145). Serum bilirubin is normally almost all unconjugated. In liver disease, an increase is usually accompanied by other liver biochemistry abnormalities. Differentiation between conjugated and unconjugated bilirubin is only necessary in congenital disorders of bilirubin metabolism (usually Gilbert's disease) or to exclude haemolysis.

- Aminotransferases. These enzymes (referred to as transaminases) are contained in hepatocytes and leak into the blood following liver cell damage. Two are assayed:

  - *Aspartate aminotransferase* (AST) is primarily a mitochondrial enzyme (80%; 20% in cytoplasm) and is also present in the heart, muscle, kidney and brain. High levels are seen in hepatic necrosis, myocardial infarction, muscle injury and congestive cardiac failure.

  - *Alanine aminotransferase* (ALT) is a cytosolic enzyme, more specific to the liver so that a rise only occurs with liver disease.

    The ALT/AST ratio is a useful clinical indicator. In viral hepatitis, ALT > AST unless cirrhosis is present, when AST > ALT. In alcoholic liver disease and steatohepatitis the AST is often greater than the ALT. Thus in patients with viral hepatitis, an AST/ALT ratio >1 indicates cirrhosis, and in patients without cirrhosis in whom AST > ALT, alcohol or obesity should be considered the most likely cause.

- *Alkaline phosphatase (ALP)*. This is present in hepatic canalicular and sinusoidal membranes, bone, intestine and placenta. The origin can be determined by electrophoretic separation of isoenzymes or bone-specific monoclonal antibodies. However, if the γ-GT is also abnormal, the ALP is presumed to come from liver.

    Serum ALP is raised in both intrahepatic and extrahepatic cholestatic disease of any cause due to increased synthesis. In cholestatic jaundice, levels may be four to six times the normal level. Raised levels also occur, usually without jaundice, with hepatic infiltrations (e.g. metastasis) and cirrhosis. The highest serum levels (>1000 IU/L) occur with hepatic metastasis and primary biliary cirrhosis.

- *γ-Glutamyl transpeptidase*. This is a microsomal enzyme present in liver and many other tissues. Activity can be induced by drugs such as phenytoin, warfarin and alcohol. If the ALP is normal, a raised serum γ-GT can be a useful guide to alcohol intake. However, mild elevation of γ-GT is common, even with minimal alcohol consumption, but it is raised in fatty liver disease. In the absence of other liver function test abnormalities, a slightly raised γ-GT can safely be ignored.

- *Total proteins and globulin fraction*. The globulin fraction is often raised in autoimmune hepatitis and a fall indicates successful therapy.

- *Additional blood investigations*
  - *Haematological*. Thrombocytopaenia is a common finding in cirrhosis, often aggravated by alcohol. Excessive use of alcohol causes red blood cell macrocytosis.

Approach to interpretation of abnormal liver biochemistry

A predominant elevation of serum aminotransferases indicates hepatocellular injury. Elevation of serum bilirubin and alkaline phosphatase in excess of aminotransferases indicates a cholestatic disorder such as primary biliary cirrhosis, primary sclerosing cholangitis or extrahepatic bile duct obstruction. An isolated rise in bilirubin is most likely due to Gilbert's disease. The approach to investigating elevated serum bilirubin is discussed under 'Jaundice'. A careful history (alcohol consumption, exposure to hepatotoxic drugs, risk factors for chronic liver disease), physical examination (particularly features of chronic liver disease), simple laboratory tests (viral hepatitis, metabolic and autoimmune liver disease, Table 4.1) and an ultrasound (US) examination of the liver are the first steps for patients with a persistent elevation of serum aminotransferases. A liver biopsy may subsequently be necessary.

OTHER INVESTIGATIONS IN LIVER AND BILIARY DISEASE

Imaging with abdominal US and computed tomography (CT) is widely used in the investigation of liver and biliary disease. US is usually performed first and is a more useful test for lesions in the gall bladder and bile duct. Colour Doppler ultrasound will demonstrate vascularity within a lesion and the direction of portal and hepatic vein blood flow.

Hepatic stiffness (transient elastography) Using a US transducer, a vibration of low frequency and amplitude is passed through the liver, the velocity of which correlates with hepatic stiffness. Stiffness (kPa) increases with

Table 4.1 Causes of chronic liver disease and cirrhosis

Cause	Non-invasive markers of aetiology
Common	
Alcohol	History of excess alcohol, ↑ serum γ-GT, ↑ MCV
Hepatitis B ± D	HBsAg ± HBeAg/DNA in serum
Hepatitis C	HCV antibodies and HCV RNA in serum
Others	
Primary biliary cholangitis	Serum antimitochondrial antibodies, ↑ serum IgM
Secondary biliary cirrhosis	Dilated extrahepatic ducts on imaging
Autoimmune hepatitis	Serum autoantibodies, ↑ serum IgG
Haemochromatosis	Family history, ↑ serum ferritin, ↑ transferrin saturation, *HFE* gene
Budd–Chiari syndrome	Presence of known risk factors, caudate lobe hypertrophy, abnormal flow in major hepatic veins on US
Wilson's disease	<40 years old, ↓ serum caeruloplasmin, ↓ serum total copper, ↑ 24-h urinary copper excretion, Kayser–Fleischer rings
Drugs	Drug history, e.g. methotrexate
α₁-Antitrypsin (AAT) deficiency	Young age, associated emphysema, ↓ serum AAT
Cystic fibrosis (CF)	Presence of extrahepatic manifestations of CF
NAFLD	Features of the metabolic syndrome, hyperechoic liver on US
Sclerosing cholangitis: primary (PSC) and secondary	Most PSC patients have IBD and serum p-ANCA multifocal stricturing and dilatation of bile ducts on cholangiography (either MRCP or ERCP)
Metabolic storage diseases	Presence of extrahepatic features
Idiopathic (cryptogenic)	Absence of any identifiable cause including on liver biopsy

AAT, α₁-antitrypsin; CF, cystic fibrosis; ERCP, endoscopic retrograde cholangiopancreatography; γ-GT, γ-glutamyl transpeptidase; HBeAg, Hepatitis B e antigen; HBsAg, hepatitis B surface antigen; IBD, inflammatory bowel disease; IgG, immunoglobulin G; IgM, immunoglobulin M; HCV, hepatitis C virus; MCV, mean corpuscular volume; MRCP, magnetic resonance cholangiopancreatography; NAFLD, non-alcoholic fatty liver disease; pANCA, peripheral antineutrophilic cytoplasmic antibody; PSC, primary sclerosing cholangitis; US, ultrasound.

worsening liver fibrosis (sensitivity and specificity 80–95% compared to liver biopsy). It cannot be used in the presence of ascites and morbid obesity, and it is affected by inflammatory tissue and congestion.

Endoscopic ultrasound (EUS) A small high-frequency ultrasound probe is incorporated into the tip of an endoscope and placed by direct vision into the gut lumen. The close proximity of the probe to the pancreas and biliary tree permits high-resolution ultrasound imaging, which enables pancreatic tumour staging. Needle aspiration provides cytological/histological tissue and may also be used to drain pancreatic and peripancreatic fluid collections.

Computed tomography (CT) examination During or immediately following i.v. contrast injection, both arterial and portal venous phases are enhanced, enabling precise characterization of a lesion and its vascular supply.

Magnetic resonance imaging (MRI) produces cross-sectional images without radiation. It is the most sensitive investigation of focal liver disease.

Magnetic resonance cholangiopancreatography (MRCP) involves manipulation of data acquired by MRI to visualize the 'water-filled' bile and pancreatic ducts. This non-invasive technique has replaced diagnostic (but not therapeutic) endoscopic retrograde cholangiopancreatography (ERCP).

Upper gastrointestinal (GI) endoscopy is used for diagnosis and treatment of varices, detection of portal hypertensive gastropathy and associated lesions such as peptic ulcers.

ERCP outlines the biliary and pancreatic ducts. It involves the passage of an endoscope into the second part of the duodenum and cannulation of the ampulla. Contrast is injected into both systems and the patient is screened radiologically. Therapeutic ERCP is used to remove common bile duct stones or drain the biliary system by passing a tube (stent) through an obstruction. Pancreatitis is the most common complication following ERCP but cholangitis is also seen. Broad-spectrum antibiotics should be given prophylactically to patients with suspected biliary obstruction or history of cholangitis.

Percutaneous transhepatic cholangiography (PTC) Under local anaesthesia, a fine flexible needle is passed into the liver and contrast injected slowly to outline the whole of the biliary tree. PTC is performed if ERCP fails or is likely to be technically difficult. In difficult cases, ERCP and PTC may be combined, PTC showing the biliary anatomy above the obstruction and ERCP the more distal anatomy. The main complications are bleeding and cholangitis with septicaemia. Prophylactic antibiotics should be administered.

Liver biopsy Liver biopsy (Table 4.2) is almost always performed as a day case under US guidance. Histological examination of the liver is valuable in the differential diagnosis of diffuse or localized parenchymal disease. Contraindications include an uncooperative patient, a prolonged prothrombin time (by 3–5 seconds), platelet count $<50 \times 10^9$/L, extrahepatic cholestasis and suspected haemangioma. The mortality rate is less than 0.02% when performed by experienced operators. A transjugular approach is used when liver histology is essential for management but coagulation abnormalities or ascites prevent a

Table 4.2 Indications and contraindications for liver biopsy

Indications
Liver disease
Unexplained hepatomegaly
Some cases of jaundice
Persistently abnormal liver biochemistry
Occasionally in acute hepatitis
Chronic hepatitis
Cirrhosis of unknown cause
Drug-related liver disease
Infiltrations
Tumours: primary or secondary
Infections (e.g. tuberculosis)
Storage disease (e.g. glycogen storage)
Pyrexia of unknown origin

Usual contraindications to percutaneous needle biopsy
Uncooperative patient
Prolonged prothrombin time (by >3 s)
Platelets $<80 \times 10^9$/L
Ascites
Extrahepatic cholestasis – dilated bile ducts on ultrasound scan

percutaneous approach. Assessment of liver fibrosis and cirrhosis is made by histopathological examination of a liver biopsy specimen. Disadvantages of liver biopsy are sampling error and its invasive nature. Most complications of liver biopsy occur within 24 hours (usually in the first 2 hours). Complications include biliary peritonitis and bleeding into the peritoneum or into the bile duct (haemobilia).

Markers of liver fibrosis An accurate assessment of fibrosis is critical for appropriate management of many liver disorders. A variety of different systems have been developed to assess the extent of liver fibrosis. These range from simple algorithms using standard haematological and biochemical tests (e.g. AST to platelet ratio index score) to measurements of liver function analysed with commercial algorithms (FibroTest) or measurements of matrix metalloproteins (enhanced liver fibrosis test). In general, these markers have been developed for chronic hepatitis C but may be applied to other liver disorders. The current assays have a high sensitivity/specificity for the detection of cirrhosis but are less effective at detecting intermediate levels of fibrosis. Combining mechanical, non-invasive tests for fibrosis, such as transient elastography and fibrosis markers, enables assessment of fibrosis without liver biopsy. Imaging (US, CT and MRI) will detect advanced liver disease such as nodularity and portal hypertension but will not assess the earlier stages of fibrosis.

SYMPTOMS AND SIGNS OF LIVER DISEASE

Acute liver disease, such as viral hepatitis, may be asymptomatic or present with generalized symptoms of lethargy, anorexia and malaise in the early stages with jaundice developing later.

Chronic liver disease may also be asymptomatic, only discovered by an incidental finding of abnormal liver biochemistry. Some patients with chronic liver disease may present at a late stage with complications of cirrhosis such as:

- Ascites with abdominal swelling and discomfort
- Haematemesis and melaena due to bleeding oesophageal varices
- Confusion and drowsiness due to hepatic encephalopathy.

Patients presenting this way are often extremely unwell and a detailed history may not be possible. However, physical examination will often reveal the signs of chronic liver disease (Fig. 4.1).

Pruritus (itching) occurs in cholestatic jaundice from any cause, but is particularly common in primary biliary cirrhosis when it may be the only symptom at presentation. Pruritus may occur in association with other systemic and skin diseases.

JAUNDICE

Jaundice (icterus) is a yellow discoloration of the sclerae and skin as a result of a raised serum bilirubin. It is usually detectable clinically when the bilirubin exceeds 50 μmol/L (3 mg/dL).

Bilirubin is derived predominantly from the breakdown of haemoglobin in the spleen and is carried in the blood bound to albumin. Unconjugated bilirubin is conjugated in the liver by glucuronyl transferase to bilirubin glucuronide, and this is excreted via the bile duct into the small intestine in bile. In the terminal ileum, conjugated bilirubin is converted to urobilinogen and excreted in the faeces (as stercobilinogen, which is responsible for the pigmentation of faeces) or reabsorbed and excreted by the kidneys (Fig. 4.2).

For clinical and diagnostic purposes, three major categories of jaundice can be considered:

- Haemolytic jaundice
- Congenital hyperbilirubinaemias – impaired conjugation of bilirubin or bilirubin handling by the liver. Other than raised bilirubin, liver biochemistry is normal.
- Cholestatic jaundice – failure of bile secretion by the liver or bile duct obstruction. Liver biochemistry is abnormal.

Haemolytic jaundice

Increased breakdown of red blood cells leads to increased production of bilirubin, which usually results in mild jaundice (68–102 μmol/L or 4–6 mg/dL), as

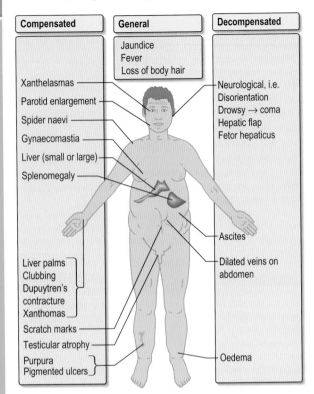

Compensated	General	Decompensated
	Jaundice Fever Loss of body hair	
Xanthelasmas Parotid enlargement Spider naevi Gynaecomastia Liver (small or large) Splenomegaly		Neurological, i.e. Disorientation Drowsy → coma Hepatic flap Fetor hepaticus
		Ascites
Liver palms Clubbing Dupuytren's contracture Xanthomas Scratch marks Testicular atrophy Purpura Pigmented ulcers		Dilated veins on abdomen Oedema

Spider naevi, telangiectases that consist of a central arteriole with radiating small vessels found in the distribution of superior vena cava; **liver palms** (palmer erythema), reddening of palms at the thenar and hypothenar eminences is a non-specific change indicative of a hyperdynamic circulation; **fetor hepaticus,** a distinctive musty, sweet breath odour in severe liver disease.

Fig. 4.1 Physical signs in chronic liver disease.

the liver can usually handle the increased bilirubin derived from haemolysis. Unlike the conjugated hyperbilirubinaemia of cholestatic jaundice, unconjugated bilirubin is not water soluble and therefore does not pass into the urine. Urinary urobilinogen is increased. Causes include haemolytic anaemia, e.g. sickle cell disease. Investigations will show features of haemolysis, with raised serum unconjugated bilirubin and an otherwise normal liver biochemistry.

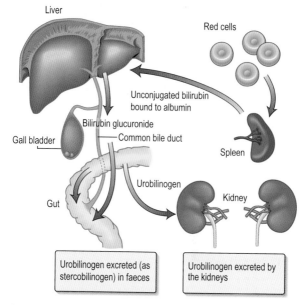

Fig. 4.2 Pathways in bilirubin metabolism.

Congenital hyperbilirubinaemia

The most common congenital hyperbilirubinaemia is Gilbert's syndrome, which affects 2–7% of the population. It is asymptomatic and is usually picked up by an incidental finding of a slightly raised serum bilirubin (17–102 μmol/L, 1–6 mg/dL). Mutations in the gene coding for UDP-glucuronyl transferase lead to reduced enzyme activity and reduced conjugation of bilirubin with glucuronic acid. Genetic testing is possible in these cases. Diagnosis is based on the findings of unconjugated hyperbilirubinaemia with otherwise normal liver biochemistry, full blood count, smear and reticulocyte count (thus excluding haemolysis) and the absence of signs of liver disease. The patient should be reassured that no further investigation or treatment is necessary.

Other congenital abnormalities of bilirubin metabolism (Crigler–Najjar, Dubin–Johnson and Rotor's syndromes, benign recurrent intrahepatic cholestasis) are rare.

Cholestatic jaundice

This can be divided into the following (Fig. 4.3):

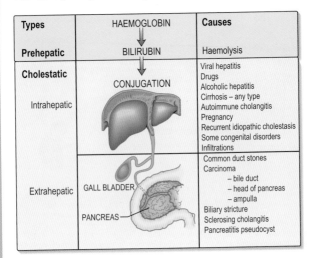

Types	HAEMOGLOBIN	Causes
Prehepatic	↓ BILIRUBIN	Haemolysis
Cholestatic Intrahepatic	↓ CONJUGATION	Viral hepatitis Drugs Alcoholic hepatitis Cirrhosis – any type Autoimmune cholangitis Pregnancy Recurrent idiopathic cholestasis Some congenital disorders Infiltrations

Extrahepatic	GALL BLADDER
	
	PANCREAS
		Common duct stones
		Carcinoma
		    – bile duct
		    – head of pancreas
		    – ampulla
		Biliary stricture
		Sclerosing cholangitis
		Pancreatitis pseudocyst

Fig. 4.3 Causes of jaundice.

- Intrahepatic cholestasis caused by hepatocellular swelling in parenchymal liver disease or abnormalities at a cellular level of bile excretion
- Extrahepatic cholestasis resulting from obstruction of bile flow at any point distal to the bile canaliculi.

In both types, there is jaundice with pale stools and dark urine and the bilirubin is conjugated. However, intrahepatic and extrahepatic cholestatic jaundice must be differentiated as their management is quite different.

Investigations

An outline of the approach to the investigation of jaundice is shown in Fig. 4.4.

- Serum liver biochemistry will confirm jaundice. The AST tends to be high early in the course of hepatitis with a smaller rise in alkaline phosphatase. Conversely, in extrahepatic obstruction, the alkaline phosphatase is elevated, with a smaller rise in the AST.
- US examination shows dilated bile ducts in extrahepatic cholestasis and may identify the level of obstruction and its cause (e.g. gallstones, tumours).
- Serum viral markers for hepatitis A or hepatitis B are present in acute viral hepatitis. Antibodies to hepatitis C virus develop late in the course of acute infection but hepatitis C virus (HCV) RNA is usually detectable by 1–2 weeks.
- Other tests – prothrombin time may be prolonged as a result of vitamin K malabsorption and is corrected by administration of vitamin K. Serum autoantibodies are present in autoimmune liver disease.

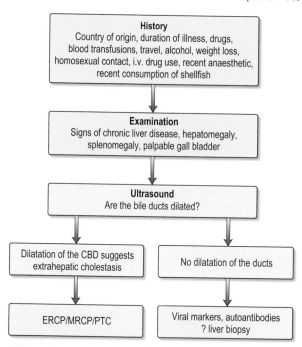

ERCP = endoscopic retrograde cholangiopancreatography
MRCP = magnetic resonance cholangiopancreatography
PTC = percutaneous transhepatic cholangiogram

Fig. 4.4 Approach to the investigation of cholestatic jaundice. The order of investigation is influenced by the age of the patient and hence the likely cause of jaundice. A young person is most likely to have intrinsic liver disease, e.g. viral hepatitis, and it may be more appropriate to organize tests to exclude these conditions before proceeding to US. CBD, common bile duct; ERCP, endoscopic retrograde cholangiopancreatography; i.v., intravenous; MRCP, magnetic resonance cholangiopancreatography; PTC, percutaneous transhepatic cholangiogram.

HEPATITIS

The pathological features of hepatitis are liver cell necrosis and inflammatory cell infiltration. Hepatitis is divided into acute and chronic types on the basis of clinical and pathological criteria.

Acute hepatitis is most commonly caused by one of the hepatitis viruses (Fig. 4.5). This is usually self-limiting, with a return to normal structure and

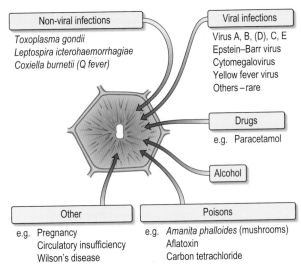

Non-viral infections

Toxoplasma gondii
Leptospira icterohaemorrhagiae
Coxiella burnetii (Q fever)

Viral infections

Virus A, B, (D), C, E
Epstein–Barr virus
Cytomegalovirus
Yellow fever virus
Others – rare

Drugs

e.g. Paracetamol

Alcohol

Other

e.g. Pregnancy
Circulatory insufficiency
Wilson's disease

Poisons

e.g. *Amanita phalloides* (mushrooms)
Aflatoxin
Carbon tetrachloride

Fig. 4.5 Causes of acute parenchymal damage.

function. Occasionally, there is progression to massive liver cell necrosis. Clinically, the patient may be jaundiced, with an enlarged and tender liver, and there is laboratory evidence of hepatocellular damage with raised serum aminotransferase levels. Disease severity is assessed by the prothrombin time and serum bilirubin. Alcoholic hepatitis is distinguished from other causes of acute hepatitis by characteristic laboratory abnormalities.

Chronic hepatitis is defined as sustained inflammatory disease of the liver lasting more than 6 months (Table 4.3). Chronic viral hepatitis is the principal cause of chronic liver disease, cirrhosis and hepatocellular carcinoma (HCC) world-wide.

Viral hepatitis

The different features of common forms of viral hepatitis are summarized in Table 4.4. All cases must be notified to the appropriate public health authority. This allows contacts to be traced and data provided on disease incidence.

Hepatitis A

Epidemiology

Hepatitis A (HAV) is the most common type of acute viral hepatitis. It occurs world-wide and particularly affects children and young adults. Spread is

Table 4.3 Causes of chronic hepatitis
Viral
Hepatitis B ± D
Hepatitis C
Autoimmune
Drugs
Methyldopa
Nitrofurantoin
Isoniazid
Ketoconazole
Hereditary
Wilson's disease
Others
Inflammatory bowel disease
Alcohol

faecal–oral and arises from the ingestion of contaminated food (e.g. shellfish, clams) or water. The virus is excreted in the faeces of infected individuals for about 2 weeks before onset of illness and for up to 7 days afterwards. It is most infectious just before the onset of jaundice.

Clinical features

After an average incubation period of 28 days, the viraemia causes non-specific prodromal symptoms such as nausea, anorexia and distaste for cigarettes. After 1 or 2 weeks, some patients become jaundiced, with dark urine and pale stools, and the prodromal symptoms improve. There is moderate hepatomegaly and the spleen is palpable in 10% of cases. Occasionally, lymphadenopathy and skin rash are present. The illness is self-limiting and usually over in 3–6 weeks. Rarely, there is fulminant hepatitis, coma and death.

Investigations

- Liver biochemistry shows raised ALT and raised bilirubin when jaundice develops.
- Blood count may show a leucopenia with relative lymphocytosis and a high erythrocyte sedimentation rate (ESR). The prothrombin time is prolonged in severe cases.
- Acute HAV infection is diagnosed by immunoglobulin (Ig)M anti-HAV in the serum; the presence of IgG anti-HAV indicates previous infection.

Table 4.4 Some features of viral hepatitis

Virus	A RNA	B DNA	D RNA	C RNA	E RNA
Transmission (main sources)	Faecal–oral Saliva	*Blood/blood products Sexual Vertical Saliva	*Blood/blood products Saliva	*Blood/blood products	Faecal–oral
Incubation	2–6 weeks	1–5 months	1–3 months	2–6 months	3–8 weeks
Chronic liver disease	No	Yes	Yes	Yes	No**
Liver cancer	No	Yes	Rare	Yes	No
Mortality (acute)	<0.5%	<1%	<1%	<1%	1–2% (pregnant women 10–20%)

*Blood/blood products includes transfusion of infected blood or blood products or by contaminated needles used by drug addicts, tattooists or acupuncturists.
** Chronic hepatitis in immunosuppressed patients.

Differential diagnosis

This includes other causes of jaundice and in particular other types of viral and drug-induced hepatitis.

Management

There is no specific treatment. Hospital admission is not usually necessary and avoidance of alcohol is advised only when the patient is ill.

Prophylaxis

- *Active immunization* with an inactivated strain of the virus is given to travellers to areas of high prevalence (Africa, Asia, South America, Eastern Europe and the Middle East), patients with chronic liver disease (in whom the disease is more severe) and persons at risk of occupational exposure (staff and residents of homes with severe learning difficulties and workers at risk of exposure to untreated sewage).

Control of hepatitis also depends on good hygiene. Travellers to high-risk areas should drink only boiled or bottled water and avoid suspicious food.

- *Passive immunization* with immunoglobulin is given to close contacts of confirmed cases of hepatitis A to prevent infection.

Hepatitis B

Epidemiology

Hepatitis B virus (HBV) is present world-wide and is particularly prevalent in parts of Africa, the Middle and Far East. Vertical transmission from mother to child during parturition is the most common method of transmission world-wide. HBV is also spread through blood and blood products, sexual intercourse (particularly men who have sex with men) and by horizontal transmission in children through minor abrasions or close contact with other children.

Viral structure

The infective virion or Dane particle is a 42-nm particle comprising an inner core or nucleocapsid surrounded by an outer envelope of surface protein (hepatitis B surface antigen, HBsAg). This surface coat is excessively produced by the infected hepatocytes and can exist separately from the whole virion in serum and body fluid.

The HBV genome is variable, and genetic sequencing can be used to define different HBV genotypes, i.e. A–H. These genotypes may influence the chance of responding to interferon treatment (A > B; C > D) but all genotypes respond equally well to nucleoside analogues.

Mutations occur in the various reading frames of the HBV genome. These mutants can emerge in patients with chronic HBV infection (escape mutants) or can be acquired by infection. *HBsAg mutants* are produced by alterations in the 'a' determinants of the HBsAg proteins with usually a substitution of glycine for arginine at position 145. This results in changes in the antibody binding domain and may confer resistance to the vaccine.

In patients with some HBV genotypes (particularly D), a mutation in the *pre-core region* occurs when a guanosine (G) to adenosine (A) change creates a stop codon that prevents the production of hepatitis B e antigen (HBeAg). The synthesis of hepatitis B core antigen (HBcAg) is unaffected. This mutation may be associated with HBeAg-negative disease but other mutations in the core promoter region can also lead to HBeAg-negative disease. To detect infectivity, HBV DNA must always be measured as no eAg should be present.

Acute HBV infection

HBV penetrates the hepatocyte and in immunocompetent adults there is a strong cellular immune response to the foreign HBV proteins expressed by hepatocytes. This response leads to clearance of the infection in 99% of infected adults and is marked by the disappearance of HBsAg from the serum, the development of antibodies to surface antigen (anti-HBs) and immunity to subsequent infection (Fig. 4.6A and Table 4.5). Acute infection may be asymptomatic or produce symptoms and signs similar to those seen in hepatitis A. Occasionally it is associated with a rash or polyarthritis affecting the small joints. One per cent of patients develop fulminant liver failure. Investigation

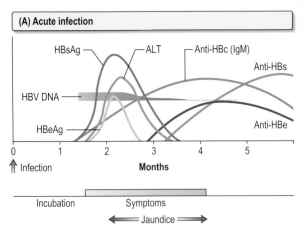

Fig. 4.6 Time course of the events and serological changes seen following infection with hepatitis B virus. ALT, alanine aminotransferase; anti-HBc, anti-hepatitis B core antibody; anti-HBe, anti-hepatitis e antibody; anti-HBs, anti-hepatitis B surface antibody; HBeAg, hepatitis B e antigen; HBsAg, Hepatitis B surface antigen; HBV, hepatitis B virus; IgM, immunoglobulin M.

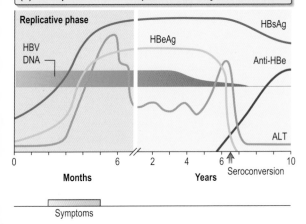

(B) Development of chronic hepatitis followed by seroconversion

Replicative phase

HBsAg

HBeAg

HBV
DNA

Anti-HBe

ALT

0   6   2   4   6   10
Months   **Years**   Seroconversion

Symptoms

(A) **Acute infection.**
Antigens
HBsAg appears in the blood from about 6 weeks to 3 months after an acute infection and then disappears.
HBeAg rises early and usually declines rapidly.
Antibodies
Anti-HBs appears late and indicates immunity.
Anti-HBc is the first antibody to appear and high titres of IgM anti-HBc suggest an acute and continuing viral replication. It persists for many months. **IgM** anti-HBc may be the only serological indicator of recent HBV infection in a period when HBsAg has disappeared and anti-HBs is not detectable in the serum.
Anti-HBe appears after the anti-HBc and its appearance relates to a decreased infectivity, i.e. a low risk.

(B) **Development of chronic hepatitis followed by seroconversion.**
HBsAg persists and indicates a chronic infection (or carrier state).
HBeAg persists and correlates with increased severity and infectivity and the development of chronic liver disease. When anti-HBe develops (seroconversion) the Ag disappears and there is a rise in ALT.
HBV DNA suggests continual viral replication. For **mutants**, see text.

Fig. 4.6, cont'd

is generally the same as for hepatitis A. There is no specific therapy for *acute* HBV infection and management is supportive.

Chronic HBV infection

The persistence of HBsAg in the serum for *more than 6 months* after acute infection defines chronic infection. Progression from acute to chronic infection

Table 4.5 Serologic markers of hepatitis B infection

	HBsAg	anti-HBc	anti-HBs	IgM anti-HBc
Susceptible to infection	Negative	Negative	Negative	Negative
Immune due to natural infection	Negative	Positive	Positive	Negative
Immune due to hepatitis B vaccination	Negative	Negative	Positive	Negative
Acutely infected	Positive	Positive	Negative	Positive
Chronically infected	Positive	Positive	Negative	Negative

anti-HBc, anti-hepatitis B core antibody; anti-HBs, anti-hepatitis B surface antibody; HBsAg, hepatitis B surface antigen; IgM, immunoglobulin M.

depends on several factors including the virulence of the virus, and the immunocompetence and age of the patient. When HBV infection is acquired at birth (vertical transmission) or early childhood, there is a high level of immunological tolerance. Cellular immune response to hepatocyte-membrane HBV proteins does not occur and chronic infection is the norm. This *immune tolerant phase* is characterized by minimal hepatic inflammatory activity and normal or near-normal serum ALT despite positive HBeAg and high levels of HBV replication. This phase may persist for two to three decades before an *immune clearance* phase that lasts for a variable period of time occurs. This is characterized by high HBV DNA levels as before but it is an active hepatitis that might lead to fibrosis and cirrhosis with elevated serum ALT. This phase ends with clearance of HBeAg and the development of anti-HBe (HBeAg seroconversion). There is also a marked decrease in serum HBV DNA and normalization of serum ALT *(the inactive HBsAg carrier state)*.

In the immune clearance phase, some patients will develop viral mutations (see above) that do not produce HBeAg but continue to replicate at a high level, with progressive liver damage and fluctuating serum levels of aminotransferases *(reactivation phase)*. Acquisition of infection later in life is associated with a very short immune tolerance phase or none at all. Most patients clear the virus (see acute infection) and only a small percentage will progress to chronic infection (Fig. 4.6B).

Table 4.5 summarizes the serological markers of HBV infection at various stages.

Treatment of chronic infection: whom to treat

Patients who present with detectable HBsAg and clinical and/or epidemiological factors suggestive of chronic infection can be considered for treatment without waiting for the 6-month period that defines chronicity. In HBsAg-positive individuals, there is a strong relationship between ongoing HBV replication and the risk of progression of chronic liver disease to cirrhosis, HCC or both. Treatment is given to patients most likely to develop progressive liver disease. Thus patients with chronic HBV infection (HBsAg-positive), high serum levels of HBV DNA ($\geq 20\,000$ IU per mL) and elevated serum ALT should be given antiviral treatment (see below). If cirrhosis is present, treatment should be given independent of ALT or HBV DNA levels. Antiviral therapy is not used for inactive HBV carriers (normal ALT and HBV DNA ≤ 2000 IU/mL) who are at low risk for progressive liver disease. Patients who lie outside these categories may require treatment if significant inflammation or necrosis is found in the liver biopsy or if there are increases in serum ALT.

All patients need long-term follow-up with annual assessment of hepatitis B serology and liver biochemistry, as transition to an active phase is common. The lifetime risk of malignancy is increased in all HBsAg-positive patients.

Antiviral agents

The aim of therapy is to prevent disease progression and, ideally, to eliminate HBsAg. Interferon is an immunostimulator which induces an immune response leading to prolonged remission after discontinuation of therapy. Alternatively, entecavir and tenofovir are oral nucleotides that suppress viral replication. Long-term viral suppression has been shown to reverse fibrosis and even patients with cirrhosis respond with reversion of the fibrosis. Resistance is rarely seen with these agents, and older, more resistance-prone drugs like lamivudine are no longer recommended. A small proportion of patients develop an immune response leading to loss of HBeAg and very rarely, loss of HBsAg. However, the majority of patients who commence oral antiviral agents will require very prolonged treatment, perhaps for life. Immunosuppression, which may occur during chemotherapy, aggravates all phases of HBV. Reactivation of HBV is common in such patients and has a high mortality rate. It is essential that all patients who are due to receive chemotherapy are screened for HBsAg, and those who have chronic HBV should receive prophylactic antiviral therapy such as tenofovir or entecavir.

Hepatitis B and HIV co-infection

Routes of infection are similar for HBV and the human immunodeficiency virus (HIV) and rates of co-infection are 10–20%. All patients with chronic HBV infection should have a test for HIV antibody and vice versa. Testing should be repeated if there is ongoing risk of HIV, particularly before antiviral treatment for HBV is contemplated. HIV infection makes it more likely that an individual exposed to HBV will develop chronic infection and this will progress to more severe liver disease. Treatment of co-infection is complex and best managed in a specialist unit.

Prophylaxis

The avoidance of high-risk factors (needle sharing, sex workers and multiple male homosexual partners) and counselling of patients who are potentially infective are key aspects of prevention. Active immunization with a recombinant yeast vaccine is universal in most developed countries. In the UK it is only recommended for those at increased risk, e.g. healthcare workers, homosexual and bisexual men, sex workers, intravenous drug users, people with haemophilia, haemodialysis patients, partners and household contacts of infected individuals. The immunity that develops after active immunization lasts for over 10 years. Combined prophylaxis (i.e. active immunization and passive immunization with specific antihepatitis B immunoglobulin) is given to non-immune individuals after high-risk exposure, e.g. needle-stick injury from a carrier, newborn babies of HBsAg-positive mothers and HBV-negative sexual partners of HBsAg-positive patients.

Hepatitis D (delta or δ agent)

This is caused by the hepatitis D virus (HDV) which is an incomplete RNA particle enclosed in a shell of HBsAg and belongs to the Deltaviridae family. It is unable to replicate on its own but is activated by the presence of HBV. Diagnosis is by finding HDV RNA or IgM anti-HDV in the serum. It is common in some parts of the world including Eastern Europe (Romania, Bulgaria), North Africa and the Brazilian rainforest. Hepatitis D viral infection can occur as a co-infection with HBV. It is clinically indistinguishable from an acute icteric HBV infection but a biphasic rise of serum aminotransferases may be seen. Superinfection results in an acute flare-up of previously quiescent chronic HBV infection. A rise in serum AST or ALT may be the only indication of infection. Diagnosis is by finding HDV RNA or serum IgM anti-HDV at the same time as IgG anti-hepatitis B core antibody (anti-HBc). Active HBV DNA synthesis is reduced by delta superinfection and patients are usually negative for HBeAg with low HBV DNA. Acute hepatic failure can follow both types of infection but is more common after co-infection.

Chronic hepatitis D is an infrequent chronic hepatitis but spontaneous resolution is rare. Between 60% and 70% of patients will develop cirrhosis more rapidly than with HBV infection alone. In 15% of cases, the disease is rapidly progressive with development of cirrhosis in a few years. Treatment for patients with active liver disease is with pegylated α-2a interferon for 12 months, although response rates are very low.

Hepatitis C

The prevalence rate of infection ranges from 0.4% in Europe to 1–3% in Southern Europe (possibly linked to intramuscular injections of vaccines or other medicines), 6% in Africa, and in Egypt the rates are as high as 19% due to parenteral antimony treatment for schistosomiasis. The virus is transmitted by blood and blood products and was common in persons with haemophilia treated before screening of blood products was introduced. The incidence in intravenous drug users is high (50–60%). The low rate of HCV infection in high-risk groups such as men who have sex with men, sex workers and attendees at sexually transmitted infection (STI) clinics suggests a limited role for sexual transmission. Vertical transmission from a healthy mother to child can occur, but is rare (~5%). Other routes of community-acquired infection (e.g. close contact) are extremely rare. In 20% of cases the exact mode of transmission is unknown. An estimated 240 million people are infected world-wide.

Hepatitis C virus

HCV is a single-stranded RNA virus of the Flaviviridae family with six genotypes which differ in geographical distribution. Genotypes 1a and 1b account for 70% of cases in the USA and 50% in Europe.

Most acute infections are asymptomatic, with about 10% of patients having a mild flu-like illness with jaundice and a rise in serum aminotransferases. Some 85–90% of asymptomatic patients develop chronic liver disease. A higher percentage of symptomatic patients 'clear' the virus with only 48–75% going on to develop chronic liver disease.

Chronic hepatitis C infection

Patients with chronic hepatitis C infection are usually asymptomatic, the disease being discovered only following a routine biochemical test when mild elevations in the aminotransferases (usually ALT) are noticed (50%). The elevation in ALT may be minimal and fluctuating while some patients have a persistently normal ALT (25%), the disease being detected when checking for HCV antibodies (e.g. in blood donors). Non-specific malaise and fatigue are common in chronic infection and often reverse following viral clearance. Extrahepatic manifestations are seen, including arthritis, cryoglobulinaemia with or without glomerulonephritis and porphyria cutanea tarda. There is a higher incidence of diabetes and association with lichen planus, sicca syndrome and non-Hodgkin's lymphoma.

Chronic HCV infection causes slowly progressive fibrosis. After 20 years of infection, 16% of patients would have developed cirrhosis. Factors associated with rapid progression of HCV fibrosis include excessive alcohol consumption, co-infection with HIV, obesity, diabetes and infection with genotype 3. Once cirrhosis has developed, some 3–4% per year will develop decompensated cirrhosis and approximately 1% will develop liver cancer.

Diagnosis is made by finding HCV antibody in the serum. A small proportion of patients with spontaneous clearance will have undetectable HCV RNA in serum (measured by polymerase chain reaction [PCR]) but most patients who are antibody positive will be viraemic and the level of viraemia varies from a few thousands to several millions. Disease progression is not influenced by the viral load but treatment outcome is less effective in those with high levels of viraemia.

The HCV genotype should be characterized in patients who are to be given treatment and assessment of fibrosis (either by liver biopsy or non-invasive methods) is important. The aim of treatment is to eliminate HCV RNA from the serum in order to stop the progression of active liver disease and prevent the development of hepatocellular carcinoma. A clinical cure is determined by a sustained virological response (SVR), defined by a negative HCV RNA using PCR, 6 months after the end of therapy.

Treatment for HCV infection is undergoing a revolution with treatments changing from interferon-based regimes to all-oral combination regimes of directly acting antiviral agents. The latter are expensive and are not available in all countries. However, new and less costly all-oral regimes are expected and it is to be hoped that in the near future, all patients can be cured without interferon, which is associated with numerous side effects. The direct acting antiviral regimes for HCV target different viral replication enzymes. Inhibitors of the NS3 protease enzyme, the NS5A replication complex initiator and the NS5B polymerase are now available. In clinical trials, these agents have shown SVR rates of 90–95% following 8–12 weeks of treatment. These oral regimes are almost side-effect free although they have not yet been widely used so their full side-effect profile has not yet been clearly defined.

Hepatitis E[nd]

Hepatitis E virus (HEV) is an RNA virus which causes enteral (epidemic or waterborne) hepatitis, similar to hepatitis A, particularly in developing countries (Table 4.4). Diagnosis is by detection of IgG and IgM anti-hepatitis E virus (anti-HEV) in the serum or HEV RNA in serum or stools.

Acute hepatic failure

This is hepatic failure with encephalopathy, a neuropsychiatric condition which develops as a consequence of liver disease. It develops in *less than 2 weeks* in a patient with a previously normal liver or in patients with an acute exacerbation of underlying liver disease. Cases that evolve at a slower pace (*2–12 weeks*) are called subacute hepatic failure. It is an infrequent complication of acute liver damage from any cause (Fig. 4.5) and occurs as a result of massive liver cell necrosis. In the UK, viral hepatitis and paracetamol overdose are the most common causes. Presentation is with hepatic encephalopathy (Table 4.6) of varying severity, accompanied by severe jaundice and a marked coagulopathy. The complications include cerebral oedema, hypoglycaemia, severe bacterial and fungal infections, hypotension and renal failure (hepatorenal syndrome). Most patients should be managed with supportive treatment in a specialist liver unit (Table 4.7). Emergency liver transplantation offers life-saving treatment, depending on the cause, and transplantation offered solely based on severity (grade IV encephalopathy), of which 80% might otherwise die.

Table 4.6 Clinical grading of hepatic encephalopathy

Grade	Neurological findings
0	No alteration in consciousness, intellectual function, personality or behaviour
1	Daytime somnolence, short attention span, mild asterixis*
2	Lethargic, drowsiness, disorientated usually in time, inappropriate behaviour, obvious asterixis*
3	Asleep but rousable, confusion, incomprehensible speech
4	Coma

Asterixis (liver flap), involuntary flapping movements of the hand when the arm is extended and wrist held in a backward position.

Table 4.7 Transfer criteria for patients with acute liver injury to specialized units

INR >3.0
Presence of hepatic encephalopathy
Hypotension after resuscitation with fluid
Metabolic acidosis
Prothrombin time (seconds) > interval (hours) from overdose (paracetamol cases)

INR, international normalized ratio.

Alcohol use

Drink-related problems have increased in recent years. In the UK, approximately one in five male admissions to acute medical wards is directly or indirectly the result of alcohol. Over the past 20 years, admissions to psychiatric hospitals for the treatment of alcohol-related problems have increased 25-fold. Excessive alcohol use is the leading cause of preventable hypertension with increased risk of myocardial infarction and stroke. There is a steady rise in recorded alcohol consumption in developing countries but these data are also likely to conceal heavy drinking in some localities and among populations. Associated with this is an increase in alcohol-related problems including trauma, violence, various cancers and alcohol-associated organ damage.

Alcohol dependence is defined by a physical dependence on or addiction to alcohol. The key feature of alcohol dependence is a lack of control over alcohol use, demonstrated by a compulsive need to drink and the inability to cut down or stop drinking. Guidelines for safe drinking limits are 21 units weekly for males and 14 units weekly for females. A slightly higher intake is probably unlikely to lead to harm, but more than 36 units per week in men and 24 units in women increases the risk to health. Units of alcohol in a drink are calculated by a simple equation:

Units of alcohol in a drink = volume (1)
$$\times \text{\% alcohol by volume (ABV)}$$

e.g. a 0.75-L bottle of whisky which is 40% ABV contains 30 units of alcohol.

In general, 1 unit = a measure of spirits, a glass of wine or half a pint of standard-strength beer.

Screening for problem drinking

An elevated serum γ-GT and raised red cell mean corpuscular volume (MCV) are useful screening tests for excessive alcohol use and are helpful in monitoring progress. Blood and urine alcohol levels are sometimes measured to demonstrate high intake.

Consequences of alcohol use and dependence

Physical complications These usually occur after a long period of heavy drinking, e.g. 10 years. Problems are generally seen earlier in women than in men. Damage is the result of direct tissue toxicity and the effects of malnutrition and vitamin deficiency which often accompany excessive alcohol use:

- *Cardiovascular:* a direct toxic effect on the heart leads to a cardiomyopathy and arrhythmias
- *Neurological:* acute intoxication leads to ataxia, falls and head injury with intracranial bleeds. Long-term complications include polyneuropathy, myopathy, cerebellar degeneration, dementia and epilepsy.

Wernicke's encephalopathy (WE) is the result of vitamin B_1 (thiamine) deficiency. It can also occur in severe starvation and prolonged vomiting. The classic triad of WE (confusion, ataxia and ophthalmoplegia) occur in a minority of patients. Mental changes are the most common (acute confusion, drowsiness, pre-coma and coma), whereas ataxia and ophthalmoplegia occur in less than one-third of patients. The diagnosis is clinical. A high index of suspicion and a low threshold for making presumptive diagnosis is necessary. Treatment is urgent and is with an intravenous injection of B-complex vitamins (e.g. two pairs of ampoules of high potency vitamins three times daily for 3 days, followed by one pair of ampoules daily for 5 days). This may reverse some of the early changes. Inappropriately managed, WE is fatal in 20% of patients. Many survivors will develop long-term brain damage (Korsakoff's syndrome) with a gross defect of short-term memory associated with confabulation. Patients at risk of WE (significant weight loss, signs of undernutrition, alcohol withdrawal symptoms requiring hospital admission) should be treated prophylactically with one pair of ampoules of high potency B vitamins daily for 3–5 days followed by oral B vitamins on discharge. Administration of glucose may exacerbate the acute loss of thiamine and it is essential that thiamine is given before glucose.

- *Gastrointestinal:* liver damage, acute and chronic pancreatitis, oesophagitis and an increased incidence of oesophageal carcinoma.
- *Haematological:* thrombocytopenia (alcohol inhibits platelet maturation and release from bone marrow), a raised MCV and anaemia caused by dietary folate deficiency.
- *Psychiatric complications:* there is an increased incidence of depression and deliberate self-harm among patients with alcohol dependence. Attempted suicide must always be taken seriously and a psychiatric referral made.
- *Social complications:* marital and sexual difficulties, employment problems, financial difficulties and homelessness.

Alcohol withdrawal Most heavy drinkers will experience some form of withdrawal symptoms if they attempt to reduce or stop drinking. No patient should ever be advised to stop drinking immediately in view of the potentially life-threatening complications of alcohol withdrawal without appropriate detoxification:

- Mild, early features occur within 6–12 hours and include tremor, nausea and sweating. Treatment is with a reducing dose of chlordiazepoxide (see Emergency Box 4.1).
- Major features usually occur later, within 2–3 days, but may take up to 2 weeks.
- Generalized tonic–clonic seizures.
- Delirium tremens is a potentially fatal severe alcohol withdrawal syndrome. There is fever, marked tremor, tachycardia, agitation and visual hallucinations ('pink elephants'). Treatment must be given urgently (see Emergency Box 4.1).

✚ Emergency Box 4.1

Management of alcohol withdrawal in hospital

- Prevent or treat established Wernicke's encephalopathy by administration of intravenous vitamin B complex. Give before administration of glucose-containing intravenous fluids.
- Correct dehydration and electrolyte imbalance. Hypophosphataemia and hypomagnesaemia are common.
- Chlordiazepoxide 30 mg four times daily decreasing to zero over 7 days. With very heavy alcohol intake and severe withdrawal symptoms, the dose can be increased up to 60 mg four times a day, then decreased to zero over 10 days.
- Oxazepam is the drug of choice for alcohol detoxification in patients with severe liver disease as it is not metabolized by the liver.

Alcohol detoxification is sometimes carried out in the community under the care of a specialist team. The patient attends daily for medication and monitoring. Exclusion criteria for community detoxification are inadequate social support, severe liver disease, concurrent medical or psychiatric illness or a previous history of delirium tremens or alcohol withdrawal fits.

After alcohol withdrawal, it is essential that relapse is prevented. This involves local alcohol services, specialist psychiatry and the alcohol nurse specialist. 'Brief interventions' refers to 10–15 minutes of counselling, with feedback about drinking, advice, goal setting, and follow-up contact (one or more discussions lasting 10–15 minutes with a clinician or specialist nurse). Oral acamprosate, a γ-aminobutyric acid (GABA) analogue, reduces relapses by 50%. Naltrexone is a pure opioid receptor antagonist that modifies the effects of alcohol by blunting its pleasurable effects and reducing the craving. It reduces relapse rates as compared with placebo.

Autoimmune hepatitis

This is a progressive inflammatory liver condition with a female preponderance. Approximately 40% of autoimmune hepatitis (AIH) patients have a family history of autoimmune disease (e.g. pernicious anaemia, thyroiditis and coeliac disease) and at least 20% have concomitant autoimmune disease or develop it during follow-up.

Aetiology

The pathogenesis of AIH is incompletely understood, although increasing evidence suggests that genetic susceptibility, molecular mimicry and impaired immunoregulatory networks contribute to the initiation and perpetuation of the autoimmune attack. Liver damage is thought to be mediated primarily by T cell mediated events ($CD4^+$ T-cells) against liver antigens, producing a progressive necroinflammatory process leading to fibrosis and cirrhosis.

Clinical features

The onset is often insidious, with anorexia, malaise, nausea and fatigue. Twenty-five per cent of cases present as an acute hepatitis, with rapidly progressive liver disease. The signs of chronic liver disease are often present, with palmar erythema, spider naevi, hepatosplenomegaly and jaundice. Features of other autoimmune diseases may be present.

Investigations

Circulating autoantibodies (antinuclear, smooth muscle, soluble liver antigen, liver/kidney microsomal antibodies) are present in most patients. There is hypergammaglobulinaemia (particularly IgG), and serum bilirubin and aminotransferases are elevated. Liver histology will show the non-specific changes of chronic hepatitis with interface hepatitis and often cirrhosis.

Treatment

Prednisolone 30 mg is given daily for at least 2 weeks, followed by a gradual reduction to a maintenance dose of 5–15 mg daily. Azathioprine should be added (1–2 mg/kg daily) as a steroid-sparing agent, and in some as sole long-term maintenance therapy. Levels of thiopurine methyltransferase should be obtained. Other agents that have been used in resistant cases include budesonide (in non-cirrhotic patients), mycophenolate, ciclosporin and tacrolimus.

Prognosis

Steroid and azathioprine therapy induces remission in over 80% of cases. This response indeed forms part of the diagnostic criteria. Treatment is life-long in most cases although withdrawal may be considered after 2–3 years of biochemical remission. Liver transplantation is performed if treatment fails, although the disease may recur. Hepatocellular carcinoma occurs less frequently than in viral-induced cirrhosis.

NON-ALCOHOLIC FATTY LIVER DISEASE

NAFLD is now the commonest cause of chronic liver disease in many developed countries. It is often detected on routine abdominal ultrasound examination with steatosis found in up to a third.

Non-alcoholic steatohepatitis (NASH) cirrhosis is now the third commonest indication for liver transplantation in the USA. Risk factors for NAFLD are obesity, hypertension, type 2 diabetes and hyperlipidaemia and NAFLD is considered the liver component of the metabolic syndrome. Most are asymptomatic but hepatomegaly may be present. Mild increases in serum aminotransferases and/or γ-GT (with ALT > AST) are frequently the sole liver biochemistry abnormalities. Elastography is used to evaluate the degree of fibrosis but may not be technically possible in the morbidly obese and liver biopsy may be necessary.

All NAFLD patients require lifestyle advice aimed at weight loss, increased physical activity, and attention to cardiovascular risk factors. A reduction in body weight >7–9% has been associated with reduced steatosis, hepatocellular injury and hepatic inflammation. Weight loss following bariatric surgery leads to reduced hepatic steatosis, steatohepatitis and fibrosis.

The yearly cumulative incidence of HCC is 2.6% in patients with NASH cirrhosis and US surveillance should be performed 6-monthly.

CIRRHOSIS

Cirrhosis results from necrosis of liver cells followed by fibrosis and nodule formation. The end result is impairment of liver cell function and gross distortion of the liver architecture leading to portal hypertension.

Aetiology

The causes of cirrhosis are shown in Table 4.1. Alcohol is the most common cause in the Western world but hepatitis B and C are more common causes world-wide.

Pathology

Histologically, two types are described:

- Micronodular cirrhosis: uniform, small nodules up to 3 mm in diameter. This type is often caused by ongoing alcohol damage or biliary tract disease.
- Macronodular cirrhosis: nodules of variable size and normal acini may be seen within large nodules. This type is often seen following chronic viral hepatitis.

There is also a mixed type, with both small and large nodules.

Clinical features

These are secondary to portal hypertension and liver cell failure (Fig. 4.1). Cirrhosis with the complications of encephalopathy, ascites or variceal haemorrhage is designated decompensated cirrhosis. Cirrhosis without any of these complications is termed compensated cirrhosis.

Investigations

These are performed to assess the severity of liver disease, identify the aetiology and screen for complications.

Severity

- Liver biochemistry may be normal. In most cases there is at least a slight elevation of the serum alkaline phosphatase and aminotransferases.
- Full blood count shows thrombocytopenia in most patients at diagnosis with leukopenia and anaemia developing later.
- Liver function: Prothrombin time and serum albumin are the best indicators of liver function.
- Serum electrolytes: A low sodium concentration indicates severe liver disease secondary to either impaired free water clearance or excess diuretic therapy. An elevated serum creatinine is associated with a worse prognosis.
- Serum α-fetoprotein (AFP): This is normally undetectable after fetal life, but raised levels may occur in chronic liver disease. A level greater than 200 ng/mL is strongly suggestive of the presence of a HCC.

Aetiology

Cirrhosis develops in response to chronic liver injury from any cause which is often apparent from the history and the laboratory investigations (Table 4.1). A liver biopsy may be performed to confirm the severity and type of liver disease.

Further investigations

Oesophageal varices are sought with endoscopy. Primary prophylaxis is offered to those with varices to reduce bleeding. A US is useful for detection of HCC and to assess the patency of the portal and hepatic veins. A dual energy X-ray absorptiometry (DXA) scan is performed for osteoporosis.

Management

Cirrhosis is irreversible and frequently progresses. Management is that of the complications seen in decompensated cirrhosis as they arise. Correcting the underlying cause, e.g. venesection for haemochromatosis and abstinence from alcohol for alcoholic cirrhosis may halt the progression of liver disease. Screening for HCC (measurement of serum AFP and US every 6 months) is performed to identify tumours at an early stage. Liver transplantation should be considered in patients with end-stage cirrhosis. Patients should also be offered influenza immunization.

Prognosis

This is variable and depends on the aetiology and presence of complications. The severity and prognosis of liver disease can be graded according to the modified Child–Pugh classification (dependent on five variables: encephalopathy, ascites, prothrombin time, serum bilirubin and albumin) or the MELD score (modification of end-stage liver disease dependent on serum bilirubin, creatinine, and the international normalized ratio [INR]). Overall, the 5-year survival rate is approximately 50%.

COMPLICATIONS AND EFFECTS OF CIRRHOSIS

Portal hypertension

The portal vein is formed by the union of superior mesenteric (from the gut) and splenic vein (from the spleen) and transports blood to the liver. It accounts for 75% of hepatic vascular inflow; 25% is via the hepatic artery. Blood vessels enter the liver via the hilum (porta hepatis) and blood passes into the hepatic sinusoids via the portal tracts and leaves the liver through the hepatic veins to join the inferior vena cava. The normal portal pressure is 5–8 mmHg. The inflow of portal blood to the liver can be partially or completely obstructed at a number of sites, leading to high pressure proximal to the obstruction and the diversion of blood into portosystemic collaterals, e.g. at the gastro-oesophageal junction (varices) where they are superficial and liable to rupture, causing massive gastrointestinal haemorrhage (p. 168).

The main sites of obstruction are:

- Prehepatic, due to blockage of the portal vein before the liver
- Intrahepatic, resulting from distortion of the liver architecture
- Posthepatic, due to venous blockage outside of the liver (rare).

Table 4.8 Complications and effects of cirrhosis

Portal hypertension and gastrointestinal haemorrhage
Ascites
Portosystemic encephalopathy
Acute kidney injury (hepatorenal syndrome)
Hepatopulmonary syndrome
Hepatocellular carcinoma
Bacteraemias, infection
Malnutrition
Osteoporosis

Aetiology

The most common cause (Table 4.9) of portal hypertension is cirrhosis.

Clinical features

The only evidence of portal hypertension may be splenomegaly in a patient with clinical signs of chronic liver disease. The common presenting features are:

- Gastrointestinal bleeding from oesophageal or less commonly gastric varices
- Ascites
- Hepatic encephalopathy.

Variceal haemorrhage

Most patients with cirrhosis will eventually develop varices but only a third will bleed from them. Bleeding is often massive and mortality is as high as 50%.

Table 4.9 Causes of portal hypertension

Prehepatic	Portal vein thrombosis
Intrahepatic	Cirrhosis
	Alcoholic hepatitis
	Idiopathic non-cirrhotic portal hypertension
	Schistosomiasis
	Veno-occlusive disease
Posthepatic	Budd–Chiari syndrome
	Right heart failure (rare)
	Constrictive pericarditis
	Inferior vena caval obstruction

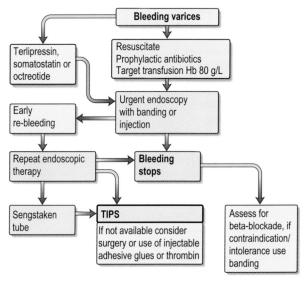

Fig. 4.7 Management of gastrointestinal haemorrhage due to oesophageal varices and transjugular intrahepatic portosystemic shunt. TIPS, transjugular intrahepatic portosystemic shunting.

Management

The general management of varices is summarized in Fig. 4.7.

Active bleeding Patients should be resuscitated and undergo urgent gastroscopy to confirm the diagnosis and exclude bleeding from other sites.

- Endoscopic therapy is the treatment of choice and will stop bleeding in 80% of cases bleeding from oesophageal varices. The common endoscopic methods are band ligation (small elastic bands are placed over the varices) or sclerotherapy (injection of a sclerosant solution, e.g. ethanolamine, into the varices).

- Pharmacological treatment is used for emergency control of bleeding while waiting for endoscopy. Terlipressin, a synthetic analogue of vasopressin, restricts portal inflow by splanchnic arterial constriction. It is given by i.v. bolus injection (2 mg 6-hourly) but is contraindicated in patients with ischaemic heart disease. An i.v. infusion of 250–500 μg/h somatostatin lowers portal pressure by a similar mechanism but is less effective. It is used when there are contraindications to terlipressin.

- Balloon tamponade with a Sengstaken–Blakemore tube is used if the medical or endoscopic treatment described above has failed or is contraindicated or if there is exsanguinating haemorrhage. The gastric balloon is inflated and pulled back against the gastro-oesophageal junction to prevent cephalad variceal blood flow to the bleeding point. It can have serious complications such as aspiration pneumonia, oesophageal rupture and mucosal ulceration. To reduce complications, the airway should be protected and the tube left in situ for no longer than 12 hours. It is removed just before endoscopy.

- Transjugular intrahepatic portosystemic shunting (TIPS) is used when there is a second re-bleed after treatment. A metal stent is passed over a guidewire in the internal jugular vein. The stent is then pushed into the liver substance under radiological guidance to create a shunt between the portal and hepatic veins, lowering portal pressure.

- Surgery (oesophageal transection and ligation of varices) is occasionally necessary if bleeding continues in spite of all the above measures.

- Additional treatment: Patients require high-dependency/intensive care unit nursing. Antibiotic prophylaxis such as cefotaxime is given to prevent infection, reduce re-bleeding and prevent early mortality. Lactulose is given to prevent portosystemic encephalopathy and sucralfate to reduce oesophageal ulceration, a complication of endoscopic therapy.

Prevention of recurrent variceal bleeding Following an episode of variceal bleeding, there is a high risk of recurrence (60–80% over a 2-year period), and treatment is given to prevent further bleeds (secondary prophylaxis). The main options are:

- Oral propranolol (in a dose sufficient to reduce the resting pulse rate by 25%) lowers portal pressure but some patients are intolerant of treatment because of side effects. Propranolol is also given to patients with varices who have never bled (primary prophylaxis).

- Repeat variceal banding every 2 weeks until the varices are obliterated. Varices may recur, so follow-up endoscopy is required.

- TIPS or occasionally a surgical portosystemic shunt is performed if endoscopic or medical therapy fails. Hepatic encephalopathy is a complication of both procedures. Liver transplantation should always be considered when there is poor liver function.

Ascites

This is the presence of fluid in the peritoneal cavity. Cirrhosis is the commonest cause (Table 4.10).

Aetiology

In cirrhosis, peripheral arterial vasodilatation (mediated by nitric oxide and other vasodilators) leads to a reduction in effective blood volume, with activation of

Table 4.10 Causes of ascites

Transudate	Exudate
Portal hypertension, e.g. cirrhosis	Peritoneal carcinomatosis
Hepatic outflow obstruction	Peritoneal tuberculosis
Budd–Chiari syndrome	Pancreatitis
Hepatic veno-occlusive disease	Nephrotic syndrome
Cardiac failure	Lymphatic obstruction (chylous ascites)
Tricuspid regurgitation	
Constrictive pericarditis, Meig's syndrome*	

*Meig's syndrome is the triad of benign ovarian fibroma, ascites and pleural effusion.

the sympathetic nervous system and renin–angiotensin system, thus promoting renal salt and water retention. The formation of oedema is encouraged by hypoalbuminaemia and mainly localized to the peritoneal cavity as a result of the portal hypertension.

Clinical features

There is fullness in the flanks with shifting dullness. Tense ascites is uncomfortable and produces respiratory distress. A pleural effusion (usually right-sided) and peripheral oedema may also be present.

Investigations

A diagnostic aspiration of 10–20 mL of ascitic fluid should be carried out in all patients and the following performed:

- Albumin: An ascitic albumin concentration of 11 g/L or more below the serum albumin suggests a transudate; a value of <11 g/L suggests an exudate (Table 4.10)
- A neutrophil count >250 cells/mm^3 in cirrhotic ascites indicates underlying (usually spontaneous) bacterial peritonitis
- Gram stain and culture for bacteria and acid-fast bacilli
- Cytology for malignant cells
- Amylase to exclude pancreatic ascites.

Management

Treatment depends on the cause. The management of ascites due to portal hypertension is described below. In other cases, ascites will improve with treatment of the underlying condition.

Diuretics The management of ascites resulting from cirrhosis is based on a step-wise approach, starting with dietary sodium restriction 40 mmol/day and oral spironolactone 100 mg daily, increasing the dosage gradually to 500 mg daily if necessary. Furosemide 20–40 mg daily is added if the response is poor. The aim of treatment is to lose about 0.5 kg of body weight each day because the maximum rate of transfer of fluid from the ascitic to the vascular compartment is only about 700 mL/day. Too rapid diuresis causes intravascular volume depletion and hypokalaemia which can precipitate encephalopathy. Efficacy and side effects of treatment are monitored by body weight, serum creatinine and sodium. A rising creatinine level or hyponatraemia indicates inadequate renal perfusion and the need for temporary cessation of diuretic therapy (if sodium <128 mmol/L). This approach to treating ascites is effective in over 90% of patients.

Paracentesis is used in patients with tense ascites or those who are resistant to standard medical therapy. All the ascites can be removed over several hours providing rapid symptom relief. Intravenous infusion of albumin (8 g/L removed) administered immediately after paracentesis increases the circulating volume (ascites reaccumulates at the expense of the circulating volume).

TIPS is occasionally used for resistant ascites.

Complications

Spontaneous bacterial peritonitis (SBP) occurs in 8% of cirrhotic patients with ascites and has a mortality rate of 10–15%. The most common infecting organism is *Escherichia coli*. Clinical features may be minimal and the diagnosis should be suspected in any patient with cirrhotic ascites who deteriorates. Diagnostic aspiration should always be performed and empirical antibiotic therapy with a third-generation cephalosporin, e.g. intravenous cefotaxime, is started if the ascitic fluid neutrophil count is $\geq$250 cells/mm^3. Antibiotics can subsequently be adjusted on the basis of culture results. Antibiotic prophylaxis with oral norfloxacin is indicated in patients after one episode or in patients at high risk (ascites protein <10 g/dL or severe liver disease). SBP is also an indication for referral to a liver transplant centre.

Portosystemic encephalopathy

Portosystemic encephalopathy (PSE) is a neuropsychiatric syndrome which occurs with advanced hepatocellular disease, either chronic (cirrhosis) or acute (fulminant hepatic failure). It is also seen in patients following surgical or TIPS shunts.

Pathophysiology

The mechanisms are unclear but are believed to involve 'toxic' substances normally detoxified by the liver, bypassing the liver via the collaterals and gaining

Table 4.11 Factors precipitating portosystemic encephalopathy

High dietary protein
Gastrointestinal haemorrhage (i.e. a high protein load)
Constipation
Infection including spontaneous bacterial peritonitis
Fluid and electrolyte disturbance (spontaneous or diuretic-induced)
Sedative drugs, e.g. opiates, diazepam
Portosystemic shunt operations and TIPS
Any surgical procedure
Progressive liver damage
Development of hepatocellular carcinoma

TIPS, transjugular intrahepatic portocaval shunt.

access to the brain. Ammonia plays a major role and is produced from breakdown of dietary protein by gut bacteria. In chronic liver disease, there is an acute-on-chronic course with acute episodes precipitated by a number of possible factors (Table 4.11).

Clinical features

An acute onset often has a precipitating cause; the patient becomes increasingly drowsy and eventually comatose (Table 4.6). There is increased tone and hyperreflexia. Chronically, the patient may be irritable; confused; with slow, slurred speech and a reversal of the sleep pattern, with the patient sleeping during the day and restless at night. The signs are fetor hepaticus (a sweet smell to the breath), a flapping tremor of the outstretched hand (asterixis), inability to draw a five-pointed star (constructional apraxia) and a prolonged trail-making test (the ability to join numbers and letters within a certain time). Serial attempts are easily compared and used to monitor patient progress.

Differential diagnosis

None of the manifestations of hepatic encephalopathy are specific to this disorder. Alternative diagnosis such as other metabolic or toxic encephalopathies or intracranial mass lesions may present similarly and should be considered.

Investigations

The diagnosis is clinical. An electroencephalogram (EEG) (showing δ waves), visual evoked potentials and arterial blood ammonia are sometimes used in difficult diagnostic cases or to follow patients (ammonia).

Management

The aims of management are to identify and treat any precipitating factors (Table 4.11) and to minimize the absorption of nitrogenous material, particularly ammonia, from the gut. This is achieved by the following:

- Laxatives: Oral lactulose (10–30 mL three times daily) is an osmotic purgative that reduces colonic pH and limits ammonia absorption. It may be given via a nasogastric tube if the patient is comatose. The dose should be titrated to result in two to four soft stools daily.
- Antibiotics are given to reduce the number of bowel organisms and hence the production of ammonia. Rifaximin is mainly unabsorbed and well tolerated. Oral metronidazole (200 mg four times daily) is also used.
- Maintenance of nutrition with adequate calories: Protein is initially restricted but increased after 48 hours as encephalopathy improves.

Prognosis

Prognosis depends on the underlying liver disease.

Hepatorenal syndrome

This is the development of acute kidney injury in a patient who usually has advanced liver disease, either cirrhosis or alcoholic hepatitis. Marked peripheral vasodilatation leads to a fall in systemic vascular resistance and effective hypovolaemia. This in turn results in vasoconstriction of the renal circulation with markedly reduced renal perfusion. The diagnosis is made on the basis of oliguria, a rising serum creatinine (over days to weeks), a low urine sodium (<10 mmol/L), absence of other causes of acute kidney injury, lack of improvement after volume expansion (if necessary) and withdrawal of diuretics. Prognosis is poor, and renal failure will often respond only if liver function improves. Albumin infusion and terlipressin have been used with some success.

Hepatopulmonary syndrome

Intrapulmonary vascular dilatation in patients with advanced liver disease causes hypoxaemia. In severe cases, patients are breathless on standing. Diagnosis is by echocardiogram and the changes improve with liver transplantation.

LIVER TRANSPLANTATION

Indications for liver transplantation include acute or chronic liver failure of any cause. Triggers for referral in chronic liver disease include progressive jaundice, diuresis-resistant ascites, an episode of spontaneous bacterial peritonitis and some cases of HCC. Careful selection of patients is crucial. Psychological assessment and education of patients and their families is essential before transplantation. Absolute contraindications are: active sepsis outside the liver and biliary tree, malignancy outside the liver, liver metastases (excluding neuroendocrine) and lack of psychological commitment by the patient.

With rare exceptions, patients over 65 years are not offered transplant. A 6-month abstinence rule prior to transplantation applies to patients with alcohol-related liver disease. The aim is for long-term abstinence after transplantation and possible improvement of liver function to avoid transplantation. Graft rejection is reduced by immunosuppressive agents such as ciclosporin. Early complications include haemorrhage, sepsis and acute rejection (<6 weeks), which is reversible with methylprednisolone. Late complications include recurrence of disease (hepatitis B and C, autoimmune liver disease), chronic rejection (the 'vanishing bile duct syndrome') and the consequences of immune suppression (malignancy, cardiovascular disease, diabetes mellitus). Overall, the 5-year survival rate after liver transplantation is 70–85%.

TYPES OF CHRONIC LIVER DISEASE AND CIRRHOSIS

Alcoholic cirrhosis

See alcoholic liver disease.

Primary biliary cholangitis

Primary biliary cholangitis (PBC) is a chronic disorder in which there is progressive destruction of intrahepatic bile ducts causing cholestasis, eventually leading to cirrhosis.

Epidemiology

It affects predominantly women in the age range 40–50 years.

Aetiology

An inherited abnormality of immunoregulation leads to a T-lymphocyte-mediated attack on bile duct epithelial cells. It is thought that disease expression results from an environmental trigger, possibly infective, in a genetically susceptible individual. Antimitochondrial antibodies (AMAs) are present in most (>95%) patients, but their role in disease pathogenesis is unclear.

Clinical features

Pruritus, with or without jaundice, is the single most common presenting complaint. In advanced disease, there is, in addition, hepatosplenomegaly and xanthelasma (PBC is a cause of secondary hypercholesterolaemia). Asymptomatic patients on routine examination or screening may be found to have hepatomegaly, a raised serum alkaline phosphatase or autoantibodies. Patients with advanced disease may have steatorrhoea and malabsorption of fat-soluble vitamins due to decreased biliary secretion of bile acids, resulting in low concentrations of bile acids in the small intestine. Autoimmune disorders such as Sjögren's syndrome, scleroderma and rheumatoid arthritis occur with increased frequency.

Investigations

- A raised serum alkaline phosphatase is often the only abnormality in liver biochemistry.
- Serum AMAs are found in more than 95% of patients and a titre of 1:160 or greater makes the diagnosis highly likely. M2 antibody is specific. Other non-specific antibodies such as antinuclear factor may also be present.
- Serum IgM may be high.
- Liver biopsy shows loss of bile ducts, lymphocyte infiltration of the portal tracts, granuloma formation in 40% of cases and, at a later stage, fibrosis and eventually cirrhosis.
- A US scan is sometimes performed in the jaundiced patient to exclude extrahepatic biliary obstruction.

PBC is almost certainly present if the serum alkaline phosphatase and IgM concentrations are both raised and the antimitochondrial antibody test is positive. Liver biopsy provides information about disease stage and prognosis but is not essential to make the diagnosis.

Management

Treatment, which is for life, is with ursodeoxycholic acid (10–15 mg/kg daily by mouth), a naturally occurring dihydroxy bile acid. It slows disease progression and reduces the need for liver transplantation. The mechanism of action is incompletely understood. It should be given early in the asymptomatic phase. Pruritus may be helped by cholestyramine and malabsorption of fat-soluble vitamins (A, D and K) is treated by supplementation. Obeticholic acid is now being used.

Liver transplantation is indicated in patients with advanced disease (serum bilirubin persistently >100 μmol/L).

Prognosis

Asymptomatic patients may show a near-normal life expectancy. In symptomatic patients with jaundice, there is a steady downhill course with death in approximately 5 years without transplantation.

Secondary biliary cirrhosis

Cirrhosis can result from months of prolonged large duct biliary obstruction. Causes include bile duct strictures, CBD stones and sclerosing cholangitis. US examination followed by MRCP is performed to outline the ducts. ERCP may then be necessary to treat the cause, e.g. stone removal.

Hereditary haemochromatosis

Hereditary haemochromatosis (HH) is an autosomal recessive disorder which is prevalent among Caucasians. It affects 1 in 400 in the population of which approximately 10% are gene carriers. There is excessive iron deposition in various organs eventually leading to fibrosis and functional organ failure.

Aetiology

HH is characterized by an abnormal increase in iron absorption from the upper small intestine. In most cases, HH is due to a mutation in the gene *HFE* on the short arm of chromosome 6. The normal HFE protein is expressed in the small intestine and plays a role in the regulation of iron absorption. Two missense mutations of the *HFE* gene account for most cases of HH. This involves a change of cysteine at position 282 for tyrosine (C282Y mutation) or a change of histidine at position 63 to aspartate (H63D mutation). Human leucocyte antigen (HLA)-A3, -B7 and -B14 occur with increased frequency in patients with HH compared with the general population. In a minority of patients, iron overload is due to defects in other proteins involved in iron metabolism.

Clinical features

Most patients are diagnosed when elevated serum iron or ferritin levels are noted on routine biochemistry or screening is performed because a relative is diagnosed with HH. Presentation may also be with symptoms and signs of iron loading in parenchymal organs (Table 4.12). There is a reduced incidence of overt disease in women because of extra iron losses associated with menstruation and a smaller dietary intake of iron.

Table 4.12 Clinical presentation of haemochromatosis

Health screening (often symptomatic)

Abnormal liver biochemistry
Abnormal iron studies
Familial and/or population screening

Symptomatic disease due to iron deposition in:

Liver: hepatomegaly, lethargy
Pancreas: diabetes mellitus
Myocardium: cardiomegaly, heart failure, conduction disturbances
Pituitary: loss of libido, impotence
Joints: arthralgia
Skin: hyperpigmentation

Investigations

- Serum liver biochemistry is often normal even with cirrhosis.
- Serum iron is elevated and total iron-binding capacity (TIBC) reduced. Transferrin saturation (serum iron/TIBC) is >45% (normal <33%).
- Serum ferritin reflects iron stores and is usually greatly elevated (often >500 µg/L).
- Genotyping (by PCR reaction using whole blood samples) for mutation analysis of the *HFE* gene is performed in patients with elevated ferritin and transferrin saturation.
- Patients with abnormal iron studies and mutations of the *HFE* gene are treated by phlebotomy without the need for liver biopsy. Assessment of the degree of fibrosis is performed by non-invasive tests or liver biopsy in patients who are predicted to have significant hepatic injury (abnormal liver biochemistry or serum ferritin >1000 µg/L). Liver biopsy and measurement of hepatic iron content is performed if the diagnosis is in doubt.

Causes of secondary iron overload, such as multiple transfusions, must be excluded. In addition, in alcoholic liver disease, hepatic iron stores may increase. The precise reason is unknown but the hepatic iron concentration does not reach the very high levels seen in haemochromatosis.

Management

Excess tissue iron is removed by venesection: 500 mL of blood (containing 250 mg of iron) are removed twice-weekly until iron stores are normalized (as assessed by serum ferritin and transferrin saturation). This may need to be continued for up to 2 years, and then three or four venesections per year are required life-long to prevent reaccumulation of iron. Surveillance for HCC is performed in patients with cirrhosis.

Genotyping to detect *HFE* mutations and iron studies should be performed on first-degree relatives of affected individuals.

Prognosis

The major complication is the development of HCC in patients with cirrhosis. This can be prevented by venesection before cirrhosis develops. Life expectancy will then be the same as for the normal population.

Wilson's disease (hepatolenticular degeneration)

This is a rare, recessively inherited disorder. Mutations in the *ATP7B* gene on chromosome 13 result in decreased secretion of copper into the biliary system and reduced incorporation of copper into procaeruloplasmin, the precursor of caeruloplasmin. Copper accumulates in the liver (leading to fulminant hepatic failure and cirrhosis), basal ganglia of the brain (Parkinsonism and eventually dementia), cornea (greenish-brown rings called Kayser–Fleischer rings) and renal tubules. Diagnosis is made by demonstrating low total serum copper and caeruloplasmin, increased 24-hour urinary copper excretion and increased copper in a liver biopsy specimen. Treatment is with penicillamine or trientene (to chelate copper) or zinc (reduces copper absorption). Liver transplantation is offered to those with end-stage liver disease or fulminant hepatic failure. First-degree relatives are screened and homozygotes should be treated.

α_1-Antitrypsin deficiency

This is a rare cause of cirrhosis. Mutations in the α_1-antitrypsin *(α_1-AT)* gene on chromosome 14 lead to reduced hepatic production of α_1-AT, which normally inhibits the proteolytic enzyme, neutrophil elastase. The genetic variants of α_1-AT are characterized by their electrophoretic mobilities as medium (M), slow (S) or very slow (Z). The normal genotype is PiMM. Most patients with clinical disease are homozygote for Z (PiZZ) and develop chronic liver disease (due to accumulation of the abnormal protein within the liver) and early-onset emphysema due to proteolytic lung damage. Diagnosis is made by demonstrating low serum levels of serum α_1-AT and confirmed by genotype assessment. On liver histology, α_1-AT-containing globules are seen in hepatocytes. Treatment is for chronic lung and liver disease. Intravenous augmentation therapy with plasma-derived α_1-AT is used but this not widely available. Patients should be advised to stop smoking.

Alcohol and the liver

Alcohol is the most common cause of chronic liver disease in the Western world. Alcoholic liver disease occurs more commonly in men, usually in the fourth and fifth decades, although patients can present in their 20s with advanced disease. Although alcohol acts as a hepatotoxin, the exact mechanism leading to hepatitis and cirrhosis is unknown. As only 10–20% of persons who drink excessively develop cirrhosis, genetic predisposition and immunological mechanisms have been suggested.

There are three major pathological lesions and clinical illnesses associated with excessive alcohol intake.

Fatty change

This is the most common biopsy finding in alcoholic individuals. Regular alcohol use, even for a few weeks, can result in fatty liver (steatosis), a disorder in which hepatocytes contain macrovesicular droplets of triglycerides. Symptoms are usually absent, and on examination, there may be hepatomegaly.

Laboratory tests are often normal, although an elevated MCV often indicates heavy drinking. The γ-GT level is usually elevated. The fat disappears on cessation of alcohol intake, but with continued drinking it may progress to fibrosis and cirrhosis.

Alcoholic hepatitis

Alcoholic hepatitis generally occurs after years of heavy drinking and may coexist with cirrhosis. Histologically, in addition to steatosis (see above), there are ballooned (swollen) hepatocytes that often contain amorphous eosinophilic material called Mallory bodies, surrounded by neutrophils. There may be fibrosis and foamy degeneration of hepatocytes.

Clinical features

The cardinal sign of alcoholic hepatitis is a rapid onset of jaundice. Other symptoms and signs are nausea, anorexia, right upper quadrant pain, encephalopathy, fever, ascites and tender hepatomegaly.

Investigations

- Full blood count shows leucocytosis, elevated MCV and often thrombocytopenia (results from bone marrow hypoplasia and/or hypersplenism associated with portal hypertension).
- Serum electrolytes are frequently abnormal with hyponatraemia. An elevated serum creatinine is an ominous sign and may predict the development of hepatorenal syndrome.
- Liver biochemistry shows elevated AST and ALT with a disproportionate rise in AST (usually AST : ALT ratio >2) and the absolute values for AST and ALT usually <500 IU/L; higher values suggest acute hepatitis due to another cause. The bilirubin may be markedly elevated, 300–500 μmol/L, reflecting the severity of the illness. Serum albumin is low and prothrombin time prolonged.
- Microscopy and culture of blood, urine and ascites is performed to search for an underlying infection.
- US (liver and biliary) is useful to identify biliary obstruction and HCC, which may also be present.
- Liver biopsy (often via the transjugular approach because of abnormal clotting) is not always required. Diagnosis is usually made on the basis of clinical presentation, neutrophilia, elevated INR and liver biochemistry profile.

Management

Patients with severe alcoholic hepatitis require supportive treatment and adequate nutritional intake must be maintained, if necessary, via a nasogastric tube. Corticosteroids (40 mg per day for 4 weeks) reduce the inflammatory process and are indicated if Maddrey's discriminant function is ≥ 32, indicating severe disease

[4.6 × (prothrombin time above control in seconds)

+ bilirubin (mg/dL)]

Bilirubin mmol/L ÷ 17 to convert to mg/dL

Steroids are contraindicated if renal failure, infection or bleeding is present. Pentoxifylline, a phosphodiesterase inhibitor with many effects including modulation of tumour necrosis factor (TNF)-α transcription, also reduces mortality, which it is thought to do mainly by the prevention of hepatorenal syndrome.

Alcoholic cirrhosis

This represents the final stage of liver disease from alcohol abuse. There is destruction of liver architecture and fibrosis with regenerating nodules giving rise to micronodular cirrhosis. Although patients may be asymptomatic, they often present with one of the complications of cirrhosis and there are usually signs of chronic liver disease. Investigation is as for cirrhosis in general. Management is directed at the complications of cirrhosis and patients are advised to stop drinking for life. Abstinence from alcohol improves the 5-year survival rate.

PRIMARY SCLEROSING CHOLANGITIS

Primary sclerosing cholangitis (PSC) is a chronic cholestatic liver disease characterized by a progressive obliterating fibrosis of intra and extrahepatic ducts, leading to cirrhosis. The cause is unknown. More than 75% of cases have ulcerative colitis, which may be asymptomatic. Patients are often diagnosed during an asymptomatic phase. Routine blood tests in a patient with inflammatory bowel disease reveal abnormal liver biochemistry, often a raised alkaline phosphatase. Patients present with symptoms such as pruritus, jaundice or cholangitis. Sixty per cent of patients have myeloperoxidase antineutrophilic cytoplasmic antibodies (ANCA). Diagnosis is usually by MRCP or liver biopsy. Treatment is usually limited to management of complications arising from chronic liver disease and eventually liver transplantation. Extrahepatic strictures may be amenable to dilatation at ERCP. High-dose ursodeoxycholic acid (30 mg/kg) may slow down disease progression. Cholangiocarcinoma (bile duct cancer) occurs in up to 15% of patients. Sclerosing cholangitis, secondary to *Cryptosporidium* infection, is seen in patients with acquired immune deficiency syndrome (AIDS).

BUDD–CHIARI SYNDROME

In this condition, occlusion of the hepatic vein obstructs venous outflow from the liver and the resulting congestion within the liver lead to hypoxic damage and necrosis of hepatocytes.

Aetiology

Common causes include a hypercoaguable state associated with myeloproliferative disorders, malignancy, oral contraceptives and inherited thrombophilias. The cause is unknown in 20% of cases.

Clinical features

Clinical manifestations depend on the extent and rapidity of the hepatic vein occlusion and whether a venous collateral circulation has developed. Right upper quadrant pain, hepatomegaly, jaundice and ascites are typical features. Acute disease may also present with fulminant hepatic failure. Cirrhosis may develop in the chronically congested liver, resulting in portal hypertension and the development of varices and other features of portal hypertension. A clinical picture similar to Budd–Chiari may develop in right-sided cardiac failure, inferior vena cava obstruction or constrictive pericarditis.

Investigations

Doppler US is the initial investigation of choice. This will show abnormal flow in the major hepatic veins or inferior vena cava, thickening, tortuosity, and dilatation of the walls of the hepatic veins. Non-specific findings include hepatomegaly, splenomegaly, ascites and caudate lobe hypertrophy. If the US is normal but clinical suspicion is high, CT or MRI may demonstrate abnormalities. Liver biopsy is often unnecessary in making a diagnosis but it will show centrizonal congestion, necrosis and haemorrhage.

Treatment

The goals of therapy are three-fold:

- To restore hepatic venous drainage. This is usually only feasible in the acute state and it entails thrombolysis, angioplasty and stent insertion or TIPS.
- Treatment of complications related to ascites and portal hypertension.
- Detection of the underlying hypercoagulable disorder and prevention of further clot formation.

LIVER ABSCESS

Liver abscesses are pyogenic, amoebic or hydatid.

Aetiology

The cause of pyogenic liver abscess is often unknown although biliary sepsis or portal pyaemia from intra-abdominal sepsis may be responsible. Other causes include trauma, bacteraemia or direct extension from, for example, a perinephric abscess. The organisms most commonly found include *E. coli* and

Streptococcus milleri but anaerobes such as *Bacteroides* are also seen. An amoebic abscess results from the spread of *Entamoeba histolytica* from the bowel to the liver via the portal venous system.

Clinical features

There are non-specific symptoms of fever, lethargy, weight loss and abdominal pain. The liver may be enlarged and tender and there may be consolidation or effusion in the right side of the chest. Patients with amoebic liver abscess often do not give a history of dysentery.

Investigations

- Laboratory abnormalities reflect the non-specific findings of infection, including anaemia, raised ESR and low albumin. Serum alkaline phosphatase is usually raised and bilirubin often normal.
- A US will show single or multiple rounded lesions that are hypoechoic in relation to the surrounding liver. CT is diagnostic and shows the abscesses as non-enhancing cavities with a surrounding rim of inflammation that are enhanced in relation to the rest of the liver.
- Serological tests for amoebae, e.g. complement-fixation test or enzyme-linked immunosorbent assay (ELISA), are almost always positive in amoebic liver abscess.

Management

Amoebic liver abscess diagnosed on the basis of clinical and radiological features (migrants from and travellers to endemic countries who have a single abscess in the right lobe of the liver) is treated with metronidazole (800 mg three times daily by mouth for 10 days) without the need for aspiration of the abscess.

Pyogenic abscess should have percutaneous aspiration under radiological control and usually a pigtail catheter is inserted for continuous drainage. The initial antibiotic regime (intravenous metronidazole and cefuroxime) is subsequently adjusted, depending on the organisms obtained from the aspirate.

LIVER DISEASE IN PREGNANCY

Viral hepatitis is the most common cause of jaundice in pregnancy. Three types of liver disease are specific to pregnancy: intrahepatic cholestasis (presenting with pruritus, elevated liver enzymes and increased serum bile acids), acute fatty liver of pregnancy (a severe fulminating illness with jaundice, vomiting and hepatic coma) and haemolysis (occasionally producing jaundice) which occurs in pre-eclamptic toxaemia. The three conditions present most commonly in the third trimester and resolve with delivery of the baby.

LIVER TUMOURS

The most common malignant liver tumours are metastatic, particularly those from the gastrointestinal tract, breast or bronchus. Primary liver tumours are either benign or malignant. Liver cysts and haemangiomas are common and may be confused with tumours on initial imaging. They usually need no further treatment.

Hepatocellular carcinoma (hepatoma)

HCC is the fifth most common cancer world-wide. The wide geographical distribution of HCC is probably due to regional variations in exposure to hepatitis B and C virus and environmental pathogens.

Aetiology

The majority of HCCs occur in patients with chronic liver disease or cirrhosis, especially viral hepatitis. Other aetiological factors include aflatoxin (a metabolite of a fungus found in groundnuts), androgenic steroids and possibly the contraceptive pill.

Clinical features

Weight loss, anorexia, fever, ascites and abdominal pain occur. The rapid development of these features in a patient with cirrhosis is highly suggestive of HCC. Due to surveillance by serum AFP estimation and liver US, asymptomatic HCC is increasingly found in asymptomatic patients with known cirrhosis. A focal lesion in the liver in a patient with cirrhosis is highly likely to be HCC.

Investigations

- Serum AFP may be raised but is normal in at least a third of patients.
- US or CT scan shows large filling defects in 90% of cases.
- MRI or angiography is useful in cases where there is doubt in diagnosis.
- Biopsy is only performed when there is a doubt in diagnosis as there is a risk of tumour seeding in the percutaneous needle biopsy tract. For instance, in a patient with cirrhosis and a liver mass greater than 2 cm in diameter, the lesion is almost certainly HCC and biopsy is not indicated.

Management

Surgical resection or liver transplantation is occasionally possible. Percutaneous ablation therapy using ethanol injection or high-frequency US probes will produce necrosis of the tumour. Transarterial chemoembolization involves the injection of a chemotherapeutic agent and Lipiodol into the hepatic artery. It is used in the treatment of large unresectable tumours. Chemotherapy given intravenously has a very limited role.

Prognosis

Overall, the median survival is only 6–20 months.

Benign liver tumours

The most common are haemangiomas, usually found incidentally on liver US or CT scan. They require no treatment. Hepatic adenomas are less common, and they are associated with the use of oral contraceptives. Resection is required if there are symptoms (e.g. pain, intraperitoneal bleeding).

GALLSTONES

Gallstones are present in 10–20% of the population. They are most common in women, and the prevalence increases with age.

Pathophysiology

Gallstones are of two types:

- *Cholesterol gallstones* account for 80% of all gallstones in the Western world. Cholesterol is held in solution by the detergent action of bile salts and phospholipids with which it forms micelles and vesicles. Cholesterol gallstones only form in bile which has an excess of cholesterol, either because there is a relative deficiency of bile salts and phospholipids or a relative excess of cholesterol (supersaturated or lithogenic bile). The formation of cholesterol crystals and gallstones in lithogenic bile is promoted by factors that favour nucleation such as mucus and calcium. Gallstone formation is further promoted by reduced gall bladder motility and stasis. The mechanism of cholesterol gallstone formation in patients with risk factors (Table 4.13) is frequently

Table 4.13 Risk factors for cholesterol gallstones

Increasing age
Sex (F > M)
Family history
Multiparity
Obesity ± metabolic syndrome
Rapid weight loss
Diet (e.g. high in animal fat/low fibre)
Ileal disease or resection (leading to bile salt loss)
Diabetes mellitus
Acromegaly treated with octreotide
Liver cirrhosis

multifactorial (cholesterol supersaturation, nucleation factors and reduced gall bladder motility).

* *Pigment stones* consist of bilirubin polymers and calcium bilirubinate. They are seen in patients with chronic haemolysis (e.g. hereditary spherocytosis and sickle cell disease) in which bilirubin production is increased and cirrhosis. Pigment stones may also form in the bile ducts after cholecystectomy and with duct strictures.

Clinical presentation

Most gallstones never cause symptoms and cholecystectomy is not indicated in asymptomatic cases. The complications are summarized in Fig. 4.8.

Biliary pain

Biliary pain (colic) is the term used for the pain associated with the temporary obstruction of the cystic duct or CBD by a stone.

Clinical features

There are recurrent episodes of severe and persistent pain in the upper abdomen which subsides after several hours. The pain may radiate to the right shoulder and the right subscapular region and is often associated with vomiting. Examination is often normal.

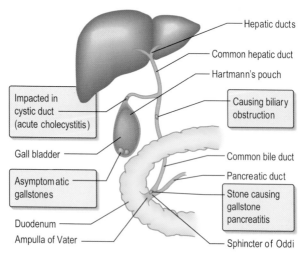

Fig. 4.8 The complications of gallstones.

Investigations

The diagnosis is usually made on the basis of a typical history and a US showing gallstones. Increases of serum alkaline phosphatase and bilirubin during an attack support the diagnosis of biliary pain. The absence of inflammatory features (fever, white cell count and local peritonism) differentiates this from acute cholecystitis.

Management

The treatment is with analgesics and elective cholecystectomy. Abnormal liver biochemistry or a dilated CBD on ultrasonography is an indication for pre-operative MRCP. CBD stones identified on imaging are removed at ERCP or sometimes at the same time as cholecystectomy.

Acute cholecystitis

Acute cholecystitis follows the impaction of a stone in the cystic duct or neck of the gall bladder. Very occasionally, acute cholecystitis may occur without stones (acalculous cholecystitis).

Clinical features

The initial clinical features are similar to those of biliary colic. However, over a number of hours, it progresses to severe pain localized in the right upper quadrant associated with a fever, tenderness and muscle guarding. The tenderness is worse on inspiration (Murphy's sign). Complications include empyema (pus) and perforation with peritonitis. The diagnosis of acute cholecystitis is usually straightforward. The differential diagnosis is from other causes of severe right upper quadrant pain.

Investigations

- White cell count shows leucocytosis.
- Serum liver biochemistry may be mildly abnormal.
- Abdominal US shows gallstones and a distended gall bladder with a thickened wall. There is focal tenderness directly over the visualized gall bladder (sonographic Murphy's sign).

Management

The initial treatment is conservative, with nil by mouth, intravenous fluids, pain relief and intravenous antibiotics such as cefotaxime. Cholecystectomy is usually performed within 48 hours of the acute attack and always if complications (see above) develop.

Chronic cholecystitis

Chronic inflammation of the gall bladder is often found in association with gallstones. On US examination, this may appear as a small shrunken gall bladder.

There is no evidence that this produces any symptoms and cholecystectomy is not indicated. Chronic right hypochondrial pain and fatty food intolerance are likely to be functional in origin and gallstones an incidental finding.

Acute cholangitis

This is an infection of the biliary tree and most often occurs secondary to CBD obstruction by gallstones (choledocholithiasis). Other causes are benign biliary strictures following biliary surgery or associated chronic pancreatitis, PSC, HIV cholangiopathy and patients with biliary stents. Bile duct obstruction due to cancer of the head of pancreas or bile duct (cholangiocarcinoma) can also cause cholangitis and this is more likely after ERCP. In the Far East, parts of Eastern Europe and the Mediterranean, biliary parasites can cause blockage and cholangitis.

Clinical features

The classic description of cholangitis with fever, jaundice and right upper quadrant pain (Charcot's triad) is not always present, although most patients often have fever with rigours. Jaundice is cholestatic in type and therefore urine is dark, the stools are pale and the skin may itch. Elderly patients may present with non-specific symptoms such as confusion and malaise.

Investigations

- White cell count shows leucocytosis.
- Blood cultures are positive (*E. coli*, *Enterococcus. faecalis*, sometimes anaerobes) in about 30% of patients.
- Liver biochemistry shows a cholestatic picture with raised serum bilirubin and alkaline phosphatase.
- US shows a dilated CBD and may show the cause of the obstruction.
- MRCP can further assess the site and cause of obstruction.
- ERCP is the definitive investigation and will also allow biliary drainage. It will show the site of obstruction and the cause. Bile can be sampled for culture and cytology (if a malignant cause is suspected).

Management

Treatment of acute cholangitis includes resuscitation and volume replacement in shocked patients, pain relief, treatment of infection with appropriate intravenous antibiotics and relief of obstruction by biliary drainage. Bacterial infection may be polymicrobial and a suitable antibiotic regimen is a third-generation cephalosporin such as cefotaxime (ciprofloxacin if allergic) plus metronidazole. An alternative regimen is amoxicillin, gentamicin (with appropriate monitoring) and metronidazole. In endemic areas, primary parasite infection must also be treated.

Biliary drainage and/or clearance are usually achieved at ERCP with or without sphincterotomy. The urgency of this procedure depends on the clinical condition of the patient and the initial response to antibiotics. Stones can be removed from the CBD and a stent can be placed in the biliary tree if stones cannot be removed to relieve obstruction, such as in patients with cancer of the head of pancreas or CBD. Antibiotics are continued after biliary drainage until symptom resolution, usually in 7–10 days.

Common bile duct stones (choledocholithiasis)

CBD stones may also be asymptomatic with no features of cholangitis and present with abnormal liver biochemistry, usually with a cholestatic picture. US will show gall bladder stones and may show the obstructed CBD containing a stone. MRCP is more sensitive than transabdominal US and it is sometimes performed if there is a high index of suspicion and US is negative. An alternative technique for imaging the biliary system is endoscopic US.

THE PANCREAS

The pancreas has both endocrine and exocrine functions. The islets of Langerhans secrete several hormones directly into the blood stream (endocrine function) of which insulin and glucagon play crucial roles in the regulation of blood sugar. The pancreatic acinar cells produce pancreatic enzymes (lipase, colipase, amylase and proteases) which pass via the main pancreatic duct into the duodenum and are involved in the digestion of fat, carbohydrate and protein in the small intestine.

Pancreatitis

Pancreatitis is divided into *acute* and *chronic*. Acute pancreatitis occurs in the backdrop of a normal pancreas and the pancreas returns functionally and structurally to normal after the episode. It occurs as isolated or recurrent attacks. In chronic pancreatitis, there is continuous inflammation with irreversible structural changes. In practice, it is not always possible to clearly separate acute from chronic forms because the acute causes (if untreated) may eventually lead to chronic pancreatitis and there may be relapses of the chronic condition (acute-on-chronic pancreatitis).

Acute pancreatitis

Acute pancreatitis is a disease of increasing incidence and it is associated with significant morbidity and mortality. Most patients will recover from the attack with only general supportive treatment, but 25% will develop severe acute pancreatitis with multiorgan failure. About 20% of these patients may die. The causes of acute pancreatitis are stated in Table 4.14.

Table 4.14 Causes of pancreatitis

Acute	Chronic
Gallstones*	Alcohol*
Alcohol*	Tropical
Infections (e.g. mumps, Coxsackie B)	Autoimmune (IgG4-related)
Pancreatic tumours	Idiopathic
Drugs: azathioprine, oestrogens, corticosteroids, didanosine	Hereditary: trypsinogen and inhibitory protein defects, cystic fibrosis
Iatrogenic: post-surgical, post-ERCP	
Metabolic: hypercalcaemia, hypertriglyceridaemia	
Miscellaneous: trauma, scorpion bite, cardiac surgery	
Idiopathic (unknown cause)	

*Commonest causes in the Western world.
ERCP, endoscopic retrograde cholangiopancreatography.

Pathogenesis

It is thought that the final common pathway, whatever is the initiating cause, is a marked elevation in intracellular calcium, leading to activation of intracellular proteases and the release of pancreatic enzymes. Acinar cell injury and necrosis follows, which promotes migration of inflammatory cells from the microcirculation into the interstitium. Release of a variety of mediators and cytokines leads to a local inflammatory response and sometimes a systemic inflammatory response that can result in single or multiple organ failure.

Clinical features

There is usually epigastric or upper abdominal pain radiating through to the back, associated with nausea and vomiting. On examination, there is epigastric or general abdominal tenderness, guarding and rigidity. However, other manifestations (coma, multiorgan failure) may dominate the clinical picture, causing a delay in diagnosis. Ecchymoses around the umbilicus (Cullen's sign) or in the flanks (Grey Turner's sign) indicate severe necrotizing pancreatitis.

Investigation

The purpose of investigation is to make a diagnosis, assess the severity and determine the aetiology.

- *Blood tests:* A raised serum amylase or lipase, in conjunction with the appropriate history and clinical signs, strongly indicate a diagnosis of acute pancreatitis. A normal level of serum amylase occurs if the patient presents late, at which time urinary amylase or serum lipase levels may still be raised. Serum amylase may also be moderately raised in other abdominal conditions, such as acute cholecystitis, perforated peptic ulcer and intestinal ischaemia, but very high levels (over three times the normal level) are diagnostic of pancreatitis. Full blood count, C-reactive protein (CRP), urea and electrolytes, liver biochemistry, plasma calcium and arterial blood gases are also measured on admission and after 24 and 48 hours. These are used to assess the severity of pancreatitis (Table 4.15).

- *Radiology:* An erect chest X-ray is performed to exclude perforated peptic ulcer as the cause of the pain and raised amylase. Abdominal US is performed as a screening test to look for gallstones as a cause of pancreatitis and may show swelling of the inflamed pancreas. A contrast-enhanced spiral CT scan or MRI is performed in all but the mildest attack of pancreatitis to confirm diagnosis, identify the presence and extent of pancreatic necrosis (associated with organ failure and higher mortality) and identify peripancreatic fluid collections. It is performed after 72 days, as early CT may underestimate the severity of pancreatitis.

Management

The management of acute pancreatitis is summarized in Fig. 4.9. Assessment of severity is essential; those predicted to have severe pancreatitis with a protracted course can then be managed in a high-dependency or intensive care unit with vigorous fluid resuscitation, correction of metabolic abnormalities and administration of therapies to improve outcome. Most attacks of pancreatitis are mild with only minimal or no pancreatic necrosis and without systemic complications. These patients usually recover within 5–7 days and need general supportive care only. In contrast, severe pancreatitis is

Table 4.15 Glasgow criteria for severity*

Age	>55 years
White blood cell count	$>15 \times 10^9$/L
Blood glucose	>10 mmol/L
Serum urea	>16 mmol/L
Serum albumin	<30 g/L
Serum aminotransferase	>200 U/L
Serum calcium	<2 mmol/L
Lactate dehydrogenase	<600 U/L
P_aO_2	<8.0 kPa (60 mmHg)

Three or more factors present during the first 48 hours predict a severe episode and a poor prognosis.

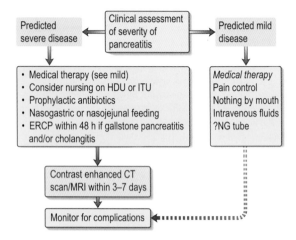

Fig. 4.9 The management of acute pancreatitis. ERCP, endoscopic retrograde cholangiopancreatography; HDU, high-dependency unit; ITU, intensive care unit; MRI, magnetic resonance imaging; NG, nasogastric.

associated with failure of one or more organ systems, such as renal or respiratory failure, and impaired coagulation with disseminated intravascular coagulation. Severe attacks are usually associated with pancreatic necrosis on CT scan. Several scoring systems are in use to predict those patients with severe pancreatitis: Glasgow criteria (Table 4.15), Ranson's criteria and the acute physiology and chronic health evaluation score (APACHE). Obesity and a CRP >200 mg/L in the first 4 days are also associated with a worse outcome.

General supportive care

Early fluid replacement is essential, and in severe pancreatitis 5 L or more of crystalloid daily may be required to maintain adequate urine output (>0.5 mL/kg body weight/hour). Supplemental oxygen is given and requirements are guided by pulse oximetry and arterial blood gases. Low molecular weight heparin is given for deep vein thrombosis prophylaxis. Electrolyte and metabolic abnormalities are corrected and a sliding scale of insulin may be necessary for good control of blood sugar levels. Pain is controlled by pethidine and tramadol and a patient-controlled system of administration is necessary if there is persistent pain. Morphine is avoided because it increases sphincter of Oddi pressure and may aggravate pancreatitis. In patients with a predicted severe episode, there is little likelihood of oral nutrition for a number of weeks. Nutrition is provided via a nasogastric tube or a naso-jejunal tube (placed endoscopically) for patients who are intolerant of nasogastric feeding due to exacerbation of pain or nausea and vomiting.

Therapies to reduce the severity or frequency of complications

Broad-spectrum antibiotics such as cefuroxime or aztreonam reduce the risk of infection of the necrotic pancreas and they are given from the outset. Early ERCP (within 48–72 hours) and sphincterotomy improves the outcome in patients with biliary pancreatitis, evidence of cholangitis or a high suspicion of a CBD stone (dilated CBD or CBD stone seen on US or jaundice). They can also be done when pancreatitis is predicted to be severe. Surgical treatment is sometimes required for very severe necrotizing pancreatitis, particularly if it is infected or complications such as pancreatic abscesses or pseudocysts occur.

Complications

Acute complications include hyperglycaemia, hypocalcaemia, renal failure and shock.

Chronic pancreatitis

Inappropriate activation of enzymes within the pancreas leads to precipitation of protein plugs within the duct lumen, forming a nidus for calcification. Subsequent duct blockage leads to ductal hypertension and further pancreatic damage. This together with cytokine activation leads to pancreatic inflammation, irreversible morphological change and/or permanent impairment of function. The commonest cause of chronic pancreatitis in most developed countries is excess alcohol. Other causes are tropical chronic pancreatitis, heredity, autoimmune causes and cystic fibrosis.

Clinical features

Epigastric abdominal pain, either intermittent or constant radiating through to the back, is the commonest symptom. There may be severe weight loss as a result of anorexia. Diabetes and steatorrhoea may develop due to endocrine (insulin) and exocrine (lipase) insufficiency. Occasionally, jaundice is the presenting symptom. This is due to obstruction of the CBD during its course through the fibrosed head of pancreas. The differential diagnosis is pancreatic carcinoma, which also presents with pain and weight loss and may develop on the backdrop of chronic pancreatitis. Carcinoma should be considered when there is a short history and localized ductal abnormalities on imaging.

Investigations

The diagnosis of chronic pancreatitis is made by imaging (to demonstrate structural changes in the gland) and metabolic studies which demonstrate functional abnormalities.

- *Radiology:* A plain abdominal X-ray will show pancreatic calcification in some cases. US and CT scan may show calcifications, ductal dilatation, irregular consistency, an outline of the gland and fluid collections. CT is a more sensitive test than US. MRCP and endoscopic US are sometimes used if the diagnosis is not confirmed with other imaging tests. ERCP is usually reserved for therapeutic (e.g. pancreatic stent placement) rather than diagnostic purposes.

- *Functional assessment:* These tests are insensitive in early pancreatic insufficiency. Faecal elastase, measured on a single, random stool sample, is reduced. Other tests rely on measuring decreased concentrations of the products of synthetic compounds such as fluorescein dilaurate (pancreolauryl) or N-benzoyl-L-tryosyl-p-amino benzoic acid (NBT-PABA). They appear in the urine after oral administration and intraluminal hydrolysis by pancreatic esterases and gut absorption. Serum amylase is not useful in the diagnosis of chronic pancreatitis but it may be raised during an acute episode of pain. A raised blood sugar indicates diabetes mellitus.

Treatment

The patient should be advised to stop taking alcohol. The pain may require opiates for control but they have an attendant risk of addiction. Surgical resection combined with drainage of the pancreatic duct into the small bowel (pancreaticojejunostomy) is of value for severe disease with intractable pain. Pancreatic strictures or stones are sometimes amenable to endoscopic treatment with ERCP. Persistent pseudocysts are drained endoscopically into the stomach or by surgical drainage. Pancreatic enzyme supplements are useful for those with steatorrhoea and may reduce the frequency of attacks of pain in those with recurrent symptoms. Diabetes requires appropriate treatment with diet, oral hypoglycaemics or insulin.

CARCINOMA OF THE PANCREAS

Epidemiology

Pancreatic cancer is the fifth most common cause of cancer death in the Western world. Men are affected more commonly than women, and the incidence increases with age, with most cases occurring in patients over 60 years. Most are adenocarcinomas of ductal origin.

Aetiology

Heredity (a dominant susceptibility gene in some families and other susceptibility genes in defined syndromes) and environmental factors (smoking and obesity in particular) both contribute. Chronic pancreatitis is also pre-malignant, particularly in patients with hereditary pancreatitis.

Clinical features

Cancer affecting the head of the pancreas or ampulla of Vater presents with painless jaundice as a result of obstruction of the common duct and weight loss. On examination, there is jaundice with characteristic scratch marks and a distended, palpable gall bladder (Courvoisier's law: if the gall bladder is palpable in a case of painless jaundice, it is not due to gallstones). In gallstone disease, chronic inflammation and fibrosis prevent distension of the gall bladder. There may be a central abdominal mass.

Cancer of the body or tail presents with abdominal pain, weight loss and anorexia. Diabetes may occur and there is an increased risk of thrombophlebitis. However, patients may also present with non-specific symptoms, e.g. an elderly patient with dyspepsia and change in bowel habit.

Investigations

Diagnosis is made by US (which demonstrates dilated bile ducts and a mass lesion) and/or contrast-enhanced spiral CT; the latter is a more sensitive test particularly for body and tail tumours and is almost always necessary to stage the cancer. MRI and endoscopic US is used for staging (endoscopic US) and for diagnosis in difficult cases. ERCP is usually restricted to palliative treatment (e.g. bile duct stenting in a jaundiced patient) but may provide a source for cytology in making the diagnosis. The tumour marker, CA19-9, is sensitive but not specific for diagnosis. Serial measurements are more frequently used to monitor response to treatment.

Management

Optimal management is by a multidisciplinary team approach with the involvement of the palliative care team for advanced disease, particularly to help with management of pain. Surgical resection offers the only hope of cure, but few patients have resectable disease at diagnosis. Tumour adherence or invasion into adjacent structures, particularly major blood vessels (locally advanced disease), makes complete resection difficult, and these patients are treated with combined chemotherapy and radiotherapy. Gemcitabine and 5-Fluorouracil improve survival in advanced disease. It also increases survival when used as an adjuvant therapy to pancreatic resection. Palliative treatment is often necessary to relieve obstructive jaundice (usually by endoscopic placement of a stent across the obstructed distal CBD), gastric outflow obstruction, and pain in patients with unresectable pancreatic cancer.

Prognosis

Overall, the prognosis is very poor. For the few patients who have had surgical resection with curative intent, the 3-year survival is 30–40%. The median survival for treated patients with locally advanced disease is 8–12 months, and for patients with metastatic disease it is 3–6 months.

Cancer of the bile ducts

Like pancreatic cancer, cholangiocarcinoma is also a disease of the elderly with a poor prognosis. It occurs more frequently in patients with primary sclerosing cholangitis, congenital bile duct abnormality and infections with liver flukes, e.g. *Clonorchis sinensis*. Presentation is usually with jaundice secondary to bile duct obstruction or with metastatic disease. Imaging by US, CT or MRI shows a bile duct stricture, a hilar mass or multiple metastases.

NEUROENDOCRINE TUMOURS OF THE PANCREAS

Islet cell tumours are rare and usually produce their clinical effects by secretion of hormones (Table 4.16). Non-functioning tumours present with pain and weight loss. Circulating hormone concentrations, e.g. gastrin, can be measured in the serum. High levels help to make the diagnosis. Most neuroendocrine tumours express large numbers of somatostatin receptors and radiolabelled somatostatin analogue scanning (^{111}In-labelled octreotide) provides a means of tumour localization. Endoscopic US is also used for tumour localization. Treatment is by excision of the primary tumour if possible. Symptomatic treatment (e.g. high-dose proton pump inhibitors for gastrinomas) and chemotherapy or hepatic artery embolization are used for patients with hepatic metastases.

Table 4.16 Clinical syndromes resulting from neuroendocrine tumours

Tumour	Secreted hormone	Symptoms	Symptom control
Gastrinoma (Zollinger–Ellison syndrome)	Gastrin	Duodenal ulceration – recurrent and severe Diarrhoea – hypersecretion of gastric acid inhibits digestive enzymes	High-dose proton pump inhibitors
VIPoma	Vasoactive intestinal polypeptide	Severe watery diarrhoea and hypokalaemia due to stimulation of intestinal water and electrolyte secretion	Octreotide
Glucagonoma	Glucagon	Migratory necrolytic dermatitis, weight loss, diabetes mellitus, deep venous thrombosis	Octreotide
Somatostatinoma	Somatostatin	Diabetes mellitus, gallstones, diarrhoea/steatorrhoea	Octreotide

5 Haematological disease

Blood consists of red cells, white cells, platelets and plasma. Plasma is the liquid component of blood which contains soluble fibrinogen and in which the other components are suspended. Serum is what remains after the formation of the fibrin clot.

Haemopoiesis is the formation of blood cells. The haemopoietic system includes the bone marrow, liver, spleen, lymph nodes and thymus. There is huge turnover of cells with the red cells surviving 120 days, platelets around 7 days but granulocytes only 7 hours. The bone marrow is the only source of blood cells during normal childhood and adult life. Pluripotent stem cells give rise to:

- Lymphoid stem cells, which give rise to pre-T cells (and then T suppressor, T helper and natural killer cells) and pre-B cells (and then B cells and plasma cells).
- Mixed myeloid progenitor cells (CFU_{GEMM}), which give rise to colony-forming units committed to the production of red cells, platelets, monocytes, neutrophils, eosinophils and basophils. Production is stimulated by growth factors such as erythropoietin (red cells), thrombopoietin (platelets), neutrophils (granulocyte colony stimulating factor [G-CSF]) and interleukin-5 (eosinophils). Other factors such as tumour necrosis factor (TNF) are inhibitory.

Reticulocytes are young red cells recently released from the bone marrow and still contain RNA. They are larger than mature red cells and normally represent 0.5–2.5% of total circulating red blood cells. The reticulocyte count gives a guide to the erythroid activity in the bone marrow and there is normally an increase with haemorrhage, haemolysis and after treatment with specific haematinics in deficiency states.

ANAEMIA

The principal function of haemoglobin (Hb) is to deliver oxygen to the tissues from the lungs. Hb is a tetramer consisting of two pairs of globin polypeptide chains. A haem group, consisting of a single molecule of protoporphyrin IX bound to a single ferrous ion (Fe^{2+}) is linked covalently at a specific site to each globin chain. Oxygenation and deoxygenation of Hb occur at the haem iron.

Anaemia is present when there is a decrease in the level of Hb in the blood below the reference range for the age and sex of the individual. Reduction of Hb is usually accompanied by a fall in red cell count (RCC) and packed cell volume (PCV, haematocrit), although an increase in plasma volume (as with massive splenomegaly) may cause anaemia with a normal RCC and PCV ('dilutional anaemia').

Table 5.1 Normal values for adult peripheral blood

	Male	Female
Hb (g/L)	135–175	115–160
PCV (haematocrit, L/L)	0.4–0.54	0.37–0.47
RCC (10^{12}/L)	4.5–6.0	3.9–5.0
MCV (fL)	80–96	
MCH (pg)	27–32	
MCHC (g/L)	320–360	
RDW (%)	11–15	
WCC (10^9/L)	4.0–11.0	
Platelets (10^9/L)	150–400	
ESR (mm/h)[9]	<20	
Reticulocytes	0.5–2.5% (50–100 × 109/L)	

ESR, erythrocyte sedimentation rate; Hb, haemoglobin; MCH, mean corpuscular haemoglobin; MCHC, mean corpuscular haemoglobin concentration; MCV, mean corpuscular volume of red cells; PCV, packed cell volume; RCC, red cell count; RDW, red blood cell distribution width (an increase indicates greater variation in red cell size with both large and small red cells); WCC, white cell count.

The normal values for these indices are given in Table 5.1, all of which are measured using automated cell counters as part of a routine full blood count (FBC). Anaemia should also be evaluated with the white blood cell and platelet counts, reticulocyte count (indicating marrow activity) and the blood film (abnormal red cell morphology may indicate the diagnosis).

Clinical features

Symptoms depend on the severity and speed of onset of anaemia. A very slowly falling level of Hb allows for haemodynamic compensation and enhancement of the oxygen-carrying capacity of the blood, and thus patients with anaemia may be asymptomatic. In general, elderly people tolerate anaemia less well than young people. The symptoms are non-specific and include fatigue, faintness and breathlessness. Angina pectoris and intermittent claudication may occur in those with coexistent atheromatous arterial disease. On examination the skin and mucous membranes are pale; there may be a tachycardia and a systolic flow murmur. Cardiac failure may occur in elderly people or those with compromised cardiac function.

Classification of anaemia (Table 5.2)

Anaemia is not a final diagnosis, and a cause should be sought. Causes are classified according to the measurement of red blood cell size (mean corpuscular volume [MCV]). This classification is useful because the type of anaemia

Table 5.2 Classification of the anaemias based on the mean corpuscular volume (MCV)

Small cells (microcytes) Low MCV (<80 fL)	Normal-sized cells Normal MCV	Large cells (macrocytes) High MCV (>96 fL)
Iron deficiency	Acute blood loss	Megaloblastic
Anaemia of chronic disease	Anaemia of chronic disease	Vitamin B_{12} deficiency
Thalassaemia	Combined deficiency, e.g. iron and folate	Folate deficiency
Sideroblastic anaemia	Marrow infiltration/ fibrosis	Normoblastic
	Endocrine disease	Alcohol
	Haemolytic anaemias	↑ Reticulocytes, e.g. haemorrhage, haemolysis
		Liver disease
		Hypothyroidism
		Drug therapy, e.g. azathioprine

indicates the underlying causes and necessary investigations. Irrespective of the cause, most patients with chronic anaemia do not require blood transfusion and the appropriate management, unless severely anaemic, is treatment of the underlying cause.

Microcytic anaemia

Microcytosis usually reflects a decreased Hb content within the red blood cell and is then often associated with a reduction in the mean corpuscular Hb (MCH) and mean corpuscular Hb concentration (MCHC), producing a hypochromic appearance on the blood film. The causes of microcytic anaemia are listed in Table 5.2: α- or β-thalassaemia minor (p. 212) is associated with a microcytosis usually in the absence of anaemia.

Iron deficiency

Iron is necessary for the formation of haem and iron deficiency is the most common cause of anaemia world-wide. The average daily diet in the UK contains 15–20 mg of iron, although normally only 10% of this is absorbed, mainly in the duodenum. Body iron content is regulated by alteration in intestinal iron absorption. Factors that promote intestinal absorption include gastric acid, iron deficiency and increased erythropoietic activity. Elimination of iron is fixed at 1 mg/day and occurs through shedding of skin and mucosal cells and excretion in sweat, urine and faeces. In women there is an additional loss during menses, and pre-menopausal women may often border on iron deficiency. There are two forms of dietary iron:

- Non-haem iron forms the main part of dietary iron and is derived from fortified cereals and vegetables. It is dissolved in the low pH of the stomach and reduced from the ferric to the ferrous form by a brush border ferrireductase before transportation across the mucosal cells.
- Haem iron is derived from Hb and myoglobin in red or organ meats. Haem iron is better absorbed than non-haem iron.

Iron is transported in the plasma bound to the protein transferrin, which is synthesized in the liver and normally about one-third saturated with iron (Fig. 5.1). Most of the body's iron content is incorporated into Hb in developing erythroid precursors and mature red cells. Most of the remaining body iron is stored as ferritin and haemosiderin in hepatocytes, skeletal muscle and reticuloendothelial macrophages.

Causes of iron deficiency

Causes of iron deficiency are:

- Blood loss
- Increased demands such as growth and pregnancy

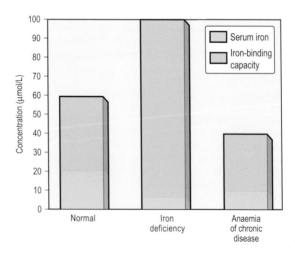

Fig. 5.1 Serum iron and total iron-binding capacity (transferrin) in normal subjects, iron deficiency anaemia and anaemia of chronic disease.

- Decreased absorption, e.g. small bowel disease or post-gastrectomy
- Poor intake; this is rare in developed countries.

Most iron deficiency is due to blood loss, usually from the uterus or gastrointestinal tract. On a world-wide basis, hookworm is a common cause of intestinal blood loss and iron deficiency. In women of childbearing age, menstrual blood loss, pregnancy and breast-feeding contribute to iron deficiency.

Clinical features

Symptoms and signs are the result of anaemia (p. 198) and of decreased epithelial cell iron, which causes brittle hair and nails, atrophic glossitis and angular stomatitis.

Investigations

- Blood count and film. The red cells are microcytic (MCV <80 fL) and hypochromic (MCH <27 pg). There is anisocytosis (variation in size) and poikilocytosis (variation in shape).
- Serum ferritin reflects iron stores and is low. However, ferritin is an acute-phase reactant, and in the presence of inflammatory or malignant disease, levels may be within the normal range in the presence of iron deficiency.
- Serum iron is low and the total iron-binding capacity (TIBC) is high, resulting in a transferrin saturation (serum iron divided by TIBC) $<19\%$ (Fig. 5.1).
- Serum soluble transferrin receptor number increases in iron deficiency.
- Bone marrow examination is generally unnecessary.

Iron deficiency is almost always the result of chronic, often occult, gastrointestinal blood loss in men and in post-menopausal women, and further investigation of the gastrointestinal tract is required to determine the cause of the blood loss (see p. 89). Iron deficiency anaemia in pre-menopausal women is usually the result of menstrual blood loss. In this group the only investigation necessary is serology for coeliac disease, and endoscopic investigation only if there are intestinal symptoms or a family history of colorectal cancer (two first-degree relatives or one <45 years of age).

Differential diagnosis

This is from other causes of a microcytic/hypochromic anaemia (Table 5.2). In thalassaemia, sideroblastic anaemia and anaemia of chronic disease, the iron stores are normal or increased.

Management

- Find and treat the underlying cause.
- Oral iron, e.g. ferrous sulphate or ferrous gluconate (p. 243). A response to iron treatment is characterized by an increase in the reticulocyte count

followed by an increase in Hb at a rate of about 10 g/L every week until the Hb concentration is normal.

- Parenteral iron (deep intramuscular or intravenous infusion) is rarely necessary and used only when patients are intolerant or there is a poor response to oral iron, e.g. severe malabsorption.

Sideroblastic anaemia

Sideroblastic anaemia is a rare disorder of haem synthesis characterized by a refractory anaemia with hypochromic cells in the peripheral blood and ring sideroblasts in the bone marrow. Ring sideroblasts are erythroblasts with iron deposited in mitochondria and reflect impaired utilization of iron delivered to the developing erythroblast. It may be inherited or acquired (secondary to myelodysplasia, alcohol excess, lead toxicity, isoniazid). Treatment is to withdraw the causative agents and some cases respond to pyridoxine (vitamin B_6).

Anaemia of chronic disease

This occurs in patients with chronic inflammatory diseases (such as Crohn's disease and rheumatoid arthritis), chronic infections (such as tuberculosis), malignancy and chronic kidney disease. There is a normochromic, normocytic or microcytic anaemia. Characteristic laboratory findings include low serum iron levels, low serum iron-binding capacity (Fig. 5.1) and increased or normal serum ferritin. The mechanisms responsible for these effects include decreased release of iron from bone marrow to developing erythroblasts, inadequate erythropoietin response to the anaemia and high levels of hepcidin expression. Hepcidin binds to the export transport protein, ferroportin, in the iron-absorbing cells in the duodenum, thereby causing its degradation, with a consequent reduction in the transport of iron from duodenal cells into the plasma. Treatment of anaemia of chronic disease is that of the underlying cause and sometimes recombinant erythropoietin (p. 398).

Macrocytic anaemia

Macrocytosis is a rise in mean cell volume of the red cells above the normal range. Macrocytic anaemia can be divided into megaloblastic and non-megaloblastic types, depending on the bone marrow findings. In practice, macrocytosis is usually investigated without performing a bone marrow examination. The initial investigation is measurement of serum B_{12} and red cell folate.

Megaloblastic anaemia

Megaloblastic anaemia is characterized by the presence in the bone marrow of developing red blood cells with delayed nuclear maturation relative to that of the cytoplasm *(megaloblasts)*. The underlying mechanism is defective DNA synthesis, which may also affect the white cells (causing hypersegmented neutrophil nuclei with six lobes, and sometimes leucopenia) and platelets (causing thrombocytopenia). The most common cause of megaloblastic anaemia is deficiency of vitamin B_{12} or folate, both of which are necessary for the synthesis of DNA (Table 5.2).

Vitamin B_{12} deficiency

Animal products (meat and dairy products) provide the only dietary source of vitamin B_{12} for humans. The daily requirement is 1 μg, which is easily supplied by a balanced Western diet (containing 5–30 μg daily). Vitamin B_{12} is liberated from protein complexes in food by gastric acid and pepsin and binds to a vitamin B_{12}-binding protein ('R' binder) derived from saliva. Free B_{12} is then released by pancreatic enzymes and becomes bound to intrinsic factor, which, along with H^+ ions, is secreted from gastric parietal cells. This complex is delivered to the terminal ileum, where vitamin B_{12} is absorbed and transported to the tissues by the carrier protein transcobalamin II. Vitamin B_{12} is stored in the liver, where there is sufficient supply for 2 or more years. About 1% of an oral dose of B_{12} is absorbed 'passively' without the need for intrinsic factor, mainly through the duodenum and ileum. The causes of vitamin B_{12} deficiency are listed in Table 5.3.

Pernicious anaemia

Pernicious anaemia is an autoimmune condition in which there is atrophic gastritis (plasma and lymphoid cell infiltration in the fundus) with loss of parietal cells and hence failure of intrinsic factor production and vitamin B_{12} malabsorption.

Table 5.3 Vitamin B_{12} deficiency – causes
Low dietary intake
Vegans
Impaired absorption
Stomach
Pernicious anaemia
Gastrectomy
Congenital deficiency of intrinsic factor
Small bowel
Ileal disease or resection, e.g. Crohn's disease
Coeliac disease
Tropical sprue
Bacterial overgrowth
Fish tapeworm *(Diphyllobothrium latum)*
Abnormal utilization
Congenital transcobalamin II deficiency (rare)
Nitrous oxide (inactivates B_{12})

There is also achlorhydria. It is the most common cause of vitamin B_{12} deficiency in adults in Western countries.

Epidemiology

This disease is common in elderly people and many cases are undiagnosed. It is more common in women and in people with fair hair and blue eyes. There is an association with other autoimmune diseases, particularly thyroid disease, Addison's disease and vitiligo.

Clinical features

The onset of pernicious anaemia is insidious, with progressively increasing symptoms of anaemia. There may be glossitis (a red sore tongue), angular stomatitis and mild jaundice caused by excess breakdown of Hb. Neurological features can occur with very low levels of serum B_{12} and include a polyneuropathy caused by symmetrical damage to the peripheral nerves and posterior and lateral columns of the spinal cord (subacute combined degeneration of the cord). The latter presents with progressive weakness, ataxia and eventually paraplegia if untreated. Dementia and visual disturbances due to optic atrophy may also occur. There is a higher incidence of gastric carcinoma with pernicious anaemia than in the general population.

Investigation of B_{12} deficiency

- Blood count and film. There is a macrocytic anaemia (MCV often >110 fL) with hypersegmented neutrophil nuclei and, in severe cases, leucopenia and thrombocytopenia.
- Serum vitamin B_{12} is low, frequently <50 ng/L (normal >160 ng/L).
- Red cell folate may be reduced because vitamin B_{12} is necessary to convert serum folate to the active intracellular form.
- Serum autoantibodies. Parietal cell antibodies (not specific) are present in 90% and intrinsic factor antibodies (specific to the diagnosis) in 50% of patients with pernicious anaemia.
- Serum bilirubin may be raised as a result of excess breakdown of Hb, due to ineffective erythropoiesis in the bone marrow.
- In most cases, the cause is apparent from the history and autoantibody screen. A small bowel barium follow-through (to look at the terminal ileum) and distal duodenal biopsies (to look for coeliac disease) may be necessary in some patients.
- Bone marrow examination shows a hypercellular bone marrow with megaloblastic changes. This is not necessary in straightforward cases.

Differential diagnosis

Vitamin B_{12} deficiency must be differentiated from other causes of megaloblastic anaemia, principally folate deficiency, but this is usually clear from the blood levels of these two vitamins. Pernicious anaemia should be distinguished from other causes of vitamin B_{12} deficiency (Table 5.3).

Management

Treatment is with intramuscular hydroxocobalamin (vitamin B_{12}, p. 244) or oral B_{12} 2 mg per day.

Folate deficiency

Folate is found in green vegetables and offal such as liver and kidney. It is absorbed in the upper small intestine. The daily requirement for folate is 100–200 µg and a normal mixed diet contains 200–300 µg. Body stores are sufficient for about 4 months, but folate deficiency may develop much more rapidly in patients who have a poor intake and excess utilization of folate, for example patients in intensive care. The main cause of folate deficiency is poor intake, which may occur alone or in combination with excessive utilization or malabsorption (Table 5.4).

Clinical features

Symptoms and signs are the result of anaemia. Unlike B_{12} deficiency, there is no neuropathy.

Investigations

Red cell folate is low (normal range 160–640 µg/mL) and is a more accurate guide to tissue folate than serum folate, which is also usually low (normal range 4.0–18 µg/L). If the history does not suggest dietary deficiency as the cause, further investigations such as endoscopic small bowel biopsy should be performed to look for small bowel disease.

Management

The underlying cause must be treated and folate deficiency corrected by giving oral folic acid 5 mg daily for 4 months (p. 243); higher daily doses may be necessary with malabsorption. In megaloblastic anaemia of

Table 5.4 Causes of folate deficiency	
Poor intake	Old age, poverty, alcohol excess (also impaired utilization), anorexia
Malabsorption	Coeliac disease, Crohn's disease, tropical sprue
Excess utilization	Physiological: pregnancy, lactation, prematurity
	Pathological: chronic haemolytic anaemia, malignant and inflammatory diseases, renal dialysis
Drugs	Phenytoin, trimethoprim, sulfasalazine, methotrexate

undetermined cause, folic acid alone must not be given, as this will aggravate the neuropathy of vitamin B_{12} deficiency. Prophylactic folic acid is given to patients with chronic haemolysis (5 mg weekly).

Prevention of neural tube defects with folic acid To prevent first occurrence of neural tube defects, women should be advised to take folate supplements (at least 400 µg/day) before conception and during pregnancy. Larger doses (5 mg daily) are recommended for mothers who already have an infant with a neural tube defect.

Differential diagnosis

A raised MCV with macrocytosis on the peripheral blood film can occur with a normoblastic rather than a megaloblastic bone marrow (Table 5.5). The most common cause of macrocytosis in the UK is alcohol excess. The exact mechanism for the large red cells in each of these conditions is uncertain, but in some it is thought to be due to altered or excessive lipid deposition on red cell membranes.

Anaemia caused by marrow failure (aplastic anaemia)

Aplastic anaemia is defined as *pancytopenia* (deficiency of all cell elements of the blood) with *hypocellularity* (aplasia) of the bone marrow. It is an uncommon but serious condition which may be inherited but is more commonly acquired. There is a reduction in the number of pluripotent stem cells together with a fault in those remaining or an immune reaction against them so that they are unable

Table 5.5 Causes of macrocytosis other than megaloblastic anaemia

Physiological
Pregnancy
Newborn

Pathological
Alcohol excess
Liver disease
Reticulocytosis (e.g. due to haemolysis)
Hypothyroidism
Haematological disorders:
Myelodysplastic syndrome
Sideroblastic anaemia
Aplastic anaemia
Drugs:
Hydroxycarbamide (hydroxyurea)
Azathioprine
Cold agglutinins

to repopulate the bone marrow. Failure of only one cell line may also occur, resulting in isolated deficiencies, e.g. red cell aplasia.

Aetiology

Aplastic anaemia can be induced by a variety of disorders (Table 5.6). Many drugs have been associated with the development of aplastic anaemia, and this occurs as a predictable dose-related effect (e.g. chemotherapeutic agents) or as an idiosyncratic reaction (e.g. chloramphenicol, phenytoin, non-steroidal anti-inflammatory agents).

Clinical features

Symptoms are the result of the deficiency of red blood cells, white blood cells and platelets, and include anaemia, increased susceptibility to infection and bleeding. Physical findings include bruising, bleeding gums and epistaxis. Mouth infections are common.

Investigations

- Blood count shows pancytopenia with low or absent reticulocytes.
- Bone marrow examination shows a hypocellular marrow with increased fat spaces.

Differential diagnosis

This is from other causes of pancytopenia (Table 5.7). A bone marrow trephine biopsy is essential for assessment of the bone marrow cellularity.

Management

Treatment includes withdrawal of the offending agent, supportive care and some form of definitive therapy (see later). Blood and platelet transfusions

---

Table 5.6 Causes of aplastic anaemia

Congenital, e.g. Fanconi's anaemia
Idiopathic acquired (67% of cases)
Cytotoxic drugs and radiation
Idiosyncratic drug reaction, e.g. phenytoin, carbamazepine, carbimazole, NSAIDs
Chemicals: benzene, insecticides
Infections, e.g. EBV, HIV, hepatitis, tuberculosis
Paroxysmal nocturnal haemoglobinuria
Miscellaneous, e.g. pregnancy

EBV, Epstein-Barr virus; HIV, human immunodeficiency virus; NSAIDs, non-steroidal anti-inflammatory drugs.

Table 5.7 Causes of pancytopenia

Aplastic anaemia (Table 5.6)
Drugs
Megaloblastic anaemia
Bone marrow infiltration or replacement: lymphoma, acute leukaemia,
   myeloma, secondary carcinoma, myelofibrosis
Hypersplenism
Systemic lupus erythematosus
Disseminated tuberculosis
Paroxysmal nocturnal haemoglobinuria
Overwhelming sepsis

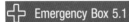

Emergency Box 5.1

Assessment and treatment of suspected neutropenic sepsis

Suspect neutropenic sepsis in a neutropenic patient (neutrophil count
$<1 \times 10^9$/L) who is pyrexial or has new-onset confusion, tachycardia,
hypotension, dyspnoea or hypothermia.

Assessment

- History and physical examination including mucous membranes, oropharynx
  (?thrush, erythema), surgical sites and intravenous lines

Investigations

- Bloods: Full blood count and differential white cell count, C-reactive protein,
  urea and electrolytes, liver biochemistry, clotting, blood cultures
- Radiology: Chest X-ray. Consider further imaging if localizing signs, e.g.
  computed tomography (CT) scan of abdomen and pelvis
- Microbiology: Microscopy and culture of peripheral blood (as above) and
  taken from central lines, sputum, urine, stool (if diarrhoea)

Antibiotics

- Seek expert help from microbiologist and oncologist
- Start empirical intravenous antibiotic treatment, e.g. piperacillin
  and aminoglycoside, to cover Gram-negative organisms and
  Pseudomonas
- Add vancomycin if clinical deterioration, fever persists or suspected
  methicillin-resistant *Staphylococcus aureus* (MRSA) infection
- Subsequent treatment is adjusted on the basis of cultured organisms and
  clinical progress
- Swap to oral antibiotics when apyrexial for 48 hours and continue for
  10–14 days

are used cautiously in patients who are candidates for bone marrow transplantation (BMT) to avoid sensitization. Patients with severe neutropenia (absolute neutrophil count <500 cells/μL) are at risk of serious infections with bacteria, fungi (e.g. *Candida* and aspergillosis) and viruses (herpesvirus). Fever in a neutropenic patient is a medical emergency (Emergency Box 5.1).

The course of aplastic anaemia is very variable, ranging from a rapid spontaneous remission to a persistent, increasingly severe pancytopenia, which may lead to death through haemorrhage or infection. Features that indicate a poor prognosis are neutrophil count $<0.5 \times 10^9$/L, platelet count $<20 \times 10^9$/L and a reticulocyte count of $<40 \times 10^9$/L.

In those patients who do not undergo spontaneous recovery the options for treatment are as follows:

- BMT from a human leucocyte antigen (HLA)-identical sibling donor is the treatment of choice for patients under 40 years of age.
- Immunosuppressive therapy with antilymphocyte globulin and ciclosporin is used for patients over the age of 40 years in whom BMT is not indicated because of the high risk of graft-versus-host disease.

HAEMOLYTIC ANAEMIA

Haemolytic anaemia results from increased destruction of red cells with a reduction of the circulating lifespan (normally 120 days). There is a compensatory increase in bone marrow activity with premature release of immature red cells (reticulocytes, p. 197).

Red cell destruction may be intravascular (within the blood vessels) but is more commonly extravascular (within the reticuloendothelial system, mainly the spleen). The causes of haemolytic anaemia in adults are listed in Table 5.8.

Intravascular haemolysis is suggested by

- **Raised levels of plasma Hb** as red cells are broken down.
- **Positive Schumm's test:** Hb appears in the plasma as the oxidized form, methaemoglobin, which dissociates into ferrihaem and globin. Binding of ferrihaem to albumin forms *methaemalbumin* and this can be detected in the plasma (Schumm's test).
- **Very low or absent haptoglobins:** Free Hb binds to plasma *haptoglobins;* the bound complex is rapidly removed by the liver, leading to low plasma haptoglobin levels.
- **Haemosiderinuria:** Unbound Hb appears in the urine as *haemoglobinuria*. Some Hb is broken down in the renal tubular cells and appears as *haemosiderin* in the urine.

Table 5.8 Causes of haemolytic anaemia

Inherited	Acquired
Red cell membrane defect	Immune
Hereditary spherocytosis	Autoantibodies
Hereditary elliptocytosis	Alloimmune
	Drug-induced antibodies
Hb abnormalities	
Thalassaemia	Non-immune
Sickle cell disease	Paroxysmal nocturnal haemoglobinuria
	Mechanical destruction: microangiopathic
Metabolic defects	Haemolytic anaemia, damaged artificial
G6PD deficiency	heart valves, march haemoglobinuria
Pyruvate kinase deficiency	Secondary to systemic disease, e.g. liver
Pyrimidine kinase	failure
deficiency	Infections, e.g. malaria
	Drugs/chemicals
	Hypersplenism

G6PD, glucose-6-phosphate dehydrogenase deficiency.

Fig. 5.2 shows an approach to investigating the patient with suspected haemolytic anaemia.

INHERITED HAEMOLYTIC ANAEMIAS

Inherited haemolytic anaemias are due to defects in one or more components of the mature red blood cell:

- Cell membrane
- Hb
- Metabolic machinery of the red blood cell.

Membrane defects

Hereditary spherocytosis

This is the most common inherited haemolytic anaemia in northern Europeans, and is inherited in an autosomal dominant manner. A defect in the red cell membrane causes an increased permeability to sodium; the red cells become spherical in shape, are more rigid and less deformable than normal red cells, and are destroyed prematurely in the spleen. The most common cause of

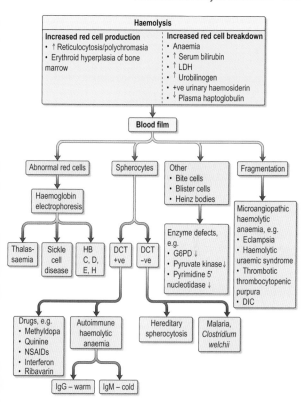

Fig. 5.2 An approach to investigation of suspected haemolytic anaemia. DCT, direct Coombs' test; DIC, disseminated intravascular coagulation; G6PD, glucose-6-phosphate dehydrogenase; IgG, immunoglobulin G; IgM, immunoglobulin M; LDH, lactate dehydrogenase; NSAIDs, non-steroidal anti-inflammatory drugs.

hereditary spherocytosis is a deficiency of the red cell structural membrane protein *spectrin*.

Clinical features

The clinical severity varies from symptom-free carrier to severe haemolysis with anaemia, jaundice and splenomegaly. As in many haemolytic anaemias, the course of the disease may be interrupted by aplastic, haemolytic and megaloblastic crises. Aplastic anaemia usually occurs after infections, particularly with erythro(parvo)virus, whereas megaloblastic anaemia is the result of folate depletion caused by hyperactivity of the bone marrow. Chronic haemolysis may lead to the development of pigment gallstones.

Investigations

- Blood count demonstrates reticulocytosis and anaemia, which is usually mild.
- The blood film shows spherocytes and reticulocytes.
- Haemolysis is evident (e.g. the serum bilirubin and urinary urobilinogen will be raised).

The diagnosis is usually straightforward and made on the basis of clinical features, family history, laboratory investigation (as above) and exclusion of other causes of haemolytic anaemia, particularly autoimmune haemolytic anaemia.

Management

Splenectomy is indicated in hereditary spherocytosis to relieve symptoms due to anaemia or splenomegaly. This is usually postponed until after childhood to minimize the risk of overwhelming infections (p. 226).

Hereditary elliptocytosis

Hereditary elliptocytosis is similar to spherocytosis, but the red cells are elliptical in shape. It is milder clinically and usually does not require splenectomy.

Haemoglobin abnormalities

Normal adult Hb is made up of haem and two polypeptide globin chains, α and β. The haemoglobinopathies can be classified into two subgroups: *abnormal chain production* or *abnormal chain structure* of the polypeptide chains (Table 5.9).

Thalassaemia

In normal Hb there is balanced (1 : 1) production of α and β chains. The thalassaemias are a group of disorders arising from one or multiple gene defects, resulting in a reduced rate of production of one or more globin chains. The imbalanced globin chain production leads to precipitation of globin chains within red cells or precursors. This results in cell damage, death of red cell precursors in the bone marrow (ineffective erythropoiesis) and haemolysis. The thalassaemias affect people throughout the world. There are two main types:

- α-Thalassaemia: reduced α chain synthesis
- β-Thalassaemia: reduced β chain synthesis.

β-Thalassaemia In homozygous β-thalassaemia there is little or no β chain production, resulting in excess α chains. These combine with whatever

Table 5.9 Types of haemoglobin

	Hb	Structure	Comment
Normal	A	$\alpha_2\beta_2$	97% of adult haemoglobin (Hb)
	A_2	$\alpha_2\delta_2$	2% of adult Hb; elevated in β-thalassaemia
	F	$\alpha_2\gamma_2$	Normal Hb in foetus from 3rd to 9th month; increased in β-thalassaemia
Abnormal chain production	H	β_4	Found in α-thalassaemia, biologically useless
	Barts	γ_4	Found in α-thalassaemia, biologically useless
Abnormal chain structure	S	$\alpha_2\beta_2$	Substitution of valine for glutamic acid in position 6 of β chain
	C	$\alpha_2\beta_2$	Substitution of lysine for glutamic acid in position 6 of β chain

δ and γ chains are produced, leading to increased Hb A_2 and Hb F. There are three main clinical forms of β-thalassaemia:

- *β-Thalassaemia minor (trait)*. This is the asymptomatic heterozygous carrier state. Anaemia is mild or absent, with a low MCV and MCH. Iron stores and serum ferritin levels are normal.
- *β-Thalassaemia intermedia*. This includes patients with moderate anaemia (Hb 70–100 g/L) that does not require regular blood transfusions. Splenomegaly, bone deformities, recurrent leg ulcers and gallstones are other features. This may be caused by a combination of homozygous β- and α-thalassaemias.
- *β-Thalassaemia major (homozygous β-thalassaemia)*. This presents in the first year of life with severe anaemia *(Cooley's anaemia),* failure to thrive and recurrent infections. Hypertrophy of the ineffective bone marrow leads to bony abnormalities: the thalassaemic facies, with an enlarged maxilla and prominent frontal and parietal bones. Resumption of haemopoiesis in the spleen and liver (extramedullary haemopoiesis), the chief sites of red cell production in fetal life, leads to hepatosplenomegaly.

Investigations

In homozygous disease, blood count and film show a hypochromic/microcytic anaemia, raised reticulocyte count and nucleated red cells in the peripheral circulation.

The diagnosis is made by Hb electrophoresis, which shows an increase in Hb F and absent or markedly reduced Hb A.

Management

In homozygous patients, the mainstay of treatment is blood transfusion, aiming to keep the Hb above 100 g/L, thus suppressing ineffective erythropoiesis, preventing bony abnormalities and allowing normal development. Long-term folic acid supplements are required. Iron overload caused by repeated blood transfusions may lead to damage of the endocrine glands, liver, pancreas and heart, with death in the second decade from cardiac failure. Treatment with iron-chelating agents (subcutaneous desferrioxamine, oral deferasirox or deferiprone) decreases iron loading. Ascorbic acid 200 mg daily is also given as it increases the urinary excretion of iron in response to desferrioxamine. BMT has been used in some cases of thalassaemia.

α-Thalassaemia The clinical manifestations of this disorder vary from a mild anaemia with microcytosis to a severe condition incompatible with life. There are four α-globin genes per cell. The manifestations depend on whether one, two, three or all four of the genes are deleted, and thus whether a chain synthesis is partial or completely absent. In the most severe form, where there is complete absence of α-globin (Hb Barts), infants are stillborn (hydrops fetalis).

Sickle syndromes

Sickle syndromes are a family of haemoglobin disorders in which the sickle β-globin gene is inherited (Table 5.9). The sickle β gene is spread widely throughout Africa (25% carry the gene), India, the Middle East and Mediterranean countries. In the homozygous state *(sickle cell anaemia)* both genes are abnormal (Hb SS), whereas in the heterozygous state *(sickle cell trait,* Hb AS) only one chromosome carries the abnormal gene. Inheritance of the *HbS* gene from one parent and *HbC* from the other parent gives rise to Hb SC disease, which tends to run a milder clinical course than sickle cell disease but with more thromboses.

In the deoxygenated state Hb S molecules are insoluble and polymerize. This results in increased rigidity of the red cells, causing the classic sickle appearance (Fig. 5.3). Sickling can produce:

- Premature destruction of red cells (haemolysis)
- Obstruction of the microcirculation (vaso-occlusion), leading to tissue infarction.

Sickling is precipitated by hypoxia, dehydration, infection, acidosis and cold.

Sickle cell anaemia

Clinical features

As the production of Hb F is normal, the disease is usually not manifest until Hb F decreases to adult levels at about 6 months of age. There is extreme

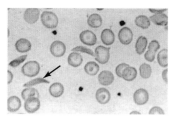

Fig. 5.3 Sickle cells (arrowed) and target cells ('Mexican hat cells').

phenotypic variation, with some patients having few or no symptoms and others having recurrent crises and a markedly reduced life expectancy.

Vaso-occlusion In early childhood, acute pain in the hands and feet (dactylitis) is due to occlusion of the small vessels and avascular necrosis of bone marrow. In adults, bone pain most commonly affects the long bones, ribs, spine and pelvis. The frequency of attacks varies from daily to perhaps once a year.

Anaemia Most patients have a steady-state Hb of 60–80 g/L with a high reticulocyte count (10–20%). They often do not have symptoms of anaemia because Hb S releases oxygen to the tissues more easily than normal Hb. A rapid fall in the Hb can occur due to:

- Splenic sequestration. The spleen becomes engorged with red cells, leading to an acute fall in Hb and rapid enlargement of the spleen. Liver sequestration can also occur.
- Bone marrow aplasia most commonly due to erythrovirus B19 infection, which destroys erythrocyte precursors
- Further haemolysis due to drugs or acute infection.

Long-term problems Avascular necrosis of bones results in shortened, deformed bones in children. Other complications of vaso-occlusion include splenic atrophy (resulting in susceptibility to infection with pneumococcus, *Salmonella* species and *Haemophilus*), retinal ischaemia (which may precipitate proliferative sickle retinopathy and visual loss) and cerebral infarction (causing fits and strokes). Transcranial Doppler ultrasound measures mean velocity of blood flow in the large intracranial vessels and is used to screen for patients at high risk of stroke and offer them prophylactic transfusion. Sequestration of red cells within the corpora cavernosa causes priapism (prolonged painful erections) and eventual impotence. Chronic haemolysis is associated with increased formation of pigment gallstones. Other complications of sickle cell disease include chronic kidney disease, leg ulcers, osteomyelitis, pulmonary hypertension and acute chest syndrome. Acute chest syndrome is a medical emergency and is characterized by fever, cough, dyspnoea and pulmonary infiltrates on the chest X-ray. It is caused by infection, fat embolism from necrotic bone marrow or pulmonary infarction due to sequestration of sickle cells.

Investigations

Sickle cell disease is diagnosed by screening in the neonate (using cord blood or the heel prick test), in the fetus of at-risk couples through prenatal diagnosis and in children and adults from high-risk areas before undergoing surgery. In Africa many patients are still diagnosed only when they present with complications.

- Blood count. Hb (60–80 g/L) is low with a high reticulocyte count.
- Blood film shows sickled erythrocytes (Fig. 5.3).

Diagnosis is made with Hb electrophoresis showing 80–95% Hb SS and absent Hb A. In addition, sickling can be induced in vitro with sodium dithionite.

Management

Precipitating factors should be avoided or treated promptly. Transfusions are not routinely given in steady-state anaemia. Folic acid is given to all patients with haemolysis. Pneumococcal and influenza vaccination is given routinely and daily penicillin, 500 mg orally.

Most patients with a painful crisis are managed in the community, but hospital admission is necessary when the pain is not controlled by non-opiate analgesia such as paracetamol and non-steroidal anti-inflammatory drugs, or if there are complications (Table 5.10). Many patients carry cards with details of their ideal analgesic regimen. The management of a painful sickle crisis is summarized in Emergency Box 5.2.

Blood transfusions are given only in certain situations including after transient ischaemic attacks and stroke, acute chest syndrome, splenic sequestration crisis and aplastic crises, as well as before elective operation and during pregnancy.

Table 5.10 Complications of sickle cell anaemia requiring inpatient management

Pain – uncontrolled by non-opiate analgesia
Swollen painful joints
Acute sickle chest syndrome or pneumonia
Mesenteric sickling and bowel ischaemia
Splenic or hepatic sequestration
Central nervous system deficit
Cholecystitis (pigment stones)
Cardiac arrhythmias
Renal papillary necrosis resulting in colic or severe haematuria
Hyphema (layer of red cells in anterior chamber of eye) or retinal detachment
Priapism

✚ Emergency Box 5.2

Management of an acute painful sickle cell crisis in opioid-naïve adults

- **Analgesia**
  - Morphine 0.1 mg/kg i.v./subcutaneously (s.c.) every 20 minutes until pain controlled, then 0.05–0.1 mg/kg i.v./s.c./p.o. every 2–4 hours. Consider patient-controlled analgesia (PCA).
  - Give adjuvant non-opioid analgesia: paracetamol, ibuprofen, diclofenac.
- **Prescribe** laxatives routinely and other adjuvants as necessary:
  - Laxatives: lactulose 10 mL twice daily, senna two to four tablets daily
  - Anti-pruritics: hydroxyzine 25 mg twice daily
  - Antiemetics: cyclizine 50 mg three times daily
  - Anxiolytic: haloperidol 1–3 mg oral/intramuscularly (i.m.) as required
  - Antibiotics: e.g. cefotaxime and clarithromycin in acute chest syndrome.
- **Oxygen,** 60% by face mask if arterial oxygen saturation <95%
- **Rehydration,** encourage oral fluids 60 mL/kg/24 hours. Give i.v. or nasogastric fluids if insufficient intake orally
- **Investigations** in all patients: full blood count, reticulocyte count, urea and electrolytes – repeat daily. In others, depending on clinical circumstances: liver biochemistry, blood and urine cultures, chest X-ray, arterial blood gases (if saturations <95%), ultrasound of abdomen
- **Monitor** pain, sedation, vital signs, respiratory rate and oxygen saturations every 30 minutes until the pain is controlled and stable and then every 2 hours
- **Examine** daily: the respiratory system for the acute chest syndrome, and the abdomen for increase in liver or spleen size which may indicate a sequestration crisis

Hydroxycarbamide (hydroxyurea) raises the concentration of fetal Hb and is used in some patients with recurrent painful crises. BMT from a HLA-matched sibling is used in some patients with severe disease.

Sickle cell trait

In the heterozygous state, Hb AS, the blood count and film are normal. There are usually no symptoms unless there are extreme circumstances leading to hypoxia, such as flying in a non-pressurized aircraft.

Metabolic red cell disorders

A number of red cell enzyme deficiencies may produce haemolytic anaemia, the most common of which is glucose-6-phosphate dehydrogenase (G6PD) deficiency.

Glucose-6-phosphate dehydrogenase deficiency

G6PD is a vital enzyme in the hexose monophosphate shunt, which maintains glutathione in the reduced state. Glutathione protects against oxidant injury in the red cell. G6PD deficiency is a common heterogeneous X-linked trait found predominantly in African, Mediterranean and Middle Eastern populations.

G6PD deficiency causes neonatal jaundice, chronic haemolytic anaemia and acute haemolysis precipitated by the ingestion of fava beans and a number of common drugs such as quinine, sulphonamides, quinolones and nitrofurantoin. Diagnosis is by direct measurement of enzyme levels in the red cell. Treatment involves the avoidance of precipitating factors, and transfusion if necessary.

ACQUIRED HAEMOLYTIC ANAEMIA

Autoimmune haemolytic anaemia

Acquired haemolytic anaemia is due to immunological destruction of red blood cells mediated by autoantibodies directed against antigens on the patient's red blood cells. Autoimmune haemolytic anaemia is classified according to whether the antibody reacts best at body temperature *(warm antibodies)* or at lower temperatures *(cold antibodies)* (Table 5.11). Immunoglobulin (Ig) G or IgM

Table 5.11 Features of autoimmune haemolytic anaemia

	Warm	Cold
Temperature at which antibody attaches best to red cell	37°C	Lower than 37°C
Type of antibody	IgG	IgM
Direct Coombs' test	Strongly positive	Positive
Primary condition	Idiopathic	Idiopathic
Secondary causes	Autoimmune disorders, e.g. SLE	Infections, e.g. *Mycoplasma* spp. Infectious mononucleosis
	Lymphomas	Lymphomas
	CLL	Paroxysmal cold
	Carcinomas	Haemoglobinuria (rare)
	Many drugs, e.g. methyldopa	

CLL, chronic lymphocytic leukaemia; IgG, immunoglobulin G; IgM, immunoglobulin M; SLE, systemic lupus erythematosus.

antibodies attach to the red cell, resulting in extravascular haemolysis through sequestration in the spleen, or in intravascular haemolysis through activation of complement. The autoimmune haemolytic anaemias are diagnosed on the basis of a positive direct antiglobulin (Coombs') test. This is a test for antibodies or complement attached to the surface of red blood cells. The red blood cells of the patient are reacted with antiserum or monoclonal antibodies prepared against the various immunoglobulins and the third component of complement (C3d). If either or both of these are present on the red cell surface, agglutination of red cells will be detected.

'Warm' autoimmune haemolytic anaemia

Clinical features

This anaemia occurs at all ages in both sexes, with a variable clinical picture ranging from mild haemolysis to life-threatening anaemia. It may be primary or secondary (Table 5.11).

Investigation

There is evidence of haemolysis (p. 209) and direct Coombs' test is positive.

Management

High-dose steroids (e.g. prednisolone 1 mg/kg daily) induce remission in 80% of cases. Splenectomy is useful in those failing to respond to steroids. Occasionally, immunosuppressive drugs such as azathioprine and rituximab are beneficial.

'Cold' autoimmune haemolytic anaemia

Clinical features

IgM antibodies (cold agglutinins) attach to red cells in the cold peripheral parts of the body and cause agglutination and complement-mediated intravascular haemolysis. After certain infections (e.g. *Mycoplasma*, Epstein–Barr virus), there is increased synthesis of cold agglutinins (normally produced in insignificant amounts) and transient haemolysis. A chronic idiopathic form occurs in elderly people, with recurrent haemolysis and peripheral cyanosis.

Investigation

There is evidence of haemolysis (p. 209), and direct Coombs' test is positive. Examination of a peripheral blood film at room temperature shows red cell agglutination.

Management

Treatment is usually that of the underlying condition and avoiding exposure to cold.

Drug-induced haemolysis

Two types of mechanisms have been identified:

- In the most common form, the drug may associate with structures on the red cell membrane and thus be part of the antigen in a haptenic reaction. There is severe complement-mediated intravascular haemolysis which resolves quickly after drug withdrawal.
- The drug may induce a subtle alteration of one component of the red cell membrane, rendering it antigenic. There is extravascular haemolysis and a protracted clinical course.

The mechanisms for drug-induced haemolytic anaemia probably also apply to drug-induced thrombocytopenia and neutropenia.

Non-immune haemolytic anaemia

Paroxysmal nocturnal haemoglobinuria

There is an inability to produce the glycosylphosphatidylinositol (GPI) anchor, which tethers several proteins to the cell membrane. Deficiency of two of these proteins, CD59 (membrane inhibitor of reactive lysis) and CD55 (decay-accelerating factor), renders the red cell exquisitely sensitive to the haemolytic action of complement. The clinical manifestations of this rare disease are related to abnormalities in haemopoietic function, including intravascular haemolysis, venous thrombosis and bone marrow aplasia. Haemoglobinuria typically manifests as dark urine at night and in the morning on waking. Progression to myelodysplasia and acute leukaemia can also occur. Paroxysmal nocturnal haemoglobinuria should be considered in any patient with chronic or episodic haemolysis. Diagnosis is made by demonstrating deficiency of the GPI-anchored proteins on haematopoietic cells by flow cytometry. Treatment is supportive (e.g. with blood transfusions) and with eculizumab, a monoclonal antibody that binds to the C5 component of complement, prevents its activation and reduces haemolysis. BMT has been successful in selected patients.

Mechanical haemolytic anaemia

Red cells may be injured by physical trauma in the circulation. Examples of this form of haemolysis include:

- Leaking prosthetic heart valves: damage to red cells in their passage through the heart
- March haemoglobinuria: damage to red cells in the feet from prolonged marching
- Microangiopathic haemolysis: fragmentation of red cells in abnormal microcirculation caused by malignant hypertension, haemolytic-uraemic syndrome or disseminated intravascular coagulation (DIC).

MYELOPROLIFERATIVE DISORDERS

In these disorders there is uncontrolled clonal proliferation of one or more of the cell lines in the bone marrow, namely erythroid, myeloid and megakaryocyte lines. Myeloproliferative disorders include polycythaemia vera, essential thrombocythaemia, myelofibrosis (all of which have a mutation of the gene Janus kinase 2, *JAK-2*) and chronic myeloid leukaemia. These disorders are grouped together as there can be transition from one disease to another; for example, polycythaemia vera can lead to myelofibrosis, and they may also transform into acute leukaemia. They occur principally in middle-aged and elderly people. They differ from the acute leukaemias (also clonal proliferation of a single cell line), where the cells also do not differentiate normally but where there is progressive accumulation of immature cells.

Polycythaemia

Polycythaemia is defined as an increase in Hb, PCV and RCC. These measurements are all concentrations and are therefore directly dependent on plasma volume as well as red blood cell mass. The production of red cells by the bone marrow is normally regulated by the hormone erythropoietin, which is produced in the kidney. The stimulus for erythropoietin production is tissue hypoxia.

In *absolute polycythaemia* there is an increase in the red cell mass. Primary polycythaemia is due to an acquired or inherited mutation leading to an abnormality within red blood progenitors. It includes polycythaemia vera and rare familial variants. Secondary polycythaemia is caused by an erythropoietin response to chronic hypoxia or by an erythropoietin-secreting tumour (Fig. 5.4).

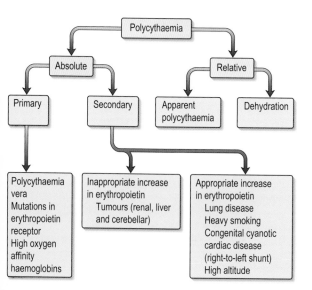

Fig. 5.4 The causes of polycythaemia.

Relative or apparent polycythaemia (Gaisböck's syndrome) occurs in middle-aged obese men and is associated with smoking, increased alcohol intake and hypertension. The PCV is normal but plasma volume is decreased.

Polycythaemia vera

Polycythaemia vera arises from a single haematopoietic progenitor cell and leads to excessive proliferation of red cells and a variable increase in platelets and myeloid cells. *JAK-2* mutations, present in over 95% of patients, lead to constitutive activation of its tyrosine kinase activity, which plays a pivotal role in cell proliferation and survival.

Clinical features

Symptoms and signs are the result of hypervolaemia and hyperviscosity. Typical symptoms include headache, vertigo, tinnitus, visual disturbance, angina pectoris, intermittent claudication, pruritus and venous thrombosis. Physical signs include a plethoric complexion and hepatosplenomegaly as a result of extramedullary haemopoiesis. Splenomegaly, if present, reliably distinguishes polycythaemia vera from secondary polycythaemia. There is an increased risk of haemorrhage as a result of friable haemostatic plugs, and an increased risk of gout caused by increased cell turnover and uric acid production.

Investigations

A blood count showing raised white cell and platelet counts is suggestive of polycythaemia vera as opposed to other causes of polycythaemia. The diagnosis is made by demonstrating evidence of increased red cell volume (Hb >185 g/L in men and >165 g/L in women) and a gain of function mutation in *JAK-2* (e.g. V617F) with at least one of:

- Erythroid hyperplasia, with increased numbers of megakaryocytes and granulocytes on bone marrow examination
- Serum erythropoietin levels below normal
- Erythroid colony formation in vitro in the absence of exogenous erythropoietin.

Management

There is no cure, and treatment is given to maintain a normal blood count and to prevent the complications of the disease, particularly thrombosis and haemorrhage.

- Venesection to maintain PCV <0.45 L/L. Regular venesection (e.g. 3-monthly) may be all that is needed in many patients.
- Chemotherapy. Hydroxycarbamide (hydroxyurea) and busulfan are used to reduce the platelet count. Subcutaneous α-interferon injections are also effective.
- Low-dose aspirin with the above treatments is used for patients with recurrent thrombotic episodes.

- ***Anagrelide*** inhibits megakaryocyte differentiation and is useful for thrombolysis.
- Radioactive phosphorus (^{32}P) is only given to patients over 70 years of age because of the increased risk of leukaemic conversion with its use.
- Allopurinol is given to decrease uric acid levels.

Secondary polycythaemia

Secondary polycythaemia presents with similar clinical features to primary polycythaemia, although the white cell and platelet counts are usually normal and the spleen is not enlarged. In patients with tumours the primary disease must be treated to lower the level of erythropoietin. In hypoxic patients, oxygen therapy (p. 520) may reduce the Hb, and a small-volume phlebotomy (400 mL) may help those with severe symptoms. Smokers should be advised to stop smoking.

Essential thrombocythaemia

Patients have normal Hb levels and white cell count but elevated platelet count. Platelet size and function are abnormal, and presentation may be with bleeding or thrombosis. Differential diagnosis is from secondary causes of a raised platelet count and other myeloproliferative disorders (Table 5.12). There is no global gold standard diagnostic test but, in general, an otherwise well person with a platelet count of $>1000 \times 10^9$/L will have essential thrombocythaemia. Busulfan, hydroxycarbamide (hydroxyurea), anagrelide or interferon alfa are used to reduce platelet production.

Table 5.12 Differential diagnosis of a raised platelet count

Reactive thrombocytosis
Autoimmune rheumatic disorders
Chronic infections
Inflammatory bowel disease
Malignancy
Haemorrhage
Surgery
Splenectomy and functional hyposplenism
Primary thrombocythaemia
Polycythaemia vera
Myelofibrosis
Myelodysplasia

Myelofibrosis (myelosclerosis)

Myelofibrosis is characterized by haemopoietic stem cell proliferation associated with marrow fibrosis (abnormal megakaryocyte precursors release fibroblast-stimulating factors, such as platelet-derived growth factor).

Clinical features

There is an insidious onset of weakness, weight loss and lethargy. Bleeding occurs in the thrombocytopenic patient. There is hepatomegaly and massive splenomegaly caused by extramedullary haemopoiesis. The most common causes of death are transformation to acute myeloid leukaemia, progression of myelofibrosis, cardiovascular disease and infection.

Investigations

- Blood count shows anaemia. The white cell and platelet counts are high initially, but fall with disease progression as a result of marrow fibrosis.
- Blood film examination shows a leucoerythroblastic picture (immature red cells caused by marrow infiltration) and 'teardrop'-shaped red cells.
- Bone marrow is usually unobtainable by aspiration ('dry tap'); trephine biopsy shows increased fibrosis.
- The Philadelphia chromosome is absent; this and the bone marrow appearance helps to distinguish myelofibrosis from chronic myeloid leukaemia, which may present similarly.
- *JAK2 mutation* is present in approximately half of the cases.

Management

- Transfusions are given for anaemia and allopurinol to decrease serum uric acid levels.
- Historically, symptomatic splenomegaly was managed using hydroxycarbamide, busulfan, radiotherapy or splenectomy. However, splenectomy is associated with significant morbidity and mortality in myelofibrosis and the other treatments are largely ineffective.
- A promising development is the targeted therapy with JAK inhibitors. Ruxolitinib results in substantial spleen reduction, improved life expectancy and reduction in symptoms.
- Allogeneic stem cell transplantation may offer hope of a cure for younger patients.

Myelodysplasia

Myelodysplasia is a group of acquired bone marrow disorders caused by a defect in stem cells. There is progressive bone marrow failure, which may evolve into acute myeloid leukaemia. The myelodysplastic syndromes are predominantly diseases of the elderly, and may be diagnosed on a routine full blood count or when patients present with anaemia, infection or bleeding due to pancytopenia. The diagnosis is made on the basis of characteristic blood film and bone marrow appearances. The paradox of peripheral pancytopenia and a hypercellular bone marrow reflects premature cell loss by apoptosis.

Supportive treatment (red cell and platelet transfusions) is given to elderly patients with symptomatic disease. For younger patients, intensive chemotherapy (as used for acute myeloblastic leukaemia) or allogeneic BMT are used. Lenalidomide (a thalidomide analogue) is used in the treatment of early-stage disease.

THE SPLEEN

The spleen, situated in the left hypochondrium, is the largest lymphoid organ in the body. Its main functions are phagocytosis of old red blood cells, immunological defence and to act as a 'pool' of blood from which cells may be rapidly mobilized. Pluripotent stem cells are present in the spleen and proliferate in severe haematological stress *(extramedullary haemopoiesis)*, e.g. haemolytic anaemia.

Splenomegaly

Causes of splenomegaly are given in Table 5.13. The spleen is only palpable once it has almost doubled in size. Splenomegaly may cause hypersplenism,

Table 5.13 Causes of splenomegaly

Massive (extending into right iliac fossa)	Moderate
Chronic myeloid leukaemia	Lymphoma
Myelofibrosis	Leukaemia
Chronic malaria	Myeloproliferative disorders
Kala-azar	Haemolytic anaemia
Gaucher's disease (rarely)	Acute infection, e.g. endocarditis, typhoid
	Chronic infection, e.g. tuberculosis, brucellosis
	Parasitic, e.g. malaria
	Rheumatoid arthritis
	Sarcoidosis
	Systemic lupus erythematosus
	Storage diseases, e.g. Gaucher's
	Tropical splenomegaly

which results in pancytopenia, increased plasma volume and haemolysis. Splenectomy is performed mainly for:

- Trauma
- Idiopathic thrombocytopenic purpura
- Haemolytic anaemias
- Hypersplenism.

Complications after splenectomy are an increased platelet count (thrombophilia) in the short term and overwhelming infection in the long term, particularly with *Streptococcus pneumoniae*, *H. influenzae* and the meningococci. Pneumoccocal, *Haemophilus*, meningococcal group C and influenza vaccination is given before elective splenectomy. Meningococcal polysaccharide vaccine is given for travellers to Africa and Saudi Arabia. In addition, the patient is given lifelong penicillin V 500 mg twice daily or erythromycin if they are allergic to penicillin.

BLOOD TRANSFUSION

The components of whole blood are prepared by differential centrifugation of blood collected from volunteer donors.

- Blood components, such as red cell and platelet concentrates, fresh frozen plasma (FFP) and cryoprecipitate, are prepared from single donors.
- Blood components such as coagulation factor concentrates, albumin and immunoglobulin are prepared using plasma from many donors as the starting material.

Whole blood is rarely used, even for acute blood loss. Use of the required component is a more effective use of a scarce resource.

Red cell concentrates The plasma is removed from whole blood and replaced with an additive solution. Storage is at 4°C with a shelf-life of 35 days and transfusion should be completed within 4 hours of removal from cold storage. Red cell concentrates are used for acute bleeds in combination with crystalloid or colloid and correction of anaemia. Transfusion of red cells in addition to colloid is usually only necessary when >30% (>1500 mL in an adult) of circulating volume has been lost. This degree of blood loss is manifest by reduced systolic and diastolic blood pressure, pulse rate >120/min, slow capillary refill and respiratory rate >20/min. The patient will be pale and may be anxious and aggressive. Transfusion may be required for lesser degrees of blood loss that are superimposed on a pre-existing anaemia or reduced cardiorespiratory reserve capacity. Transfusion of red cells is rarely necessary for correction of chronic anaemia (where the underlying cause should be treated) unless the anaemia is severe and life-threatening.

Platelet concentrates are stored at between +20°C and +24°C. Cold storage causes irreversible platelet aggregation. Platelets are used to treat or prevent bleeding in patients with severe thrombocytopenia. They are not used in stable chronic thrombocytopenia without bleeding. For platelet transfusion, the

ABO and RhD group of the patient must be known and the same bedside checks and monitoring procedures as for red cell transfusion must be used. Usually 1 unit (250 mL of plasma containing $>40 \times 10^9$/L platelets) is given, and the platelet count should rise by $>20 \times 10^9$/L.

Fresh frozen plasma is separated from blood cells and frozen for storage. It contains all the coagulation factors and is used in acquired coagulation factor deficiencies.

Cryoprecipitate is the supernatant obtained after thawing of FFP at 4°C. It contains factor VIII : C, von Willebrand factor (vWF) and fibrinogen and is used in DIC where the fibrinogen level is very low (<1.0 g/L).

Factor VIII and IX concentrates are used for the treatment of haemophilia and von Willebrand disease where recombinant factor concentrates are unavailable.

Albumin (4.5% and 20%) are given to patients with acute severe hypoalbuminaemia and to patients with liver disease and nephrotic syndrome (20% solution) who are fluid overloaded and resistant to diuretics.

Immunoglobulins are used in patients with hypogammaglobulinaemia to prevent infection and in patients with idiopathic thrombocytopenic purpura. Specific immunoglobulin, e.g. anti-hepatitis B, is used after exposure of a non-immune patient to infections.

Blood groups

The blood groups are determined by antigens on the surface of red cells. The ABO and rhesus (Rh) systems are the two major blood groups. In the ABO groups, individuals produce antibodies against the antigen that are not present on their own red cells (Table 5.14). If red cells carrying A or B antigens are transfused to someone who has antibodies to these then a severe immune reaction will occur leading to shock and DIC (p. 238), which may be fatal within minutes to hours. Patients with blood group AB can receive blood of any other ABO group and are known as universal recipients. Most of the population carry RhD antigens (Rh + ve) on their red cells and they can receive any RhD type blood. RhD –ve patients should receive RhD –ve blood. Exposure to RhD + ve blood through transfusion or pregnancy will lead to development of anti-D.

Table 5.14 The ABO system: antigens and antibodies

Blood group	Red cell antigen	Antibody in patient's plasma
A	A	Anti-B
B	B	Anti-A
AB	AB	No antibodies to A or B
O	No A or B	Anti-A and anti-B

Blood groups O and A are the most common in the UK.

Procedure for blood transfusion

Compatibility testing is performed by the transfusion service in order to select donor blood of the correct ABO and Rh group for the recipient and to screen the patient's serum or plasma for antibodies against other red cell antigens (such as Kell and Duffy) that may cause a transfusion reaction. After a massive bleed when immediate transfusion is necessary, O RhD −ve blood can be given without any transfusion investigations being undertaken. It should need to be used only on rare occasions.

Many hospitals have guidelines for the ordering of blood for elective surgery. Operations in which blood is required only occasionally can be classified as 'group and save', in order to conserve blood usage. In this case, ABO and Rh testing is performed along with the antibody screen. Should blood unexpectedly be required during the course of the procedure, compatible units can be released within a matter of minutes after an immediate spin cross-match, whereby the patient's serum or plasma is incubated with the donor red cells to confirm compatibility.

Blood transfusion is a potentially hazardous procedure, which should only be undertaken when the benefits outweigh the risks. Stringent procedures need to be followed to ensure that the correct blood is given to the correct patient and that any adverse reactions are dealt with promptly and efficiently (Table 5.15). The temperature, pulse rate and blood pressure should be recorded before the start of each unit, 15 minutes after the start and at hourly intervals during the transfusion. A temperature rise of 1°C or greater above baseline may indicate an acute haemolytic transfusion reaction due to blood group incompatibility and is an indication to stop the transfusion.

Complications of transfusing red blood cells

- ABO incompatibility is the most serious complication. It usually results from simple clerical errors, leading to the incorrect labelling and identification of the correct patient receiving the correct blood at the correct time. Within minutes of starting the transfusion there is pyrexia, rigors, dyspnoea, hypotension, loin and back pain. Intravascular haemolysis leads to dark urine. The transfusion must be stopped and the donor units returned to the blood transfusion laboratory for testing with a new blood sample from the patient. Emergency treatment may be needed to maintain the blood pressure (p. 578). Autoimmune haemolysis may develop about a week after transfusion in patients alloimmunized by previous transfusions in whom the antibody level is too low to be detected during compatibility testing.

- Febrile reactions are usually the result of anti-leucocyte antibodies in the recipient acting against transfused leucocytes, leading to the release of pyrogens. These reactions are less common since the introduction of leucocyte-depleted blood.

Table 5.15 Care of the patient receiving a blood transfusion or blood products

1 Taking the blood sample for cross-matching

Identify patient positively by asking their surname, forename, date of birth

Confirm ID details on hospital wrist band match those on transfusion request form

Label sample tube after blood has been added

Label sample tube with patient identification (full name, date of birth, hospital number), patient location, date of sample and signature of person taking blood

2 Procedure for patient identification before transfusion

Check the blood bag is not leaking or wet and has a compatibility label attached

Check patient identity (full name, sex, date of birth, hospital number) matches that on the blood transfusion request form and compatibility label attached to the blood pack. This is now usually done by a handheld computer reading a barcode on the patient's wristband and the compatibility label and ensuring a match.

Check intravenous fluid prescription chart

3 Blood checks

Check expiry date of the blood on compatibility label and blood bag

Check blood group and blood pack donation number on blood transfusion request form, blood pack and compatibility label

Record the blood pack donation number on intravenous fluid prescription chart

Date, time and signature on blood transfusion request form, compatibility label, intravenous fluid prescription chart

- Anaphylactic reactions are seen in patients lacking IgA but who produce anti-IgA that reacts with IgA in the transfused blood. This is a medical emergency (p. 576). Urticarial reactions are treated by slowing of the infusion and giving intravenous antihistamines, e.g. chlorphenamine (chlorpheniramine) 10 mg intravenously (i.v.).

- Transmission of infection has decreased now that donated blood is tested for hepatitis B surface antigen and antibodies to hepatitis C, human immunodeficiency virus (HIV)-1 and human T-cell lymphotropic virus (HTLV)-1. Cytomegalovirus (CMV)-seronegative blood is given to immunosuppressed patients who are susceptible to acquiring CMV infection.

- Heart failure may occur, particularly in elderly people and those having large transfusions.

- Complications of massive transfusion (>10 units within 24 hours) include hypocalcaemia, hyperkalaemia and hypothermia. Bleeding may occur as a result of depletion of platelets and clotting factors in stored blood.

- Post-transfusion purpura is rare. Antibodies develop against the human platelet antigen 1a, leading to immune destruction of the patient's own platelets and thrombocytopenia 2–12 days after a blood transfusion.

Concerns about the safety of blood transfusion have led to increased interest in strategies for avoiding or reducing the use of donor blood. These include artificial Hb solutions and autologous blood transfusion. The latter is more popular in developing countries and involves collection of blood from the donor/patient either pre-operatively or by intraoperative blood salvage.

THE WHITE CELL

The five types of leucocytes (white cells) found in peripheral blood are neutrophils, eosinophils and basophils (which are all called granulocytes) and lymphocytes and monocytes. *Leucocytosis* and *leucopenia* describe an increase ($>11 \times 10^9$/L) and a decrease ($<4.0 \times 10^9$/L), respectively, in the total circulating white cells.

Neutrophils

The prime function of neutrophils is to ingest and kill bacteria, fungi and damaged cells.

Neutrophil leucocytosis ($>10 \times 10^9$/L) occurs in bacterial infection, tissue necrosis, inflammation, corticosteroid therapy, myeloproliferative disease, acute haemorrhage, haemolysis, leukaemoid reaction (excessive leucocytosis characterized by the presence of immature cells in the peripheral blood) and leucoerythroblastic anaemia (immature red and white cells appear in the peripheral blood in marrow infiltration, e.g. malignancy, myeloid leukaemia, severe anaemia). A 'left shift' describes the presence of immature white cells (promyelocytes, myelocytes and metamyelocytes) in the peripheral blood and occurs with infection and in leukoerythroblastic anaemia.

Neutropenia is a decrease in circulating neutrophils in the peripheral blood ($<1.5 \times 10^9$/L). Causes include race (in black Africans), viral infection, severe bacterial infection, megaloblastic anaemia, pancytopenia, drugs (marrow aplasia or immune destruction) and inherited abnormalities. An absolute neutrophil count of $<0.5 \times 10^9$/L is regarded as severe neutropenia and may be associated with life-threatening infections. The management of neutropenic sepsis is summarized in Emergency Box 5.1.

Monocytes

Monocytes are precursors of tissue macrophages. Monocytosis (normal range 0.04–0.44 $\times 10^9$/L, 1–6% of total white cells) occurs in chronic bacterial infections (e.g. tuberculosis), myelodysplasia and malignancy, particularly chronic myelomonocytic leukaemia.

Eosinophils

Eosinophils play a part in allergic responses and in the defence against infections with helminths and protozoa. Eosinophilia (normal range 0.04–0.44×10^9/L, 1–6% of total white cells) occurs in asthma and allergic disorders, parasitic infections (e.g. *Ascaris*), skin disorders (urticaria, pemphigus and eczema), malignancy and the hyper-eosinophilic syndrome (restrictive cardiomyopathy hepato-splenomegaly and very high eosinophil count).

Lymphocytes

There are two types: T and B lymphocytes. Lymphocytosis occurs in response to viral infection, chronic infections (e.g. tuberculosis and toxoplasmosis), chronic lymphocytic leukaemia and some lymphomas.

HAEMOSTASIS AND THROMBOSIS

A bleeding disorder is suggested when the patient has unexplained (i.e. no history of trauma) bruising or bleeding, or prolonged bleeding in response to injury or surgery, e.g. after tooth extraction.

Haemostasis

Haemostasis is the process of blood clot formation at the site of vessel injury. When a blood vessel wall breaks, the haemostatic response must be quick, localized to the site of injury, and carefully regulated. Abnormal bleeding or a propensity to non-physiological thrombosis (i.e. thrombosis not required for haemostatic regulation) may occur when specific elements of these processes are missing or dysfunctional.

Haemostasis is a complex process and depends on interactions between the vessel wall, platelets and coagulation and fibrinolytic mechanisms.

- *Vessel wall* Platelet adhesion and thrombus formation is inhibited on the intact endothelium by its negative charge and also by antithrombotic factors (thrombomodulin, heparin sulphate, prostacyclin, nitric oxide, plasminogen activator). Injury to vessels leads to immediate vasoconstriction, thus reducing blood flow to the injured area, and endothelial damage results in loss of antithrombotic properties.
- *Platelets* Intimal injury and exposure of subendothelial elements leads to *platelet adherence*, via the platelet membrane receptor glycoprotein (Gp) Ib, to collagen and vWF in the subendothelial matrix. GpIIb/IIIa receptor on the platelet surface is then exposed forming a second binding site for vWF. Deficiency of GpIb or vWF leads to congenital bleeding disorders: Bernard–Soulier disease and von Willebrand's disease, respectively. Following adhesion, platelets spread along the subendothelium and *release*

the contents of their cytoplasmic granules containing adenosine diphosphate (ADP), serotonin, thromboxane A_2, fibrinogen and other factors. ADP leads to a conformational change in the GpIIb/IIIa receptor allowing it to bind to fibrinogen, a dimer that acts as a bridge between platelets and so binds them into aggregates *(platelet aggregation)*. During aggregation, platelet membrane receptors are exposed, providing a surface for the interaction of coagulation factors and ultimately the formation of a stable haemostatic plug.

• *Coagulation* Coagulation involves a series of enzymatic reactions leading to the conversion of soluble plasma fibrinogen to fibrin clot (Fig. 5.5). The local generation of fibrin enmeshes and reinforces the platelet plug. Coagulation is initiated by tissue damage. This exposes tissue factor (TF) which binds to factor VII and this complex has the dual effect of converting factor X to factor Xa ('a' indicates active) and factor IX to factor IXa. Generation of factor Xa alone is insufficient to allow haemostasis to proceed to completion. Factor VIII consists of a molecule with coagulant activity (VIII : C) associated with vWF, which prevents premature breakdown of VIII : C. Factor VIII increases the activity of factor IXa by about 200 000-fold. All of the coagulation factors

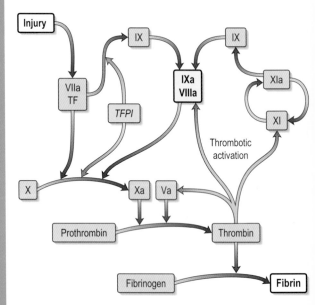

Fig. 5.5 Coagulation mechanism. The in vivo pathway begins with the activation of factor X by the complex formed by factor VIIa and tissue factor. Factor XI is activated by thrombin. TF, tissue factor; TFPI, tissue factor pathway inhibitor.

are synthesized in the liver and vWF is synthesized by endothelial cells and megakaryocytes. The vitamin K-dependent enzymes are prothrombin and factors VII, IX and X.

- *Physiological limitation of coagulation* Coagulation would lead to dangerous occlusion of blood vessels if it was not limited to the site of injury by protective mechanisms. Antithrombin binds to and forms complexes with coagulation factors, thereby inactivating them. Its activity is increased by heparin. Activated protein C inactivates factors V and VIII and this is enhanced by the cofactor, protein S. Inherited deficiency or abnormality of these natural anticoagulant proteins is termed *thrombophilia* and places the patient at increased risk of venous thromboembolism (p. 240).

- *Fibrinolysis* Fibrinolysis is a normal haemostatic response that helps to restore vessel patency after vascular damage. The plasma protein plasminogen is converted to plasmin by activators (principally tissue plasminogen activator, tPA) released from endothelial cells. Plasmin breaks down fibrin and fibrinogen into fragments collectively known as fibrin degradation products (FDPs), which include D-dimers.

Bleeding disorders are therefore the result of a defect in vessels, platelets or the coagulation pathway (Table 5.16).

Table 5.16 Classification of bleeding disorders

Blood vessel defect

Hereditary
    Hereditary haemorrhagic telangiectasia
    Connective tissue disorders, e.g. Marfan's, Ehlers–Danlos syndromes
Acquired
    Severe infections, e.g. meningococcal, typhoid
    Drugs: steroids, sulphonamides
    Allergic: Henoch–Schönlein purpura, autoimmune rheumatic disorders
    Others: scurvy, senile purpura, easy bruising syndrome

Platelet defect

Thrombocytopenia (Table 5.17)
Platelet dysfunction
    Inherited, e.g. Bernard–Soulier syndrome
    Acquired: renal and liver disease, paraproteinaemias, platelet inhibitory drugs,
      e.g. aspirin

Coagulation defect

Hereditary: haemophilia A or B, von Willebrand's disease
Acquired: anticoagulant treatment, liver disease, disseminated intravascular
    coagulation

Investigation of bleeding disorders

The nature of the defect and therefore the most appropriate initial investigations may be suggested by the history and examination, e.g. family history, intercurrent disease, alcohol consumption, drugs.

Vascular/platelet bleeding is characterized by bruising of the skin and bleeding from mucosal membranes. Bleeding into the skin is manifest as petechiae (small capillary haemorrhages, a few millimetres in diameter) and superficial ecchymoses (larger areas of bleeding).

Coagulation disorders (e.g. haemophilia A and B) are typically associated with bleeding after injury or surgery, spontaneous haemarthroses (bleeding into joints) and muscle haematomas. The most common cause of abnormal bleeding is thrombocytopenia.

- Platelet count and blood film will show the number and morphology of platelets and any blood disorder such as leukaemia.
- Coagulation tests are abnormal with deficiencies or inhibitors of the clotting factors. If the abnormal result is corrected by the addition of normal plasma to the patient's plasma in the assay, then the result is abnormal as a result of deficiency and not of inhibitors.
  - The prothrombin time (PT) is prolonged with abnormalities of factors VII, X, V, II or I, liver disease, or if the patient is on warfarin. The international normalized ratio (INR) is the ratio of the patient's PT to a normal control when using the international reference preparation. The advantage of the INR over the PT is that it uses international standards and thus anticoagulant control in different hospitals across the world can be compared.
  - The activated partial thromboplastin time (APTT) is prolonged with deficiencies or inhibitors of one or more of the following factors: XII, XI, IX, VIII, X, V or I (but not factor VII). Heparin prolongs the APTT.
  - Thrombin time (TT) is prolonged with fibrinogen deficiency, dysfibrinogenaemia (normal levels but abnormal function), heparin treatment or DIC.
- The normal ranges of these tests vary from laboratory to laboratory.
- The bleeding time is a measure of the interaction of platelets with the blood vessel wall and is abnormal in von Willebrand's disease, in blood vessel defects, and when there is a decrease in the number or function of platelets.

These tests will localize the site of the problem. Further specialized investigations (e.g. platelet aggregation studies and measurement of fibrinogen, FDPs and individual clotting factors), will be necessary to identify the exact haemostatic defect correctly.

Platelet disorders

Platelet disorders are the result of thrombocytopenia (platelet count $<150 \times 10^9$/L; Table 5.17) or disorders of platelet function, e.g. those occurring with aspirin treatment and uraemia. Congenital abnormalities of platelet number (e.g. Fanconi's anaemia, Wiskott–Aldrich syndrome) or function (e.g. Bernard–Soulier syndrome) are all extremely rare.

Mild thrombocytopenia can be artefactual and due to platelet clumping or a blood clot in the sample. This is excluded by asking the haematologist to confirm an unexpectedly low count by manual differentiation. Spontaneous bleeding from skin and mucous membranes is unlikely to occur with platelet counts above 20×10^9/L. Increased destruction or decreased production can be differentiated by bone marrow examination, which will show, respectively, increased or decreased numbers of megakaryocytes (platelet precursors). Platelet transfusion is usually indicated when the platelet count is very low ($<10 \times 10^9$/L) or to maintain a platelet count of $>50 \times 10^9$/L in the presence of active bleeding or prior to an invasive procedure.

Table 5.17 Causes of thrombocytopenia

Impaired production	Excessive destruction
Bone marrow failure	Immune
Megaloblastic anaemia	Autoimmune – ITP
Leukaemia	Secondary immune (SLE, CLL, viruses, drugs, e.g. heparin)
Myeloma	Post-transfusion purpura
Myelofibrosis	Other
Myelodysplasia	Disseminated intravascular coagulation
Solid tumour infiltration	Thrombotic thrombocytopenic purpura
Aplastic anaemia (Table 5.6)	Haemolytic uraemic syndrome
HIV infection	Sequestration
	Hypersplenism
	Dilutional
	Massive transfusion

CLL, chronic lymphocytic leukaemia; ITP, immune thrombocytopenic purpura; SLE, systemic lupus erythematosus.
Thrombocytopenia due to impaired production is selective megakaryocyte depression (drugs, chemicals) or more often also associated with failure of red and white cell production.

Immune thrombocytopenic purpura (ITP)

There is immune destruction of platelets.

- *ITP in children* often follows viral infection. There is rapid onset of purpura, which is usually self-limiting.
- *ITP in adults* is usually less acute than in children and is characteristically seen in young women. It may occur with other autoimmune disorders, e.g. systemic lupus erythematosus and thyroid disease, in patients with chronic lymphatic leukaemia and after infection with some viruses, e.g. HIV. There is a fluctuating course, with easy bruising, epistaxis and menorrhagia. Major haemorrhage is rare.

Investigation

There is thrombocytopenia with normal or increased megakaryocytes on bone marrow examination. The detection of platelet autoantibodies (present in 60–70%) is not essential for diagnosis, which often depends on exclusion of other causes of excessive destruction of platelets.

Management

Patients with platelet counts greater than 30×10^9/L require no treatment unless they are about to undergo a surgical procedure. Platelet transfusions are reserved for intracranial or other extreme haemorrhage.

First-line therapy Oral corticosteroids 1 mg/kg body weight produces a response in two-thirds of patients but relapse is common when the dose is reduced. Intravenous immunoglobulin (i.v. IgG) is useful where a rapid rise in platelet count is desired, especially before surgery.

Second-line therapy is splenectomy, to which the majority of patients respond. In cases where splenectomy is not successful, possible treatments include high-dose corticosteroids, i.v. IgG and immunosuppressive agents such as rituximab. Thrombopoietin receptor agonists, such as romiplostim and eltrombopag, drive increased platelet production and may be used in refractory ITP.

Thrombotic thrombocytopenic purpura (TTP)

Widespread adhesion and aggregation of platelets lead to microvascular thrombosis and profound thrombocytopenia. This occurs due to deficiency of ADAMTS 13, a protease which is normally responsible for degradation of vWF. ADAMTS 13 deficiency is congenital, sporadic or autoantibody mediated (pregnancy, systemic lupus erythematosus, infection, drug treatment [e.g. clopidogrel]). There is florid purpura, fever, fluctuating cerebral dysfunction and haemolytic anaemia with red cell fragmentation, often accompanied by renal failure. The coagulation screen is usually normal but lactate dehydrogenase levels are markedly raised as a result of haemolysis. Treatment is with plasma exchange (to remove the antibody to ADAMTS 13), methylprednisolone and rituximab. Platelet concentrates are contraindicated.

Inherited coagulation disorders

Inherited disorders usually involve a deficiency of only one coagulation factor, whereas acquired disorders involve a deficiency of several factors.

Haemophilia A

This is the result of a deficiency of factor VIII (p. 232). It is inherited as an X-linked recessive, affecting 1 in 5000 males.

Clinical features

Clinical features depend on the plasma levels of factor VIII.

- *Levels < 1 IU/dL* (severe disease) are associated with frequent spontaneous bleeding into muscles and joints that can lead to a crippling arthropathy.
- *Levels 1–5 IU/dL* are associated with severe bleeding following injury and occasional apparently spontaneous episodes.
- *Levels >5 IU/dL* produce mild disease with bleeding only with trauma or surgery.

Cerebral haemorrhage is much more frequent than in the general population.

Investigations

There is a prolonged APTT and reduced plasma level of factor VIII. The PT, bleeding time and vWF are normal.

Management

- Intravenous infusion of recombinant factor VIII concentrate is the treatment of choice and is used in preference to plasma-derived concentrates where possible. It is given as prophylaxis, e.g. before and after surgery, or to treat an acute bleeding episode. Patients with severe haemophilia are given prophylaxis three times weekly from early childhood to prevent permanent joint damage. Many patients also have a supply of factor VIII concentrate at home to inject at the first sign of bleeding.
- Synthetic vasopressin (desmopressin) – intravenous, subcutaneous or intranasal administration – raises the level of factor VIII and is used to treat some patients with mild haemophilia.
- Patients should be vaccinated against hepatitis A and B and encouraged to take part in exercise regimens that avoid contact sport.

Complications

Recurrent bleeding into joints leads to deformity and arthritis. The risk of infection (hepatitis C and HIV) from multiple transfusions of plasma-derived clotting factor concentrates has been virtually eliminated because of the exclusion of high-risk blood donors, screening of donors and heat treatment of factor VIII concentrates. Ten per cent of people with haemophilia develop antibodies to factor VIII, and may need massive doses to overcome this. Recombinant factor VIIa is also used to 'bypass' the inhibitor.

Haemophilia B (Christmas disease)

This is the result of a deficiency of factor IX, and affects 1 in 30 000 males. Inheritance and clinical features are the same as for haemophilia A. Treatment is with factor IX concentrates. Desmopressin is ineffective.

von Willebrand's disease

vWF contributes to platelet adhesion to damaged subendothelium and stabilization of factor VIII in plasma. Deficiency of vWF leads to defective platelet function (p. 228) and factor VIII deficiency (p. 232).

Clinical features

Types 1 and 2 are mild forms, with autosomal dominant inheritance, and characterized by mucosal bleeding (nose bleeds and gastrointestinal bleeding) and prolonged bleeding after dental treatment or surgery.

Type 3 patients (recessively inherited) have more severe bleeding, but rarely experience the joint and muscle bleeds seen in haemophilia A.

Investigations

Prolonged bleeding time reflects a defect in platelet adhesion. There is a prolonged APTT, normal PT and decreased plasma levels of VIII : C and vWF.

Management

This depends on the severity of the bleeding, and includes treatment with desmopressin and factor VIII concentrates, which contain vWF.

Acquired coagulation disorders

Vitamin K deficiency

Vitamin K is needed for the formation of active factors II, VII, IX and X. Deficiency occurs with malnutrition, malabsorption and with warfarin treatment (an inhibitor of vitamin K synthesis). There is an increase in PT and APTT. Treatment is with phytomenadione (vitamin K, p. 244).

Disseminated intravascular coagulation (DIC)

DIC involves widespread generation of fibrin within blood vessels, caused by initiation of the coagulation pathway. Consumption of platelets and coagulation factors occurs, as well as secondary activation of fibrinolysis, leading to production of FDPs, which contribute to bleeding by inhibiting fibrin polymerization.

Aetiology

DIC results from massive activation of the clotting cascade. The major initiating factors are the release or expression of tissue factor, extensive damage to vascular endothelium exposing tissue factor or enhanced expression of tissue factor by monocytes in response to cytokines. The most common causes are sepsis, major trauma and tissue destruction (surgery, burns), advanced cancer and obstetric complications (amniotic fluid embolism, abruptio placentae). DIC occurs in most cases of acute promyelocytic leukaemia due to generation of procoagulant substances in the blood.

Clinical features

The presentation varies from no bleeding at all to complete haemostatic failure, with bleeding from venepuncture sites and the nose and mouth. Thrombotic events may occur as a result of vessel occlusion by platelets and fibrin.

Investigations

The diagnosis is suggested by the history (e.g. severe sepsis, trauma, malignancy), the clinical presentation and the presence of severe thrombocytopenia. It is confirmed by finding a prolonged PT, APTT and TT, decreased fibrinogen and elevated FDPs. The blood film shows fragmented red cells. In mild cases with compensatory increase of coagulation factors, the only abnormality may be an increase in the FDPs, or in the D-dimer fragment reflecting accelerated fibrinolysis.

Management

- Treat the underlying condition.
- Platelets concentrates (to maintain count $>50 \times 10^9$/L), FFP, cryoprecipitate and red cell concentrates are indicated in patients who are bleeding.

Liver disease

Liver disease results in a number of defects of haemostasis: vitamin K deficiency in cholestasis, reduced synthesis of clotting factors, thrombocytopenia and functional abnormalities of platelets. DIC may occur in acute liver failure.

THROMBOSIS

A thrombus is defined as a solid mass formed in the circulation from the constituents of the blood during life. Fragments of thrombi (emboli) may break off and block vessels downstream.

Arterial thrombosis

Arterial thrombosis is usually the result of atheroma, which forms particularly in areas of turbulent blood flow, such as the bifurcation of arteries. Platelets adhere to the damaged vascular endothelium and aggregate in response to ADP and thromboxane A_2. This may stimulate blood coagulation, leading to complete occlusion of the vessel, or embolization resulting in distal obstruction. Arterial emboli may also form in the left ventricle after myocardial infarction, in the left atrium in mitral valve disease, or on the surface of prosthetic valves.

Prevention

Prevention of arterial thrombosis is achieved by minimizing risk factors associated with atherosclerosis (p. 446) and with antiplatelet drugs.

- Aspirin (p. 245) irreversibly inhibits cyclo-oxygenase, reducing platelet production of thromboxane A_2 (p. 232). It is the most commonly used antiplatelet drug.
- Dipyridamole inhibits phosphodiesterase-mediated breakdown of cyclic AMP, which prevents platelet activation.
- Clopidogrel (p. 245) and prasugrel block platelet aggregation and prolong platelet survival by inhibiting the binding of ADP to its platelet receptor.
- Antibodies (e.g. abciximab), peptides (e.g. eptifibatide) and non-peptide antagonists (e.g. tirofiban) block the receptor of GpIIb/IIIa, inhibiting the final common pathway of platelet aggregation (p. 232). They are used as an adjunct in invasive coronary artery intervention and as primary medical therapy in coronary artery disease. Excessive bleeding has been a problem.
- Epoprostenol is a prostacyclin which is used to inhibit platelet aggregation during renal dialysis (with or without heparin) and is also used in primary pulmonary hypertension.

Treatment

Treatment is with thrombolytic therapy (p. 251). Streptokinase is a purified fraction of the filtrate obtained from cultures of haemolytic streptococci. It forms a complex with plasminogen, which activates other plasminogen molecules to form plasmin. Tissue-type plasminogen activators such as alteplase (t-PA), tenecteplase (TNK-PA) and reteplase (r-PA) are produced using recombinant gene technology. Unlike streptokinase, they are not antigenic and do not produce allergic reactions, though they have a slightly higher risk of intracerebral haemorrhage. The use of thrombolytic therapy in myocardial infarction, pulmonary embolism and ischaemic stroke is discussed on pages 455, 476, and 751, respectively.

Venous thrombosis

Unlike arterial thrombosis, venous thrombosis usually occurs in normal vessels, often in the deep veins of the leg. It originates around the valves as red thrombi consisting of red cells and fibrin. Propagation occurs, inducing a risk of embolization to the pulmonary vessels. Chronic venous obstruction in the leg results in a permanently swollen leg which is prone to ulceration (post-phlebitic syndrome). Heparin (p. 247) and warfarin (p. 248) are the two drugs used most frequently in the prevention and treatment of thromboembolism.

Prevention

About 25 000 people in the UK die from preventable, hospital-acquired venous thromboembolism every year. All patients should be assessed on admission to hospital for their risk of developing venous thromboembolism. Prophylactic measures include early mobilization, leg elevation and compression stockings. Thromboprophylaxis with low molecular weight heparin (LMWH) is indicated in medical inpatients (i.e. non-surgical) with any of the risk factors listed in Table 5.18. Recent long-distance, sedentary travel is an additional risk factor to consider in outpatients presenting with suspected venous thromboembolism. Prophylaxis of venous thromboembolism in surgical patients depends on the type of surgery and other risk factors (Table 5.18). Patients undergoing minor surgery (anaesthetic <60 min) with no risk factors for venous thrombosis are not usually given LMWH. Patients undergoing major surgery (anaesthetic >60 min) but without risk factors for venous thrombosis or patients undergoing minor surgery but with risk factors are at moderate risk and should receive LMWH (20 mg, p. 247). Patients undergoing major surgery and with risk factors are at high risk and should receive LWMH (40 mg).

Treatment

Clinical features and investigation of deep venous thrombosis (DVT) and pulmonary embolism (PE) are discussed on pages 488 and 473, respectively.

Table 5.18 Risk factors for venous thromboembolism in hospital inpatients

Age >60 years
One or more significant medical comorbidities, e.g. heart disease, respiratory failure, acute infectious disease
Obesity (body mass index >30 kg/m^2)
Major abdominal/pelvic surgery
Active cancer
Pregnancy
Use of oestrogen containing contraceptive/hormone replacement therapy
Significant immobility
Varicose veins with phlebitis
Hyperosmolar hyperglycaemic states (p. 680)
Personal history or first-degree relative with a history of venous thromboembolism
Thrombophilia (p. 233)
Inflammatory bowel disease
Nephrotic syndrome

Treatment of established thromboembolism

- Obtain objective evidence of thrombosis as soon as possible; heparin treatment is often started on the basis of clinical suspicion.
- Perform a coagulation screen and platelet count before starting treatment to exclude a pre-existing thrombotic tendency.
- LMWH (p. 247). Where feasible, selected patients can be safely treated as outpatients.
- Warfarin (p. 248) is started at the same time as heparin.
- The dose of warfarin is adjusted to maintain the INR, usually at two to three times the control value.
- Heparin is overlapped with warfarin for a *minimum* of 5 days and continued until the INR is in the therapeutic range (Table 5.19).
- Major side effects of heparin therapy are bleeding and thrombocytopenia. The platelet count should be measured in all patients receiving heparin for more than 5 days.

Anticoagulation for 6 weeks is sufficient for patients after their first thrombosis with a precipitating cause, provided there are no persisting risk factors. Long-term anticoagulation is required for those with repeated episodes or continuing risk factors.

Other anticoagulant drugs

- Fondaparinux – a synthetic pentasaccharide that inhibits factor X and is similar to the LMWHs.
- Hirudins are direct thrombin inhibitors. Bivalirudin is used in percutaneous coronary interventions and lepirudin is used for anticoagulation in patients with heparin-induced thrombocytopenia (p. 247).
- Dabigatran (direct thrombin inhibitor) and rivaroxaban (inhibitor of factor X) are both given orally and an option for the prophylaxis of venous thromboembolism after total hip or knee replacement surgery.

Table 5.19 Indications for oral anticoagulation and target international normalized ratio (INR)

Target INR	
2.5	Pulmonary embolism, deep vein thrombosis, symptomatic inherited thrombophilia, atrial fibrillation, cardioversion, mural thrombus, cardiomyopathy
3.0	Prevention of embolisation after insertion of mechanical prosthetic aortic valves
3.5	Recurrence of venous thromboembolism while on warfarin therapy, antiphospholipid syndrome, prevention of embolisation after insertion of mechanical prosthetic mitral valves, coronary artery graft thrombosis

THERAPEUTICS

Oral iron

Reference nutrient intake is 8.7 mg for men, 14.8 mg for women.

Indications

Treatment of iron deficiency, prophylaxis in patients with risk factors for iron deficiency, e.g. malabsorption, menorrhagia, pregnancy and post-gastrectomy. Adding a 250 mg ascorbic acid tablet at the time of iron administration enhances the degree of iron absorption (iron is best absorbed as the ferrous [Fe^{2+}] ion in a mildly acidic environment). Iron and folic acid combination preparations are used in pregnancy for women who are at risk of developing iron and folic acid deficiency.

Preparations and dose

Ferrous sulphate Tablets: 200 mg (65 mg iron).
  Treatment: One tablet three times daily – continue for 3 months following normal Hb result (the total duration of therapy should be for 6 months); prophylactic: One tablet daily.
  Ferrous gluconate Tablets 300 g (35 mg iron).
  Treatment: Two to six tablets daily in divided doses.

Side effects

Constipation and diarrhoea. Nausea and epigastric pain are related to the amount of elemental iron ingested and are lower with preparations containing a low elemental iron content, e.g. ferrous gluconate.

Cautions/contraindications

Avoid long-term use unless indicated; excretion of iron is fixed at 1–2 mg of iron per day through gastrointestinal loss, and prolonged use may result in iron overload.

Folic acid

Reference nutrient intake is 200 µg/day.

Indications

Folate-deficient megaloblastic anaemia, prevention of folic acid deficiency in chronic haemolytic states, renal dialysis and pregnancy, prevention of neural tube defects.

Preparations and dose

Folic acid Tablets: 400 µg, 5 mg; Syrup: 400 µg/mL, 2.5 mg/mL; Injection: 15 mg/mL.

Folate deficiency: 5 mg daily for 4 months, maintenance 5 mg daily.

To prevent first neural tube defect: 400 µg daily before conception and during pregnancy.

To prevent recurrence of neural tube defect: 5 mg daily before conception and during pregnancy.

Side effects

Very rarely allergic reactions.

Cautions/contraindications

Folic acid should not be used in undiagnosed megaloblastic anaemia unless vitamin B_{12} is administered concurrently, otherwise neuropathy may be precipitated.

Vitamin B_{12}

Reference nutrient intake is 1.5 µg/day.

Indications

Vitamin B_{12} deficiency.

Preparations and dose

Hydroxocobalamin Injection: 1 mg/mL.

Vitamin B_{12} deficiency without neurological involvement: 1 mg intramuscularly three times a week for 2 weeks then 1 mg every 3 months lifelong.

Vitamin B_{12} deficiency with neurological involvement: 1 mg intramuscularly daily for 6 days then 1 mg every 2 months.

Cyanocobalamin Tablets: 50 µg; Liquid: 35 µg/5 mL.

Vitamin B_{12} deficiency of dietary origin: 50–150 µg or more daily taken between meals.

Side effects

Itching, fever, nausea, dizziness, anaphylaxis after injection. Hypokalaemia, sometimes fatal, is due to intracellular potassium shift on anaemia resolution after treatment of severe vitamin B_{12} deficiency.

Cautions/contraindications

Contraindicated if hypersensitivity to hydroxocobalamin or any component of preparation.

Vitamin K

Mechanism of action

Vitamin K is a fat-soluble vitamin necessary for the production of blood clotting factors and proteins necessary for the normal calcification of bone; reference nutrient intake 1 µg/kg body weight.

Indications

Water-soluble form used to prevent deficiency in patients with fat malabsorption (especially biliary obstruction or hepatic disease); intravenous form for excessive anticoagulation with warfarin and in patients with prolonged INR (due to fat malabsorption) prior to invasive procedures (e.g. endoscopic retrograde cholangiopancreatography [ERCP] or liver biopsy) or in whom there is bleeding.

Preparations and dose

Phytomenadione Vitamin K_1 tablets: 10 mg; Injection: 10 mg/mL.

Oral Excessive anticoagulation (INR >8.0): 0.5–2.5 mg.

IV Excessive anticoagulation and major bleeding (any INR value): 5 mg over 10 minutes together with prothrombin complex concentrate or FFP (15 mL/kg).

Menadiol sodium phosphate

Water-soluble tablets: 10 mg For prevention of vitamin K deficiency in patients with fat malabsorption: 10 mg daily.

Side effects

Anaphylaxis with i.v. preparation.

Cautions/contraindications

Caution with menadiol in G6PD deficiency and vitamin E deficiency (risk of haemolysis).

Drugs affecting haemostasis

Antiplatelet agents

- Aspirin, dipyridamole
- Clopidogrel, prasugrel, ticagrelor
- Glycoprotein GP11b/111a inhibitor.

Mechanism of action

Decrease platelet aggregation and inhibit thrombus formation in the arterial circulation, where anticoagulants have little effect. Aspirin irreversibly inhibits the enzyme cyclo-oxygenase, reducing production of thromboxane A_2, a stimulator of platelet aggregation. Dipyridamole inhibits phosphodiesterase-mediated breakdown of cyclic adenosine monophosphate (AMP), which leads to impaired platelet activation by multiple mechanisms. It has largely been superseded by clopidogrel in the secondary prevention of stroke. Clopidogrel is a pro-drug that is metabolized by the liver, partly by cytochrome P450 2C19, before it is biologically active. It blocks binding of ADP to platelet receptors and thus inhibits activation of the GpIIb/IIIa complex and platelet activation. Prasugrel, a novel thienopyridine, is similar to clopidogrel. Glycoprotein GpIIb/IIIa inhibitors (e.g. abciximab, eptifibatide, tirofiban) prevent platelet aggregation by blocking the binding of fibrinogen to receptors on platelets. They are used as an adjunct to percutaneous coronary intervention in selected patients with acute coronary syndromes.

Preparations and dose

Aspirin Tablets: 75 mg, 300 mg, also as a dispersible form.

Secondary prevention of thrombotic cerebrovascular or cardiovascular disease: 300 mg chewed followed by maintenance dose of 75 mg daily.

Primary prevention when estimated 10-year cardiovascular risk is $\geq$20% (p. 447), provided that blood pressure is controlled.

After coronary artery bypass grafting: 75 mg daily.

In combination with clopidogrel – see below.

Atrial fibrillation (selected cases, p. 431): 75 mg daily.

Transient musculoskeletal pain and pyrexia (see Chapter 7).

    Clopidogrel Tablets: 75 mg, 300 mg.

Where aspirin is contraindicated for the prevention of atherosclerotic events in patients with history of ischaemic stroke, myocardial infarction or established peripheral artery disease: 75 mg daily.

Following coronary artery stent insertion: 300 mg daily, then 75 mg daily with aspirin 75 mg daily. Continue clopidogrel for 6 weeks; 12 months if a drug-eluting stent. Continue aspirin indefinitely.

Acute coronary syndrome: 300 mg, then 75 mg daily in addition to aspirin and other treatments. Continue clopidogrel for 12 months.

Side effects

An increased risk of bleeding is the main risk with all antiplatelet agents. Aspirin causes peptic ulceration. Patients with a past history of ulceration must be co-prescribed a proton pump inhibitor (PPI) with aspirin, to prevent recurrent ulceration. In patients with a history of peptic ulcer bleeding while taking aspirin, co-administration of a PPI is associated with a reduced rate of re-bleeding compared with administration of clopidogrel alone.

    The effects of aspirin and clopidogrel last for the duration of the platelet life i.e. 7–10 days. For surgical interventions: stop aspirin if indicated for primary prevention and continue if indicated for secondary prevention. Clopidogrel is likely to have been given for a high-risk indication, e.g. to prevent coronary stent thrombosis, and should not be stopped perioperatively without prior discussion with the cardiology team. However, the risk of bleeding perioperatively is high if clopidogrel is continued, and non-urgent surgery should be delayed until such time that clopidogrel can be stopped. For urgent surgery, excessive and uncontrolled bleeding is treated with platelet transfusion.

Cautions/contraindications

Active bleeding, haemophilia and other bleeding disorders are contraindications. Aspirin also causes bronchospasm and must be prescribed with caution to patients with asthma. Aspirin interacts with a number of other drugs, and its interaction with warfarin is a special hazard (refer to *National Formulary* for details). Drugs that inhibit CYP2C19 (fluoxetine, moclobemide, voriconazole, fluconazole, ticlopidine, ciprofloxacin, cimetidine, carbamazepine, oxcarbazepine and chloramphenicol) reduce the efficacy of clopidogrel and should be avoided.

Thrombin inhibitors

- Heparin
- Fondaparinux
- Bivalirudin.

Mechanism of action

Unfractionated heparin is not a single substance but a mixture of polysaccharides which binds to and activates antithrombin (AT), which inactivates thrombin and other proteases involved in blood clotting, particularly factor Xa. Usually, LMWH is used, due to its superior bioavailability and longer half-life. Fondaparinux binds to AT and inhibits only factor Xa. Bivalirudin is a direct thrombin inhibitor.

Indications

LMWH, produced by the enzymatic or chemical breakdown of the heparin molecule, is almost always used for the prevention and treatment of DVT and pulmonary embolism, myocardial infarction and acute coronary syndromes. For patients at high risk of bleeding, unfractionated heparin (which requires monitoring by measurement of APPT) is more suitable than LMWH because its effect can be terminated rapidly by stopping the infusion. Refer to national formulary for dosing for unfractionated heparin.

Preparations and dose

LMWH *Enoxaparin – Injection: 20 mg, 40 mg, 60 mg, 80 mg, 100 mg, 120 mg, 150 mg.*

Prophylaxis of thromboembolism by subcutaneous injection:

Surgical patients: moderate risk 20 mg daily until the patient is fully mobile with first dose 2 hours before surgery; high risk 40 mg daily until the patient is fully mobile with first dose 12 hours before surgery. Extended treatment (after hospital discharge) for 4–6 weeks is recommended in high-risk patients after major cancer/gynaecological/orthopaedic surgery.

Medical patients: 40 mg daily.

In all patients, reduce dose to 20 mg if body weight <50 kg or creatinine clearance is <30 mL/min.

Treatment of DVT and pulmonary embolism: 1.5 mg/kg (150 units/kg) by subcutaneous injection every 24 hours, usually for at least 5 days and until oral anticoagulation is established.

Unstable angina and non-ST-segment elevation myocardial infarction (NSTEMI): 1 mg/kg (100 units/kg) by subcutaneous injection every 12 hours usually for 2–8 days.

Side effects

- Haemorrhage
- Thrombocytopenia, which is immune mediated and does not usually develop until after 5–14 days after first exposure; it may be complicated by thrombosis. Platelet counts are recommended for patients receiving heparin for more than 5 days. Heparin should be stopped immediately and not repeated in those who develop thrombocytopenia or a 50% reduction of platelet count.
- Hyperkalaemia due to aldosterone secretion
- Osteoporosis after prolonged use

Cautions/contraindications

Contraindicated with active bleeding, acquired or inherited bleeding disorders, thrombocytopenia (platelets $<75 \times 10^9$/L), recent cerebral haemorrhage, severe liver disease, severe untreated hypertension (>230/120 mmHg), recent surgery to eye or nervous system, history of heparin-induced thrombocytopenia, lumbar puncture/epidural within the past 4 hours or expected within the next 12 hours, acute stroke (discuss with stroke consultant).

Oral anticoagulants

Mechanism of action

Warfarin, a coumarin, inhibits vitamin K-dependent γ-carboxylation of coagulation factors II, VII, IX and X, thus leading to biologically inactive forms. Monitoring is by measurement of the INR.

Indications

Prophylaxis of embolization in atrial fibrillation, cardioversion, dilated cardiomyopathy and mechanical prosthetic aortic or mitral valve insertion; prophylaxis and treatment of venous thrombosis and pulmonary embolism (see Table 5.19 for specific INR targets). Warfarin takes at least 48–72 hours for the anticoagulant effect to develop fully. All patients starting warfarin should be given an anticoagulant treatment booklet (advice on treatment, recording of INR and dosing) and be advised to avoid cranberry juice (increases INR).

Preparations and dose

Warfarin Tablets: 1 mg, 3 mg, 5 mg.

For rapid anticoagulation in venous thromboembolism, starting dose is 10 mg on days 1 and 2 with subsequent doses adjusted according to the INR. A lower dose (5 mg) is used in patients >60 years, body weight <50 kg, baseline INR >1.4 or patients taking interacting drugs which inhibit the metabolism of warfarin. Slow induction of warfarin (1 mg daily for a week) is used for patients in atrial fibrillation with subsequent dosing dependent on the INR.

Maintenance dose – usually 3–9 mg daily by mouth taken at the same time each day. Daily monitoring of the INR in the early days of treatment, then at longer intervals depending on response.

Side effects

Skin necrosis in patients with protein C or protein S deficiency, occurs soon after starting treatment.

Haemorrhage; management is based on the INR and whether there is major or minor bleeding:

- Major bleeding (intracranial, intraperitoneal, intraocular, muscular compartment syndrome *or* life-threatening from any orifice); stop warfarin, give vitamin phytomenadione (vitamin K_1) 5 mg by slow i.v. injection, and prothrombin complex concentrate 30–50 units/kg *or* FFP (15 mL/kg).
- INR >8, no bleeding or minor bleeding, stop warfarin. Give vitamin K, 500 µg by slow i.v. injection or 5 mg by mouth if there are risk factors for bleeding.
- Any other INR > target range, stop warfarin and restart when INR <5.

Contraindications

- Underlying abnormalities of haemostasis (e.g. haemophilia, thrombocytopenia)
- Hypersensitivity to warfarin or any of the excipients
- After an ischaemic stroke for 2–14 days depending on the size of infarct and blood pressure
- Surgery – stop warfarin 3 days prior to surgery if there is a risk of severe bleeding. In most instances, warfarin can be restarted post-operatively as soon as the patient starts oral intake. Warfarin does not need to be stopped before tooth extraction provided INR <3.
- Severe uncontrolled hypertension
- Active peptic ulceration

- Severe liver disease
- Pregnancy – teratogenic in first trimester and risk of placental or fetal haemorrhage in third trimester. Warfarin can be used during breast-feeding.

Drug interactions Many drugs interact with warfarin (check national formulary for full list) and the patient's INR should be measured frequently whenever any drug is added to, or withdrawn from, the patient's therapeutic regimen. Warfarin activity is particularly *increased* by alcohol, allopurinol, amiodarone, aspirin and other NSAIDs, omeprazole, ciprofloxacin, clofibrate, co-trimoxazole, dipyridamole, macrolide antibiotics such as erythromycin, metronidazole, statins, tamoxifen and levothyroxine. Warfarin activity is particularly *decreased* by carbamazepine, rifampicin, rifabutin, griseofulvin and some herbal remedies, e.g. St John's wort. Warfarin activity may be *increased* or *decreased* by phenytoin, corticosteroids and colestyramine. Other drugs co-administered with warfarin increase the risk of bleeding and should be avoided, i.e. antiplatelet drugs (p. 250), NSAIDs and the antidepressant drugs serotonin selective reuptake inhibitors.

Novel oral anticoagulants (NOACs)

Mechanism of action

These orally active drugs directly inhibit either thrombin (e.g. dabigatran) or factor Xa (e.g. rivaroxaban, apixaban, edoxaban). NOACs have a much broader therapeutic window than warfarin, have fewer drug interactions (aside from stronger inducers and inbitors of P-glycoprotein and CYP3A4) and offer the prospect of fixed drug dosing without the need for regular monitoring. Dose amendment is recommended with some NOACs in relation to patient age, weight and renal/liver function. If monitoring is required, specific drug levels must be measured as INR is not helpful.

Indications

Dagibatran, apixaban and rivaroxaban are licensed for prevention of stroke in atrial fibrillation, treatment of venous thromboembolism and prevention of thrombosis in hip and knee replacement surgery.

Preparations and dose

Dabigatran Capsules: 75 mg, 150 mg.

Atrial fibrillation – usual dose 150 mg b.d., reduced to 75 mg b.d. if the creatinine clearance is <30 mL/min. It is not recommended if the creatinine clearance is <15 mL/min.

Treatment of DVT or PE – 150 mg b.d. Not recommended if the creatinine clearance is <30 mL/min.

Prevention of DVT or PE after joint replacement – 110 mg p.o. 1–4 hours after surgery and after hemostasis has been achieved on the 1st day, then 220 mg o.d. for 28–35 days. It is not recommended if the creatinine clearance is < 30 mL/min.

Apixaban Tablets: 2.5 mg, 5 mg.

Atrial fibrillation 5 mg b.d.

Treatment of DVT or PE – 10 mg b.d. for 1 week then reduce to 5 mg b.d.

Prevention of DVT or PE after joint replacement – Give 2.5 mg p.o. 12–24 hours after surgery. Continue at a dose of 2.5 mg b.d. for 12 days after knee replacement and for 35 days after hip replacement.

Dose adjustments are needed for age, creatinine clearance and body weight. See the national formulary for full details.

Rivaroxaban Tablets: 10 mg, 15 mg, 25 mg.

Atrial fibrillation – 20 mg o.d.

Treatment of DVT or PE – 15 mg b.d. for 21 days with food, then 20 mg o.d. for 6 months.

Prevention of DVT or PE after joint replacement – Give 10 mg o.d. starting 12–24 hours after surgery. Continue 12 days after knee replacement and for 35 days after hip replacement.

For all indications, avoid if creatinine clearance is < 30 mL/min

Side effects

NOACs have higher rates of gastrointestinal haemorrhage but lower rates of intracranial haemorrhage than warfarin. Specific antidotes are now available. If bleeding occurs on these new agents that requires anticoagulant reversal, this can be partially achieved using prothrombin complex concentrates. All agents have relatively short half-lives (< 14 hours) and will wear out of the circulation relatively quickly.

Contraindications

Patients with significant hepatic dysfunction or renal impairment may not be good candidates for these drugs due to their hepatic and renal excretion.

Fibrinolytic drugs

Mechanism of action

Fibrinolytic drugs hydrolyse a peptide bond in plasminogen to yield the active enzyme, plasmin, which promotes clot lysis.

Indications

- Acute myocardial infarction within 12 hours of symptom onset
- Selected cases of venous thromboembolism
- Acute ischaemic stroke within 4.5 hours of symptom onset.

Preparations and dose

Alteplase Injection: 10 mg (5.8 million units), 20 mg (11.6 million units) and 50 mg (29 million units)/vial.

Acute myocardial infarction within 12 hours of symptom onset: 15 mg by i.v. injection, followed by i.v. infusion of 50 mg (in patients <65 kg, 0.75 mg/kg) over 30 minutes, then 35 mg (<65 kg, 0.5 mg/kg) over 60 minutes. For acute myocardial infarction, 6–12 hours within symptom onset 10 mg by i.v. injection, followed by i.v. infusion of 50 mg over 60 minutes, then four infusions each of 10 mg over 30 minutes; maximum total dose 1.5 mg/kg in patients <65 kg.

Massive pulmonary embolism with hypotension: 10 mg by i.v. injection over 1–2 minutes, followed by i.v. infusion of 90 mg over 2 hours; max 1.5 mg/kg in patients <65 kg.

Acute ischaemic stroke, 900 µg/kg (max 90 mg) over 60 minutes by i.v. infusion; initial 10% given by i.v. injection. Start as soon as possible ('time is brain') and given up to 4.5 hours after symptom onset.

Streptokinase Injection: 1.5 million international units.

Myocardial infarction: 1.5 million units over 60 minutes.

In selected cases of DVT, pulmonary embolism, acute arterial thromboembolism, central retinal venous or arterial thrombosis: by i.v. infusion 250 000 units over 30 minutes, then according to clinical condition.

Side effects

The main disadvantage is the indiscriminate activation of plasminogen both in clots and in the circulation, leading to an increased risk of haemorrhage. Other side effects are cardiac arrhythmias during reperfusion of the myocardium, hypotension and allergic reactions (bronchospasm, urticaria) with streptokinase.

Contraindications

Gastrointestinal or genitourinary bleeding (within the previous 21 days), aortic dissection, severe uncontrolled hypertension (systolic blood pressure >180 mmHg, diastolic blood pressure >110 mmHg), intracranial aneurysm, recent major trauma/surgery/head injury (within the previous 14 days) or invasive diagnostic procedure (within the last 7–10 days), recent stroke (other than acutely in ischaemic stroke), bleeding disorders, pregnancy or recent obstetric delivery, INR >1.7 if on warfarin.

6 Malignant disease

Malignant disease is common and is the second most common cause of death after cardiovascular disease. Most tumours arise from genetic mutations within a single population of precursor stem cells and over subsequent cell divisions there is an accumulation of further abnormalities. The genes most commonly affected are those that control cell cycle checkpoints, DNA repair and DNA damage recognition, apoptosis, differentiation and growth signalling. Gene mutations may be:

- Germline – e.g. mutations in *BRCA1* and *BRCA2* account for most cases of familial breast cancer. The protein product of these mutated genes is unable to bind to the DNA repair enzyme Rad51 to make it functional in repairing DNA breaks.
- Somatic – in response to environmental carcinogens, e.g. smoking.

DIAGNOSIS OF MALIGNANCY

The diagnosis of malignancy is made by:

- *Screening* in an asymptomatic person with the aim of detecting cancer at an earlier stage than symptomatic presentation and hopefully a better outcome. This is undertaken by population screening or individual screening of at-risk individuals. In the UK, population screening programmes are established for breast, cervical and colon cancer. Individual screening programmes are established for persons with a higher-than-average risk, usually because of family history, e.g. colonoscopy in persons with a family history of colon cancer at a young age.
- *Surveillance* in a patient with a disease that places them at higher risk of developing malignancy, e.g. liver ultrasound and measurement of serum α-fetoprotein in a patient with cirrhosis with the aim of detecting hepatocellular carcinoma at an earlier stage than symptomatic presentation.
- *Investigation* in a symptomatic patient. Symptoms are the result of:
  - The primary tumour
  - Metastases
  - The coagulopathy of cancer may cause deep venous thromboses and pulmonary emboli, particularly in association with cancers of the pancreas, stomach and breast.
  - Paraneoplastic symptoms. These are a consequence of the cancer but are not due to the local presence of the cancer and may be mediated by hormones or cytokines secreted by the cancer (e.g. ectopic adrenocorticotropic hormone [ACTH] secretion in small cell lung cancer)

or an immune response directed against the cancer, e.g. dermatomyositis.

- Non-specific effects such as weight loss, tiredness and lethargy.

Investigations

- *To confirm the presence of malignancy in a patient with suspicious symptoms or signs.* This is by radiological imaging (with the specific test depending on the site) and biopsy of a suspicious lesion (e.g. at endoscopy) with histological examination and tissue tumour markers. Serum tumour markers (Table 6.1) are intracellular proteins or cell surface glycoproteins released into the circulation and may be present in higher than usual concentration in patients with cancer. In many cases they are requested inappropriately as most tumour markers are neither sensitive nor specific for a particular malignancy and can also be raised in benign conditions. Serum tumour markers are mainly used in monitoring response to treatment. Biopsy is necessary to confirm the tissue diagnosis and to inform treatment decisions.
- *To stage the cancer once diagnosed.* Staging the cancer will divide the patients into groups of different prognoses, which can guide treatment selection. The staging systems vary according to tumour type and may be site specific (see Hodgkin's lymphoma) or the TNM (tumour, node, metastasis) classification which can be adapted for application to most common cancers.
- *To assess a patient's suitability for treatment*, their general state of health ('performance status') needs to be considered. Performance status is of great prognostic significance and reflects the effects of the cancer on the patient's functional capacity.

Table 6.1 Serum tumour markers

α-Fetoprotein	Hepatocellular carcinoma and non-seminomatous germ cell tumour of the gonads
β-Human chorionic gonadotrophin (β-hCG)	Choriocarcinomas, germ cell tumours (testicular) and lung cancer
Prostate-specific antigen (PSA)	Prostate cancer
Carcinoembryonic antigen (CEA)	Colorectal cancer. May also be raised in other gastrointestinal malignancies
CA-125	Ovarian cancer. May also be raised in breast, cervical, endometrial and gastrointestinal malignancies
CA19-9	Upper gastrointestinal malignancies
CA15-3	Breast cancer
Osteopontin	Many cancers including mesothelioma

Cancer treatment

The management of patients with cancer must be coordinated by a multidisciplinary team (MDT), which may include a surgeon, oncologist, radiologist, histopathologist, physician, specialist nurse and other healthcare workers, e.g. dietician. Discussion with the patient about the treatment plan at each step will allow them to make a fully informed choice about their management.

In some solid tumours, treatment (chemotherapy, radiotherapy or hormone) is given after the primary treatment, e.g. surgical resection, where dissemination is undetectable but patients are at risk of micrometastases. This is called *adjuvant* therapy. *Neoadjuvant therapy* is given before the primary treatment to shrink the tumour in order to improve the efficacy of the local excision and to treat micrometastases as soon as possible. If effective, these treatments should lead to an increased chance of cure or overall disease-free survival.

Chemotherapy

There are many chemotherapy drugs in common use. These drugs directly damage DNA and/or RNA and kill cells by promoting apoptosis and sometimes cell necrosis. They therefore affect not only tumour cells, but also the rapidly dividing normal cells of the bone marrow, gastrointestinal tract and germinal epithelium.

Side effects include tiredness, bone marrow suppression (leading to anaemia, thrombocytopenia and neutropenia), mucositis (causing mouth ulceration), hair loss (alopecia) and sterility. Side effects are much more directly dose related than anticancer effects. To minimize side effects, chemotherapy is given at intervals to allow some recovery of normal cell function between cycles. Nausea and vomiting may be severe with some drugs, such as cisplatin, and are related to the direct actions of cytotoxic agents on the brainstem chemoreceptor trigger zone. Antiemetics such as metoclopramide (p. 136) and domperidone (p. 136) are used initially, but the serotonin 5-hydroxytryptamine type 3 (5-HT$_3$) antagonists (ondansetron and granisetron) combined with dexamethasone are used for severe vomiting. Chemotherapy drugs may themselves cause cancer, particularly acute leukaemia presenting years after treatment. Some side effects are specific to one class of drug, e.g. cardiotoxicity with the anthracyclines (such as doxorubicin) and neurotoxicity and nephrotoxicity with cisplatin.

Radiotherapy

Radiation induces strand breaks in DNA and apoptosis. The complications of radiotherapy depend on the radiosensitivity of normal tissue in the path of the radiation field. There may be damage to the skin (erythema and desquamation), gut (nausea, mucosal ulceration and diarrhoea), testes (sterility) and bone marrow (anaemia, leucopenia). General side effects are lethargy and loss of energy.

Endocrine therapy

This is used in the treatment of breast and prostate cancer to block the effects of oestrogens and androgens which may act as growth factors. Tamoxifen is a mixed agonist and antagonist of oestrogen on the oestrogen receptor and is used as an adjuvant therapy in breast cancer and in advanced metastatic breast disease. Aromatase inhibitors, e.g. anastrozole, letrozole and exemestane, block the conversion of androgens (synthesized by the adrenal glands) to estrone in the subcutaneous fat of post-menopausal women. They have greater efficacy than tamoxifen in the treatment of metastatic breast cancer and equal efficacy in the adjuvant setting. Gonadotropin-releasing hormone (GnRH) agonists (e.g. goserelin), which lower levels of circulating androgens, and androgen receptor blockers (e.g. flutamide), are both used in the treatment of prostate cancer.

Biological therapy

This group includes a range of protein molecules, from small peptide chemokines and larger cytokines to complex antibody molecules, made available by genetic engineering.

- Interferons, such as interferon alfa, have antiproliferative activity and stimulate humoral and cell-mediated immune responses to the tumour.
- Interleukins have widespread activity in coordinating cellular activity in many organs. Interleukin 2 is used in renal cell carcinoma and melanoma.
- Tyrosine kinase inhibitors (imatinib, sunitinib, sorafenib) have diverse effects on cell growth, differentiation and metabolism.
- Anti-growth factor agents, e.g. bevacizumab (antivascular endothelial growth factor receptor) and cetuximab (antiepidermal growth factor receptor), are added to chemotherapy to improve response.
- Anti-CD20 (rituximab) inhibits CD20 on B cells, which normally plays a role in the development and differentiation of B cells into plasma cells. Anti-CD52 (alemtuzumab) inhibits CD52 expressed on T and B lymphocytes and monocytes.
- Immune checkpoint inhibitors interfere with the relationship between T cells and tumour cells to overcome the common problem of immune tolerance. Ipilimumab is a monoclonal antibody used in the treatment of melanoma. The inhibitors of the programmed death (PD-1) receptor are used in metastatic melanoma.
- Proteasome inhibitors cause apoptosis in cancer cells. Bortezomib (the first of these agents to reach clinical practice) is used in myeloma and some types of non-Hodgkin's lymphoma (NHL).
- Haemopoietic growth factors such as erythropoietin and granulocyte colony-stimulating factor (G-CSF) are used to treat anaemia or to reduce the duration of neutropenia following chemotherapy.

MYELOABLATIVE THERAPY AND HAEMOPOIETIC STEM CELL TRANSPLANTATION

Myeloablative therapy is the term used for treatment that employs high-dose chemotherapy or chemotherapy plus radiation, with the aim of clearing the bone marrow completely of both benign and malignant cells. Without bone marrow replacement or 'transplantation', the patient would die of bone marrow failure. Approaches to restore bone marrow function include the following:

- *Allogeneic* bone marrow transplantation (BMT): Bone marrow or peripheral blood stem cells *from another individual*, usually a human leucocyte antigen (HLA)-identical sibling, are infused intravenously following myeloablative therapy. Immunosuppression is required to prevent host rejection and graft-versus-host disease (GVHD). The latter is a syndrome in which donor T lymphocytes infiltrate the skin, gut and liver, causing a maculopapular rash, diarrhoea and liver necrosis. This occurs in 30–50% of transplant recipients and is potentially fatal in some cases. Following allogeneic BMT the blood count usually recovers within 3–4 weeks. The mortality rate is 20–40%, depending on the person's age, and is often a result of infection or GVHD.

- *Autologous* (the patient acts as his or her own source) stem cells: These are collected from bone marrow or peripheral blood before myeloablative chemotherapy and stored and reinfused afterwards. The main advantage is the short time for blood count recovery because peripheral blood progenitor cells are more differentiated. This technique has been particularly effective in relapsed leukaemias, lymphomas, myeloma and germ cell tumours.

- *Syngeneic:* Donor cells are taken from an identical twin.

- *From umbilical cord blood:* This is increasingly being used for adult and childhood leukaemia.

Oncological emergencies

These arise as a result of the tumour itself or as a complication of treatment.

Neutropenic sepsis is the most common cause of attendance in the emergency department for any cancer patient and must be always considered in any patient who is unwell within a month of chemotherapy. This is discussed on page 208.

Superior vena cava syndrome can arise from any upper mediastinal mass but is most commonly associated with lung cancer and lymphoma. Presentation is with difficulty breathing and/or swallowing, oedematous facies and arms, and venous congestion in the neck with dilated veins in the upper chest and arms. Treatment is with immediate steroids, vascular stents, radiotherapy and chemotherapy for sensitive tumours.

Acute tumour lysis syndrome occurs as a result of treatment producing massive and rapid breakdown of tumour cells, leading to increased serum level of urate, potassium and phosphate with secondary hypocalcaemia. It is most commonly seen as a complication of treatment of acute leukaemia and high-grade lymphoma unless preventive measures are taken. Hyperuricaemia and hyperphosphataemia result in acute kidney injury through urate and calcium phosphate deposition in the renal tubules. Prevention and treatment is with allopurinol (p. 299), rasburicase (urate oxidase) and high fluid loads, e.g. 4–5 L daily by intravenous (i.v.) infusion prior to, and continuing during, chemotherapy.

Spinal cord compression (p. 782), hypercalcaemia (p. 656), pulmonary embolus (p. 475) and raised intracranial pressure (p. 776) are discussed elsewhere.

The leukaemias

The leukaemias are malignant neoplasms of the haemopoietic stem cells, characterized by diffuse replacement of the bone marrow by neoplastic cells. In most cases, the leukaemic cells spill over into the blood, where they may be seen in large numbers. The cells may also infiltrate the liver, spleen, lymph nodes and other tissues throughout the body. They are relatively rare diseases with an overall incidence of 10 per 100 000 per year.

General classification The characteristics of leukaemic cells can be assessed by light microscopy, expression of cytosolic enzymes and expression of surface antigens. These will reflect the lineage and degree of maturity of the leukaemic clone. Thus leukaemia can be divided into acute or chronic on the basis of the speed of evolution of the disease. Each of these is then further subdivided into myeloid or lymphoid, according to the cell type involved:

- Acute myeloid leukaemia (AML)
- Acute lymphoblastic leukaemia (ALL)
- Chronic myeloid leukaemia (CML)
- Chronic lymphocytic leukaemia (CLL).

Aetiology

In most cases the aetiology is unknown, though several factors are associated.

- Chemicals, e.g. benzene compounds used in industry
- Drugs, e.g. AML occurs after treatment with alkylating agents (e.g. melphalan)
- Radiation exposure can induce genetic damage to haemopoietic precursors and increased incidences of leukaemia have been seen in survivors of Hiroshima and Nagasaki and in patients treated with ionizing radiation.
- Viruses, e.g. human T cell lymphotropic retrovirus type 1 (HTLV-1) is associated with some types of leukaemia
- Genetic factors are suggested by the increased incidence in patients with chromosomal disorders (e.g. Down's syndrome) and in identical twins of affected patients. Chromosomal abnormalities have been described in

patients with leukaemia. The earliest described was the Philadelphia (Ph) chromosome, found in 97% of cases with CML and some patients with ALL. In the Ph chromosome the long arm of chromosome 22 is shortened by reciprocal translocation to the long arm of chromosome 9 (t(9;22)). The protein product of the resulting 'fusion' gene, *BCR-ABL*, has tyrosine kinase activity, and enhanced phosphorylating activity compared with the normal protein, resulting in altered cell growth, stromal attachment and apoptosis.

The leukaemic cells of most patients with acute promyelocytic leukaemia (APML) have the translocation t(15;17) involving the retinoic acid receptor alpha *(RARa)* on chromosome 17 and the promyelocytic leukaemia gene *(PML)* on chromosome 15. The resulting PML-RARa fusion protein shows reduced sensitivity to retinoic acid and prevents differentiation of myeloid cells.

Acute leukaemia

The acute leukaemias are characterized by a clonal proliferation of myeloid or lymphoid precursors with reduced capacity to differentiate into more mature cellular elements. There is accumulation of leukaemic cells in the bone marrow, peripheral blood and other tissues, with a reduction in red cells, platelets and neutrophils.

Epidemiology

Both types of acute leukaemia can occur in all age groups, but ALL is predominantly a disease of childhood, whereas AML is seen most frequently in older adults (middle-aged and elderly).

Clinical features

These are the result of marrow failure: anaemia, bleeding and infection, e.g. sore throat and pneumonia. Sometimes there is peripheral lymphadenopathy and hepatosplenomegaly.

Investigations

A definitive diagnosis is made on the peripheral blood film and a bone marrow aspirate. The various subtypes (Table 6.2) are classified on the basis of morphology and immunophenotyping, and cytogenetic studies of blast cells. Auer rods (a rod-like conglomeration of granules in the cytoplasm) within blast cells are pathognomonic of AML. If the patient has a fever, blood cultures and chest radiograph are essential.

- Blood count shows anaemia and thrombocytopenia. The white cell count is usually raised, but may be normal or low.
- Blood film shows characteristic leukaemic blast cells.
- Bone marrow aspirate usually shows increased cellularity, with a high percentage of abnormal lymphoid or myeloid blast cells.

Table 6.2 World Health Organization classification of acute leukaemia

A. AML (acute myeloid leukaemia)

1. AML with recurrent cytogenetic abnormalities (including acute promyelocytic leukaemia with t(15;17) or variants
2. AML with multilineage dysplasia (often secondary to a pre-existing MDS)
3. AML and MDS, therapy-related, occurring after chemotherapy or radiotherapy
4. AML – not otherwise categorized

B. ALL (acute lymphoblastic leukaemia)

1. Precursor B cell acute lymphoblastic leukaemia
2. Burkitt cell leukaemia
3. Precursor T cell acute lymphoblastic leukaemia

MDS, myelodysplastic syndrome.

- Lumbar puncture and cerebrospinal fluid examination are performed after blasts have been cleared from peripheral blood in all patients with ALL and AML with monoblast/monocytic component as the risk of central nervous system (CNS) involvement is high.

Management

The initial requirement of therapy is to return the peripheral blood and bone marrow to normal (complete remission) with 'induction chemotherapy' tailored to the particular leukaemia and the individual patient's risk factors. The risk of failure of treatment is based on the cytogenetic pattern. Successful remission induction is always followed by further treatment (consolidation), the details being determined by the type of leukaemia and the patient's risk factors (and the patient's tolerance of treatment). Recurrence is almost invariable if 'consolidation' therapy is not given.

Supportive care Before starting treatment the following need to be performed:

- Correction of anaemia, thrombocytopenia and coagulation abnormalities by administration of blood, platelets and blood products
- Treatment of infection with i.v. antibiotics
- Prevention of the acute tumour lysis syndrome (p. 257).

Treatment

Acute myeloid leukaemia

Complete remission is usually achieved in about 80% of patients under the age of 60 years with no significant comorbidity, in whom treatment is offered with curative intent.

Low risk of treatment failure (based on the cytogenetic pattern)

- A moderately intensive combination of i.v. chemotherapy, e.g. cytosine arabinoside (cytarabine) and daunorubicin, is given at intervals to allow marrow recovery in between. This is followed by consolidation therapy with a minimum of four cycles of treatment given at 3–4-week intervals.

Intermediate risk

- Consolidating chemotherapy to induce remission followed by sibling-matched allogeneic bone marrow transplantation, despite its attendant risks.

High risk of treatment failure

- This is only curable with allogeneic transplantation but unfortunately 'high risk' is more common with advancing age when the toxicity of this treatment increases greatly.

Acute promyelocytic leukaemia

APML is a variant of AML that is specifically associated with disseminated intra-vascular coagulation (DIC; p. 238), which may worsen when treatment is started. It is conventional to combine chemotherapy for APML with all-*trans*-retinoic acid (ATRA), which causes differentiation of promyelocytes and rapid reversal of the bleeding tendency caused by DIC. Successful remission induction is followed by maintenance ATRA. Remission induction therapy as in other forms of AML is also necessary for long-term survival.

Prognosis Complete remission occurs in at least 90% of younger adults with APML and at least 70% will expect to be cured. The management of recurrence is undertaken on an individual basis, since the overall prognosis is very poor despite the fact that second remissions may be achieved. Long survival following recurrence is rarely achieved without allogeneic transplantation.

Acute lymphoblastic leukaemia

The principles of treatment differ in detail from that for AML. Remission induction is undertaken with combination chemotherapy including vincristine, dexa-methasone, asparaginase and daunorubicin. Details of consolidation will be determined by the anticipated risk of failure but is usually with intensive che-motherapy and then maintenance therapy for 2 years to reduce the risk of dis-ease recurrence. Unlike AML, ALL has a propensity to involve the CNS, so treatment also includes prophylactic intrathecal drugs, methotrexate or cyto-sine arabinoside (cytarabine). Cranial irradiation is used in those at very high risk or in those with symptoms.

The prognosis in children with ALL is excellent, with almost all achieving complete remission and with 80% being alive and disease free at 5 years. The results in adults are not as good, the prognosis getting worse with advanc-ing years. Overall, about 70–80% achieve complete remission with only about 30% being cured.

Chronic myeloid leukaemia

Clinical features

CML occurs most commonly in middle age and is characterized by the presence of the Ph chromosome. There is an insidious onset, with fever, weight loss, sweating and symptoms of anaemia. Massive splenomegaly is characteristic.

Untreated, this chronic phase lasts 3–4 years. This is usually followed by blast transformation, with the development of acute leukaemia (usually acute myeloid) and, commonly, rapid death. Less frequently, CML transforms into myelofibrosis, death ensuing from bone marrow failure.

Investigations

- Blood count usually shows anaemia and a raised white cell count (often $>100 \times 10^9$/L). The platelet count may be low, normal or raised.
- Bone marrow aspirate shows a hypercellular marrow with an increase in myeloid progenitors. The Ph chromosome and the *BCR-ABL* oncogene are shown by cytogenetics and reverse transcriptase polymerase chain reaction (RT-PCR).

Management

Imatinib, a tyrosine kinase inhibitor that specifically blocks the enzymatic action of the BCR-ABL fusion protein, is first-line treatment for the chronic phase. Imatinib produces a complete haematological response in over 95% of patients, and 70–80% of these have no detectable *BCR-ABL* transcripts in the blood. Event-free, and overall, survival appear to be better than for other treatments. Imatinib can be continued indefinitely.

In the acute phase (blast transformation) most patients have only a short-lived response to imatinib, and other chemotherapy as for acute leukaemia is used in the hope of achieving a second chronic phase.

Chronic lymphocytic leukaemia

CLL, the most common form of leukaemia, is an incurable disease of older people, characterized by an uncontrolled proliferation and accumulation of mature B lymphocytes.

Clinical features

CLL usually follows an indolent course. Early CLL is generally asymptomatic and isolated peripheral blood lymphocytosis is frequent. Symptoms are a consequence of bone marrow failure: anaemia, infections and bleeding. An autoimmune haemolysis contributes to the anaemia. Some patients may be asymptomatic, the diagnosis being a chance finding on the basis of a blood count performed for a different reason. There may be lymphadenopathy and, in advanced disease, hepatosplenomegaly.

Investigations

- Blood count shows a raised white cell count with lymphocytosis ($>5 \times 10^9$/L). There may be anaemia and thrombocytopenia.
- Blood film shows small lymphocytes of mature appearance with 'smear or smudge cells', an artefactual finding due to cell rupture while the film is being made.
- Bone marrow reflects peripheral blood usually heavily infiltrated with lymphocytes.
- Immunophenotyping is essential to exclude reactive lymphocytosis and other lymphoid neoplasms.
- Cytogenetics to characterize the specific mutation can be helpful in assessing prognosis.

Management

The decision to treat depends on the stage of the disease and more recently on cytogenetic markers. Early-stage disease is treated expectantly whereas advanced-stage disease is always treated immediately. Other indications for treatment include anaemia, recurrent infections, splenic discomfort and progressive disease.

Combination therapy with fludarabine, cyclophosphamide and rituximab (p. 256) has become standard first-line therapy and can induce complete remission. For older patients, chlorambucil usually reduces lymphocytosis, lymphadenopathy and splenomegaly to palliate the disease. Alemtuzumab (p. 256) is used in patients in whom there is disease progression after treatment with fludarabine. New generation anti-CD20 monoclonal antibodies, such as Ofatumumab and Obinutuzumab, are also used in fludarabine- or alemtuzumab-refractory CLL or in combination with chlorambucil.

Prognosis

The median survival from diagnosis is very variable and correlates closely with disease stage at diagnosis and cytogenetic findings, e.g. patients with either 11q or 17p deletions (the sites of two tumour suppressor genes) are at high risk of not responding to initial treatment and rapid progression. In other patients there is near-normal life expectancy.

THE LYMPHOMAS

The lymphomas are B- and T-cell malignancies of the lymphoid system. They are the fifth most common malignancy in the Western world (more common than leukaemia) and are increasing in incidence for reasons that are unclear. The disease is classified on the basis of histological appearance into Hodgkin's and NHL.

Hodgkin's lymphoma

Hodgkin's lymphoma is primarily a disease of young adults. Previous infection with Epstein–Barr virus (EBV) is thought to play a role in pathogenesis in some patients.

Clinical features

Painless lymph node enlargement (often cervical nodes) is the most common presentation. These lymph nodes have a rubbery consistency on examination. There may be hepatosplenomegaly. Systemic 'B' symptoms are fever, drenching night sweats and weight loss (>10% in previous 6 months). Other constitutional symptoms such as pruritus, fatigue, anorexia and alcohol-induced pain at the site of the enlarged lymph nodes also occur.

Investigations

- Blood count may be normal or show a normochromic, normocytic anaemia.
- The erythrocyte sedimentation rate (ESR) is usually raised and is an indicator of disease activity.
- Liver biochemistry may be abnormal, with or without liver involvement.
- Serum lactate dehydrogenase (LDH) if raised is an adverse prognostic marker.
- Chest X-ray may show mediastinal widening from enlarged nodes.
- Diagnosis is by lymph node biopsy and histological examination showing Reed–Sternberg cells (binucleate or multinucleate malignant B lymphocytes) in a background rich in benign small lymphocytes and histiocytes.
- Disease staging is by computed tomography (CT) scan, which may show intrathoracic, abdominal and pelvic nodes. Positron emission tomography (PET) (p. 828) is becoming a standard investigation.

Differential diagnosis

This includes any other cause of lymphadenopathy (Table 6.3). Persistently enlarged lymph nodes must always be excised for histological and microbiological examination for diagnostic purposes.

Management

Treatment is given with curative intent. The choice of treatment depends on:
- Stage (Table 6.4)
- Involved sites
- 'Bulk' of lymph nodes involved
- Presence of 'B' symptoms.

Table 6.3 Differential diagnosis of lymphadenopathy

Localized	Generalized
Local infection Pyogenic infection, e.g. tonsillitis Tuberculosis	Infection Epstein–Barr virus Cytomegalovirus *Toxoplasma* sp. Tuberculosis HIV infection
Lymphoma	Lymphoma
Secondary carcinoma	Leukaemia
	Systemic disease Systemic lupus erythematosus Sarcoidosis Rheumatoid arthritis Drug reaction, e.g. phenytoin

HIV, human immunodeficiency virus.

Table 6.4 Staging classification of Hodgkin's lymphoma

Stage	Definition
I	Involvement of a single lymph node region or a single extralymphatic organ or site
II	Involvement of two or more lymph node regions on the same side of the diaphragm, or localized involvement of an extralymphatic organ or site and of one or more lymph node regions on the same side of the diaphragm
III1	Involvement of lymph node regions on both sides of the diaphragm, which may also be accompanied by involvement of the spleen (IIIS) or by localized involvement of an extralymphatic organ (IIIE) or site or both (IIISE)
IV	Diffuse or disseminated involvement of one or more extralymphatic organs or tissues, with or without associated lymph node involvement

Each stage can also be graded A (no 'B' symptoms) or B (with 'B' symptoms), X (bulky disease) or E (involvement of a single extranodal site that is contiguous or proximal to the known nodal site).

- *'Early' stage disease* (Stage IA, IIA with no bulk) is treated with brief chemotherapy (ABVD, doxorubicin, bleomycin, vinblastine, dacarbazine) followed by involved field irradiation.
- *Advanced disease* (all other stages) is treated with cyclical combination chemotherapy (eight cycles of ABVD) with irradiation at sites of bulk disease. PET/CT is used to detect disease activity after treatment and to distinguish between active tumour (PET-positive) and necrosis or fibrosis (PET-negative) in residual masses. Irradiation, with its attendant complications, can be omitted in PET-negative masses after chemotherapy.

Prognosis is related to the stage of disease at presentation, with a 5-year survival rate of over 90% in stage I declining to 60% in stage IV. The presence of B symptoms indicates more severe disease with a worse prognosis.

Non-Hodgkin's lymphoma

These are malignant tumours of the lymphoid system classified separately from Hodgkin's lymphoma. There is a malignant clonal expansion of lymphocytes, which occurs at different stages of lymphocyte development. Most (80%) are of B cell origin. In general, neoplasms of non-dividing mature lymphocytes are indolent, whereas those of proliferating cells (e.g. lymphoblasts, immunoblasts) are much more aggressive. The B and T/natural killer (NK) cell lymphomas are each further divided on this basis, e.g. precursor B cell lymphoma, and then again subdivided based on cytogenetics and immunophenotyping. The aetiology is unknown in most cases but some are associated with a specific infection, e.g. *Helicobacter pylori*, and gastric mucosa-associated lymphoid tissue (MALT) lymphoma. Immune suppression, immunosuppressant drugs (particularly as used for solid organ transplantation) and human immunodeficiency virus (HIV) infection are all associated with an increased incidence of lymphoma.

Clinical features

Presentation is rare before the age of 40 years. Most patients present with painless peripheral lymph node enlargement. Systemic symptoms as in Hodgkin's lymphoma may occur. Extranodal involvement is more common than in Hodgkin's lymphoma and almost any organ in the body can be involved. Bone marrow infiltration leads to anaemia, recurrent infections and bleeding. Skin involvement with T cell lymphoma presents as mycosis fungoides and Sézary syndrome.

Investigations

- Blood count may show anaemia. An elevated white cell count or thrombocytopenia suggests bone marrow involvement. The ESR may be raised.
- Liver biochemistry may be abnormal if the liver is involved.
- Serum lactate dehydrogenase and β_2-microglobulin are prognostic indicators.

- Chest X-ray, CT, PET and gallium scans are of help in staging.
- Bone marrow aspiration and trephine biopsy will confirm marrow involvement.
- Lymph node biopsy is required for definitive diagnosis and subtype classification.

Management

Treatment depends on the lymphoma type and stage (similar to Hodgkin's lymphoma). *Diffuse large B cell lymphoma* is the most common lymphoma and first-line treatment is with cyclical combination chemo-immunotherapy (CHOP + R, cyclophosphamide, hydroxydaunorubicin, vincristine, prednisolone and rituximab) with field irradiation for those with bulky disease. Between 60% and 70% of those with early-stage disease will achieve a cure with this regimen.

- *Primary gastric lymphoma* in many cases is associated with *H. pylori* infection. Treatment to eradicate the infection (p. 89) is usually all that is required provided there is no evidence of disease outside the stomach. This is followed by close endoscopic surveillance.
- *Burkitt's lymphoma* occurs mainly in African children and is associated with EBV infection. Jaw tumours are common, usually with gastrointestinal involvement. Treatment is with cyclical combination chemotherapy.

THE PARAPROTEINAEMIAS

Multiple myeloma

Multiple myeloma is a malignant disease of the plasma cells of bone marrow, accounting for 1% of all malignant disease. There is clonal proliferation of bone marrow plasma cells usually capable of producing monoclonal immunoglobulins (paraproteins), which in most cases are immunoglobulin (Ig) G or IgA. The paraproteinaemia may be associated with excretion of light chains in the urine (Bence Jones protein) which are either kappa or lambda; sometimes there are light chains without a paraproteinaemia.

Clinical features

The peak age of presentation is 60 years. There is:

- *Bone destruction* – increased osteoclastic activity causes bone pain (back ache is the most common presenting symptom), osteolytic lesions, pathological fractures, spinal cord compression and hypercalcaemia.
- *Bone marrow infiltration* with plasma cells resulting in anaemia, infections and bleeding.
- *Acute kidney injury* has multiple causes: deposition of light chains in the tubules, hypercalcaemia, hyperuricaemia and amyloid deposition in the kidneys.

Paraproteins may form aggregates in the blood, which greatly increase the viscosity, leading to blurred vision, gangrene and bleeding. Infections are also due to a reduction in the normal polyclonal immunoglobulin levels (immune paresis).

Investigations

Two out of three diagnostic features should be present:

- Paraproteinaemia on serum protein immunofixation or Bence Jones protein in the urine
- Radiological evidence (CT, MRI) of lytic bone lesions
- An increase in bone marrow plasma cells on bone marrow aspirate or trephine biopsy.

Other essential investigations are as follows:

- Blood count, which may show anaemia, thrombocytopenia and leucopenia. The ESR is almost always high.
- Serum biochemistry may show evidence of renal failure and hypercalcaemia. The alkaline phosphatase is usually normal.
- Serum β_2-microglobulin and albumin are used in prognosis.

Management

With good supportive care and chemotherapy with autologous stem cell transplantation, median survival is now 5 years, with some patients surviving to 10 years. Young patients receiving more intensive therapy may live longer. However, myeloma remains incurable.

Supportive therapy includes correction of anaemia with blood transfusion or erythropoietin, prompt treatment of infections and treatment of bone pain with radiotherapy or high-dose dexamethasone. Acute kidney injury (p. 386) and hypercalcaemia (p. 656) may be corrected by adequate hydration alone. Progression of bone disease is reduced by bisphosphonates, e.g. zoledronate, which inhibit osteoclastic activity. Hyperviscosity is treated by plasmapheresis together with systemic therapy.

Initial treatment typically consists of an alkylator (cyclophosphamide or melphalan), steroid (prednisolone or dexamethasone) and novel agent (bortezomib or thalidomide). Lenalidomide is a thalidomide analogue, which is also used for relapsed myeloma. It has greater potency than thalidomide with less toxicity. Younger patients (<65–70 years) are treated with high-dose melphalan with peripheral blood stem cell rescue.

Monoclonal gammopathy of undetermined significance

This is usually seen in older patients, where a raised level of paraprotein (usually IgA) is found in the blood, but without other features of myeloma. Patients are often asymptomatic and no treatment is required. Follow-up is necessary as 20–30% go on to develop multiple myeloma over a 25-year period.

PALLIATIVE MEDICINE AND SYMPTOM CONTROL

Palliative care describes the multidisciplinary approach to patients with advanced end-stage disease. Patients with advanced cancer and chronic non-malignant disease, e.g. organ failure (heart, lung and kidney), neurological disease and HIV infection, all benefit from this approach, which aims to achieve the best possible quality of life. It includes management of symptoms, access to support services, involving patients and family in their care and helping them to make decisions about end-of-life care.

Management of pain

The approach to successful management of pain includes an assessment of patient characteristics (mood, previous problems with analgesia, fear of opioids) and the likely aetiology of the pain. Pain can be controlled in most patients using a simple step-wise approach (the World Health Organization [WHO] analgesic ladder) that guides the choice of analgesia according to pain severity (Fig. 6.1). Morphine is the most commonly used strong opioid and where possible it should be given regularly by mouth.

- *Dose titration of morphine* is with a normal release formulation with a rapid onset and duration of action, e.g. 5–10 mg morphine elixir or tablets every 4 hours (depending on body weight, renal function and use of other weak opioids) with extra doses allowed for 'breakthrough pain' as often as necessary. The daily requirements can be assessed after 24 hours and the regular dose adjusted as necessary.

- *Maintenance of pain relief* is with a controlled-release morphine preparation. When the stable dose requirement is established by titration the morphine can be changed to a controlled-release preparation, e.g. 20 mg morphine elixir 4-hourly = 60 mg of a twice-daily preparation or 120 mg of a once-daily preparation. Side effects of morphine include nausea and vomiting (see p. 270), constipation (lactulose and senna should be co-prescribed), confusion, drowsiness and nightmares.

As pain may be due to different physical aetiologies, an appropriate adjuvant analgesic may be needed in addition to, or instead of, traditional drug treatments:

- Adjuvant analgesics include non-steroidal anti-inflammatory drugs (pain, p. 321) and bisphosphonates (p. 323) used in addition to opioids, for bone pain

- Tricyclic antidepressants (e.g. amitriptyline 10–75 mg daily) and antiepileptics (e.g. gabapentin 600–2400 mg daily or pregabalin 150 mg increasing to 600 mg daily) for neuropathic pain

- Steroids, e.g. dexamethasone (p. 664) for the headache of raised intracranial pressure or liver capsule pain.

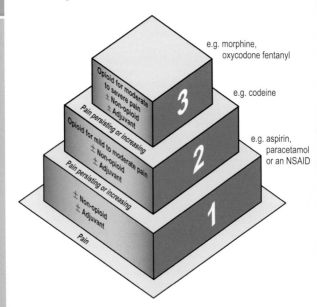

Fig. 6.1 The World Health Organization (WHO) three-step analgesic ladder is a framework for the prescription of analgesic drugs. The ladder attempts to meet the ceiling effect of analgesic drugs to the degree of pain present. If pain is severe or analgesia ineffective, then an ascent of the ladder is recommended. NSAID, non-steroidal anti-inflammatory drug.

Palliation of nausea and vomiting

Nausea and vomiting are common symptoms and successful management involves identifying the likely cause and the nerve pathway activated by the trigger:

- Chemoreceptor trigger zone in the floor of the fourth ventricle where dopamine and serotonin type 3 (5-HT$_3$) receptors are stimulated by drugs and metabolites
- Vomiting centre in the brainstem where histamine type 1, acetylcholine and 5-hydroxytryptamine type 2 (5-HT$_2$) receptors receive sensory input from higher centres, from visceral and serosal stretch receptors and from the VIIIth cranial nerve (p. 738)
- Afferents from stretch receptors on the liver capsule, peritoneum and bowel input to the vomiting centre.

Nausea and vomiting associated with chemotherapy or opioids is treated with haloperidol (1.5–3 mg daily) or metoclopramide (10–20 mg three times daily by mouth or subcutaneously), both of which block dopamine type 2 receptors. When the risk of nausea and vomiting is high, a specific 5-HT$_3$ antagonist (e.g. ondansetron 8 mg orally or by slow i.v. injection) is used. Vomiting due to gastric distension is treated with metoclopramide but vomiting due to complete bowel obstruction is best treated with physical measures to relief the obstruction (e.g. stent insertion or defunctioning colostomy in large bowel obstruction) and an antispasmodic, e.g. hyoscine hydrobromide, at the end of life.

Care of the dying patient

The dying patient requires appropriate care in their last hours or days of life. Most people express a wish to die in their own homes, provided their symptoms are controlled and their carers are supported. However, patients may die in any setting so all healthcare professionals should be proficient in end-of-life care, including the management of symptoms such as pain, agitation, vomiting, breathlessness and respiratory secretions. Reports of inadequate hospital care have led to the development of integrated pathways of care for the dying. Pathways act as prompts of care, including psychological, social, spiritual and carer concerns in those who are diagnosed as dying. The decision that a patient is dying is reached by a multiprofessional team through careful assessment of the patient and exclusion of reversible causes of deterioration.

7 Rheumatology

Musculoskeletal problems are common and usually short-lived and self-limiting. They account for about one in five consultations in primary care. Recognition and early treatment of rheumatic conditions help to reduce the incidence of chronic pain disorders in non-inflammatory conditions and allow early referral for specialist care in inflammatory arthritis to achieve better symptom control and prevention of long-term joint damage. Pain, stiffness and swelling are the most common presenting symptoms of joint disease and may be localized to a single joint or affect many joints.

THE NORMAL JOINT

There are three types of joints – fibrous, fibrocartilaginous and synovial. Fibrous and fibrocartilaginous joints include the intervertebral discs, the sacroiliac joints, the pubic symphysis and the costochondral joints. Little movement occurs at such joints. Synovial joints include the ball-and-socket joints (e.g. hip) and the hinge joints (e.g. interphalangeal). In synovial joints the opposed cartilaginous articular surfaces move painlessly over each other, stability is maintained during use and the load is distributed across the surface of the joint (Fig. 7.1).

MUSCULOSKELETAL SYMPTOMS

Arthralgia describes joint pains when the joint appears normal on examination. *Arthritis* is the term used when there is objective evidence of joint inflammation (swelling, deformity or an effusion).

In a patient presenting with joint pains, the history and examination must assess the distribution of joints affected (e.g. is the pain symmetrical, axial or peripheral), the presence of morning stiffness (>30 minutes in inflammatory arthropathies), aggravating and relieving factors, past medical history and family history. Table 7.1 lists the likely causes of joint pains based on the age and sex of the patient.

Pain in or around a single joint may arise from the joint itself (articular problem) or from structures surrounding the joint (periarticular problem). Enthesitis (inflammation at the site of attachment of ligaments, tendons and joint capsules), bursitis and tendinitis are all causes of periarticular pain. Pain arising from the joint may be the result of a mechanical problem (e.g. torn meniscus) or an inflammatory problem.

The causes of a large-joint monoarthritis include osteoarthritis, gout, pseudogout, trauma and septic arthritis. Disseminated gonococcal infection is a

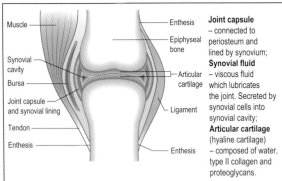

Muscle — Enthesis

— Epiphyseal bone

Synovial cavity —

Bursa —

Joint capsule and synovial lining —

Tendon —

Enthesis —

— Articular cartilage

— Ligament

— Enthesis

Joint capsule – connected to periosteum and lined by synovium;
Synovial fluid – viscous fluid which lubricates the joint. Secreted by synovial cells into synovial cavity;
Articular cartilage (hyaline cartilage) – composed of water, type II collagen and proteoglycans.

Creates a smooth highly compressible structure which acts as a shock absorber and distributes loads over the joint surface;
Enthesis – point at which ligaments and tendons (both stabilize joints) insert into bone;
Epiphyseal bone abuts the joint and differs structurally from the shaft (metaphysis).

Fig. 7.1 Anatomy and physiology of a normal synovial joint.

Table 7.1 Differential diagnosis of polyarticular arthritis in adults in the UK

Age	Predominantly males		Predominantly females
Young	Reactive arthritis		Systemic lupus erythematosus
	Ankylosing spondylitis		Rheumatoid arthritis
			Sjögren's syndrome
		Psoriatic arthropathy Enteropathic arthropathy	
Middle age	Gout	Osteoarthritis	Rheumatoid arthritis
Elderly		Osteoarthritis Polymyalgia rheumatica Pseudogout	

Any age: *Lyme disease, endocarditis, acute hepatitis B infection, human immunodeficiency virus infection, parvovirus.*
Uncommon arthropathies: *malignancy (hypertrophic pulmonary osteoarthropathy), rheumatic fever, Henoch–Schönlein purpura, Behçet's syndrome.*

common cause of acute non-traumatic monoarthritis or oligoarthritis in young adults. Less common causes are rheumatoid arthritis (RA), the spondyloarthropathies, tuberculous infection and haemarthrosis (e.g. in haemophilia, or on warfarin). Acute monoarthritis requires urgent investigation and treatment (p. 301). The key investigation is synovial fluid aspiration with Gram stain and culture and analysis for crystals in gout and pseudogout.

If the patient presents with stiffness, it is necessary to establish whether it is localized or generalized, whether it affects the limb girdles or periphery and whether it is worse first thing in the morning or after activity. If joint swelling is present, the distribution of joints affected can be helpful. In certain rheumatological conditions, the presence of extra-articular features can also clarify the diagnosis.

COMMON INVESTIGATIONS IN MUSCULOSKEKETAL DISEASE

Blood tests

Simple blood tests will usually show evidence of a non-specific acute-phase response with inflammatory arthritides and autoimmune rheumatic conditions. Normochromic, normocytic anaemia is common, though hypochromic, microcytic anaemia may be present, indicating iron deficiency, often due to nonsteroidal anti-inflammatory drug (NSAID)-induced gastrointestinal bleeding. Thrombocytopenia may be a feature of systemic lupus erythematosus (SLE). Erythrocyte sedimentation rate (ESR) and C-reactive protein (CRP) are the most widely used indicators of the acute-phase response and are frequently used to monitor disease activity. A raised alkaline phosphatase may indicate bony disease (p. 140).

Autoantibodies (see rheumatoid factor [p. 286] and Table 7.2) may be non-specific and found in normal individuals. At high titre ($>$1:160) their disease specificity increases and they help to establish a diagnosis in patients with clinical features suggestive of an autoimmune disease. They can sometimes be used to monitor disease activity and provide prognostic data, e.g. seropositive RA (i.e. cyclic citrullinated peptide antibodies [anti-CCP] or rheumatoid factor are present) is associated with more erosive joint disease and extra-articular manifestations than seronegative RA.

Imaging

Plain X-rays may show fractures, deformity, soft tissue swelling, decreased bone density, osteolytic and osteosclerotic areas suggestive of metastases, joint erosions, joint space narrowing and new bone formation. X-rays may be normal in early inflammatory arthritis but are used as a baseline for later comparison.

Table 7.2 Autoantibodies and disease associations

Antibody	Disease
Anti citrullinated peptide antibodies (ACPA); rheumatoid factor	High specificity for rheumatoid arthritis
Antinuclear antibodies	Non-specific – autoimmune disease, infections, normal individuals
Anti-dsDNA	SLE
Anti-histone	Drug-induced lupus
Anti-topoisomerase I (Scl-70)	Diffuse cutaneous SSc
Anti-centromeric	Limited SS
Anti-Ro (SS-A)	Primary SS, SLE
Anti-La (SS-B)	Primary SS, SLE
Anti-Smith (Sm)	SLE
Anti-U1-RNP	SLE, overlap syndrome
Anti-Jo-1	Polymyositis, dermatomyositis
Cytoplasmic ANCA	Granulomatosis with polyangiitis (formerly known as Wegener's granulomatosis)
Perinuclear ANCA	Microscopic polyarteritis, eosinophilic granulomatosis with polyangiitis (formerly known as Churg–Strauss syndrome)
Antiphospholipid	Antiphospholipid syndrome, SLE

ds, double-stranded; SLE, systemic lupus erythematosus; SS, Sjögren's syndrome; RNP, ribonucleoprotein; SSc, systemic scleroderma; ANCA, antineutrophil cytoplasmic antibody.

Bone scintigraphy (isotope bone scan) uses a tracer (^{99}Tc-bisphosphonate), which, following intravenous injection, localizes to sites of increased bone turnover and blood circulation. 'Hot spots' are non-specific and occur in osteomyelitis, septic arthritis, malignancy, Paget's disease and following surgery or trauma. It is best used in combination with other anatomical imaging techniques.

Ultrasound is useful for assessment of soft tissue and periarticular changes, such as hip joint effusion, Baker's cyst and inflamed/damaged tendons. It is sometimes used to assess bone density (at the heel), as a screening procedure prior to dual energy X-ray absorptiometry (DXA) and is increasingly being used to examine the shoulder and other structures during movement.

Magnetic resonance imaging (MRI) is particularly useful in the investigation of articular disease and spinal disorders. It is not indicated in patients with uncomplicated mechanical low back pain.

DXA measures bone mineral density (BMD) in the diagnosis and monitoring of osteoporosis (p. 316).

Arthroscopy is a direct means of visualizing the inside of a joint, particularly the knee or shoulder. Biopsies can be taken, surgery performed in certain conditions (e.g. repair or trimming of meniscal tears) and loose bodies removed.

Synovial fluid analysis

A needle is inserted into a joint for three main reasons: aspiration of synovial fluid for diagnosis or to relieve pressure, and injection of corticosteroid or local anaesthetic. The most common indications for joint aspiration are evaluation for sepsis in a single inflamed joint (p. 301) and confirmation of gout and pseudogout by polarized light. Synovial fluid should be analysed for colour, viscosity, cell count, culture, glucose and protein.

Investigation of suspected muscle disease

Suspected muscle disease may be investigated by rheumatologists or neurologists. This is covered on p. 740–741.

COMMON REGIONAL MUSCULOSKELETAL PROBLEMS

Inflammatory arthritis or osteoarthritis causes pain in one or more joints. This section describes specific regional problems. The diagnosis of most of these conditions is usually clinical and initial treatment is with painkillers, e.g. paracetamol and NSAIDs. Physiotherapy and local steroid injections are used in some cases.

Pain in the neck and shoulder is often due to muscular spasm. There is unilateral or bilateral pain which may radiate upwards to the occiput and often is associated with tension headaches. Nerve root compression by cervical disc prolapse or spondylotic osteophytes causes unilateral neck pain radiating to interscapular and shoulder regions (see below). It is associated with pins and needles and neurological signs in the arms. Pain in the neck may also be caused by RA, ankylosing spondylitis or fibromyalgia (chronic widespread muscle pain often in young women with no underlying cause; large psychological overlay in some patients). Polymyalgia rheumatica (p. 310) causes pain and stiffness in the shoulder girdle.

Rotator cuff injury and inflammation is one of the most common causes of *shoulder pain.* The rotator cuff muscles (supraspinatus, infraspinatus, subscapularis, teres minor) are positioned around the shoulder joint. They stabilize the joint and help with movement. The muscular tendons join to form the rotator cuff tendon, which inserts into the humerus. Rotator cuff tendinitis, impingement and tears cause shoulder pain with a painful arc (between 70 and 120°) on shoulder abduction in the former two and prevention of active abduction (in the first 90°) in the latter. Adhesive capsulitis ('frozen' shoulder) causes severe shoulder pain with all movements, leading to the 'frozen phase' where there is loss of all shoulder movements but little pain. Ultrasound examination is the best investigation to differentiate between these causes.

Elbow pain occurs due to inflammation of the insertion site of the wrist extensor tendon into the lateral epicondyle (tennis elbow) or the wrist flexor tendon into the medial epicondyle (golfer's elbow). There is local tenderness and pain radiates into the forearm on using the affected muscles.

Hip problems Pain arising from the hip joint itself is felt in the groin, lower buttock and anterior thigh, and may radiate to the knee. Occasionally and inexplicably, hip arthritis causes pain only in the knee. Fracture of the femoral neck (pain in the hip, usually after a fall, leg shortened and externally rotated) or avascular necrosis of the femoral head (severe hip pain in a patient with risk factors, p. 318) will often be suspected from the history and examination. Pain over the trochanter which is worse going up stairs and when abducting the hip can be due to trochanteric bursitis or a tear of the gluteus medius tendon at its insertion into the trochanter. MRI will differentiate the two. Meralgia paraesthetica (lateral cutaneous nerve of thigh compression) causes numbness and increased sensitivity to light touch over the anterolateral thigh. It is usually self-limiting.

The knee is a frequent site of sports injuries that lead to torn menisci and cruciate ligaments. These injuries may be associated with bleeding into the joint (haemarthrosis). The knee is also frequently involved in inflammatory arthritides, osteoarthritis and pseudogout. An associated effusion causes swelling, stiffness and pain, with the 'bulge sign' and 'patellar tap' on examination. In a few patients with an effusion there is a connection to a bursa, forming a cyst *(Baker's cyst)* in the popliteal fossa. This may rupture *(ruptured popliteal or Baker's cyst)* and the escape of fluid into the soft tissue of the popliteal fossa and upper calf causes sudden and severe pain, swelling and tenderness. It may be confused with a deep venous thrombosis (DVT) and is diagnosed on ultrasonography. Treatment is with analgesics, rest with the leg elevated, aspiration and injection of corticosteroids into the knee joint.

BACK PAIN

Lumbar back pain

Lumbar back pain is a common symptom experienced by most people at some time in their lives. Only a few patients have a serious underlying disorder. Mechanical back pain is a common cause in young people. It starts suddenly, is often unilateral, and may be helped by rest. It may arise from the facet joints, spinal ligaments or muscle. The history, physical examination and simple investigations will also often identify the minority of patients with other causes of back pain (Table 7.3).

Table 7.3 Causes of lumbar back pain

Causes		History and examination
Mechanical	Lumbar disc prolapse Osteoarthritis Fractures Spondylolisthesis Spinal stenosis	Often sudden onset Pain worse in the evening Morning stiffness is absent Exercise aggravates pain
Inflammatory	Ankylosing spondylitis Infection (see below)	Gradual onset Pain worse in the morning Morning stiffness is present Exercise relieves pain
Serious causes	Metastases Multiple myeloma Tuberculosis osteomyelitis Bacterial osteomyelitis Spinal and root canal stenosis	Age <20 or >50 years* Constant pain without relief* History of TB, HIV, carcinoma, steroid use* Systemically unwell: fever, weight loss* Localized bone tenderness* Bilateral signs in the legs* Neurological deficit involving more than one root level* Bladder, bowel or sexual function deficits*
Others	Osteomalacia, Paget's disease, referred pain from pelvic abdominal disease	

TB, tuberculosis.
*Indicates the 'red flags' in a patient with lumbar back pain. Onset of thoracic pain is also a 'red flag'.

The age of the patient helps in deciding the aetiology of back pain because certain causes are more common in particular age groups. These are illustrated in Table 7.4.

Investigations

A detailed history and physical examination (Table 7.3) will lead to the diagnosis in many cases. The key points are age, speed of onset, the presence of motor or sensory symptoms, involvement of the bladder or bowel, the presence of stiffness and the effect of exercise. Young adults with a history suggestive of mechanical back pain and with no physical signs do not need further investigation.

- Full blood count, ESR and serum biochemistry (calcium, phosphate, alkaline phosphatase) are required only when the pain is likely to be due to malignancy, infection or a metabolic cause. Prostate-specific antigen should be measured if secondary prostatic disease is suspected.

Table 7.4 Low back pain – disorders most commonly found in specific age groups

15–30 years	30–50 years	50 years and over
Mechanical	Mechanical	Degenerative joint disease
Prolapsed intervertebral disc	Prolapsed intervertebral disc	Osteoporosis
		Paget's disease
Ankylosing spondylitis	Degenerative joint disease	Malignancy
Spondylolisthesis	Malignancy	Myeloma
Fractures (all ages)	Fractures (all ages)	Fractures (all ages)
Infective lesions (all ages)	Infective lesions (all ages)	Infective lesions (all ages)

- Spinal X-rays are only indicated if there are 'red flag' symptoms and signs (Table 7.4) which indicate a high risk of more serious underlying problems.
- Bone scans (p. 276) show increased uptake with infection or malignancy.
- MRI is useful when neurological symptoms and signs are present. It is useful for the detection of disc and cord lesions. Computed tomography (CT) scans demonstrate bone pathology more effectively.

Management

The treatment depends on the cause. Mechanical back pain is managed with analgesia, brief rest and physiotherapy. Patients should stay active within the limits of their pain. Exercise programmes reduce long-term problems.

INTERVERTEBRAL DISC DISEASE

Acute disc disease

Prolapse of the intervertebral disc results in acute back pain (lumbago), with or without radiation of the pain to areas supplied by the sciatic nerve (sciatica). It is a disease of younger people (20–40 years) because the disc degenerates with age and in elderly people is no longer capable of prolapse. In older patients, sciatica is more likely to be the result of compression of the nerve root by osteophytes in the lateral recess of the spinal canal.

Clinical features

There is a sudden onset of severe back pain, often following a strenuous activity. The pain is often clearly related to position and is aggravated by movement.

Muscle spasm leads to a sideways tilt when standing. The radiation of the pain and the clinical findings depend on the disc affected (Table 7.5), the lowest three discs being those most commonly affected.

Investigations

Investigations are of very limited value in acute disc disease and X-rays are often normal. MRI is usually reserved for patients in whom surgery is being considered (see later).

Management

Treatment is aimed at the relief of symptoms and has little effect on the duration of the disease. In the acute stage, treatment consists of bed rest on a firm mattress, analgesia and occasionally epidural corticosteroid injection in severe disease. Surgery is only considered for severe or increasing neurological impairment, e.g. foot drop or bladder symptoms. Physiotherapy is used in the recovery phase, helping to correct posture and restore movement.

Chronic disc disease

Chronic lower back pain is associated with 'degenerative' changes in the lower lumbar discs and facet joints. Pain is usually of the mechanical type

Table 7.5 Symptoms and signs of common root compression syndromes produced by lumbar disc prolapse

Root lesion	Pain	Sensory loss	Motor weakness	Reflex lost	Other signs
S1	From buttock down back of thigh and leg to ankle and foot	Sole of foot and posterior calf	Plantar flexion of ankle and toes	Ankle jerk	Diminished straight leg raising
L5	From buttock to lateral aspect of leg and dorsum of foot	Dorsum of foot and anterolateral aspect of lower leg	Dorsiflexion of foot and toes	None	Diminished straight leg raising
L4	Lateral aspect of thigh to medial side of calf	Medial aspect of calf and shin	Dorsiflexion and inversion of ankle; extension of knee	Knee jerk	Positive femoral stretch test

(see above). Sciatic radiation may occur with pain in the buttocks radiating into the posterior thigh. Usually the pain is long-standing and the prospects for cure are limited. However, measures that have been found useful include NSAIDs, physiotherapy and weight reduction. Surgery can be considered when pain arises from a single identifiable level and has failed to respond to conservative measures, and fusion at this level, with decompression of the affected nerve roots, can be successful.

Mechanical problems

Spondylolisthesis

Spondylolisthesis is characterized by a slipping forward of one vertebra on another, most commonly at L4/L5. It arises because of a defect in the pars interarticularis of the vertebra, and may be either congenital or acquired (e.g. trauma). The condition is associated with mechanical pain which worsens throughout the day. The pain may radiate to one or other leg and there may be signs of nerve root irritation. Small spondylolistheses, often associated with degenerative disease of the lumbar spine, may be treated conservatively with simple analgesics. A large spondylolisthesis causing severe symptoms should be treated with spinal fusion.

Spinal stenosis

Narrowing of the lower spinal canal compresses the cauda equina, resulting in back and buttock pain, typically coming on after a period of walking and easing with rest. Accordingly, it is sometimes called spinal claudication. Causes include disc prolapse, degenerative osteophyte formation, tumour and congenital narrowing of the spinal canal. CT and MRI will demonstrate cord compression, and treatment is by surgical decompression. Rest helps, as does bending forwards, a manoeuvre that opens the spinal canal.

Neck pain

Disc disease, both acute and chronic, the latter in association with osteoarthritis, may occur in the neck as well as in the lumbar spine. The three lowest cervical discs are most often affected, and there is pain and stiffness of the neck with or without root pain radiating to the arm. Chronic cervical disc disease is known as cervical spondylosis.

OSTEOARTHRITIS

Osteoarthritis (OA) is a disease of synovial joints (Fig. 7.1) and is the most common form of arthritis.

Epidemiology

The prevalence of OA increases with age, and most people over 60 years will have some radiological evidence of it although only a proportion of these have symptoms. OA occurs world-wide, it is more common in women and there is a familial tendency to develop nodal and generalized OA. Other risk factors are obesity, a fracture through a joint, congenital joint dysplasias, pre-existing joint damage of any cause, occupation (e.g. OA of the hip in farmers and labourers) and repetitive use and injury associated with some sports.

Pathology and pathogenesis

OA is the result of active, sometimes inflammatory but potentially reparative processes, rather than the inevitable result of trauma and ageing. It is characterized by progressive destruction and loss of articular cartilage with an accompanying periarticular bone response. The exposed subchondral bone becomes sclerotic, with increased vascularity and cyst formation. Attempts at repair produce cartilaginous growths at the margins of the joint which later become calcified (osteophytes).

Several mechanisms have been suggested for the pathogenesis:

- Metalloproteinases, e.g. stromelysin and collagenase, secreted by chondrocytes degrade collagen and proteoglycans.
- Interleukin (IL)-1 and tumour necrosis factor (TNF)-α stimulate metalloproteinase production and inhibit collagen production.
- Deficiency of growth factors, such as insulin-like growth factor and transforming growth factor, impairs matrix repair.
- Osteoprotegerin (OPG), receptor activator of nuclear factor-κB (RANK) and RANK ligand (RANKL) control subchondral bone remodelling. Their levels are significantly different in OA chondrocytes. Inhibiting RANKL may prove a new therapeutic approach in OA.
- Genetic susceptibility (35–65% influence) from multiple genes rather than a single gene defect. Mutations in the gene for type II collagen have been associated with early polyarticular OA. Polymorphisms in the gene for human aggrecan have been correlated with OA of the hand in older men.

Most OA is primary, with no obvious predisposing factor. Secondary OA occurs in joints that have been damaged in some way or are congenitally abnormal.

Clinical features

Joint pain is the main symptom, made worse by movement and relieved by rest. Stiffness occurs after rest ('gelling') and in contrast to inflammatory arthritis there is only transient (<30 minutes) morning stiffness. The joints most commonly involved are the distal interphalangeal joints (DIPJs) and first

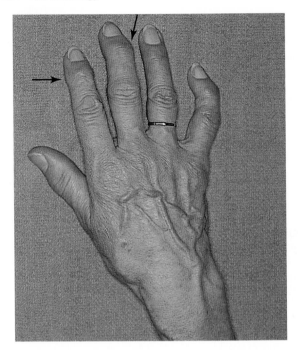

Fig. 7.2 Severe nodal osteoarthritis (OA). The distal interphalangeal joints (DIPJs) demonstrate Heberden's nodes (arrows). The middle finger DIPJ is deformed and unstable. The thumb is adducted and the bony swelling of the first carpometacarpal joint is clearly shown – 'the squared hand of nodal OA'.

carpometacarpal joint of the hands, first metatarsophalangeal joint of the foot and the weight-bearing joints – vertebrae, hips and knees. Elbows, wrists and ankles are rarely affected. On examination there is deformity and bony enlargement of the joints, limited joint movement and muscle wasting of surrounding muscle groups. Crepitus (grating) is a common finding and is probably due to the disruption of the normally smooth articulating surfaces of the joints. There may be a joint effusion. Heberden's nodes are bony swellings at the DIPJs. Bouchard's nodes are similar but occur at the proximal interphalangeal joints (PIPJs) (Fig. 7.2).

Differential diagnosis

OA is differentiated from RA by the pattern of joint involvement and the absence of the systemic features and marked early morning stiffness that occur in RA.

A chronic arthropathy (pseudo-OA) occurs, predominantly in elderly women with severe chondrocalcinosis (p. 299) but the wrists and shoulder are usually involved and the hands rarely involved. Chronic tophaceous gout (p. 297) and psoriatic arthritis affecting the DIPJs (p. 295) may mimic OA.

Investigations

- Full blood count and ESR are normal. Rheumatoid factor is negative, but positive low-titre tests may occur incidentally in elderly people.
- X-rays are only abnormal in advanced disease and show narrowing of the joint space (resulting from loss of cartilage), osteophytes, subchondral sclerosis and cyst formation.
- MRI demonstrates early cartilage changes. It is not necessary for most patients with suggestive symptoms and typical plain X-ray features.

Management

Treatment should focus on the symptoms and disability, not the radiological appearances. Patient education about the disease, non-pharmacological measures, drugs and surgery all have a role. Obese patients should be encouraged to lose weight, particularly if weight-bearing joints are affected.

- Physical measures are the keystone of OA treatment. Local strengthening and aerobic exercises improve local muscle strength, improve the mobility of weight-bearing joints and improve general aerobic fitness. Local heat or ice packs applied to an affected joint may also help. Bracing devices, joint supports, insoles for joint instability and footwear with shock-absorbing properties for lower limb OA are also used. A walking stick held on the contralateral side to the affected lower limb joint is useful. Acupuncture helps knee OA.
- Medication. Paracetamol (p. 320) has traditionally been the initial drug of choice for pain relief, with the addition of a weak opioid, e.g. dihydrocodeine (p. 321), if necessary. However, randomized trial data show that paracetamol is no more effective than placebo for back pain, with only a small benefit for hip and knee pain. NSAIDs (p. 321), e.g. ibuprofen or coxibs, are used in patients who do not respond to simple analgesia and should be used in short courses rather than on a continuous basis. NSAIDs can also be given topically. Intra-articular corticosteroid injections produce short-term improvement when there is a painful joint effusion; systemic corticosteroids are not used.
- Surgery. Total hip and knee replacement has transformed the management of severe symptomatic OA. There is reduced pain and stiffness and an associated increase in function and mobility. Complication rates are low with loosening and late bone infection being the most serious.

INFLAMMATORY ARTHRITIS

Inflammatory arthritis includes a large number of arthritic conditions in which the predominant feature is synovial inflammation. The three main subgroups of inflammatory arthritis are RA, spondyloarthritis and crystal arthritis. There is joint pain and stiffness after rest and in the morning. Morning stiffness may last several hours (cf. osteoarthritis). Blood tests often show a normochromic, normocytic anaemia and raised inflammatory markers (ESR and CRP).

Rheumatoid arthritis

RA is a chronic systemic autoimmune disorder causing a symmetrical polyarthritis.

Epidemiology

RA affects 0.5–1% of the population world-wide, with a peak prevalence between the ages of 30 and 50 years.

Aetiology and pathogenesis

Genetic and environmental factors play an aetiological role.

- *Gender.* Women before the menopause are affected three times more often than men, with an equal sex incidence thereafter suggesting an aetiological role for sex hormones.
- *Familial.* There is an increased incidence in those with a family history of RA.
- *Genetic factors.* Human leucocyte antigen (HLA)-DR4 and HLA-DRB1* 0404/0401 confer susceptibility to RA and are associated with development of more severe erosive disease. Protein tyrosine phosphatase N22 (PTPN22), STAT4 and PADI-4 have also been identified as susceptibility genes.
- *Smoking* is an environmental risk factor for seropositive RA.

The triggering antigen in RA is not known but factors produced by activated T cells (interferon, IL-2 and IL-4), macrophages (IL-1, IL-8, TNF-α, macrophage inflammatory protein), mast cells (histamine and TNF-α) and fibroblasts (IL-6, vascular cell adhesion molecule, delay accelerating factor) contribute to the ongoing synovial inflammation. Local production of rheumatoid factor (autoantibodies directed against the Fc portion of immunoglobulin [Ig]) by B cells and formation of immune complexes with complement activation also maintain the chronic inflammation.

Pathology

RA is characterized by synovitis (inflammation of the synovial lining of joints, tendon sheaths or bursae) with thickening of the synovial lining and infiltration by inflammatory cells. Generation of new synovial blood vessels is induced by angiogenic cytokines, and activated endothelial cells produce adhesion molecules, such as vascular cell adhesion molecule-1 (VCAM-1), which expedite extravasation of leucocytes into the synovium. The synovium proliferates and grows out over the surface of cartilage, producing a tumour-like mass called 'pannus'. Pannus destroys the articular cartilage and subchondral bone, producing bony erosions. This early damage justifies the use of disease-modifying drugs within 3 months of onset of the arthritis to try and induce disease remission.

Clinical features

The typical presentation is with an insidious onset of pain, early-morning stiffness (lasting more than 30 minutes) and symmetrical swelling in the proximal small joints of the hands and feet. There is spindling of the fingers caused by swelling of the PIPJs but not DIPJs. The metacarpophalangeal and wrist joints are also swollen. As the disease progresses there is weakening of joint capsules, causing joint instability, subluxation (partial dislocation) and deformity. The characteristic deformities of the rheumatoid hand are shown in Fig. 7.3. Most patients eventually have many joints involved, including the wrists, elbows, shoulders, cervical spine, knees, ankles and feet. The dorsal and lumbar spine are not involved. Joint effusions and wasting of muscles around the affected joints are early features. Less common presentations are 'explosive' (sudden onset of widespread arthritis), palindromic (relapsing and remitting monoarthritis of different large joints) or with a systemic illness with few joint symptoms initially.

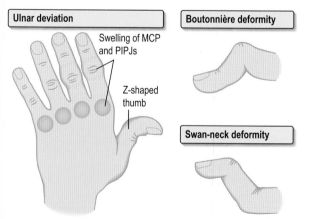

Fig. 7.3 Characteristic hand deformities in rheumatoid arthritis. MCP, metacarpophalanges; PIPJs, proximal interphalangeal joints.

In patients presenting with disproportionate involvement of a single joint, septic arthritis (p. 300) must be excluded before the symptoms are attributed to a disease flare-up.

Non-articular manifestations

Periarticular features of RA include bursitis, tenosynovitis, muscle wasting and subcutaneous nodules (rheumatoid nodules) usually over pressure points at the elbow, the finger joints and Achilles tendon. Nodules may also occur in the pleura, pericardium and lung.

Other non-articular manifestations are summarized in Table 7.6. Patients with RA also have a greater risk of infection and osteoporosis. The chronic inflammation and endothelial damage associated with RA contributes to accelerated atherosclerosis, which is partly responsible for the increased mortality rate in severe RA.

Table 7.6 Non-articular manifestations of rheumatoid arthritis

Systemic	Fever
	Fatigue
	Weight loss
Eyes	Sjögren's syndrome
	Scleritis
	Scleromalacia perforans (perforation of the eye)
Neurological	Carpal tunnel syndrome
	Atlanto-axial subluxation
	Cord compression
	Polyneuropathy, predominantly sensory
	Mononeuritis multiplex
Haematological	Lymphadenopathy
	Felty's syndrome (rheumatoid arthritis, splenomegaly, neutropenia)
	Anaemia (chronic disease, NSAID-induced gastrointestinal blood loss, haemolysis, hypersplenism)
	Thrombocytosis
Pulmonary	Pleural effusion
	Lung fibrosis
	Rheumatoid nodules
	Rheumatoid pneumoconiosis (Caplan's syndrome)
	Obliterative bronchiolitis

Table 7.6 Non-articular manifestations of rheumatoid arthritis—cont'd

Heart and peripheral vessels	Pericarditis (rarely clinically apparent)
	Pericardial effusion
	Raynaud's syndrome
Kidneys	Amyloidosis (rare)
	Analgesic nephropathy
Vasculitis	Leg ulcers
	Nail fold infarcts
	Gangrene of fingers and toes

NSAID, non-steroidal anti-inflammatory drug.

Investigations

The diagnosis of RA cannot be established by a single laboratory test and depends on the aggregation of characteristic clinical features (symmetrical peripheral polyarthritis with morning stiffness and nodules in some patients), blood tests and radiological appearances.

- Blood count. There is usually a normochromic, normocytic anaemia and thrombocytosis. The ESR and CRP are raised in proportion to the activity of the inflammatory process.
- Serum autoantibodies. ACPA (p. 286) has high specificity (90%) and sensitivity (80%) for RA and is particularly useful to distinguish early RA from acute transient synovitis. Rheumatoid factor is positive in 70% of cases and antinuclear factor at low titre in 30% (p. 286). Rheumatoid factor is not specific for RA and may occur in connective tissue diseases and some infections.
- X-ray of the affected joints shows soft tissue swelling in early disease and later joint narrowing, erosions at the joint margins and porosis of periarticular bone and cysts.
- Synovial fluid is sterile with a high neutrophil count in uncomplicated disease. In a suddenly painful joint, septic arthritis should be suspected and appropriate tests completed (p. 300).

Differential diagnosis

In the patient with symmetrical peripheral polyarthritis, prolonged morning stiffness, rheumatoid nodules and positive ACPA or rheumatoid factor, the diagnosis is straightforward. RA must be distinguished from symmetrical seronegative spondyloarthropathies; severe RA can mimic a form of psoriatic arthritis known as 'arthritis mutilans' (p. 295). In a young woman presenting with joint pains, SLE must be considered, but characteristically the joints look normal on examination in this condition. Acute viral polyarthritis (rubella, hepatitis B or parvovirus) must be considered in the differential diagnosis of early RA but these rarely last longer than 6 weeks. ACPA will be negative.

Management

No treatment cures RA; therefore the therapeutic goals are remission of symptoms, a return of full function and the maintenance of remission with disease-modifying agents. Effective management of RA requires a multidisciplinary approach, with input from rheumatologists, orthopaedic surgeons (joint replacement, arthroplasty), occupational therapists (aids to reduce disability) and physiotherapists (improvement of muscle power and maintenance of mobility to prevent flexion deformities). Patients should be advised to stop smoking to reduce the risk of cardiovascular disease.

NSAIDs and coxibs (p. 321) are effective in relieving the joint pain and stiffness of RA, but they do not slow disease progression. Individual response to NSAIDs varies considerably and it is reasonable to try several drugs in a particular patient to find the most suitable. Slow-release preparations (e.g. slow-release diclofenac) taken at night may produce dramatic relief of symptoms on the following day. Paracetamol with or without codeine or dihydrocodeine can be added for additional pain relief.

Corticosteroids suppress disease activity but the dose required is often large, with the considerable risk of long-term toxicity (p. 663). *Oral corticosteroids* are used in early disease (short-term intensive regimens) and in some patients with severe non-articular manifestations, e.g. vasculitis. *Local injection* of a troublesome joint (see below) with a long-acting corticosteroid improves pain, synovitis and effusion but repeated injections are avoided because they may accelerate joint damage. *Intramuscular* depot methylprednisolone helps to control severe disease flares.

Disease-modifying antirheumatic drugs (DMARDs) act mainly through inhibition of inflammatory cytokines and are used early (6 weeks to 6 months of disease onset) to reduce inflammation and thus slow the development of joint erosion and irreversible damage, and reduce cardiovascular risk. *Sulfasalazine* is used in patients with mild to moderate disease and for many is the drug of choice especially in younger patients and women who are planning a family. *Methotrexate* is the drug of choice for patients with more active disease. It is contraindicated in pregnancy (teratogenic) and should not be prescribed (men and women) in the 3 months prior to conception in those planning a pregnancy. Folic acid reduces side effects but may also reduce efficacy. *Leflunomide* blocks T-cell proliferation. It has a similar initial response rate to sulfasalazine but improvement continues and it is better sustained at 2 years. It is used alone or in combination with methotrexate. All drugs can have serious

Table 7.7 Side effects of disease-modifying antirheumatic drugs (DMARDs)

Drug	Side effects
Sulfasalazine	Mouth ulcers Hepatitis Male infertility (reversible)
Methotrexate	Mouth ulcers and diarrhoea Liver fibrosis Pulmonary fibrosis Renal impairment
Leflunomide	Diarrhoea Hypertension Hepatitis Alopecia
TNF-α blockers	Infusion reactions (infliximab) Infections (e.g. tuberculosis and septicaemia) Demyelinating disease Heart failure Lupus-like syndrome Autoimmune syndromes

All may cause myelosuppression (with neutropenia, thrombocytopenia and anaemia) and regular check of the full blood count is indicated together with other specific monitoring (e.g. LFTs with methotrexate and leflunomide). Rash and nausea are additional side effects of most of the drugs listed.

side effects (Table 7.7), so monitoring with blood tests is necessary. Azathioprine, gold (intramuscular or oral), hydroxychloroquine and penicillamine are used less frequently.

Biological DMARDs currently available work by the following mechanisms:

- TNF-α inhibitors (etanercept, infliximab, adalimumab, certolizumab). They vary in their mechanism of action and frequency and mode of administration. For instance, infliximab is a chimeric (human/mouse) antibody to TNF-α and is given intravenously every 8 weeks after an induction schedule. Etanercept is a soluble TNF-α receptor fusion protein that binds TNF-α and is given by self-administered subcutaneous injection
- IL-1 receptor blocker (anakinra)
- Lysis of B cells (rituximab)
- Interleukin-6 receptor antibody (tocilizumab)
- Blocks T-cell activation (abatacept).

TNF-α inhibitors are first-line treatment and slow or halt erosion formation in up to 70% of patients. They are currently used in patients who have active disease despite adequate treatment with at least two DMARDs, including methotrexate. In future the 'biologicals' will be used earlier and in more patients as the cost falls.

Prognosis

Prognosis is variable: some patients will have minimal disability after many years and others will be severely disabled, with most patients between these extremes. Prognosis can be dramatically altered with early DMARDs given under expert supervision. A poor prognosis is indicated by the following: insidious onset, female sex, increasing number of joints involved, level of disability at onset, higher inflammatory and autoimmune markers and signs of early erosive damage on imaging.

THE SERONEGATIVE SPONDYLOARTHRITIS

This title describes a group of conditions (Table 7.8) that share certain clinical features:

- A predilection for axial (spinal and sacroiliac) inflammation
- Asymmetrical peripheral arthritis
- Absence of rheumatoid factor or ACPA antibodies, hence 'seronegative'
- Inflammation of the enthesis (Fig. 7.1)
- A strong association with HLA-B27, but its aetiological relevance is unclear.

Axial spondylarthritis

This is an inflammatory disorder of the spine, affecting mainly young adults. When radiographic changes at the sacroiliac joints are present, the term 'ankylosing spondylitis' is used. It is both more common (ratio of 5:1) and more severe in men than in women.

Table 7.8 Seronegative spondyloarthritis

Axial spondylarthritis (ankylosing spondylitis)
Psoriatic arthritis
Reactive arthritis (sexually acquired, Reiter's disease, post-dysenteric reactive arthritis)
Enteropathic arthritis (ulcerative colitis/Crohn's disease)

Clinical features

The typical patient is a young man (late teens, early 20s) who presents with increasing pain and prolonged morning stiffness in the lower back and buttocks. Pain and stiffness improve with exercise but not with rest. There is a progressive loss of spinal movement. Inspection of the spine reveals two characteristic abnormalities:

- Loss of lumbar lordosis and increased kyphosis (Fig. 7.4).
- Limitation of lumbar spine mobility in both sagittal and frontal planes. Reduced spinal flexion is demonstrated by the Schober test. A mark is made

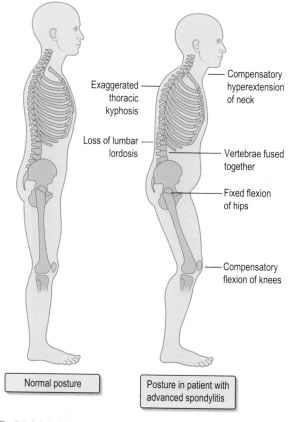

Exaggerated thoracic kyphosis

Loss of lumbar lordosis

Compensatory hyperextension of neck

Vertebrae fused together

Fixed flexion of hips

Compensatory flexion of knees

Normal posture

Posture in patient with advanced spondylitis

Fig. 7.4 Ankylosing spondylitis. The typical posture in advanced cases compared to normal posture.

at the fifth lumbar spinous process and 10 cm above, with the patient in the erect position. On bending forward, the distance should increase to >15 cm in normal individuals.

Other features include Achilles tendinitis and plantar fasciitis (enthesitis) and tenderness around the pelvis and chest wall. Reduction in chest expansion (<2.5 cm on deep inspiration measured at the fourth intercostal space) is due to costovertebral joint involvement. Non-articular features include anterior uveitis (p. 711) and, rarely, aortic incompetence, cardiac conduction defects and apical lung fibrosis.

Investigations

- ESR and CRP are often raised.
- X-rays may be normal or show erosion and sclerosis of the margins of the sacroiliac joints, proceeding to ankylosis (immobility and consolidation of the joint). In the spinal column, blurring of the upper or lower vertebral rims at the thoracolumbar junction is caused by an enthesitis at the insertion of the intervertebral ligaments. This heals with new bone formation, resulting in bony spurs (syndesmophytes). Progressive calcification of the interspinous ligaments and syndesmophytes eventually produce the 'bamboo spine' (Fig. 7.5).

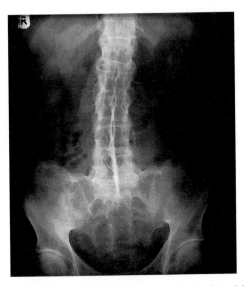

Fig. 7.5 X-ray of bamboo spine in ankylosing spondylitis. In advanced disease there is calcification of the interspinous ligaments and fusion of the facet joints as well as syndesmophytes at all levels. The sacroiliac joints fuse.

- MRI shows sacroiliitis before it is seen on plain X-ray.
- HLA-B27 testing is not usually performed.

Management

Early diagnosis and treatment is essential to prevent irreversible syndesmophyte formation and progressive calcification. With effective treatment, most patients are able to lead a normal active life and remain at work.

- Morning exercises to maintain posture and spinal mobility.
- Slow-release NSAIDs taken at night are particularly effective in relieving night pain and morning stiffness.
- Methotrexate helps the peripheral arthritis but not spinal disease. TNF-α-blocking drugs (see RA) are highly effective in active inflammatory disease and improve both spinal and peripheral joint inflammation. Early clinical studies have shown apremilast, a phosphodiesterase type 4 (PDE4) inhibitor, to be effective in spondylarthritis.

Psoriatic arthritis

Arthritis occurs in 10% of patients with psoriasis, particularly in those with nail disease (p. 811) and may precede the skin disease.

Clinical features

There are several types:

- *Distal interphalangeal arthritis*, the most typical pattern of joint involvement – dactilytis is characteristic
- *Mono- or oligoarthritis*
- *Symmetrical seronegative polyarthritis* resembling RA
- *Arthritis mutilans*, a severe form with destruction of the small bones in the hands and feet
- *Sacroiliitis* – unilateral or bilateral.

Investigations

- Routine blood tests are unhelpful in the diagnosis. The ESR is often normal.
- X-rays may show a 'pencil in cup' deformity in the interphalangeal joints (IPJs) (bone erosions create a pointed appearance and the articulating bone is concave).

Treatment

Treatment is with analgesia and NSAIDs. Local synovitis responds to intra-articular corticosteroid injections. In severe cases, methotrexate or

TNF-blocking drugs (p. 291) control both the arthritis and the skin lesions. Anti-IL-17 and PDE4 inhibitors have shown promise in clinical trials. The prognosis for joint involvement is generally better than in RA.

Reactive arthritis

Reactive arthritis is a sterile synovitis, which occurs following:

- Gastrointestinal infection with *Shigella*, *Salmonella*, *Yersinia* or *Campylobacter*
- Sexually acquired infection – non-specific urethritis in the male or cervicitis in the female due to infection with *Chlamydia trachomatis* or *Ureaplasma urealyticum*.

Persistent bacterial antigen in the inflamed synovium of affected joints is thought to drive the inflammatory process. HLA-B27 positivity increases the susceptibility to reactive arthritis.

Clinical features

The typical case is a young man who presents with an acute arthritis shortly (within 4 weeks) after an enteric or sexually acquired infection, which may have been mild or asymptomatic. The joints of the lower limbs are particularly affected in an asymmetrical pattern; the knees, ankles and feet are the most common sites.

The skin lesions resemble psoriasis. Circinate balanitis causes superficial ulcers around the penile meatus, which harden to a crust in the circumcised male. Red plaques and pustules that resemble pustular psoriasis (keratoderma blenorrhagica) are found on the palms and soles of the feet. Nail dystrophy may also occur.

Additional features are acute anterior uveitis, enthesitis (plantar fasciitis, Achilles tendonitis) and the classic triad of Reiter's syndrome (urethritis, reactive arthritis and conjunctivitis). A few patients develop sacroiliitis and spondylitis.

Investigations

The diagnosis is clinical. The ESR is raised in the acute stage. Aspirated synovial fluid is sterile, with a high neutrophil count.

Management

The acute joint inflammation responds well to NSAIDs and local corticosteroid injections. Any persisting infection is treated with antibiotics. Most patients have a single attack; relapsing cases are treated with sulfasalazine or methotrexate and TNF-blocking drugs (p. 291) in severe cases.

Enteropathic arthritis

Enteropathic arthritis is a large-joint mono- or asymmetrical oligoarthritis occurring in 10–15% of patients with ulcerative colitis or Crohn's disease. It usually parallels the activity of the inflammatory bowel disease and consequently improves as bowel symptoms improve. A HLA-B27 sacroiliitis or spondylitis occurs in 5% of patients with inflammatory bowel disease which is not related to disease activity.

CRYSTAL ARTHRITIS

Two main types of crystal – sodium urate and calcium pyrophosphate – account for the majority of crystal-induced arthritis. Neutrophils ingest the crystals and initiate a pro-inflammatory reaction.

Gout and hyperuricaemia

Gout is an inflammatory arthritis caused by hyperuricaemia and intra-articular sodium urate crystals. Hyperuricaemia and sodium urate deposition is also often asymptomatic.

Epidemiology

Gout is common. The disease is five times more common in men, occurs rarely before young adulthood (when it suggests a specific enzyme defect), and seldom occurs in pre-menopausal females. There is often a family history of gout.

Pathogenesis

Hyperuricaemia results from overproduction of uric acid or renal underexcretion (Table 7.9). Urate is derived from the breakdown of purines (adenine and guanine in DNA and RNA), which are mainly synthesized in the body. Idiopathic (primary) gout is the most common form and most patients have impaired renal excretion of uric acid.

Clinical features

Hyperuricaemia and deposition of sodium urate crystals result in four clinical syndromes:

- Acute sodium urate synovitis – acute gout
- Chronic interval gout
- Chronic polyarticular gout
- Chronic tophaceous gout
- Urate renal stone formation (p. 381).

Table 7.9 Causes of hyperuricaemia

Impaired excretion of uric acid

Chronic kidney disease (clinical gout unusual)
Drug therapy, e.g. thiazide diuretics, low-dose aspirin
Hypertension
Lead toxicity
Primary hyperparathyroidism
Hypothyroidism
Increased lactic acid production from alcohol, exercise, starvation
Glycogen storage disease type 1 (also increased production of uric acid)

Increased production of uric acid

Increased de novo purine synthesis (rare) due to:
   HGPRT deficiency (Lesch–Nyhan syndrome)
   PPS overactivity
Increased turnover of purines
Myeloproliferative disorders, e.g. polycythaemia vera
Lymphoproliferative disorders, e.g. leukaemia
Others, e.g. carcinoma, severe psoriasis

HGPRT, hypoxanthine-guanine phosphoribosyltransferase; PPS, phosphoribosyl-pyrophosphate synthetase.

Acute gout presents typically in a middle-aged male with sudden onset of severe pain, swelling and redness of the metatarsophalangeal joint of the big toe. The signs of inflammation may extend beyond the joint, giving the impression of cellulitis. The attack may be precipitated by dietary or alcoholic excess, by dehydration or by starting a diuretic. Acute attacks must be differentiated from other causes of monoarthritis, particularly septic arthritis. Presentation can also be with a polyarticular inflammatory arthritis, particularly in elderly women on long-term diuretics.

Chronic tophaceous gout presents with large, smooth, white deposits (tophi) in the skin and around the joints, particularly on the ear, the fingers and on the Achilles tendon.

Investigations

The clinical picture is often diagnostic, as is the rapid response to NSAIDs or colchicine.

- Joint fluid microscopy is the most specific and diagnostic test, revealing long, needle-shaped crystals which are negatively birefringent under polarized light. This is not usually necessary in clinical practice.
- Serum uric acid is usually raised, but may be normal during an acute attack – the levels subsequently increase and should be rechecked several

weeks after. However, the diagnosis is excluded if the serum uric acid is in the lower half of the normal range.

- Serum urea and creatinine for signs of renal impairment.

Management

Acute attacks are treated with anti-inflammatory drugs:

- NSAIDs (p. 321), e.g. diclofenac (75–100 mg immediately, then 50 mg every 6–8 hours), or coxibs, e.g. lumiracoxib 100 mg once daily. After 24–48 hours reduced doses are given for a further week.
- Colchicine (1000 µg immediately, then 500 µg every 6–12 hours) but only if NSAIDs are not tolerated or ineffective. It has a narrow therapeutic window and is extremely toxic in overdose (diarrhoea, abdominal pain, multi-organ failure).
- Corticosteroids: intramuscular or intra-articular depot methylprednisolone.

Further attacks are prevented by reducing serum uric acid levels. Obese patients should lose weight, alcohol consumption should be reduced and drugs such as thiazides and salicylates should be withdrawn. A diet which reduces total calorie and cholesterol intake and avoids purine-rich foods (offal, some fish and shellfish and spinach) is advised. Patients with frequent attacks (more than two per year) despite dietary changes or with gouty tophi or renal impairment are treated with allopurinol. Treatment is not started within 1 month after an acute attack and NSAIDs or colchicine are given for 4 weeks before and after starting allopurinol, as it may induce an acute attack. Allopurinol inhibits xanthine oxidase (an enzyme in the purine breakdown pathway) and reduces serum urate levels rapidly. Febuxostat is a non-purine analogue inhibitor of xanthine oxidase that is well tolerated and as effective as allopurinol. Anakinra blocks IL-1β and canakinumab is a human monoclonal antibody with specific cross-reactivity for IL-1β but not other members of the IL-1 family. Their cost-effectiveness in managing gout resistant to conventional agents is still subject to trials.

Asymptomatic hyperuricaemia is not usually treated unless plasma levels are very high or in patients with cancer to prevent the tumour lysis syndrome (p. 257).

Pseudogout (pyrophosphate arthropathy)

Deposition of calcium pyrophosphate dihydrate in articular cartilage and periarticular tissue produces the radiological appearance of chondrocalcinosis (linear calcification parallel to the articular surfaces). Shedding of crystals into a joint produces acute synovitis that resembles acute gout, except that it is more common in elderly women and usually affects the knee or wrist. In young people it may be associated with haemochromatosis, hyperparathyroidism, Wilson's disease or alkaptonuria (excess homogentisic acid polymerizes to produce a black/brown product deposited in cartilage and other tissues).

Investigations

- The diagnosis is made on joint fluid microscopy demonstrating small brick-shaped pyrophosphate crystals which are positively birefringent under polarized light (compare uric acid). The presence of chondrocalcinosis on X-ray is also suggestive of pseudogout.
- Blood count may show a raised white cell count.

Management

Joint aspiration with NSAIDs or colchicine forms the mainstay of treatment. Injection of local corticosteroids may also be useful once septic arthritis is excluded on joint fluid examination.

INFECTION OF BONES AND JOINTS

Infection of the joints is usually caused by bacteria and rarely by fungi. Some viruses (rubella, mumps and hepatitis B virus infections) are associated with a mild self-limiting arthritis but this is not due to direct joint involvement.

Septic arthritis

Septic arthritis is a medical emergency. Delay in treatment can result in irreversible joint destruction, long-term disability or death. It results from infection of the joint with pyogenic organisms, most commonly *Staphylococcus aureus*. Gram-negative organisms are more common in the elderly or immunosuppressed. Joints become infected by direct injury or by blood-borne infection from an infected skin lesion or other site. Risk factors for septic arthritis are prosthetic joints, pre-existing joint disease, recent intra-articular steroid injection and diabetes mellitus.

Clinical features

Classically there is a hot, painful, swollen, red joint, which has developed acutely. There may be fever and evidence of infection elsewhere. In the elderly and immunosuppressed and in RA the articular signs may be muted and a high index of suspicion is needed to make the diagnosis. In 20% of cases the septic arthritis involves more than one joint. Prosthetic joint infection may be early (within 3 months of joint infection) or delayed/late. Early infection presents with wound inflammation or discharge, joint effusion, loss of function and pain. Late disease presents with pain or mechanical dysfunction.

Management

This is summarized in Emergency Box 7.1.

✚ Emergency Box 7.1

Acute monoarthritis

Investigations

1. Joint aspiration (by ultrasound guidance if necessary) and synovial fluid analysis:
   - Appearance and white cell count (WCC)
     - Normal fluid – straw coloured, contains <3000 WCC/mm³
     - Inflammatory fluid – cloudy, contains >3000 WCC/mm³
     - Septic fluid – opaque, contains up to 75 000 WCC/mm³, mostly neutrophils
   - Urgent Gram stain (but may be negative in bacterial infection) and culture
   - Polarized light microscopy for crystals (in gout and pseudogout)
2. Bloods: Full blood count, erythrocyte sedimentation rate, C-reactive protein, blood cultures
3. X-rays of the affected joint are of no value in the diagnosis because usually normal initially. Loosening or bone loss around a previously well, fixed prosthetic implant suggests infection
4. Swab of urethra, cervix and anorectum if gonococcal infection a possibility

Treatment of acute non-gonococcal bacterial arthritis

- Initial treatment pending sensitivities: flucloxacillin 1–2 g 6 hourly i.v. (erythromycin or clindamycin if penicillin allergic) and oral fusidic acid 500 mg 8 hourly. Add gentamicin in immunosuppressed patients to cover Gram-negative organisms. Modify treatment depending on culture and sensitivity and continue with two antibiotics for 6 weeks (initial 2 weeks intravenously) and a single antibiotic for a further 6 weeks
- Adequate joint drainage: by needle aspiration, arthroscopy or open drainage. Always refer infection of a prosthetic joint to orthopaedic surgeons
- Immobilize joint in acute stages, mobilize early to avoid contractures
- NSAIDs for pain relief

Specific types of bacterial arthritis

Gonococcal arthritis involves one or several joints and occurs secondary to genital, rectal or oral infection (often asymptomatic). It is the most common cause of septic arthritis in previously fit young adults. Concomitant skin involvement is common (maculopapular pustules). The organism can usually be cultured from the bloodstream and from the joints. Culture is usually positive from the genital tract, even if the joint fluid is sterile. Treatment is with penicillin, ciprofloxacin or doxycycline for 2 weeks, and joint rest.

Meningococcal arthritis may complicate meningococcal septicaemia and presents as a migratory polyarthritis. It results from the deposition of circulating immune complexes containing meningococcal antigens. Treatment is with penicillin.

Tuberculous arthritis Approximately 1% of patients with tuberculosis have joint and also bone involvement. The hip, knee and spine (intervertebral disc) are most commonly affected. There is an insidious onset of pain, swelling and dysfunction. The patient is febrile, has night sweats and loses weight. Culture of synovial fluid, synovial biopsy or intervertebral disc biopsy (under CT guidance) is necessary to make the diagnosis. Treatment is as for tuberculosis elsewhere (p. 543) but extended to 9 months, together with initial joint rest and immobilization.

Osteomyelitis

Osteomyelitis can be due either to metastatic haematogenous spread (e.g. from a boil) or to local infection. *Staphylococcus* is the most common causative organism. Other organisms are *Haemophilus influenzae* and *Salmonella* (in sickle cell anaemia). Symptoms are fever, local pain and erythema, and sinus formation in chronic osteomyelitis. Diagnosis is usually by CT, MRI or bone scan (p. 276). Blood cultures, as well as bone biopsy and culture, can be used to identify the organism and sensitivities. Usual treatment is with flucloxacillin and fusidic acid for at least 4–6 weeks with intravenous medication initially.

AUTOIMMUNE RHEUMATIC DISEASES

Autoimmune disease is a pathological condition caused by an immune response directed against an antigen within the host, i.e. a self-antigen. Organ-specific autoimmune diseases include Graves' disease, Hashimoto's thyroiditis and type 1 diabetes mellitus. In the autoimmune rheumatic diseases (ARDs) the autoantibodies are not organ-specific. The term 'ARD' is preferable to the older term 'connective tissue disease' because the clinical effects of ARD are not limited to connective tissue (Table 7.2) and the clinical manifestations are systemic and diverse. These diseases are:

- SLE
- Antiphospholipid syndrome
- Systemic sclerosis (scleroderma)
- Polymyositis and dermatomyositis
- Sjögren's syndrome
- 'Overlap' syndromes and undifferentiated autoimmune rheumatic disease.

Systemic lupus erythematosus

SLE is an inflammatory multisystem disease characterized by the presence of serum antibodies against nuclear components.

Epidemiology

It is a disease mostly of young women, with a peak age of onset between 20 and 40 years. It affects about 0.1% of the population but is more common in African-American women, with a prevalence of 1 in 250.

Aetiology

The cause of the disease is unknown and is probably multifactorial:

- *Heredity.* There is a higher concordance rate in monozygotic (identical) twins (up to 25%) compared to dizygotic twins (3%).
- *Genetics.* Genes linked to the development of SLE include HLA-B8, -DR3 and -A1 and deficiencies of the complement genes C1q, C2 or C4.
- *Sex hormone status.* The higher incidence in pre-menopausal women and males with Klinefelter's (XXY) syndrome suggests an oestrogen hormonal effect.
- *Drugs.* Hydralazine, isoniazid, procainamide and penicillamine can cause a mild lupus-like syndrome, which often resolves after the drug is withdrawn.
- *Ultraviolet light* can trigger flares of SLE, especially in the skin.
- *Exposure to Epstein–Barr virus* has been suggested as a trigger for SLE.

Pathogenesis

Apoptotic cells and cell fragments are cleared inefficiently by phagocytes, resulting in transfer to lymphoid tissue where they are taken up by antigen-presenting cells. These self-antigens, including nuclear constituents (e.g. DNA and histones), are presented to T cells, which in turn stimulate B cells to produce autoantibodies directed against the antigens. The clinical manifestations of SLE are mediated by antibody formation and the development and deposition of immune complexes, complement activation and influx of neutrophils and abnormal cytokine production (increased blood levels of IL-10 and α-interferon).

Clinical features

Clinical manifestations are varied (Table 7.10). A symmetrical small-joint arthralgia and skin manifestations are common presenting features. Synovitis and joint effusions are uncommon and joint destruction is very rare. Non-specific features such as fever, malaise and depression can dominate the clinical picture.

Discoid lupus is a benign variant of the disease, in which only the skin is involved. There is a characteristic facial rash with erythematous plaques which progress to scarring and pigmentation.

Investigations

- Blood count usually shows a normochromic, normocytic anaemia, often with neutropenia/lymphopenia and thrombocytopenia. The ESR is

Table 7.10 Clinical features of systemic lupus erythematosus

Musculoskeletal (affected in >90%)

Small joint arthralgia
Myalgia
Aseptic necrosis of hip or knee

General

Tiredness
Fever
Depression
Weight loss

Skin (affected in 85% cases)

'Butterfly' rash – erythematous rash on cheeks and bridge of nose
Vasculitic lesions (finger tips, nail folds)
Urticaria and purpura
Photosensitivity
Alopecia

Blood

Anaemia (chronic disease and/or haemolytic)
Leucopenia/lymphopenia
Thrombocytopenia

Nervous system (affected in 60% cases)

Epilepsy
Migraine
Cerebellar ataxia
Aseptic meningitis
Cranial nerve lesions
Polyneuropathy

Lungs (affected in 50% cases)

Pleurisy/pleural effusions (exudates)
Restrictive defect (rare)

Heart and cardiovascular system (affected in 25% cases)

Pericarditis and pericardial effusions
Myocarditis leading to arrhythmias
Aortic valve lesions (rare)
Thrombosis – arterial and venous
Accelerated atherosclerosis
Raynaud's phenomenon

Kidneys (clinical involvement in 30% cases)

Glomerulonephritis

Gastrointestinal symptoms

Mouth ulcers (common, may be presenting feature)
Mesenteric vasculitis

raised but the CRP is usually normal unless the patient has a coexistent infection.

- Urea and creatinine only rise when renal disease is advanced. Low serum albumin or high urine protein/creatinine ratio are early indicators of lupus nephritis.
- Serum autoantibodies: many different autoantibodies are present in SLE (Table 7.2). Anti-dsDNA (double stranded DNA) is specific for SLE and is positive in 70% of cases.
- Serum complement C3 and C4 levels are reduced in active disease.
- Histology. Characteristic histological and immunofluorescent abnormalities (deposition of IgG and complement) are seen in biopsies from the kidney or skin.

Management

Treatment depends on the symptoms and severity of disease. Patients should be advised to avoid excessive sunlight and reduce cardiovascular risk factors, e.g. cessation of smoking.

- NSAIDs are useful for patients with mild disease and with arthralgia.
- Chloroquine and hydroxychloroquine are used for mild disease when symptoms cannot be controlled with NSAIDs, or for cutaneous disease.
- Corticosteroids form the mainstay of treatment, particularly in moderate to severe disease. The aim is to control disease activity (e.g. prednisolone 30 mg/day for 4 weeks) before gradually reducing the dose.
- Immunosuppressives (e.g. mycophenolate mofetil, azathioprine), usually in combination with corticosteroids, are used for patients with severe manifestations, e.g. renal or cerebral disease. Newer agents such as rituximab (anti-CD20, p. 256) are used in refractory cases.
- Topical steroids are used for discoid lupus.

Prognosis

The disease is characterized by relapses and remissions even in severe disease. The 10-year survival is about 90%, although much lower if there is major organ involvement.

Antiphospholipid syndrome

This syndrome is characterized by thrombosis and/or recurrent miscarriages and persistently positive blood tests for antiphospholipid antibodies (detected by the anticardiolipin, lupus anticoagulant or anti-β_2-glycoprotein I test). These antibodies are thought to play a role in thrombosis by reacting with plasma proteins and phospholipids with an effect on platelet membranes, endothelial cells and clotting compounds. Antiphospholipid syndrome occurs on its own or in association with another autoimmune rheumatic disease, most commonly SLE.

Clinical features

The major clinical features are the result of thrombosis:

- In arteries: stroke, transient ischaemic attacks, myocardial infarction
- In veins: DVT, Budd–Chiari syndrome (p. 181)
- In the placenta: recurrent miscarriages.

Other features include valvular heart disease, migraine, epilepsy, thrombocytopenia, renal impairment and accelerated atheroma.

Management

Long-term warfarin is given to patients who have had a thrombosis. Pregnant patients with antiphospholipid syndrome are given aspirin and heparin. Aspirin or clopidogrel are sometimes given as prophylaxis to patients with antiphospholipid syndrome who have no history of thrombosis.

Systemic sclerosis (scleroderma)

Systemic sclerosis (scleroderma) is a multisystem disease with involvement of the skin and Raynaud's phenomenon (p. 488) occurring early. It is three times more common in women than in men and usually presents between the ages of 30 and 50 years.

Aetiology

Pathogenesis is complex and not completely understood. Genetic predisposition, immune activation, infection and an environmental toxin initiate an endothelial cell lesion and widespread vascular damage. Increased vascular permeability and activation of endothelial cells result in upregulation of adhesion molecules (E-selectin, vascular cell adhesion molecule [VCAM], intercellular adhesion molecule-1 [ICAM-1]), cell adhesion (T and B cells, monocytes, neutrophils) and migration through the leaky endothelium and into the extracellular matrix. These cell–cell and cell–matrix interactions stimulate the production of cytokines and growth factors which mediate the proliferation and activation of vascular and connective tissue cells, particularly fibroblasts. The end result is uncontrolled and irreversible proliferation of connective tissue, and thickening of vascular walls with narrowing of the lumen.

Clinical features

Limited cutaneous scleroderma (LcSSc, 70% of cases)

This condition usually starts with Raynaud's phenomenon many years before any skin changes (of hands, face, feet and forearms). The skin is thickened, bound down to underlying structures, and the fingers taper (sclerodactyly). There is a characteristic facial appearance, with 'beaking' of the nose, radial furrowing of the lips and limitation of mouth opening (microstomia). There may be painful digital ulcers, telangiectasia and palpable subcutaneous nodules of calcium deposition in the fingers (calcinosis). CREST syndrome (Calcinosis, Raynaud's phenomenon, Esophageal involvement, Sclerodactyly, Telangiectasia) was the term previously used to describe this syndrome.

Diffuse cutaneous scleroderma (DcSSc, 30% of cases)

The skin changes develop more rapidly and are more widespread than in limited cutaneous scleroderma. There is early involvement of other organs:

- Gastrointestinal involvement with dilatation and atony in the oesophagus (heartburn and dysphagia), small intestine (bacterial overgrowth and malabsorption) and colon (pseudo-obstruction).
- Renal involvement – acute and chronic kidney disease. Acute hypertensive crisis is a complication of the renal involvement.
- Lung disease – fibrosis and pulmonary vascular disease resulting in pulmonary hypertension.
- Myocardial fibrosis leads to arrhythmias and conduction disturbances.

Investigations

The diagnosis of scleroderma is primarily based upon the presence of characteristic skin changes.

- Blood count shows a normochromic, normocytic anaemia and the ESR may be raised.
- Urea and creatinine rise with renal disease.
- Serum autoantibodies (Table 7.2). Antinuclear antibodies are often positive. Anti-topoisomerase 1 (Scl 70) and anti-RNA polymerase I and III antibodies are highly specific for patients with diffuse cutaneous scleroderma. Anticentromere antibodies occur in limited cutaneous scleroderma. Autoantibodies do not occur in all patients.
- Radiology. An X-ray of the hands may show deposits of calcium around the fingers, and there may be erosion and resorption of the tufts of the distal phalanges. High-resolution CT demonstrates fibrotic lung involvement. Barium swallow shows impaired oesophageal motility.
- Barium swallow generally confirms impaired motility.

Management

This is symptomatic and based on organ involvement. There is no specific treatment. Angiotensin-converting enzyme inhibitors are the drug of first choice to treat hypertension and to prevent further kidney damage. Pulmonary hypertension is treated with oral vasodilators, oxygen and warfarin. Pulmonary fibrosis is treated with cyclophosphamide or azathioprine combined with low-dose oral prednisolone.

Prognosis

The 10-year survival is 70% and 55% in limited cutaneous and diffuse cutaneous disease, respectively. Pulmonary fibrosis and pulmonary hypertension are the major causes of death.

Polymyositis and dermatomyositis

Polymyositis (PM) is a rare muscle disorder of unknown aetiology in which there is inflammation and necrosis of skeletal muscle fibres. When the skin is involved it is called dermatomyositis (DM). PM and DM affect adults and children and are more common in women.

Clinical features

There is symmetrical progressive muscle weakness and wasting affecting the proximal muscles of the shoulder and pelvic girdle. Patients have difficulty squatting, going upstairs, rising from a chair and raising their hands above the head. Pain and tenderness are uncommon. Involvement of pharyngeal, laryngeal and respiratory muscles can lead to dysphagia, dysphonia and respiratory failure. In dermatomyositis there are also characteristic skin changes: heliotrope (purple) discolouration of the eyelids and scaly erythematous plaques over the knuckles (Gottron's papules). Other features include arthralgia, dysphagia resulting from oesophageal muscle involvement, and Raynaud's phenomenon. DM is associated with an increased incidence of underlying malignancy.

Investigations

- Muscle biopsy is the definitive test in establishing the diagnosis and in excluding other causes of myopathy. There is inflammatory cell infiltration and necrosis of muscle cells.
- Serum muscle enzymes (creatine kinase, aminotransferases, aldolase) are elevated.
- Anti-JO antibodies (anti-tRNA synthetase) are positive.
- ESR is usually not raised.
- Electromyography (EMG) shows characteristic changes.
- MRI can demonstrate areas of muscle inflammation.

Management

Oral prednisolone is the treatment of choice: 0.5–1.0 mg/kg body weight continued for at least 1 month after myositis has become clinically and enzymatically inactive and then tapered gradually down. Immunosuppressive therapy (azathioprine, methotrexate, ciclosporin) is required if there is disease relapse on steroid tapering.

Sjögren's syndrome

Sjögren's syndrome is characterized by immunologically mediated destruction of epithelial exocrine glands, especially the lacrimal and salivary glands. It predominantly affects middle-aged women.

Clinical features

The main features are dry eyes (keratoconjunctivitis sicca) and dry mouth (xerostomia). Clinical clues are difficulty eating a dry biscuit and absence of pooling of the saliva when the tongue is lifted. It occurs as an isolated disorder (primary Sjögren's syndrome) or in association with another autoimmune disease (secondary Sjögren's syndrome), commonly rheumatoid arthritis or SLE. Other features of Sjögren's syndrome are arthritis, Raynaud's phenomenon, renal tubular defects causing diabetes insipidus and renal tubular acidosis, pulmonary fibrosis, vasculitis and an increased incidence of non-Hodgkin's B-cell lymphoma.

Investigations

- Serum autoantibodies: antinuclear (in 80% of patients), anti-Ro (60–90%) and rheumatoid factor in primary Sjögren's syndrome.
- Labial gland biopsy shows characteristic changes of lymphocyte infiltration and destruction of acinar tissue.
- A positive Schirmer test (a standard strip of filter paper is placed on the inside of the lower eyelid; wetting of less than 10 mm in 5 minutes is positive) confirms defective tear production.

Management

Treatment is symptomatic with artificial tears and saliva replacement solutions.

'Overlap' syndrome and undifferentiated autoimmune rheumatic disease

An overlap syndrome combines features of more than one ARD. Undifferentiated ARD is the term used when patients have evidence of autoimmunity and some clinical features of ARDs but not enough to make a diagnosis of any individual ARD.

SYSTEMIC INFLAMMATORY VASCULITIS

Vasculitis is inflammation of the blood vessel walls and can be seen in many diseases, including SLE, RA, polymyositis and some allergic drug reactions. The term 'systemic vasculitides' describes a group of multisystem disorders

Table 7.11 Classification of systemic vasculitis
Large (aorta and its major branches)
Giant-cell arteritis/polymyalgia rheumatica
Takayasu's arteritis
Medium (main visceral vessels, e.g. renal, coronary)
Polyarteritis nodosa
Kawasaki's disease (affects children <5 years)
Small (small arteries, arterioles, venules and capillaries)
ANCA positive
Microscopic polyangiitis
Granulomatosis with polyangiitis
Eosinophilic granulomatosis with polyangiitis
ANCA negative
Henoch–Schönlein purpura
Cutaneous leucocytoclastic vasculitis
Essential cryoglobulinaemia
ANCA, antineutrophil cytoplasmic antibodies.

in which vasculitis is the principal feature and classification is based on the size of the vessels affected (Table 7.11) and the presence or absence of antineutrophil cytoplasmic antibodies (ANCA). They are all associated with anaemia and a raised ESR and all are rare, except for giant cell (temporal) arteritis.

Polymyalgia and giant cell arteritis

Polymyalgia (PMR) and giant cell arteritis (GCA) are systemic illnesses affecting patients older than 50 years. Both are associated with the finding of GCA on temporal artery biopsy. Some patients may have symptoms and signs limited to PMR or to GCA throughout the course of their illness, whereas other patients may have manifestations of both.

Clinical features

PMR causes an abrupt onset of stiffness and intense pain in the muscles of the neck and shoulder, and hips and lumbar spine. Symptoms are worst in the morning. Significant objective weakness is uncommon. There may be constitutional symptoms, with malaise, fever, weight loss and anorexia. Arteritic involvement by inflammation is most frequently noticed in the superficial temporal arteries and causes headache, tenderness over the scalp or temple (combing the hair may be painful), and claudication of the jaw when eating. GCA affecting the vertebrobasilar, and sometimes the carotid, circulation may result in stroke. The most devastating complication of GCA is sudden loss of vision (which may be permanent) due to involvement of the ophthalmic artery. Early recognition and treatment is therefore essential.

Investigations

Treatment is started based on a clinical diagnosis and investigations showing a very high ESR (around 100 mm/h) and CRP. There is often a normochromic, normocytic anaemia. Temporal artery biopsy is performed if GCA is suspected and should be performed before or within a week of starting corticosteroids. Lesions are patchy, so a negative biopsy does not exclude the condition.

Management

Treatment is with corticosteroids, which produce a dramatic reduction in symptoms of PMR within 24–28 hours of starting treatment. Prednisolone 10–15 mg/day is given for PMR and 60 mg/day for GCA. The dose is reduced by weekly decrements of 5 mg. Once 10 mg is reached, a reduction of 1 mg every 2–4 weeks is usually sufficient. The dose is titrated against symptoms and the ESR. Prophylaxis against steroid-induced osteoporosis should be given (p. 318). The disease may relapse when steroid treatment is stopped.

Takayasu's arteritis

This is rare, except in Japan. Vasculitis involving the aortic arch and other major arteries causes hypertension, absent peripheral pulses, strokes and cardiac failure. Treatment is with corticosteroids.

Polyarteritis nodosa

Polyarteritis nodosa (PAN) predominantly affects middle-aged men. Its occasional association with hepatitis B antigenaemia suggests a vasculitis secondary to immune complex deposition. There is a necrotizing arteritis associated with microaneurysm formation, thrombosis and infarction. Clinical features include fever, malaise, weight loss, myalgia, mononeuritis multiplex, abdominal pain (resulting from visceral infarcts), myocardial infarction and heart failure (resulting from coronary arteritis), renal impairment and hypertension. The lungs are rarely involved (cf. ANCA-positive vasculitides). The diagnosis is made on angiography (microaneurysms in hepatic, intestinal or renal vessels) or biopsy of an affected organ, often the kidney. Treatment is with corticosteroids, usually in combination with immunosuppressive drugs (e.g. azathioprine).

Microscopic polyarteritis (polyangiitis)

This condition involves the lungs and the kidney, where it results in haemoptysis, haematuria, proteinuria and progressive renal failure. Other features include arthralgia and purpuric rashes. Diagnosis is by renal biopsy and measurement of serum perinuclear (p)-ANCA, present in 60% (Table 7.2). Treatment is similar to PAN.

Eosinophilic granulomatosis with polyangiitis

This is rare and characterized by a triad of asthma, eosinophilia and a systemic vasculitis affecting the peripheral nerves and skin (nodules, petechiae, purpura) but kidney involvement is uncommon. Treatment is similar to PAN.

Henoch–Schönlein purpura

This condition is most commonly seen in children and presents as a purpuric rash, mainly on the legs and buttocks. Abdominal pain, arthritis, haematuria and nephritis also occur. It is characterized by vascular deposition of IgA-dominant immune complexes, and the onset is often preceded by an acute upper respiratory tract infection. Recovery is usually spontaneous.

Cryoglobulinaemic vasculitis

Cryoglobulins are Igs and complement components that precipitate reversibly in the cold. Types include essential cryoglobulinaemia (no underlying disease) or associated with infection (e.g. hepatitis B and C, human immunodeficiency virus [HIV]) or autoimmune disease. There is involvement of the skin (purpura, arthralgia, leg ulcers), kidneys (glomerulonephritis) and nervous system (polyneuropathy). Treatment is similar to PAN.

Behçet's disease

This rare multisystem chronic disease of unknown cause is most common in Turkey, Iran and Japan. It is characterized by recurrent oral ulceration. Diagnosis is clinical and requires the presence of oral ulceration and any two of the following: genital ulcers, eye lesions (uveitis, retinal vascular lesions), skin lesions (erythema nodosum, papulopustular lesions) or a positive skin pathergy test (skin injury, e.g. needle prick, leads to pustule formation within 48 hours). Other features include arthritis, gastrointestinal ulceration with pain and diarrhoea, pulmonary and renal lesions, meningoencephalitis and organic confusional states. Treatment is with immunosuppressive therapy (steroids, azathioprine, ciclosporin) or, occasionally, thalidomide.

DISEASES OF BONE

Bone normally consists of 70% mineral and 30% organic matrix (mostly type 1 collagen fibres). The mineral component consists mostly of a complex crystalline salt of calcium and phosphate called hydroxyapatite. Although major skeletal growth occurs in childhood, adult bone is continuously being remodelled, with bone formation and resorption. Two major cell types are involved in bone remodelling:

- Osteoblasts produce matrix and regulate its mineralization. Bone resorption is regulated through the balance of the stimulatory RANKL (the **l**igand for **r**eceptor **a**ctivator of **n**uclear factor **k**appaB) and its antagonist, OPG (osteoprotegerin). Osteoblasts express receptors for parathyroid hormone (PTH), oestrogen, glucocorticoids, vitamin D, inflammatory cytokines and the transforming growth factor-β family, all of which may influence bone remodelling.
- Osteoclasts remove and resorb the mineral phase and collagen matrix in response to RANKL.

Control of calcium and bone metabolism

Vitamin D and PTH are the major factors that control plasma calcium concentration and bone turnover. Bone metabolism is also controlled by calcitonin, glucocorticoids, sex hormones, growth hormone and thyroid hormone. The effect of different bone disorders on calcium, phosphate, PTH and alkaline phosphatase (ALP) are given in Table 7.12.

Vitamin D

The metabolism and actions of vitamin D are shown in Fig. 7.6.

Table 7.12 Biochemistry results in bone disorders

	Calcium	Phosphate	ALP	PTH
Osteoporosis	N	N	N	N
Osteomalacia	↓ (may be N)	N (may be ↓)		May be raised (secondary hyperparathyroidism)
Paget's disease	N	N	↑	N
Primary hyperparathyroidism	↑	↓	N	↑
Secondary hyperparathyroidism	↓/N	N	N/↑	↑
Hypoparathyroidism	↓	↑	N	↓

↑, increased; ↓, decreased; ALP, alkaline phosphatase; N, normal; PTH, parathyroid hormone.

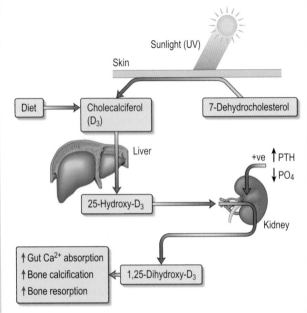

Fig. 7.6 The metabolism and actions of vitamin D. The primary source of vitamin D in humans is photoactivation in the skin of 7-dehydrocholesterol to cholecalciferol (D_3), which is then converted first in the liver to 25-hydroxyvitamin D and subsequently in the kidney to the much more active form, 1,25-dihydroxycholecalciferol [$1,25(OH)_2D_3$]. Regulation of the latter step is by parathyroid hormone, phosphate and feedback inhibition by $1,25(OH)_2D_3$. This step can also occur in lymphomatous and sarcoid tissue, resulting in the hypercalcaemia that may complicate these diseases.
Ca^{2+}, calcium; PO_4, phosphate; PTH, parathyroid hormone; UV, ultraviolet.

Parathyroid hormone

PTH is secreted from chief cells of the parathyroid gland. Plasma levels rise in response to a fall in serum ionized calcium. The effects are several, all serving to increase plasma calcium and decrease plasma phosphate:

- Increased osteoclastic resorption of bone
- Increased intestinal absorption of calcium
- Increased synthesis of $1,25\text{-}(OH)_2D_3$ (Fig. 7.6)
- Increased renal tubular reabsorption of calcium.

Hyper- and hypoparathyroidism are covered in Chapter 14 (pp. 653–658).

Osteoporosis

This reduction in bone mass and micro-architectural deterioration of bone tissue leads to bone fragility and an increased risk of fracture. Osteoporotic fractures (fragility fractures, low-trauma fractures) occur without major trauma. Osteoporosis is defined as a BMD more than 2.5 standard deviations (SDs) below the young adult mean value (T-score ≤ -2.5). Values between 1 and 2.5 SDs below the young adult mean are termed 'osteopenia'. There are additional risk factors identifiable from the history and examination which increase the fracture risk independently of BMD (Table 7.13) and thus assessment of fracture risk based solely on BMD will miss individuals at risk for fracture.

Aetiology

Osteoporosis is related to either inadequate peak bone mass and/or ongoing bone loss. Peak bone mass is achieved in early adult life and depends on genetic factors, nutritional factors, sex hormone status and physical activity. Then age-related bone loss occurs with an accelerated loss in women starting around the time of the menopause. The risk factors for osteoporosis are those that cause a reduction in peak bone mass attained in adult life or those that cause increased bone loss (Table 7.13).

Table 7.13 Risk factors for osteoporosis and fragility fracture

BMD-dependent	BMD-independent
Female sex	Increasing age
Caucasian/Asian	Previous fragility fracture
Hypogonadism	Family history of hip fracture
Immobilization	Low body mass index
Chronic liver disease	Smoking
Chronic renal disease	Alcohol abuse
Chronic obstructive pulmonary disease	Glucocorticoid therapy
Gastrointestinal disease	High bone turnover
Low dietary calcium intake	Increased risk of falling
Vitamin D insufficiency	Rheumatoid arthritis
Drugs (heparin, ciclosporin, anticonvulsants)	
Endocrine disease (Cushing's syndrome, hyperthyroidism, hyperparathyroidism)	
Other diseases (diabetes mellitus, mastocytosis, multiple myeloma)	

BMD, bone mineral density.

Clinical features

Symptoms of osteoporosis are the result of fractures, which typically occur at four sites: the thoracic and lumbar vertebrae, proximal femur and distal radius (Colles' fracture). Thoracic vertebral fractures may lead to kyphosis and loss of height ('widow's stoop').

Investigations

- DXA is the gold standard in measurement of bone density, usually of the lumbar spine and proximal femur. Osteoporosis is diagnosed when the BMD T-score falls to -2.5 or below.
- Radiology (X-rays) demonstrates fractures but is insensitive for detecting osteopenia.
- Serum biochemistry is normal (Table 7.12).
- Secondary causes of osteoporosis (Table 7.13) should be looked for by appropriate blood tests in men and pre-menopausal women.

Assessment of fracture risk

This should take into account both BMD and clinical risk factors (Table 7.13). Indications for DXA scanning are listed in Table 7.14. The Risk Factor Assessment Tool (World Health Organization [WHO] 2008) estimates the 10-year probability of hip fracture or major osteoporotic fractures combined for an untreated patient between the ages of 40 and 90 years (http://www.shef.ac.uk/FRAX/). It integrates clinical risk factors with femoral neck BMD (hip BMD may also be used in women). It is a guide only, and will not be helpful in all patients, e.g. those with low spinal BMD but normal femoral neck. In patients aged over 75 years with a fragility fracture, DXA scanning is often not necessary prior to treatment for osteoporosis. FRAX does not identify the level of fracture risk at which treatment should be started and this will vary depending partly on the

---

Table 7.14 Indications for dual-energy X-ray absorptiometry scanning

Radiographic osteopenia
Previous fragility fracture (in those aged less than 75 years)
Glucocorticoid therapy (in those aged less than 65 years)
Body mass index below 19 kg/m²
Maternal history of hip fracture
BMD-dependent risk factors in Table 7.13

In patients presenting with height loss and/or kyphosis, lateral thoracic spine X-ray is the initial investigation and shows loss of anterior vertebral body height and wedging due to fracture.
BMD, bone mineral density.

medical resources of the country. In the UK, osteoporosis treatment is cost-effective for a 4% 10-year risk of hip fracture and 3% in the USA.

Management

Prevention and treatment New vertebral fractures require bed rest for 1–2 weeks and strong analgesia. Muscle relaxants (e.g. diazepam 2 mg three times daily), subcutaneous calcitonin (50 IU daily) or intravenous pamidronate (single dose 60–90 mg) are also given for pain relief. Non-spinal fractures are treated by conventional orthopaedic means. Lifestyle advice includes stopping smoking, reducing alcohol intake, adequate intake of calcium (700–1000 mg/day, 1500 mg post-menopausally) and vitamin D (400–800 IU/day) and regular weight-bearing exercises. In the elderly, physiotherapy and assessment of home safety are performed to reduce the risk of falls. Hip protectors may reduce the risk of hip fracture in residential care.

Pharmacological intervention

- Bisphosphonates (e.g. alendronate, risedronate, zoledronate, p. 323) are first-line treatment in most patients with osteoporosis. They inhibit osteoclasts (and therefore bone resorption), increase bone mass at the hip and spine, and most have been shown to reduce fracture incidence. Optimal duration of therapy is unknown.

- Denosumab is a human monoclonal antibody to RANKL administered as a single subcutaneous injection every 6 months. It is an anti-resorptive agent which increases BMD and reduces fractures at the spine, hip and other non-vertebral sites. Adverse effects are infrequent.

- Selective oestrogen-receptor modulators (SERMs), such as raloxifene and bazedoxifene, activate oestrogen receptors on bone while having no stimulatory effect on the endometrium (cf: hormone replacement therapy [HRT], see below). They have been shown to reduce BMD loss at spine and hip, though fracture rates are reduced only in the spine. Side effects are leg cramps, flushing, increased risk of thromboembolism (similar to HRT) and stroke.

- Recombinant human parathyroid peptide 1-34 (teriparatide) and recombinant human parathyroid hormone 1-84 stimulate bone formation and are given by daily subcutaneous injection. They are indicated for severe osteoporosis or in women who are intolerant of, or fail to respond to, other therapies. They have only been shown to reduce vertebral fractures. A side effect is hypercalcaemia.

- Oestrogen therapy (HRT) is reserved for early post-menopausal women with perimenopausal symptoms. This is because of adverse effects on breast cancer and cardiovascular risk (see p. 634).

- Testosterone is given to men with biochemical evidence of hypogonadism.

- Strontium ranelate is reserved for specialist use due to concerns about cardiovascular safety.

Glucocorticoid-induced osteoporosis

Individuals requiring continuous oral glucocorticoid therapy for 3 months or more (at any dose) should be assessed for osteoporotic risk factors. Post-menopausal women, men aged over 50 years and anyone with a previous fragility fracture should receive bisphosphonate treatment without waiting for DXA scanning. Fracture risk assessment and DXA results guide treatment for other patients. Where possible, glucocorticoid doses should be minimized and consideration given to use of steroid-sparing immunosuppressants and alternative routes of steroid administration (e.g. rectal steroids for distal ulcerative colitis).

Osteonecrosis

Osteonecrosis (avascular, aseptic or ischaemic necrosis) is death of bone and marrow cells due to a reduced blood supply. The many causes include medication (glucocorticoids in over 8% of cases, bisphosphonates), alcohol abuse, sickle cell disease, trauma, radiation and HIV infection. The femoral neck is the most common site affected and presents with pain and arthropathy and bony collapse if untreated. Diagnosis is by MRI; plain X-ray will not show early changes. Treatment depends on the cause and the site affected, but joint replacement may be required.

Paget's disease

This is a focal disorder of bone remodelling in which there is increased osteoclastic bone resorption followed by formation of weaker new bone, increased local bone blood flow and fibrous tissue. The incidence increases with age; it is rare in the under 40s and affects up to 10% of adults by the age of 90 years.

Aetiology

The aetiology is unknown. The disease may result from a latent viral infection (e.g. measles or respiratory syncytial virus) in osteoclasts in a genetically susceptible host (increased risk in family members, susceptibility genes identified).

Clinical features

The most common sites are the pelvis, femur, lumbar spine, skull and tibia, although any bone can be involved. Most cases are asymptomatic, but features include the following:

- Pain in the bone or nearby joint (cartilage or adjacent bone is damaged)
- Deformities: enlargement of the skull, bowing of the tibia
- Complications: nerve compression (deafness, paraparesis), pathological fractures, rarely high-output cardiac failure (due to increased bone blood flow) and osteogenic sarcoma.

Investigations

- Serum alkaline phosphatase concentration is raised (reflects level of bone formation), often >1000 U/L, with a normal calcium and phosphate (Table 7.12). Urinary hydroxyproline excretion is raised and may be used as a marker of disease activity.
- X-rays show localized bony enlargement and distortion, sclerotic changes (increased density) and osteolytic areas (loss of bone and reduced density).
- Radionuclide bone scans show increased uptake of bone-seeking radionuclides. Appearances are similar to metastatic sclerotic carcinoma, especially from breast and prostate.

Treatment

Bisphosphonates (mainly intravenous zoledronate p. 323) inhibit bone resorption by decreasing osteoclastic activity, and form the mainstay of treatment. They are indicated for symptomatic patients and asymptomatic patients at risk of complications (e.g. fracture, nerve entrapment). Disease activity is monitored by symptoms and measurement of serum alkaline phosphatase or urinary hydroxyproline.

Osteomalacia and vitamin D deficiency

Inadequate mineralization of the osteoid framework, leading to soft bones, produces rickets during bone growth in children and osteomalacia following epiphyseal closure in adults. Osteomalacia and rickets are the clinical manifestations of profound vitamin D deficiency. The major source of vitamin D is from skin photosynthesis following ultraviolet B sunlight exposure (Fig. 7.6). A small amount is obtained from dietary sources (oily fish, egg yolks, supplemented breakfast cereals, margarine).

Aetiology

Risk factors for vitamin D deficiency include pigmented skin, use of sunscreen or concealing clothing, old age and institutionalization (particularly nursing home residents), malabsorption, short bowel, renal disease [inadequate conversion of $25\text{-}(OH)D_3$ to $1,25\text{-}(OH)_2D_3$], cholestatic liver disease and treatment with anticonvulsants, rifampicin or highly active antiretroviral treatment.

Clinical features

Proximal muscle weakness and pain are the common symptoms, but osteomalacia may be asymptomatic. Low bone density on DXA scanning or osteopenia on plain X-rays may also be a manifestation of vitamin D deficiency. Severe vitamin D deficiency may present with hypocalcaemia, tetany and seizures. Rickets in children presents with bony deformity (knock knees, bowed legs) and impaired growth.

Investigations

- Vitamin levels: serum 25-hydroxyvitamin D_3 (OHD) is low (<25 nmol/L, 10 µg/L) in osteomalacia. Serum OHD concentrations between 25 and 50 nmol/L suggest vitamin D insufficiency.
- Serum biochemistry: alkaline phosphatase is usually high. Phosphate and calcium may be normal or low. PTH is raised.
- Radiology: X-ray appearance is characteristic, showing defective mineralization and Looser's pseudofractures (low-density bands running perpendicular to the cortex, most commonly seen in the femur and pelvis).

Management

Treatment of vitamin D deficiency involves an initial loading stage to replenish stores and a subsequent maintenance phase to avoid repeat deficiency. Patients should also receive supplementary calcium of 1000–1200 mg/day. In nutritional deficiency, recommended initial replacement is with oral vitamin D 50 000 units per week for 8 weeks. Vitamin D is also available as an intramuscular injection; two doses of 300 000 units are usually enough to replenish stores. This should be followed by regular supplementation with 800–1000 units of vitamin D per day.

THERAPEUTICS

Anti-inflammatories and pain relief

Aspirin is indicated for transient musculoskeletal pain and pyrexia. In inflammatory conditions, NSAIDs are usually given. Paracetamol is similar in efficacy to aspirin, but has no demonstrable anti-inflammatory activity. It is first-line treatment in pain relief where anti-inflammatories are not routinely indicated. Codeine may be added when paracetamol alone is insufficient.

Paracetamol (acetaminophen)

Mechanism of action

Paracetamol inhibits synthesis of prostaglandins in the central nervous system and peripherally blocks pain impulse generation. It reduces pyrexia by inhibition of the hypothalamic heat-regulating centre.

Indications

Mild to moderate pain, pyrexia. NSAIDs are preferred for pain relief in the inflammatory arthritides.

Preparations and dose

Tablets, capsules, dispersible tablets: 500 mg; suspension 250 mg/mL; suppositories 60 mg, 125 mg, 250 mg, 500 mg; intravenous infusion 10 mg/mL in 50 mL or 100 mL vial.

Oral or rectal 0.5–1 g every 4–6 hours to a maximum of 4 g daily (3 g if weight <50 kg or liver disease).

IV infusion over 15 minutes: 1 g every 4–6 hours, maximum four daily; 15 mg/kg if body weight <50 kg. Mainly used post-operatively.

Side effects
Side effects are rare unless in overdose.

Cautions/contraindications
Dosing interval 6 hours or greater if estimated glomerular filtration rate <30 mL/min. Reduce dose in severe liver disease.

Compound preparations
Paracetamol (500 mg) is also available combined with a low dose of an opioid analgesic: e.g. codeine phosphate 8 mg, 15 mg or 30 mg, in tablet, dispersible tablet or capsule form. The dose of opioid may be enough to cause opioid side effects (p. 681).

Non-steroidal anti-inflammatory drugs

Mechanism of action
This mechanism is by inhibition of cyclo-oxygenase (COX), the enzyme which catalyses the synthesis of cyclic endoperoxidases from arachidonic acid to form prostaglandins. Inhibition of the COX-1 isoform in the gastrointestinal tract leads to a reduction in protective prostaglandins and predisposes to gastroduodenal damage. COX-2 is the form mainly induced in response to pro-inflammatory cytokines. The selective inhibitors of COX-2 ('coxibs' – etoricoxib and celecoxib) have a lower risk of gastroduodenal damage than the non-selective NSAIDs (e.g. ibuprofen, diclofenac).

Indications
Treatment is given in the smallest dose necessary for the shortest time.

- Pain and inflammation associated with inflammatory arthritides and severe osteoarthritis
- Crystal synovitis
- Transient musculoskeletal pain
- Pain caused by secondary bone tumours.

Preparations and dose
There are many different NSAIDs. They vary in their anti-inflammatory properties and tolerability, e.g. ibuprofen has fewer side effects than other NSAIDs but anti-inflammatory activity is weaker. Indometacin is more potent, with a higher incidence of side effects. Diclofenac and naproxen lie somewhere between these two in potency and side effects.

Two examples of non-selective NSAIDs and one coxib are listed.

Ibuprofen Tablets: 200 mg, 400 mg, 600 mg, 800 mg. Syrup: 100 mg/5 mL.

Oral Initially, 1.2–1.8 g daily in three to four divided doses after food, increased to a maximum of 2.4 g daily if necessary. Maintenance, 0.6–1.2 g daily in divided doses.

Diclofenac Tablets: 25 mg, 50 mg. Suppositories: 25 mg, 50 mg, 100 mg. Injection: 75 mg/3 mL.

Oral/rectal 75–150 mg daily in two to three divided doses.

IM 75 mg once or twice daily for up to 2 days.

Celecoxib Capsules:100 mg, 200 mg.

Oral 200 mg in one to two divided doses, increased if necessary to maximum 400 mg daily.

Side effects

Gastrointestinal toxicity The highest risk is in the elderly. Inflammation and ulceration can occur throughout the gut but clinically is most apparent in the stomach and duodenum (dyspepsia, erosions, ulceration, bleeding, perforation). Of the non-selective NSAIDs, ibuprofen is associated with the lowest risk, and piroxicam, indometacin and diclofenac with intermediate risk. NSAIDs associated with the lowest risk are generally preferred, and the lowest NSAID dose compatible with symptom relief should be prescribed. Co-prescribe proton pump inhibitors with non-selective NSAIDs in high-risk patients (>65 years, previous peptic ulceration, serious comorbidity, other medication that increases gastrointestinal risk: warfarin, aspirin, corticosteroids) to reduce gastroduodenal damage.

Other side effects Other side effects are hypersensitivity reactions (particularly rashes, bronchospasm, angio-oedema), blood disorders, fluid retention (may precipitate cardiac failure in the elderly), acute kidney injury, hepatitis, pancreatitis and exacerbation of colitis.

Cautions/contraindications

They are contraindicated in patients with a history of hypersensitivity to aspirin or any other NSAID – which includes those in whom attacks of asthma, angio-oedema, urticaria or rhinitis have been precipitated by aspirin or any other NSAID. They are also contraindicated in severe heart failure. Selective COX-2 inhibitors are contraindicated in ischaemic heart disease, cerebrovascular disease, peripheral arterial disease and moderate or severe heart failure. Avoid NSAIDs, unless absolutely necessary, in patients with active or previous gastrointestinal ulceration and in patients taking anticoagulants, corticosteroids or aspirin because of gastrointestinal risk. In patients with renal, cardiac or hepatic impairment, NSAIDs may cause a deterioration in organ function. NSAIDs may cause a flare of inflammatory bowel disease and should be avoided if possible. For interactions of NSAIDs, see *British National Formulary*.

Drugs affecting bone metabolism

Bisphosphonates

Mechanism of action

These synthetic analogues of bone pyrophosphate are adsorbed onto hydroxy-apatite crystals in bone and inhibit growth and activity of osteoclasts, thereby reducing the rate of bone turnover.

Indications

Prophylaxis and treatment of osteoporosis in combination with calcium (700–1000 mg daily, 1500 mg post-menopausally) and vitamin D (800 IU/day) supplements if dietary intake inadequate. Treatment of Paget's disease and hypercalcaemia of malignancy, treatment of osteolytic lesions and bone pain in bone metastases associated with breast cancer or multiple myeloma.

Preparations and dose

Alendronic acid Tablets: daily 10 mg; once weekly: 70 mg.

Treatment and prevention of osteoporosis: 10 mg daily at least 30 minutes before breakfast or 70 mg once weekly.

Because of severe oesophageal reactions (oesophagitis, oesophageal ulcers and strictures), patients should be advised to take the tablets with a full glass of water on rising, to take them on an empty stomach at least 30 minutes before the first food or drink of the day and to stand or sit for at least 30 minutes. Also advise patients to stop the tablets and seek medical attention if symptoms of oesophageal irritation develop.

Risedronate Tablets: 5 mg, 30 mg; once weekly: 35 mg.

Prevention and treatment of osteoporosis: 5 mg daily or 35 mg weekly.

Paget's disease: 30 mg daily for 2 months; may be repeated if necessary after at least 2 months.

Precautions for taking risedronate are as for alendronate (above). No food or drink for 2 hours after risedronate.

Disodium pamidronate Injection: 15 mg, 30 mg, 60 mg, 90 mg.

IV Patients should be hydrated first.

Hypercalcaemia of malignancy: serum calcium <3.0 mmol/L, give 15–30 mg; serum calcium >4.0 mmol/L, give 90 mg. Give as single infusion or in multiple infusions over 2–4 consecutive days. Each 60 mg must be diluted with at least 250 mL sodium chloride and given over at least 1 hour.

Osteolytic lesions and bone pain in bone metastases associated with breast cancer or multiple myeloma: 90 mg every 4 weeks (or every 3 weeks to coincide with chemotherapy in breast cancer).

Paget's disease: 30 mg once a week for 6 weeks; may be repeated every 6 months.

Zoledronic acid 4 mg/100 mL solution for infusion.

Patients should be hydrated first.

Hypercalcaemia of malignancy: give as single infusion of 4 mg zoledronic acid over at least 15 minutes.

Prevention of skeletal events (e.g. pathological fractures, spinal compression) associated with advanced malignancies involving bone: 4 mg every 3–4 weeks.

Side effects

Gastrointestinal side effects (dyspepsia, nausea, vomiting, abdominal pain, diarrhoea, constipation), influenza-like symptoms, oesophageal reactions (see above), musculoskeletal pain. With intravenous disodium pamidronate: biochemical abnormalities (hypophosphataemia, hypocalcaemia, hyper- or hypokalaemia, hypernatraemia), anaemia, thrombocytopenia, lymphocytopenia, seizures, acute kidney injury, conjunctivitis. Osteonecrosis of the jaw – greatest risk is in patients receiving intravenous bisphosphonates for cancer indications. Atypical femoral fractures are reported rarely and mainly in association with long-term treatment.

Cautions/contraindications

Correct vitamin D deficiency and hypocalcaemia before starting. Avoid risedronate and alendronate in symptomatic oesophageal disorders. Dose adjustment in severe renal impairment (see *British National Formulary*).

Calcium

Reference nutrient intake is 700 mg.

Indications

Hypocalcaemia, osteomalacia, when dietary calcium intake (with or without vitamin D) is deficient in the prevention and treatment of osteoporosis.

Preparations and dose

Calcium carbonate Chewable tablets (calcium 500 mg or Ca^{2+} 12.6 mmol). Dispersible tablets: 400 (calcium 400 mg or Ca^{2+} 10 mmol), 1000 (calcium 1 g or Ca^{2+} 25 mmol). Syrup (calcium 108.3 mg or Ca^{2+} 2.7 mmol/5 mL).

Osteoporosis and calcium deficiency: 700–1000 mg daily, syrup 55–75 mL daily.

Osteomalacia: 1000–3000 mg daily, syrup 55–155 mL daily.

Calcium gluconate Injection: 10% (calcium 89 mg or Ca^{2+} 2.2 mmol. 10 mL). 10–20 mL over 10 minutes for acute hypocalcaemia.

Side effects

Gastrointestinal disturbances; with injection, peripheral vasodilatation, fall in blood pressure, injection-site reactions.

Cautions/contraindications

Conditions associated with hypercalcaemia and hypercalciuria.

Vitamin D

Mechanism of action

Fat-soluble vitamin whose main action is to promote intestinal absorption of calcium. An oral supplement of 10 µg (400 units) prevents deficiency.

Indications

- Prevention of vitamin D deficiency in those at risk, e.g. Asians consuming unleavened bread and in elderly patients, particularly those who are housebound or live in residential or nursing homes.
- As an adjunct in the prevention and treatment of osteoporosis where dietary intake of vitamin D (and calcium) is suboptimal.
- Vitamin D deficiency caused by intestinal malabsorption, chronic liver disease and severe renal impairment.
- Hypocalcaemia of hypoparathyroidism.

Preparations and dose

Cholecalciferol Capsules: 800 units (equivalent to 20 ng of vitamin D_3).

Prevention of vitamin D deficiency: one to two capsules (800–1600 units) daily.

Vitamin D deficiency: one to four capsules (800–3200 units) daily.

Alfacalcidol 1α-Hydroxycholecalciferol capsules: 250 ng, 500 ng, 1 µg.

Vitamin D treatment in patients with chronic kidney disease: 0.25–1 µg daily.

Calcitriol 1,25-Dihydroxycholecalciferol: 250 ng, 500 ng.

Vitamin D treatment in patients with chronic kidney disease: 250–1000 ng daily.

Side effects

Symptoms of overdosage include anorexia, lassitude, nausea and vomiting, polyuria, thirst, headache and raised concentrations of calcium and phosphate in plasma and urine. All patients on pharmacological doses of vitamin D should have plasma calcium concentration checked at intervals (initially weekly) and if nausea and vomiting are present.

Cautions/contraindications

Contraindicated in hypercalcaemia and metastatic calcification.

8

Water, electrolytes and acid–base balance

WATER AND ELECTROLYTE REQUIREMENTS

In health, the volume and biochemical composition of both extracellular and intracellular fluid compartments in the body remain remarkably constant. Maintenance of the total amount depends on the balance between intake and loss. Water and electrolytes are taken in as food and water, and lost in urine, sweat and faeces. In addition, about 500 mL of water is lost daily in expired air. The reference maintenance fluid, electrolyte and nutrient intake in adults is given in Table 8.1. In certain disease states the intake and loss of water and electrolytes is altered and this factor must be taken into account when providing fluid replacements. For instance, a patient who is losing gastric secretions via a nasogastric tube will be losing additional sodium (25–80 mmol/L), potassium (5–20 mmol/L), chloride (100–150 mmol/L) and hydrogen ions (40–60 mmol/L) each day, which will need to be replaced together with the normal daily requirements.

BODY FLUID COMPARTMENTS

In a normal adult man, 50–60% of body weight is water; females have proportionately more body fat than males and total body water is about 45–50% of body weight. In a healthy 70 kg male, total body water is approximately 42 L. This is contained in three major compartments:

- Intracellular fluid (28 L, about 35% of lean body weight)
- Extracellular fluid – the interstitial fluid that bathes the cells (9.4 L, about 12%)
- Plasma (also extracellular) (4.6 L, about 4–5%).

The intracellular and interstitial fluids are separated by the cell membrane; the interstitial fluid and plasma are separated by the capillary wall.

Osmotic pressure is the primary determinant of the distribution of water among the three major compartments. Osmolality is determined by the concentration of osmotically active particles. Thus 1 mole of sodium chloride dissolved in 1 kg of water has an osmolality of 2 mmol/kg, as sodium chloride freely dissociates into two particles, the sodium ion Na^+ and the chloride ion Cl^-. One mole of urea (which does not dissociate) in 1 kg of water has an osmolality of 1 mmol/kg. Osmolarity is the osmoles of solute per litre of solution (mmol/L) and for dilute aqueous solutions is essentially equivalent to osmolality.

The intracellular fluid contains mainly potassium (K^+) (most of the cell Mg^{2+} is bound and osmotically inactive). In the extracellular compartment, sodium salts predominate in the interstitial fluid and proteins in the plasma. Body Na^+ stores are the primary determinant of extracellular fluid volume but plasma

Table 8.1 Routine fluid and electrolyte requirements

	Daily requirement
Water	25–30 mL/kg/day
Sodium	1 mmol/kg/day
Potassium	1 mmol/kg/day
Chloride	1 mmol/kg/day
Glucose	50–100 mg/day*

*For example, 5% glucose contains 5 mg glucose per 100 mL.

volume is determined by oncotic pressure as well as protein concentration. The composition of intracellular and extracellular fluids is shown in Table 8.2. The cell membrane separates the intracellular and extracellular fluid compartments and maintains, by active and passive transport mechanisms, the different electrolyte compositions within each compartment. A change in osmolality in one compartment will trigger water movement across the cell membrane to re-establish osmotic equilibrium.

Distribution of extracellular fluid

The capillary wall separating the intravascular (plasma) and interstitial spaces is freely permeable to Na^+, K^+ and glucose and, therefore, these solutes do not contribute to fluid distribution between these spaces. However,

Table 8.2 Normal adult electrolyte concentrations of intracellular and extracellular fluids

	Plasma (mmol/L)	Interstitial fluid (mmol/L)	Intracellular fluid (mmol/L)
Na^+	142	144	10
K^+	4	4	160
Ca^{2+}	2.5	2.5	1.5
Mg^{2+}	1.0	0.5	13
Cl^-	102	114	2
HCO_3^-	26	30	8
PO_4^{2-}	1.0	1.0	57
SO_4^{2-}	0.5	0.5	10
Organic acid	3	4	3
Protein	16	0	55

plasma proteins, e.g. albumin, have a limited ability to traverse the capillary bed, and act to hold water in the vascular space. The distribution of extracellular water between vascular and extravascular (interstitial) space is determined by the equilibrium between hydrostatic pressure (i.e. intracapillary blood pressure), which tends to force fluid out of the capillaries, and oncotic pressure (i.e. osmotic pressure exerted by plasma proteins), which acts to retain fluid within the vessel. The net flow of fluid outwards is balanced by 'suction' of fluid into the lymphatics, which returns it to the bloodstream (Fig. 8.1).

Oedema is defined as an increase in interstitial fluid and results from:

- Increased hydrostatic pressure, e.g. sodium and water retention in cardiac failure
- Reduced oncotic pressure, e.g. as a result of nephrotic syndrome with hypoalbuminaemia
- Obstruction to lymphatic flow
- Increased permeability of the blood vessel wall, e.g. at a site of inflammation, the cytokines lead to an increase in vascular permeability.

Inspection and palpation are usually sufficient to identify oedema. Compression of the skin of the affected area with a fingertip for 10 seconds

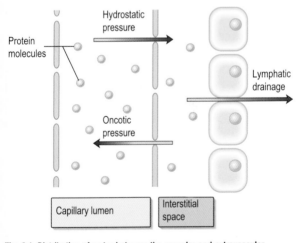

Fig. 8.1 Distribution of water between the vascular and extravascular (interstitial) spaces. This is determined by the equilibrium between hydrostatic pressure, which tends to force fluid out of the capillaries, and oncotic pressure, which acts to retain fluid within the vessel. The net flow of fluid outwards is balanced by 'suction' of fluid into the lymphatics, which returns it to the bloodstream. Similar principles govern the volume of the peritoneal and pleural spaces.

results in 'pitting'. Localized oedema is most likely to result from a local cause, e.g. venous obstruction. The location of generalized oedema, e.g. with cardiac failure, renal or liver disease, is often most prominent in the legs and feet in ambulatory patients and in the sacral region in those who are confined to bed.

Intravenous fluids in clinical practice

Intravenous fluids are frequently used in hospital to maintain fluid balance in patients unable to take fluids orally and to replenish substantial deficits or continuing losses. *Crystalloids*, e.g. sodium chloride 0.9%, contain low molecular weight salts or sugars that dissolve completely in water and pass freely between intravascular and interstitial compartments (Table 8.3). Glucose 5% is essentially free water and distributes evenly across total body water (i.e. across all three major fluid compartments) after intravenous administration;

Table 8.3 Crystalloids in general use

	Na^+ (mmol/L)	K^+ (mmol/L)	Cl^- (mmol/L)	Osmolarity (mosmol/kg)	Indication*
Normal plasma values	142	4.5	103	285–295	
Sodium chloride 0.9%	154	–	154	308	1
Sodium chloride 0.18%/glucose 4%	30	–	–	283	2
Glucose 5%	–	–	–	278	3
Hartmann's solution/Ringer's lactate solution	130	4	109	273	4

*NB: In a normal adult 1.5–2.5 L (25–35 mL/kg/24 hours) of fluid containing about 70–100 mmol sodium and 40–80 mmol potassium are required to maintain balance. Fluids are given with or without potassium chloride (depending on daily requirements and plasma levels) given as ready-mixed bags in preference to adding potassium chloride concentrate to a bag.

1. Volume expansion in hypovolaemic patients. Rarely to maintain fluid balance when there are large losses of sodium. Excessive sodium and chloride (compared to plasma) may cause hypernatraemia and hyperchloraemic metabolic acidosis, respectively.
2. Maintenance of fluid balance in normovolaemic, normonatraemic patients.
3. To replace water. Only given alone when there is no significant loss of electrolytes. Also may be alternated with sodium chloride 0.9% as an alternative to (2).
4. In fluid maintenance and replacement. Provides bicarbonate from metabolism of lactate. Also contains calcium 2 mmol/L.

very little remains in the intravascular space. Sodium chloride 0.9% remains in the extracellular space and thus about one-third of the volume infused will remain in the intravascular space. *Colloids* (e.g. dextran 70, gelatin) contain larger molecular weight substances and remain for a longer period in the intravascular space than crystalloids. Colloids are used to expand circulating volume in haemorrhage (until blood becomes available), burns and sometimes septicaemia. Although remaining in the intravascular space longer than crystalloids, comparative studies have not shown a definite advantage of colloids over crystalloids in hypovolaemic patients. Side effects of colloids are hypersensitivity reactions including anaphylactoid reactions and a transient increase in bleeding time. They have a greater sodium concentration than plasma.

Assessment and monitoring of fluid balance is made from the history (e.g. vomiting, diarrhoea), fluid balance charts (often inaccurate), daily weights, urine output and clinical observations (skin turgor, capillary refill, jugular venous pressure [JVP], pulse, lying and standing blood pressure). Invasive cardiac monitoring is also used in high-dependency patients. Measurement of central venous pressure before and after an intravenous fluid challenge is also used to assess volume status (p. 337). In the post-operative patient there is usually a short period of oliguria occurring as a physiological response to surgery. Urine output alone should not therefore be relied on to assess fluid balance in these patients. In addition, post-operatively, the ability of the kidneys to dilute the urine is impaired and there is a risk of dilutional hyponatraemia.

In the UK, the National Institute for Health and Care Excellence (NICE) has produced guidelines on intravenous fluid therapy in adults in hospital. Intravenous fluid prescriptions should be reviewed daily. Prescriptions must take into account all other sources of fluid and electrolyte intake, including oral intake, drugs and blood products. Before intravenous fluids are prescribed, clinical assessment should determine:

- The patient's fluid and electrolyte needs
- Whether fluids are needed for resuscitation, maintenance (Table 8.1), or to replace a deficit, e.g. hypovolaemia as a result of diarrhoea and vomiting
- The type of fluid needed
- The appropriate rate of fluid administration, the volume to be administered and the likely duration that intravenous fluids will be required.

Suggestions for appropriate use of the different types of fluid is indicated in Table 8.3.

REGULATION OF BODY FLUID HOMEOSTASIS

Maintenance of the effective circulating volume is essential for adequate tissue perfusion and is mainly related to the regulation of sodium balance. In contrast, maintenance of osmolality prevents changes in cell volume and is largely related to the regulation of water balance.

Regulation of extracellular volume

The regulation of extracellular volume is determined by a tight control of the balance of sodium, which is excreted by normal kidneys. Although only a small proportion of total extracellular fluid resides in the arterial circulation, it is the fullness of the arterial vascular compartment – or the so-called *effective arterial blood volume* (EABV) – that is the primary determinant of renal sodium and water excretion. The fullness of the arterial compartment depends on a normal ratio between cardiac output and peripheral arterial resistance. Thus diminished EABV is initiated by a fall in cardiac output or a fall in peripheral arterial resistance (an increase in the holding capacity of the arterial vascular tree). When the EABV is expanded, this in turn leads to an increase in urinary sodium excretion and vice versa.

Two types of volume receptors sense changes in the EABV:

- Extrarenal: in the large vessels near the heart
- Intrarenal: in the afferent renal arteriole, which controls the renin–angiotensin system via the juxtaglomerular apparatus.

A decreased effective circulating volume leads to activation of these volume receptors, which leads to an increase in sodium (and hence water) reabsorption by the kidney and expansion of the extracellular volume via stimulation of the sympathetic nervous system and activation of the renin–angiotensin system (p. 647). In contrast, atrial natriuretic peptide (ANP), produced by the atria of the heart in response to an increase in blood volume, increases sodium excretion.

Abnormalities of extracellular volume

Increased extracellular volume

Extracellular volume expansion is the result of increased sodium (and hence water) reabsorption or impaired excretion by the kidney.

Clinical features

These depend on the distribution of excess fluid within the extracellular space (i.e. between the interstitial space and intravascular compartment), which in turn depends on venous tone (which determines hydrostatic pressure), capillary permeability, oncotic pressure (mainly dependent on serum albumin) and lymphatic drainage. For instance, with hypoalbuminaemia there is a reduction in plasma oncotic pressure and predominantly interstitial volume overload. Cardiac failure leads to expansion of both compartments:

- *Interstitial volume overload* – ankle oedema, pulmonary oedema, pleural effusion and ascites

- *Intravascular volume overload* – raised jugular venous pressure, cardiomegaly and a raised arterial pressure in some cases.

This must be differentiated from local causes of oedema (e.g. ankle oedema as a result of venous damage following thrombosis), which do not reflect a disturbance in the control of extracellular volume.

Aetiology

Most causes of extracellular volume expansion are associated with renal sodium chloride retention.

- *Cardiac failure* due to a reduction in cardiac output and impaired perfusion (therefore effective hypovolaemia) of the volume receptors. The increased sympathetic activity generated by stimulation of the volume receptors also leads to release of antidiuretic hormone (ADH, vasopressin) even though plasma osmolality (see later) is unchanged.
- *Cirrhosis* is complex, but there is vasodilatation and underperfusion of the volume receptors. Hypoalbuminaemia may also contribute.
- *Nephrotic syndrome.* Sodium retention is primarily due to increased sodium reabsorption in the renal collecting tubules directly induced by the renal disease. In addition, in some patients the low plasma oncotic pressure induced by hypoalbuminaemia leads to plasma volume depletion and arterial underfilling as in cardiac failure and cirrhosis.
- *Sodium retention.* This may be as a result of renal impairment, where there is a reduction in renal capacity to excrete sodium, or due to drugs such as mineralocorticoids (aldosterone-like actions), thiazolidinediones (by upregulation of the epithelial sodium transporter channel) and non-steroidal anti-inflammatory drugs (NSAIDs). The latter inhibit synthesis of vasodilatory prostaglandins in the kidney with an increase in renal vascular resistance and an increase in water and sodium reabsorption.

Management

The underlying cause must be treated. The cornerstone of management, diuretics, increase sodium and water excretion in the kidney. There are a number of different classes of diuretic, e.g. loop diuretics such as furosemide (Table 8.4 and p. 352).

Decreased extracellular volume

Aetiology

Volume depletion occurs in haemorrhage, plasma loss in extensive burns, or loss of salt and water from the kidneys, gastrointestinal tract or skin (Table 8.5). Signs of volume depletion occur despite a normal or increased body content of sodium and water in sepsis (due to vasodilatation and increased capillary permeability) and diuretic treatment of oedematous states where mobilization of oedema lags behind a rapid reduction in plasma volume due to diuresis.

Table 8.4 The main classes of diuretics in clinical use

Class	Example	Mechanism of action	Relative potency
Loop diuretics	Furosemide Bumetanide	Reduce Na^+ and Cl^- reabsorption in ascending limb of loop of Henle	++++
Thiazides	Bendroflumethiazide Hydrochlorothiazide	Reduce sodium reabsorption in distal convoluted tubule	++
Aldosterone antagonists	Spironolactone Eplerenone	Aldosterone antagonist	+
Potassium-sparing	Amiloride	Prevent potassium exchange for sodium in distal tubule	+

Table 8.5 Causes of extracellular volume depletion

Haemorrhage

External
Concealed, e.g. leaking aortic aneurysm

Burns

Gastrointestinal losses

Vomiting
Diarrhoea
Ileostomy losses
Ileus

Renal losses

Diuretic use
Impaired tubular sodium conservation
Reflux nephropathy
Papillary necrosis
Analgesic nephropathy
Diabetes mellitus
Sickle cell disease

Clinical features

Symptoms include thirst, nausea and postural dizziness. Interstitial fluid loss leads to loss of skin elasticity ('turgor'). Loss of circulating volume causes peripheral vasoconstriction and tachycardia, a low JVP and postural hypotension. Severe depletion of circulating volume causes hypotension, which may impair cerebral perfusion, resulting in confusion and eventual coma.

Investigations

The diagnosis is usually made clinically. A central venous line allows the measurement of central venous pressure, which helps in assessing the response to treatment. Plasma urea may be raised because of increased urea reabsorption and, later, prerenal failure (when the creatinine rises as well). This is, however, non-specific. Urinary sodium is low (<20 mmol/L) if the kidneys are working normally. The urinary sodium can be misleading, however, if the cause of the volume depletion involves the kidneys, e.g. with diuretics or intrinsic renal disease.

Management

The aim of treatment is to replace what has been lost.

- Haemorrhage involves the loss of whole blood. Immediate treatment is with crystalloid or colloid until packed red cells are available.
- Loss of plasma, as in burns or severe peritonitis, should be treated with human plasma or a colloid (p. 331).
- Loss of sodium and water, as in vomiting, diarrhoea or excessive renal losses, is treated with replacement of water and electrolytes. In chronic conditions associated with mild/moderate sodium depletion, e.g. salt-losing bowel or renal disease, oral supplements of sodium chloride or sodium bicarbonate (depending on acid–base balance) may be sufficient. Glucose–electrolyte solutions are often used to restore fluid balance in patients with diarrhoeal diseases. This is based on the fact that the presence of glucose stimulates intestinal absorption of salt and water.
- In the acute situation if there have been large losses of sodium and water, patients are usually treated with intravenous sodium chloride 0.9% (Table 8.3), and replacement is assessed clinically and by measurement of serum electrolytes. Rapid infusion (1000 mL/hour) of sodium chloride 0.9% or colloid is given if the patient is hypotensive.
- Loss of water alone, e.g. diabetes insipidus, only causes extracellular volume depletion in severe cases because the loss is spread evenly over all the compartments of body water. The correct treatment is to give water. If intravenous treatment is required, water is given as glucose 5% (pure water would cause osmotic lysis of blood cells).

PLASMA OSMOLALITY AND DISORDERS OF SODIUM REGULATION

Water moves freely between compartments and the distribution is determined by the osmotic equilibrium between them. The plasma osmolality can be calculated from the plasma concentrations of sodium, urea and glucose, as follows:

$$\text{Calculated plasma osmolality (mmol)} = (2 \times \text{plasma Na}^+) \\ + [\text{urea}] + [\text{glucose}]$$

The factor of 2 applied to sodium concentration allows for associated anions (chloride and bicarbonate). The other extracellular solutes, e.g. calcium, potassium and magnesium, and their associated anions exist in very low concentrations and contribute so little to osmolality that they can be ignored when calculating the osmolality. The normal plasma osmolality is 285–300 mosmol/kg.

The *calculated* osmolality is the same as the osmolality *measured* by the laboratory, unless there is an unmeasured, osmotically active substance present. For instance, plasma alcohol or ethylene glycol concentration (substances sometimes taken in cases of poisoning) can be estimated by subtracting the calculated from the measured osmolality.

Regulation of body water content

Body water is controlled mainly by changes in the plasma osmolality. An increased plasma osmolality, sensed by osmoreceptors in the hypothalamus, causes thirst and the release of ADH from the posterior pituitary, which increases water reabsorption from the renal collecting ducts. In addition, non-osmotic stimuli may cause the release of ADH even if serum osmolality is normal or low. These include hypovolaemia (irrespective of plasma osmolality), stress (surgery and trauma) and nausea. In contrast, at a plasma osmolality of less than 275 mosmol/kg there is complete suppression of ADH secretion.

Sodium content is regulated by volume receptors, with water content adjusted to maintain a normal osmolality and a normal plasma sodium concentration. Disturbances of sodium concentration are usually caused by disturbances of water balance, rather than an increase or decrease in total body sodium.

Hyponatraemia

Hyponatraemia reflects too much water in relation to sodium; affected patients may or may not have a concurrent abnormality in sodium balance.

Hyponatraemia (serum sodium <135 mmol/L) may be the result of the following:

- Relative water excess (dilutional hyponatraemia).
- Salt loss in excess of water, e.g. diarrhoea and renal diseases.
- Rarely, pseudohyponatraemia, in which hyperlipidaemia or hyperproteinaemia results in a spuriously low measured sodium concentration. The sodium is confined to the aqueous phase but its concentration is expressed in terms of the total volume of plasma

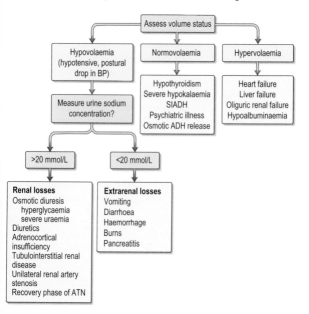

Fig. 8.2 Diagnosis of hyponatraemia. Osmotic antidiuretic hormone (ADH) release refers to unmeasured osmotically active substances stimulating osmotic release of ADH. These include glucose, mannitol, chronic alcohol abuse and sick-cell syndrome (leakage of intracellular ions). SIADH, syndrome of inappropriate ADH secretion; ATN, acute tubular necrosis; BP, blood pressure.

(i.e. water + lipid). In this situation, plasma osmolality is normal and therefore treatment of 'hyponatraemia' is unnecessary.

- Artefactual 'hyponatraemia' caused by taking blood from the drip arm into which a fluid of low sodium, e.g. 5% glucose, is being infused.

The next step is to assess whether patients are hypovolaemic, euvolaemic or hypervolaemic (Fig. 8.2).

Hyponatraemia resulting from salt loss (hypovolaemic hyponatraemia)

These patients have a deficit of both total body sodium and water, with the sodium deficit exceeding that of the water. As fluid is lost and the patient becomes hypovolaemic there is stimulation of volume receptors leading to thirst and non-osmotic release of ADH. Measurement of urinary sodium helps differentiate between renal and extrarenal sources of fluid loss (Fig. 8.2). For example, vomiting and diarrhoea are associated with avid sodium retention as the kidney responds to volume contraction by conserving sodium chloride. Diuretics are the most common cause of hypovolaemic hyponatraemia with a high urinary sodium concentration ($[Na^+]$).

Clinical features

These are usually a result of the hypovolaemia and extracellular volume depletion (p. 333). Symptoms directly related to the hyponatraemia are rare, as the loss of both sodium and water limits osmotic shifts in the brain.

Management

Restoration of extracellular volume with crystalloids or colloids interrupts non-osmotic release of ADH and normalizes serum sodium. Oral rehydration solutions (p. 134) are appropriate treatments in diarrhoeal diseases, resulting in mild hypovolaemia.

Hyponatraemia resulting from water excess (dilutional hyponatraemia)

An excess of body water relative to sodium is differentiated from hyponatraemia caused by sodium loss because there are none of the clinical features of extracellular volume depletion. This is the most common mechanism of hyponatraemia seen in hospitalized patients. The most common iatrogenic cause is overgenerous infusion of 5% glucose in post-operative patients; in this situation the hyponatraemia is exacerbated by an increased ADH secretion in response to stress.

Aetiology

Hyponatraemia is often seen in patients with severe cardiac failure, cirrhosis or the nephrotic syndrome, in which there is an inability of the kidney to excrete 'free water'. This is compounded by the use of diuretics. There is evidence of volume overload and the patient is usually oedematous. Where there is no evidence of extracellular volume overload (i.e. euvolaemic patient), causes include the syndrome of inappropriate ADH secretion (SIADH) (p. 651), Addison's disease and hypothyroidism.

Clinical features

Symptoms rarely occur until the serum sodium is less than 120 mmol/L and are more conspicuous when hyponatraemia has developed rapidly, i.e. over hours. The symptoms result from the movement of water into brain cells (cerebral oedema) in response to the fall in extracellular osmolality, and include headache, confusion, convulsions and coma. If hyponatraemia has developed slowly the brain will have adapted by decreasing intracellular osmolality, and symptoms occur at a lower serum sodium concentration, e.g. <110 mmol/L.

Investigations

Hyponatraemia in association with cardiac failure, cirrhosis or nephrotic syndrome is usually clinically obvious and no further investigation is necessary. If there is no evidence of volume overload the most probable cause is SIADH or diuretic therapy. Serum magnesium and potassium must be checked, as low levels potentiate ADH release and cause diuretic-associated hyponatraemia.

Management

The underlying cause must be corrected where possible. Most cases (those without severe symptoms) are simply managed by water restriction (to 1000 mL/day or even 500 mL/day) with a review of diuretic treatment. Management of SIADH is described on page 651. Patients with hyponatraemia developing acutely, in less than 48 hours (often a hospitalized patient on intravenous glucose), are at the greatest risk of developing cerebral oedema and should be treated more urgently (Emergency Box 8.1). Administration of desmopressin helps to avoid acute diuresis.

Vasopressin V_2 receptor antagonists, e.g. conivaptan and tolvaptan, which produce free water diuresis, may be used to treat hyponatraemia.

Central pontine myelinolysis

Over-rapid correction of the sodium concentration must be avoided, as this can result in a severe, neurological syndrome due to local areas of

---

✚ Emergency Box 8.1

Management of hyponatraemia resulting from water excess

- Treat the underlying cause.
- Restrict water intake to 500–1000 mL/day and review diuretic therapy.
- Correct magnesium and potassium deficiency.
- With acute symptomatic hyponatraemia and severe neurological signs (fits or coma):
  - Infuse hypertonic saline, e.g. 3% saline (513 mmol/L) at a rate of 1–2 mL/kg/hour; 1 mL/kg will raise plasma sodium by 1 mmol/L assuming that total body water comprises 50% of total body weight.
  - Aim to raise serum sodium by 8–10 mmol/L in the first 24 hours and 8 mmol/L in each 24-hour period thereafter.
  - Give furosemide 40–80 mg i.v. to enhance free water excretion.
  - Serum sodium should not be corrected to greater than 125–130 mmol/L.
  - Hypertonic saline is contraindicated in patients who are fluid overloaded; give 100 mL of 20% mannitol.

demyelination, called central pontine myelinolysis or the osmotic demyelination syndrome. Features of this include quadriparesis, respiratory arrest, pseudobulbar palsy, mutism and, rarely, seizures. The distribution of the areas of demyelination include most often the pons, but also, in some cases, the basal ganglia, internal capsule, lateral geniculate body and even the cerebral cortex. Diagnosis is by characteristic appearances on brain magnetic resonance imaging (MRI).

Hypernatraemia

Hypernatraemia (serum sodium >145 mmol/L) is almost always the result of reduced water intake or water loss in excess of sodium. Less commonly, it is due to excessive administration of sodium, e.g. as intravenous fluids (sodium bicarbonate or sodium chloride 0.9%) or administration of drugs with a high sodium content.

Aetiology

Insufficient fluid intake is most often found in elderly people, neonates or unconscious patients when access to water is denied or confusion or coma eliminates the normal response to thirst. The situation is exacerbated by increased losses of fluid, e.g. sweating, diarrhoea.

Water loss relative to sodium occurs in diabetes insipidus, osmotic diuresis and water loss from the lungs or skin. Usually in these situations, serum sodium is maintained because an increase in plasma osmolality is a potent stimulus to thirst; serum sodium only increases if thirst sensation is abnormal or access to water is restricted.

Clinical features

Symptoms are non-specific and include nausea, vomiting, fever and confusion.

Investigations

Simultaneous urine and plasma osmolality and sodium should be measured.

The passage of urine with an osmolality lower than that of plasma in this situation is clearly abnormal and indicates diabetes insipidus (p. 650). If urine osmolality is high, this suggests an osmotic diuresis or excessive extrarenal water loss (e.g. heat stroke).

Management

Treatment is that of the underlying cause and replacement of water, either orally if possible or intravenously with 5% dextrose. The aim is to correct sodium concentration over 48 hours, as over-rapid correction may lead to cerebral oedema. In severe hypernatraemia (>170 mmol/L), sodium chloride 0.9% (154 mmol/L) should be used to avoid too rapid a drop in serum sodium.

In addition, if there is clinical evidence of volume depletion, this implies that there is a sodium deficit as well as a water deficit, and intravenous sodium chloride 0.9% should be used.

DISORDERS OF POTASSIUM REGULATION

Dietary intake of potassium varies between 80 and 150 mmol daily, most of which is then excreted in the urine. Most of the body's potassium (3500 mmol in an adult man) is intracellular (Table 8.2). Serum levels are controlled by:

- Uptake of K^+ into cells
- Renal excretion – mainly controlled by aldosterone
- Extrarenal losses, e.g. gastrointestinal.

Hypokalaemia

This is a serum potassium concentration of <3.5 mmol/L.

Aetiology

The most common causes of hypokalaemia are diuretic treatment and hyperaldosteronism (Table 8.6). Blood taken from a drip arm may produce a spurious result.

Clinical features

Hypokalaemia is usually asymptomatic, although muscle weakness may occur if it is severe. It results in an increased risk of cardiac arrhythmias, particularly in patients with cardiac disease. Hypokalaemia also predisposes to digoxin toxicity.

Management

The underlying cause should be identified and treated where possible. Usually, withdrawal of purgatives, assessment of diuretic treatment, and replacement with oral potassium chloride supplements, preferably as a liquid or effervescent preparation (25–40 mmol/day in divided doses with monitoring of serum K^+ every 1–2 days) is all that is required (p. 345). Serum magnesium concentrations should be normalized, as hypomagnesaemia makes hypokalaemia difficult or impossible to correct. Indications for the intravenous infusion of potassium chloride include hypokalaemic diabetic ketoacidosis and severe hypokalaemia associated with cardiac arrhythmias or muscle weakness. This should be performed slowly, and replacement at rates of greater than 20 mmol/hour should only be done with electrocardiographic (ECG) monitoring and hourly measurement of serum potassium. Concentrations over 60 mmol/L should not be given via a peripheral vein because of local

Table 8.6 Causes of hypokalaemia

Increased renal excretion (spot urinary K$^+$ >20 mmol/L)	Diuretics, e.g. thiazides, loop diuretics
	Solute diuresis, e.g. glycosuria
	Hypomagnesaemia

	Increased aldosterone secretion:
	  Liver failure
	  Heart failure
	  Nephrotic syndrome
	  Cushing's syndrome
	  Conn's syndrome

	Exogenous mineralocorticoid:
	  Corticosteroids
	  Carbenoxolone
	  Liquorice

	Renal disease
	  Renal tubular acidosis: types 1 and 2
	  Renal tubular damage
	  Rare syndromes with renal potassium
	  loss, e.g. Liddle's

Gastrointestinal losses (spot urinary K$^+$ <20 mmol/L)	Prolonged vomiting,* profuse diarrhoea, villous adenoma, fistulae, ileostomies

Redistribution into cells	Increased activity of Na$^+$/K$^+$-ATPase
	  Alkalosis
	  β-Agonists
	  Insulin

	Hypokalaemic periodic paralysis (rare, episodic K$^+$ movement into cells leads to profound muscle weakness)
Reduced intake	Severe dietary deficiency
	Inadequate replacement in i.v. fluids

*Hypokalaemia, primarily due to loss of gastric acid and associated metabolic alkalosis, which leads to increased urinary loss of potassium and intracellular shift of potassium.

irritation. Ampoules of potassium should be thoroughly mixed in sodium chloride 0.9%; glucose solutions should be avoided as this may make hypokalaemia worse.

Hyperkalaemia

This is a serum potassium concentration >5.0 mmol/L. True hyperkalaemia must be differentiated from artefactual hyperkalaemia, which results from lysis of red cells during vigorous phlebotomy or in vitro release from abnormal red cells in some blood disorders, e.g. leukaemia.

Aetiology

The most common causes are renal impairment and drug interference with potassium excretion (Table 8.7). An elevated serum potassium in the absence of any of the listed causes should be confirmed before treatment, to exclude an artefactual result.

Clinical features

Hyperkalaemia usually produces few symptoms or signs, until it is high enough to cause cardiac arrest. Symptoms produced by hyperkalaemia are related to impaired neuromuscular transmission and include muscle weakness and paralysis. It may be associated with metabolic acidosis causing Kussmaul's respiration (low, deep, sighing inspiration and expiration). Hyperkalaemia may produce progressive abnormalities in the ECG (Fig. 8.3).

Management

In the absence of any underlying cause (Table 8.7) the serum potassium should be rechecked to rule out spurious hyperkalaemia unless ECG changes are present (Fig. 8.3) that warrant emergency treatment. Mild to moderate hyperkalaemia can be managed by dietary potassium restriction, restriction of drugs causing hyperkalaemia and a loop diuretic (if appropriate) to increase

Table 8.7 Causes of hyperkalaemia
Decreased excretion
Acute kidney injury Drugs (potassium-sparing diuretics, ACE inhibitors, NSAIDs, ciclosporin, heparin) Addison's disease Hyporeninaemic hypoaldosteronism (type 4 renal tubular acidosis)
Redistribution (intracellular to extracellular fluid)
Diabetic ketoacidosis Metabolic acidosis Tissue necrosis or lysis (rhabdomyolysis, tumour lysis syndrome, severe burns) Drugs (suxamethonium, digoxin toxicity) Hyperkalaemic periodic paralysis
Increased extraneous load
Potassium chloride Salt substitutes Transfusion of stored blood
ACE, angiotensin-converting enzyme; NSAID, non-steroidal anti-inflammatory drug.

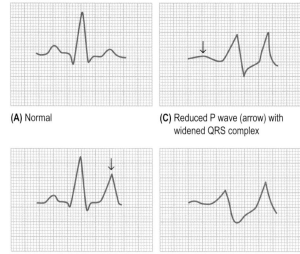

(A) Normal

(C) Reduced P wave (arrow) with widened QRS complex

(B) Tented T wave (arrow)

(D) 'Sine wave' pattern (pre-cardiac arrest)

Fig. 8.3A-D Progressive electrocardiographic changes with increasing hyperkalaemia.

urinary potassium excretion. Severe hyperkalaemia (>6.5 mmol/L) or hyperkalaemia (>6.0 mmol/L) with ECG changes (Fig. 8.3) is a medical emergency (Emergency Box 8.2).

DISORDERS OF MAGNESIUM REGULATION

Disturbance of magnesium balance is uncommon and usually associated with more obvious fluid and electrolyte disturbance. Like potassium, magnesium is mainly an intracellular cation (Table 8.2) and balance is maintained mainly via the kidney. The average daily magnesium intake is 15 mmol, about one-third of which is absorbed in the small bowel; excretion is via the kidney.

Hypomagnesaemia

Aetiology

Low serum magnesium is most often caused by loss of magnesium from the gut or kidney. Gastrointestinal causes include severe diarrhoea, malabsorption,

⊹ Emergency Box 8.2

Management of hyperkalaemia

- **Protect myocardium from hyperkalaemia** (if K⁺ >6.5 mmol/L or electrocardiographic (ECG) changes present):
  - 10 mL of 10% calcium gluconate bolus i.v. over 2–3 min with ECG monitoring
  - Repeat after 5 min if ECG changes persist
  - NB: This treatment does not alter serum K⁺
- **Drive K⁺ into cells:**
  - Soluble insulin 10 units + 50 mL 50% dextrose intravenously over 15–30 minutes and/or salbutamol nebulizer (10 mg) and/or correction of severe acidosis (pH <6.9) with 1.26% sodium bicarbonate (500 mL i.v. over 60 minutes)*
  - Effect of insulin lasts 1–2 hours; repeated doses may be necessary
- **Deplete body K⁺** (after emergency treatment):
  - Polystyrene sulphonate resin orally (15 g three times daily with laxatives) or rectally (30 g) binds potassium
  - Treat the cause
  - Stop any extra source of potassium intake or potentiating drugs, e.g. non-steroidal anti-inflammatory drugs and angiotensin-converting enzyme (ACE) inhibitors
  - Haemodialysis or peritoneal dialysis if conservative measures fail
- Monitor:
  - Blood glucose (finger-prick stick testing) hourly during and for 6 hours after insulin/dextrose infusion
  - Serum K⁺ every 2–4 hours acutely and daily thereafter

*Not to be administered through the same line as calcium salts because of a risk of precipitation.

extensive bowel resection and intestinal fistulae. Excessive renal loss of magnesium occurs with diuretics, alcohol abuse and with an osmotic diuresis such as glycosuria in diabetes mellitus.

Clinical features

Hypomagnesaemia increases renal excretion of potassium, inhibits secretion of parathyroid hormone and leads to parathyroid hormone resistance. Many of the symptoms of hypomagnesaemia are therefore due to hypokalaemia (p. 341) and hypocalcaemia (p. 656).

Management

The underlying cause must be corrected where possible and oral supplements given (magnesium chloride 5–20 mmol daily or magnesium oxide tablets 600 mg four times daily). Symptomatic severe magnesium deficiency should be treated by intravenous infusion (40 mmol of MgCl in 100 mL of sodium chloride 0.9% or dextrose 5% over 2 hours), plus a loading dose (8 mmol over 10–15 minutes) if there are seizures or ventricular arrhythmias. Take care when interpreting repeat serum concentrations after treatment – the extracellular values may appear to normalize quickly while the intracellular concentration requires longer to replenish (may require up to 160 mmol over 5 days to correct).

Hypermagnesaemia

Hypermagnesaemia is rare and is usually iatrogenic, occurring in patients with renal failure who have been given magnesium-containing laxatives or antacids. Symptoms include neurological and cardiovascular depression, with narcosis, respiratory depression and cardiac conduction defects. The only treatment usually necessary is to stop magnesium treatment. In severe cases, intravenous calcium gluconate may be necessary to reverse the cellular toxic effects of magnesium and dextrose/insulin (as for hyperkalaemia) to lower the plasma magnesium level.

DISORDERS OF ACID–BASE BALANCE

The pH (the negative logarithm of $[H^+]$) is maintained at 7.4 (normal range 7.35–7.45). The metabolism of food and endogenous body tissues produces about 70–100 mmol of H^+ each day, which is excreted by the kidneys. Bicarbonate (HCO_3^-) is the main plasma and extracellular fluid buffer. It mops up free H^+ ions and prevents increases in the H^+ concentration (Fig. 8.4). Bicarbonate is filtered at the glomerulus but is then reabsorbed in the proximal and distal renal tubule. The lungs also constantly regulate acid–base balance through the excretion of CO_2. Between production and excretion of H^+ ions there is an extremely effective buffering system maintaining a constant H^+ ion concentration inside and outside the cell. Buffers include haemoglobin proteins, bicarbonate and phosphate.

$$\text{carbonic anhydrase}$$
$$H^+ + HCO_3^- \Longleftrightarrow H_2CO_3 \Longleftrightarrow H_2O + CO_2$$

Fig. 8.4 The carbonic anhydrase reaction.

Acid–base disturbances may be caused by:

- Abnormal carbon dioxide removal in the lungs ('respiratory' acidosis and alkalosis)
- Abnormalities in the regulation of bicarbonate and other buffers in the blood ('metabolic' acidosis and alkalosis).

In general, the body compensates to some extent for changes in pH by regulating renal bicarbonate excretion and altering the respiratory rate. For instance, metabolic acidosis causes hyperventilation (via medullary chemoreceptors), leading to increased removal of CO_2 in the lungs and partial compensation for the acidosis. Conversely, respiratory acidosis is accompanied by renal bicarbonate retention, which could be mistaken for primary metabolic alkalosis.

Measurement of pH, $P_a{co_2}$ and $[HCO_3^-]$ will reveal which type of disturbance is present (Table 8.8). These measurements are made on an arterial blood sample using an automated blood gas analyser. Clinical history and examination usually point to the correct diagnosis. In complicated patients, the Flenley acid–base nomogram can be used to identify the acid–base disorder that is present when arterial hydrogen ion concentration and $P_a{co_2}$ are known (Fig. 8.5).

Respiratory acidosis

This is usually associated with ventilatory failure, with retention of carbon dioxide. Treatment is of the underlying cause.

Table 8.8 Changes in arterial blood gases

	pH	$P_a{co_2}$	HCO_3^-
Acidosis			
Metabolic	Normal or reduced	Normal or reduced	Reduced ++
Respiratory	Normal or reduced	Increased ++	Normal or increased
Alkalosis			
Metabolic	Normal or increased	Increased	Increased ++
Respiratory	Normal or increased	Reduced ++	Reduced

The pH may be at the limits of the normal range if the acidosis or alkalosis is compensated, e.g. respiratory compensation (hyperventilation) of a metabolic acidosis. The clue to the abnormality from the blood gases will be the abnormal $P_a{co_2}$ and HCO_3^-.

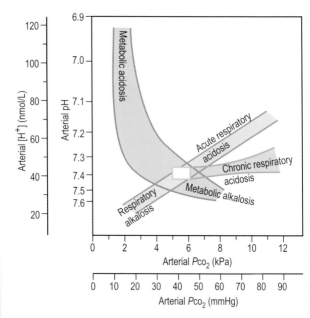

Fig. 8.5 The Flenley acid–base nomogram. The central white box shows the approximate limits of arterial pH and P_{CO_2} in normal individuals.

Respiratory alkalosis

Hyperventilation results in increased removal of carbon dioxide, resulting in a fall in P_aCO_2 and $[H^+]$.

Metabolic acidosis

This is the result of the accumulation of any acid other than carbonic acid. The most common cause is lactic acidosis following shock or cardiac arrest.

Clinical features

These include hyperventilation, hypotension caused by arteriolar vasodilatation and the negative inotropic effect of acidosis, and cerebral dysfunction associated with confusion and fits.

Differential diagnosis (the anion gap)

The first step is to identify whether the acidosis is the result of retention of HCl or of another acid. This is achieved by measurement of the anion gap. The main

Table 8.9 Causes of metabolic acidosis with a normal anion gap

Increased gastrointestinal HCO_3^- loss

Diarrhoea
Ileostomy
Ureterosigmoidostomy

Increased HCO_3^- renal loss

Acetazolamide ingestion
Proximal (type 2) renal tubular acidosis
Hyperparathyroidism
Tubular damage, e.g. drugs, heavy metals

Decreased renal H^+ excretion

Distal (type 1) renal tubular acidosis
Type 4 renal tubular acidosis

Increased HCl production

Ammonium chloride ingestion
Increased catabolism of lysine, arginine

electrolytes measured in plasma are sodium, potassium, chloride and bicarbonate. The sum of the cations, sodium and potassium, normally exceeds that of chloride and bicarbonate by 6–12 mmol/L. This anion gap is usually made up of negatively charged proteins, phosphate and organic acids. If the anion gap is normal in the presence of acidosis, it can be concluded that HCl is being retained or $NaHCO_3$ is being lost. The causes of a normal anion gap acidosis are given in Table 8.9.

If the anion gap is increased (i.e. >12 mmol/L), the acidosis is the result of an exogenous acid, e.g. salicylates or one of the acids normally present in small unmeasured quantities, such as lactate. Causes of a high anion gap acidosis are given in Table 8.10.

Lactic acidosis

Increased production of lactic acid occurs when cellular respiration is abnormal, resulting from either lack of oxygen (type A) or a metabolic abnormality (type B). The most common form in clinical practice is type A lactic acidosis, occurring in septicaemic or cardiogenic shock.

Diabetic ketoacidosis

This is a high anion gap acidosis caused by the accumulation of acetoacetic and hydroxybutyric acids.

Renal tubular acidosis

Renal tubular acidosis may occur in the absence of chronic kidney disease and is a normal anion gap acidosis. There is failure of the kidney to acidify the urine adequately. This group of disorders is uncommon and only rarely a cause of

Table 8.10 Causes of metabolic acidosis with a high anion gap

Renal failure (sulphate, phosphate)
Ketoacidosis
Diabetes mellitus Starvation Alcohol poisoning
Lactic acidosis
Type A
Shock Severe hypoxia Methanol ingestion Ethylene glycol ingestion Strenuous exercise
Type B
Acute liver failure Poisoning: ethanol, paracetamol Metformin accumulation Leukaemia, lymphoma
Drug poisoning
Salicylates

significant clinical disease. There are four types, of which type 4 (also known as hyporeninaemic hypoaldosteronism) is the most common. Typical features are acidosis and hyperkalaemia occurring in the setting of mild chronic kidney disease, usually caused by tubulointerstitial disease or diabetes. Plasma aldosterone and renin levels are low and do not respond to stimulation. Treatment is with fludrocortisone, diuretics, sodium bicarbonate and ion exchange resins for the reduction of serum potassium.

Uraemic acidosis

Reduction of the capacity to secrete H^+ and NH_4^+, in addition to bicarbonate wasting, contributes to the acidosis of chronic kidney disease. Acidosis occurs particularly when there is tubular damage, such as reflux and chronic obstructive nephropathy. It is associated with hypercalciuria and renal osteodystrophy because H^+ ions are buffered by bone in exchange for calcium. Treatment is with calcium or sodium bicarbonate, although acidosis in end-stage renal failure is only usually fully corrected by adequate dialysis.

Metabolic alkalosis

This is much less common than acidosis and is often associated with potassium or volume depletion. The main causes are persistent vomiting, diuretic therapy or hyperaldosteronism. Vomiting causes alkalosis, both by causing volume depletion and through loss of gastric acid.

Clinical features

Cerebral dysfunction is an early feature of alkalosis. Respiration may be depressed.

Management

This includes fluid replacement, if necessary, with replacement of sodium, potassium and chloride. The bicarbonate excess will correct itself.

THERAPEUTICS

Diuretics

Diuretics (Table 8.4) reduce sodium and chloride reabsorption at different sites in the nephron and thus increase urinary sodium and water loss.

Thiazide diuretics

Mechanism of action

They inhibit sodium reabsorption at the beginning of the distal convoluted tubule and reduce peripheral vascular resistance (mechanism unclear).

Indications

In low doses, they are used to reduce blood pressure; at higher doses, to relieve oedema in patients with mild chronic heart failure and good renal function.

Preparations and dose

Bendroflumethiazide Tablets: 2.5 mg, 5 mg.
    Hypertension: 2.5 mg p.o. each morning – higher doses rarely necessary.
    Oedema: initially 5–10 mg each morning.
    Metolazone Tablets: 5 mg.
Oedema resistant to other diuretics: start at 5 mg p.o. each morning and gradually increase if necessary to 20 mg daily.

Side effects

Postural hypotension, anorexia, diarrhoea, metabolic and electrolyte disturbances (hypokalaemia, hyponatraemia, hypomagnesaemia, hypercalcaemia, hyperlipidaemia, hyperuricaemia and gout). May aggravate diabetes mellitus.

Cautions/contraindications

Contraindicated in symptomatic hyperuricaemia, severe renal and hepatic impairment, hyponatraemia, hypercalcaemia and untreated hypokalaemia.

Loop diuretics

Mechanism of action

Loop diuretics stimulate excretion of sodium chloride and water by blocking the sodium–potassium–chloride channel in the thick ascending limb of the loop of Henle. Loop diuretics also increase venous capacitance and thus produce rapid clinical improvement before the diuresis in patients with acute heart failure.

Indications

Loop diuretics are given intravenously in patients with acute pulmonary oedema due to left heart failure. They are administered orally in patients with chronic heart failure and in patients with oedema associated with liver disease if aldosterone antagonists alone are ineffective. High doses may be needed with impaired renal function.

Preparations and dose

Furosemide Tablets: 20 mg, 40 mg, 500 mg. Oral solution: 20, 40, 50 mg/5 mL. Injection: 10 mg/mL.

Oral for oedema, initially 40 mg in the morning, increasing if necessary to 120 mg daily.

IV/IM initially, 20–50 mg; doses greater than 50 mg by i.v. infusion only; max. 1.5 g daily.

Bumetanide Tablets: 1 mg, 5 mg. Injection: 500 μg/mL. Liquid: 1 mg/5 mL.
1 mg bumetanide = 40 mg furosemide (frusemide) at low doses.

Oral initially 1 mg (0.5 mg in the elderly) daily, increased according to response, max. 5 mg daily.

IV 1–2 mg repeated after 20 minutes if necessary. Higher doses usually given as infusion over 30–60 minutes.

Side effects

Hypokalaemia, hypomagnesaemia, hyponatraemia, urate retention causing gout, hyperglycaemia, gastrointestinal disturbance, tinnitus and deafness with rapid i.v. administration or high doses, myalgia (bumetanide at high doses).

Cautions/contraindications

Untreated severe electrolyte disturbance, coma due to liver failure; renal failure due to nephrotoxic drugs or anuria.

Potassium-sparing diuretics and aldosterone antagonists

Mechanism of action

Potassium-sparing diuretics and aldosterone antagonists inhibit sodium reabsorption in the cortical collecting tubule. Amiloride and triamterene directly decrease sodium channel activity; spironolactone inhibits aldosterone. They have weak natriuretic activity.

Indications

Spironolactone is used in ascites and oedema associated with chronic liver disease and in low doses (25 mg) to improve survival in severe heart failure. Amiloride in combination with loop diuretics can be used as an alternative to giving potassium supplements. Amiloride may be used in patients with liver disease who are intolerant of spironolactone because of gynaecomastia.

Preparations and dose

Spironolactone Tablets: 25 mg, 50 mg, 100 mg. Suspension: 5 mg, 10 mg, 25 mg, 50 mg, 100 mg/5 mL.

Oral Heart failure: initially 25 mg daily increased to 50 mg if necessary.

Ascites in chronic liver disease: 100 mg with or without 40 mg of furosemide, increasing gradually to a maximum of 400 mg and 160 mg, respectively.

It is preferable to prescribe thiazides and potassium-sparing diuretics separately. The use of fixed drug combinations (e.g. co-amilozide 2.5/25; amiloride hydrochloride 2.5 mg, hydrochlorothiazide 25 mg) may be justified if compliance is a problem.

Disorders of serum potassium

Potassium supplementation

Indications

Potassium depletion.

Preparations and dose

Oral potassium

Kay-Cee-L Syrup: potassium chloride 7.5% (1 mmol/mL each of K^+ and Cl^-).

Sando-K Effervescent tablets: potassium bicarbonate and chloride equivalent to potassium 470 mg (12 mmol of K^+) and chloride 285 mg (8 mmol of Cl^-).

Prevention of hypokalaemia: 25–50 mmol in divided doses.

Treatment of hypokalaemia: 40–100 mmol daily depending on serum potassium and severity of any continuing loss.

Intravenous potassium Injection: 20 mmol/10 mL. Infusions: 10–40 mmol/L.

A variety of infusion fluids with concentrations of potassium between 10 and 40 mmol/L are available in 500 mL and 1 L bags. Concentrations over 60 mmol/L must be infused into a large (e.g. femoral) or central vein, as high concentrations are irritant to smaller veins. Maximum rate of i.v. potassium is usually 10–20 mmol/hour, although 40–100 mmol/hour has been given to selected patients with paralysis or arrhythmias (with ECG monitoring).

Side effects

Nausea and vomiting, oesophageal and small bowel ulceration with oral preparations; where appropriate, potassium-sparing diuretics are preferable. Cardiac arrhythmias and vein irritation with intravenous administration.

Cautions/contraindications

Caution in severe renal impairment and co-administration with drugs liable to raise the serum potassium, e.g. angiotensin-converting enzyme (ACE) inhibitors, potassium-sparing diuretics.

9 Renal disease

The kidneys are 11–14 cm in length and lie retroperitoneally on either side of the vertebral column from T12–L3. The functions of the kidneys are:

- Elimination of waste material
- Regulation of volume and composition of body fluid
- Endocrine function – production of erythropoietin, renin and vitamin D in its active form
- Autocrine function – production of endothelin, prostaglandins, renal natriuretic peptide.

The functional unit of the kidney is the *nephron*, which is composed of the glomerulus, proximal tubule, loop of Henle, distal tubule and collecting duct (Fig. 9.1). The renal artery (a branch of the abdominal aorta) supplies the kidney and divides many times to form *afferent arterioles*, each of which supplies one of the two million nephrons. The wider diameter of the afferent compared to efferent arterioles increases the pressure of blood within the glomerulus and forces water and solutes (but not red blood cells or larger molecular weight plasma proteins) out of the glomerular capillaries into Bowman's capsule forming the *glomerular filtrate* – about 170–180 L per day. The proximal renal tubules reabsorb most of the filtered solute required to maintain fluid and electrolyte balance, but elimination of potassium, water and non-volatile hydrogen ions is regulated in the distal tubules. As renal perfusion and glomerular filtration fall, reabsorption of water and sodium by the proximal tubules increases so that minimal fluid reaches the distal tubule. Hence, hypotensive or hypovolaemic patients cannot excrete potassium and hydrogen ions. Patients with distal tubular damage, e.g. caused by drugs, also cannot excrete potassium and hydrogen ions. Normally only about 1% of the original filtered volume, containing high concentrations of urea and creatinine, passes into the renal pelvis as urine.

PRESENTING FEATURES OF RENAL DISEASE

The most common diseases of the kidney and urinary tract are benign prostatic hypertrophy in men and urinary tract infection (UTI) in women. Symptoms suggesting renal tract disease are dysuria, frequency of micturition, haematuria, urinary retention and alteration of urine volume (either polyuria or oliguria). In addition there may be pain anywhere along the renal tract, from loin to groin. Non-specific symptoms, e.g. lethargy, anorexia and pruritus, may be the presenting features of chronic kidney disease (CKD). Renal disease may be asymptomatic and discovered by the incidental finding of hypertension, a raised serum urea, or proteinuria and haematuria on Stix testing.

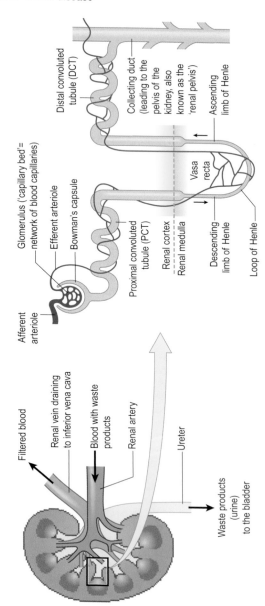

Fig. 9.1 The kidney and a nephron.

Dysuria

Dysuria (pain on micturition) is caused by:

- Inflammation involving the urethra (urethritis) or bladder (cystitis). Dysuria is common in adult women and is usually due to lower urinary tract bacterial infection (p. 372). Other causes of urethritis include infection with *Chlamydia trachomatis* or *Neisseria gonorrhoeae* (pp. 45–46).
- Inflammation involving the vagina in women or glans penis in men. Causes include infection with *Candida albicans* and *Gardnerella vaginalis*.

Polyuria and nocturia

Polyuria is an excessive urine output of greater than 2.5–3 L in 24 hours. It must be differentiated from the more common complaints of urinary frequency and nocturia (night-time urination), which are not necessarily associated with an increase in the total urine output. Causes of polyuria include polydipsia (defined as excessive thirst leading to increased fluid intake >3 L per day), solute diuresis (e.g. hyperglycaemia with glycosuria), diabetes insipidus and CKD. Nocturia is most often due to drinking before bed or, in men over 50 years, prostatic enlargement (p. 405).

Oliguria

Oliguria is a low urine output, and maintained over several hours indicates acute kidney injury (AKI, p. 386) or urinary tract obstruction. It may be 'physiological', as in patients with hypotension and hypovolaemia, where urine is maximally concentrated in an attempt to conserve water. Anuria (no urine) suggests bilateral ureteric or bladder outflow obstruction. Management of the oliguric patient involves three steps:

1. *Exclude obstruction.* The patient with outflow obstruction (acute retention of urine) is typically in great discomfort with an intense desire to micturate. The bladder is palpable as a tender mass that is dull to percussion, arising out of the pelvis. The diagnosis is confirmed by passing a urethral catheter and releasing a large volume of urine. If the patient is already catheterized, the catheter should be flushed with sterile saline to relieve any blockage. Obstruction proximal to the bladder (e.g. ureteric obstruction) is often painless, and ultrasound examination is indicated to exclude pelvicalyceal dilatation.

2. *Assess for hypovolaemia.* Once obstruction is excluded, the patient is assessed for evidence of hypovolaemia by measurement of blood pressure, pulse, jugular venous pressure (JVP) and urinary electrolytes

(p. 391). If the patient is hypovolaemic, the urine output in response to a fluid challenge (500 mL saline 0.9% intravenously over 30 minutes) is assessed.

3. *Management of established AKI* (p. 392) once obstruction and hypovolaemia have been excluded.

Haematuria

See urine dipstick testing (p. 359).

Pain

Loin/flank pain occurs in kidney infections (acute pyelonephritis), upper urinary tract obstruction and occlusion of the renal artery due to either thrombosis in situ or emboli. Chronic renal pain occurs in cystic renal disease and renal tumours. Acute severe pain radiating from the flank to the iliac fossa and testes or labium is typical of ureteric colic due to a calculus.

INVESTIGATION OF RENAL DISEASE

Once renal disease is suspected, the purpose of investigation is to determine the cause and the presence or degree of renal dysfunction. Estimation of the glomerular filtration rate (eGFR, see below) is used to determine the degree of renal dysfunction. The history and examination together with urine dipstick testing and microscopy of urine are the starting points for diagnosis.

Blood tests

The serum urea or creatinine concentration represents the dynamic equilibrium between production and elimination but levels do not rise above the normal range until there is a reduction of 50–60% in the glomerular filtration rate (GFR). The serum urea concentration is increased by a high-protein diet, increased tissue catabolism (surgery, trauma, infection) and gastrointestinal bleeding, whereas the level of creatinine is much less dependent on diet but is more related to age, sex and muscle mass. Once it is elevated, serum creatinine is a better guide to GFR than urea, although a normal level is not synonymous with a normal GFR.

Glomerular filtration rate

Measurement of the GFR is the best indicator of kidney function. Creatinine clearance is a reasonably accurate measure of GFR and is calculated using a 24-hour urine collection and a single plasma creatinine. In clinical practice the eGFR is calculated using formulae based on serum creatinine and demographics: e.g. the Cockrof–Gault equation.

Calculation of creatinine clearance using the Cockroft–Gault equation:

Men

$$\text{Creatinine clearance} = \frac{1.23 \times (140 - \text{Age}) \times (\text{Weight in kg})}{\text{Serum creatinine } (\mu\text{mol/L})}$$

Women Use the same equation but multiply by 1.04 instead of 1.23.

The modification of diet in renal disease (MDRD) is more reliable than the Cockroft–Gault equation in ethnically diverse groups of individuals (http://www.nephron.com/MDRD_GFR.cgi). Neither are validated in AKI and pregnancy. An eGFR < 60 mL/min/1.73 m^2 body surface area for more than 3 months indicates CKD.

Urine dipstick testing

Urine dipstick testing detects the presence of blood, protein, glucose, ketones, bilirubin and urobilinogen in the urine and provides a semiquantitative assessment of the amount of substance present. Dipsticks can also be used to measure urine pH, which is useful in the investigation and management of renal tubular acidosis (p. 349). Each test is based on a colour change in a strip of absorbent cellulose impregnated with the appropriate reagent. The stick is dipped briefly into a fresh specimen of urine collected in a clean container and the colour changes compared with the manufacturer's colour charts on the reagent strip container. Haematuria or proteinuria suggests renal tract disease. Dipsticks are also available for testing for urinary nitrites and leucocyte elastase to identify UTIs (p. 372).

Proteinuria

This is an excess of protein in the urine. Under normal conditions the low molecular weight proteins and albumin that are filtered by the glomerulus are almost completely reabsorbed in the proximal renal tubule. This results in a normal urinary protein excretion of less than 150 mg/day, of which only a small amount is albumin (<30 mg daily). Dipsticks are albumin specific and will detect albumin once urine levels exceed 200 mg/L (300 mg daily if urine volume is normal). Dipsticks do not detect abnormal proteins such as globulins and Bence Jones protein (immunoglobulin light chains) excreted in multiple myeloma. The causes of proteinuria are listed in Table 9.1. Persistent proteinuria detected on dipstick testing requires full investigation and should be quantified. Quantification of proteinuria is by measurement of protein and/or albumin concentration in a 'spot' urine sample (ideally an early morning specimen) and normalizing to creatinine concentration to give a urine protein-to-creatinine ratio (PCR) or the more sensitive urine albumin-to-creatinine ratio (ACR). Normal protein excretion is less than 150 mg per day (PCR < 15 mg/mmol) and nephrotic range proteinuria (p. 359) is more than 3.5 g per day (PCR > 350 mg/mmol).

Table 9.1 Causes of proteinuria

Type	Mechanism	Examples
Glomerular	Increased permeability	Glomerulopathies
Tubular*	Decreased reabsorption	Fanconi's syndrome
		Tubulointerstitial disorders
Overflow	Plasma proteins produced in excess	Multiple myeloma
		Monoclonal gammopathy
Physiological†	Increased renal haemodynamics	Acute illness
		Fever
		Intense activity
		Upright posture

*Usually <1 g per day and may be associated with other defects of proximal tubular function (e.g. glucosuria, phosphaturia, aminoaciduria).
†Mild proteinuria and not associated with underlying renal disease. Diagnosis is made by the absence of proteinuria on subsequent urine examinations when the condition, e.g. fever, resolves.

Microalbuminuria is an increase above the normal range in urinary albumin excretion that is undetectable by conventional dipsticks (i.e. 30–300 mg/day). It is an early indicator of renal disease and is widely used as a predictor of the development of nephropathy in people with diabetes. An ACR of >2.5 mg/mmol in men and >3.5 mg/mmol in women indicates microalbuminuria. Albumin excretion above 300 mg/day is overt proteinuria.

Haematuria

Haematuria is blood in the urine and is either visible (macroscopic or gross) or non-visible (microscopic), detected on urine dipstick (positive 1 + or greater).

Haematuria can arise from several sites in the kidney or urinary tract (Fig. 9.2).

- Blood that is only apparent at the start of micturition is usually due to urethral disease.
- Blood at the end of micturition suggests bleeding from the prostate or bladder base.
- Blood seen as an even discoloration throughout the urine suggests bleeding from a source in the bladder or above.

Fig. 9.3 outlines an algorithm for the investigation of haematuria. Patients should be evaluated regardless of anticoagulant or antiplatelet therapy. Transient causes such as urinary tract infection and contamination during

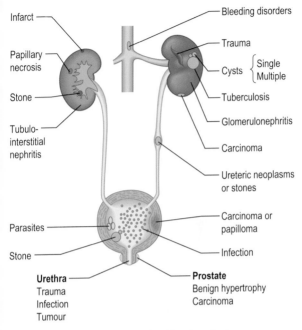

Fig. 9.2 Sites and causes of bleeding from the urinary tract.

menstruation are excluded by repeat testing. Urinary tract malignancy is more likely in patients with visible haematuria, urinary tract symptoms or those over 40 years of age; thus urological referral is usually indicated initially for appropriate imaging of the urinary tract (either ultrasound or computed tomography [CT]) and cystoscopy. All other patients are more likely to have glomerular disease (often immunoglobulin [Ig]A nephropathy) and nephrology referral is indicated if initial or subsequent testing of renal function is abnormal.

Glycosuria

Diabetes mellitus must be excluded in any patients with a positive dipstick test for glucose.

Urine microscopy

This is performed on a fresh, clean-catch, mid-stream urine specimen in all patients suspected of having renal disease.

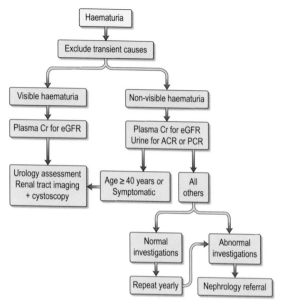

Fig. 9.3 Decision algorithm for the investigation of haematuria. Cr, creatinine; eGFR, estimated glomerular filtration rate; ACR (PCR), albumin (protein): creatinine ratio.

White cells

Ten or more white cells per cubic millimetre in fresh, unspun, mid-stream urine is abnormal, and indicates an inflammatory reaction within the urinary tract, usually a UTI. Sterile pyuria (i.e. pus cells without bacterial infection) occurs in a partially treated UTI, urinary tract tuberculosis, calculi, bladder tumour, papillary necrosis and tubulointerstitial nephritis.

Red cells

One or more red cells per cubic millimetre is abnormal and must be investigated (see haematuria).

Casts

Mucoprotein precipitated in the renal tubules results in the formation of hyaline casts. On their own these are a normal finding but the incorporation of red cells results in red cell casts, a finding pathognomonic of glomerulonephritis. White cell casts may be seen in acute pyelonephritis. Granular casts result from the disintegration of cellular debris and indicate glomerular or tubular disease.

Bacteria

Greater than 10^5 or 10^3 pathogenic organisms per mL of urine in a fresh mid-stream specimen in a symptomatic woman or man, respectively, indicates a UTI. In a woman, the diagnosis is also made with 10^2 coliform organisms per mL in the presence of pyuria (> 10 white cells/mm^3). Any growth of pathogenic organisms in urine by suprapubic aspiration is diagnostic of a UTI.

Imaging techniques

Plain X-ray is useful to identify renal calcification or radiodense calculi in the kidney, renal pelvis, line of the ureters or bladder.

Ultrasonography of the kidneys is the method of choice for assessing renal size, checking for pelvicalyceal dilatation (indicative of chronic renal obstruction), characterizing renal masses, diagnosing polycystic kidney disease, and detecting intrarenal and/or perinephric fluid (e.g. pus, blood). It has the advantage over X-ray techniques of avoiding ionizing radiation and the use of an intravascular contrast medium. Doppler ultrasonography is used to demonstrate renal artery perfusion and detect renal vein thrombosis. Bladder wall thickening can be detected in a distended bladder and an assessment of bladder emptying made by scanning after voiding.

CT is used as a first-line investigation in cases of suspected ureteric colic. It is also used to characterize renal masses that are indeterminate at ultrasonography, to stage renal, bladder and prostate tumours, and to detect 'lucent' calculi; low-density calculi which are lucent on plain films (e.g. uric acid stones), are well seen on CT. It is also used to look for retroperitoneal disease such as tumours and fibrosis, and CT angiography is used to visualize the renal arteries and veins.

Magnetic resonance imaging (MRI) is used to characterize renal masses as an alternative to CT, to stage renal, prostate and bladder cancer and also to image the renal arteries by magnetic resonance (MR) angiography with gadolinium as contrast medium. In experienced hands, its sensitivity and specificity approaches renal angiography.

Excretion urography (also known as intravenous urography [IVU] or intravenous pyelography [IVP]) has largely been replaced by ultrasonography and CT scanning.

Renal arteriography (angiography) is used in the diagnosis of renal artery disease, but MR and spiral CT angiography are being used increasingly. The technique requires cannulation of the femoral artery and injection of a contrast medium. Complications include cholesterol embolizations and contrast-induced kidney damage.

Anterograde pyelography involves percutaneous puncture of a pelvicalyceal system with a needle and the injection of contrast medium to outline the pelvicalyceal system and ureter to the level of obstruction. Drains can be sited, and stents placed during the procedure.

Retrograde pyelography under screening control allows a contrast study of the ureter from the bladder. It is invasive, commonly requires a general anaesthetic and may result in the introduction of infection.

Renal scintigraphy Renal scintigraphy involves the intravenous injection of a radiopharmaceutical (e.g. diethylenetriaminepentaacetic acid [DPTA] labelled with technetium-99m) which is extracted from the bloodstream by the kidneys and subsequent imaging on a gamma camera with computer acquisition. Isotope studies are helpful for dynamic or static studies of perfusion or excretion. It is used to detect anatomical or functional abnormalities of the kidneys or urinary tract. *Dynamic renal scintigraphy* is used to assess renal blood flow in suspected renal artery stenosis, renal function in obstruction and in detection of vesicoureteric reflux. *Static renal scintigraphy* enables assessment of the size and position of the kidneys, differential function of each kidney and parenchymal defects (scars, ischaemic areas, tumours).

Transcutaneous renal biopsy

Renal biopsy is carried out under ultrasound control in specialized centres and requires interpretation by an experienced pathologist. Microscopy is helpful in the investigation of the nephritic and nephrotic syndromes, AKI and CKD, haematuria after negative urological investigations and renal graft dysfunction. Complications include haematuria, flank pain and perirenal haematoma formation.

GLOMERULAR DISEASES

Normal glomerular structure

There are about one million renal glomeruli in each kidney, and each consists of a capillary plexus invaginating the blind end of the proximal renal tubule (Fig. 9.4). The glomerular capillaries are lined by a fenestrated endothelium, which rests on the glomerular basement membrane (GBM). External to the GBM are the visceral epithelial cells (podocytes) which only make contact with the GBM by finger-like projections, called foot processes, which are separated from one another by 'filtration pores'. This unique structure of the glomerular membrane accounts for its tremendous permeability, allowing 125–200 mL of glomerular filtrate to be formed every minute (this is the GFR). The composition of the glomerular filtrate is similar to plasma but contains only small amounts of protein (all of low molecular weight), most of which is reabsorbed in the proximal tubule. Tubular reabsorption and secretion normally substantially alter the water and electrolyte composition of the glomerular filtrate until it reaches the renal pelvis as urine.

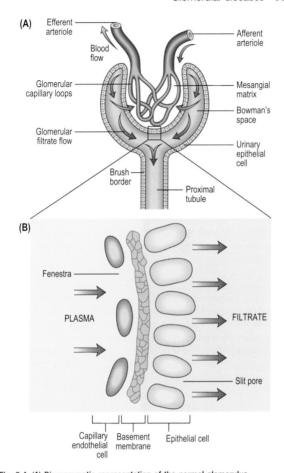

Fig. 9.4 (A) Diagrammatic representation of the normal glomerulus.
(B) Components of the glomerular membrane.
(Adapted from Read et al. 1993 Essential Medicine. Churchill Livingstone, Edinburgh; Guyton 1987 Human Physiology and Mechanisms of Disease, 4th ed. WB Saunders, London.)

Pathogenesis and terms in glomerular disease

The nomenclature for glomerular disease can be confusing, as descriptive terms (as seen on histology) overlap with clinical syndromes and more recent molecular insights into the pathogenesis of disease. If there is predominant inflammation on histology, glomerular disease may be described as a *glomerulonephritis*. If inflammation is absent, *glomerulopathy* is more correct. There remains much overlap between the two, and the terms are often (wrongly) used interchangeably. The kidneys are symmetrically involved and the renal lesion may be primary or part of a generalized disease, e.g. systemic lupus erythematosus (SLE). Glomerular disease is usually described after kidney biopsy, and commonly used important terms include:

- Focal: some, but not all, glomeruli show the lesion
- Diffuse (global): most of the glomeruli (>75%) contain the lesion
- Segmental: only a part of the glomerulus is affected (most focal lesions are also segmental, e.g. focal segmental glomerulosclerosis)
- Global: all of the glomerulus is symmetrically involved
- Proliferative: an increase in cell numbers due to hyperplasia of one or more of the resident glomerular cells with or without inflammation
- Membrane alterations: capillary wall thickening due to deposition of immune deposits or alterations in basement membrane
- Crescent formation: epithelial cell proliferation with mononuclear cell infiltration in Bowman's space.

Classification and presentation of glomerulopathies

The presence of some form of glomerular disease, as opposed to tubulo-interstitial or vascular disease, is usually suspected from the history and from one or more of the following urinary findings: haematuria (particularly if the red cells are abnormally shaped or distorted, i.e. dysmorphic), red cell casts and proteinuria, which may be in the nephrotic range (>3.5 g/day). Glomerulopathies are classified and discussed as they relate to four major glomerular syndromes:

- *Nephrotic syndrome:* massive proteinuria (>3.5 g/day), hypoalbuminaemia, oedema, lipiduria and hyperlipidaemia
- *Acute glomerulonephritis (acute nephritic syndrome):* abrupt onset of haematuria with casts or dysmorphic red cells, non-nephrotic range proteinuria, oedema, hypertension and transient renal impairment
- *Rapidly progressive glomerulonephritis:* features of acute nephritis, focal necrosis with or without crescents and rapidly progressive renal failure over weeks
- *Asymptomatic haematuria, proteinuria* (or both): these are usually incidental findings on urinary dipstick testing and may be an early indicator of renal disease. The causes and further investigation are discussed in the sections on haematuria (p. 360) and proteinuria (p. 359).

NEPHROTIC SYNDROME

There is massively increased filtration of macromolecules across the glomerular capillary wall due to structural and functional abnormalities of the glomerular podocytes.

- *Hypoalbuminaemia* (serum albumin <30 g/L) develops as a consequence of heavy *proteinuria* (>3.5 g/24 hours in adults) and increased renal catabolism of filtered protein.
- *Oedema* is primarily due to sodium retention in the renal collecting tubules, together with an increase in capillary permeability. A reduction in effective circulating volume also leads to oedema through similar mechanisms that occur in cardiac failure and cirrhosis (p. 165).
- *Hypercholesterolaemia* and *hypertriglyceridaemia* are common in nephrotic syndrome due to increased synthesis and impaired catabolism.

Aetiology

Nephrotic syndrome with 'bland' urine sediments

Membranous nephropathy and focal segmental glomerulosclerosis are the most common causes in adults and minimal-change nephropathy in children (Table 9.2). Membranous nephropathy is usually idiopathic but may occur in association with drugs (e.g. penicillamine, gold, non-steroidal anti-inflammatory drugs [NSAIDs]), autoimmune disease (e.g. SLE, thyroiditis), neoplasia (carcinoma of lung, colon, stomach, breast and lymphoma), infections (e.g. hepatitis B and C, schistosomiasis and *Plasmodium malariae*) and other causes (sarcoidosis, sickle cell disease). There is deposition of IgG and complement C3 along the outer aspect of the glomerular basement membrane. Expansion of the basement membrane appears with time as the deposits are surrounded by basement membrane and eventually undergo resorption. Focal segmental glomerulosclerosis is of unknown aetiology and is a particular common cause of nephrotic syndrome in black adults. A similar histological type occurs in human immunodeficiency virus (HIV) infection.

Minimal-change nephropathy occurs most commonly in boys under 5 years of age. It accounts for 90% of cases of nephrotic syndrome in children and 20–25% in adults. The pathogenesis is unknown; immune complexes are absent on immunofluorescence, but the increase in glomerular permeability is thought to be immunologically mediated. The glomeruli appear normal on light microscopy. On electron microscopy there is fusion of the foot processes of epithelial cells (podocytes) – a non-specific finding.

Nephrotic syndrome associated with renal amyloid (p. 698) and diabetes mellitus (p. 667) is not immune mediated. Other renal diseases, e.g. polycystic kidneys and reflux nephropathy, may cause proteinuria, but are rarely severe enough to cause the nephrotic syndrome.

Table 9.2 Glomerulopathies associated with the nephrotic syndrome

Nephrotic syndrome with 'bland' urine sediments

Primary glomerular disease:

Minimal-change glomerular disease
Membranous nephropathy
Focal segmental glomerulosclerosis
Congenital nephrotic syndrome

Secondary glomerular disease:

Amyloidosis
Diabetic nephropathy

Nephrotic syndrome with 'active' urine sediments (mixed nephrotic/nephritic)

Primary glomerular disease:

Mesangiocapillary glomerulonephritis
Mesangial proliferative glomerulonephritis

Secondary glomerular disease:

Systemic lupus erythematosus
Cryoglobulinaemic disease
Henoch–Schönlein syndrome
Idiopathic fibrillary glomerulopathy
Immunotactoid glomerulopathy
Fibronectin glomerulopathy

Nephrotic syndrome with 'active' urine sediments (mixed nephrotic/nephritic)

Mesangiocapillary (membranoproliferative glomerulonephritis) occurs with chronic infection (abscesses, infective endocarditis, infected ventriculoperitoneal shunt), cryoglobulinaemia secondary to hepatitis C infection or may be idiopathic. A different type occurs with partial lipodystrophy (loss of subcutaneous fat on the face and upper trunk). Most patients develop renal failure over several years. Mesangial proliferative glomerulonephritis presents with heavy proteinuria with minimal changes on light microscopy. There are deposits in the glomerular mesangium of IgM and complement (IgM nephropathy) or $C1_q$ ($C1_q$ nephropathy). Some patients respond to steroids but others progress to renal failure.

Clinical features

Oedema of the ankles, genitals and abdominal wall is the principal finding. The face (periorbital oedema) and arms may be involved in severe cases.

Differential diagnoses

Nephrotic syndrome must be differentiated from other causes of oedema and hypoalbuminaemia. In congestive cardiac failure there is oedema and raised JVP. In nephrotic syndrome the JVP is normal or low unless there is concomitant renal failure and oliguria. Hypoalbuminaemia and oedema occur in cirrhosis, but there are usually signs of chronic liver disease on examination (p. 175).

Investigations

Investigations are indicated to make the diagnosis, monitor progress and determine the underlying aetiology (Table 9.3).

Management

General oedema

General oedema is treated with dietary salt restriction and a thiazide diuretic, e.g. bendroflumethiazide 5 mg daily (p. 351), followed by furosemide and amiloride for unresponsive patients. Intravenous diuretics and occasionally intravenous salt-poor albumin are required to initiate a diuresis, which, once established, can usually be maintained with oral diuretics alone. Proteinuria is reduced by administration of angiotensin-converting enzyme (ACE) inhibitors or angiotensin II receptor antagonists; patients should be advised to eat a normal rather than high protein diet, which increases proteinuria. Prolonged bed rest should be avoided and long-term prophylactic anticoagulation given in view of the thrombotic tendency (see Complications). Infections are treated aggressively and patients should be offered influenza and pneumococcal vaccination (p. 515).

Specific treatment

Treatment of the underlying disease, e.g. SLE, or cessation of the offending drug, e.g. penicillamine, is usually associated with improvement in secondary glomerulopathy. Only selected patients with moderate or severe progressive idiopathic membranous nephropathy should receive specific treatment as there is a high rate of spontaneous improvement. Treatment is with cyclophosphamide or chlorambucil with prednisolone. Rituximab (p. 256) is used in resistant disease. Minimal-change nephropathy is almost always steroid responsive in children, although less commonly in adults. High-dose prednisolone therapy (60 mg/m^2/day) is given for 4–6 weeks and then tapered slowly. Further courses are given if the patient has a relapse. In patients with frequent relapses and in steroid-unresponsive patients, immunosuppressive therapy with cyclophosphamide or ciclosporin is used.

Table 9.3 Investigations indicated in glomerular disease

Investigations	Significance
Baseline measurements	
Estimated glomerular filtration rate	To determine current status, monitor progress and response to treatment
Urinary protein	
Serum urea and electrolytes	
Serum albumin	
Diagnostically useful tests	
Urine microscopy	Red cell casts indicate glomerulonephritis
Culture (swab from throat or infected skin)	Diagnosis of recent streptococcal infection
Serum antistreptolysin-O titre	
Blood glucose	Diagnosis of diabetes mellitus
Serum tests:	
Antinuclear and anti-DNA antibodies	Present in significant titre in SLE
ANCA	Positive in vasculitis
Anti-GBM antibody	Present in anti-GBM glomerulonephritis
Hepatitis B surface antigen	Hepatitis B infection
Hepatitis C antibody	Hepatitis C infection
HIV antibody	HIV infection
Cryoglobulins	Increased in cryoglobulinaemia
Chest X-ray	Cavities in Wegener's granulomatosis, malignancy
Ultrasound of kidneys	Renal size, to look for renal vein thrombosis
Renal biopsy	Diagnosis of any glomerulopathy

ANCA, antineutrophil cytoplasmic antibody; GBM, glomerular basement membrane; HIV, human immunodeficiency virus; SLE, systemic lupus erythematosus.

Complications

- *Venous thrombosis*. Loss of clotting factors in the urine predispose to thrombus formation in both peripheral and renal veins. The latter presents with renal pain, haematuria and deterioration in renal function and is diagnosed by ultrasonography.

- *Sepsis*. Loss of immunoglobulin in the urine increases susceptibility to infection, which is a common cause of death in these patients.
- *AKI* is rarely the result of progression of the underlying renal disease and more often a consequence of hypovolaemia (particularly after diuretic therapy) or renal vein thrombosis.

Acute glomerulonephritis (acute nephritic syndrome)

Acute nephritic syndrome is often caused by an immune response triggered by an infection or other disease (Table 9.4). The typical case of post-streptococcal glomerulonephritis develops in a child 1–3 weeks after a streptococcal infection (pharyngitis or cellulitis) with a Lancefield group A β-haemolytic streptococcus. The bacterial antigen becomes trapped in the glomerulus, leading to an acute diffuse proliferative glomerulonephritis.

Clinical features

The syndrome comprises:

- Haematuria (visible or non-visible) – red cell casts are typically seen in urine microscopy
- Proteinuria (usually <2 g in 24 hours)
- Hypertension and oedema (periorbital, leg or sacral) caused by salt and water retention
- Oliguria
- Uraemia.

Table 9.4 Diseases commonly associated with the acute nephritic syndrome

Post-streptococcal glomerulonephritis
Non-streptococcal post-infectious glomerulonephritis, e.g. *Staphylococcus*, mumps, *Legionella*, hepatitis B and C, schistosomiasis, malaria
Infective endocarditis
Shunt nephritis
Visceral abscess
Systemic lupus erythematosus
Henoch–Schönlein syndrome
Cryoglobulinaemia

Investigations

The history and examination will help to assess the severity of the illness and to determine any associated underlying conditions. Investigations performed in the nephritic syndrome are listed in Table 9.3. If the clinical diagnosis of a nephritic illness is clear-cut, e.g. in post-streptococcal glomerulonephritis, renal biopsy is usually unnecessary.

Management

Post-streptococcal glomerulonephritis usually has a good prognosis, and supportive measures are often all that is required until spontaneous recovery takes place. Hypertension is treated with salt restriction, loop diuretics and vasodilators. Fluid balance is monitored by daily weighing and daily recording of fluid input and output. In oliguric patients with evidence of fluid overload (e.g. oedema, pulmonary congestion and severe hypertension), fluid restriction is necessary. The management of life-threatening complications such as hypertensive encephalopathy, pulmonary oedema and severe uraemia are discussed in the appropriate chapters. In glomerulonephritis complicating SLE or the systemic vasculitides (see below), immunosuppression with prednisolone, cyclophosphamide azathioprine or rituximab improves renal function.

Rapidly progressive glomerulonephritis

There are three main causes: on a background of acute nephritic syndrome (see above), anti-glomerular basement membrane disease (which with lung involvement is called Goodpasture's syndrome, p. 552) and antineutrophilic cytoplasmic antibody (ANCA)-associated vasculitis. Investigations are listed in Table 9.3 and the management is based on general treatment of AKI (p. 386) and specific treatment directed against the causes.

URINARY TRACT INFECTION

UTI is common, particularly in women: most often occurring in a normal urinary tract, and usually as cystitis, half of all women will experience a UTI in their lifetime. Most UTIs occur in isolation and are uncommon in men and children unless there is an abnormality of the urinary tract. Between 1 and 2% of patients presenting in primary care will have a UTI. Recurrent infection causes considerable morbidity, and infection can lead to life-threatening Gram-negative septicaemia and kidney failure.

Pathogenesis

Infection is most often caused by bacteria from a patient's own bowel flora, and infection usually ascends up the urethra. In women, the short urethra makes

Table 9.5 Organisms causing urinary tract infection in domiciliary practice

Organism	Approximate frequency (%)
Escherichia coli and other 'coliforms'	68+
Proteus mirabilis	12
Klebsiella aerogenes*	4
Enterococcus faecalis*	6
Staphylococcus saprophyticus or *S. epidermidis*†	10

*More common in hospital practice.
†More common in women.

ascending infection more likely. Rarely, infection may arise from the blood-stream, lymphatics or by direct extension (e.g. from a vesicocolic fistula). For *Escherichia coli*, the presence of flagellae (for motility), aerobactin (used to acquire iron), haemolysin (to form pores) and, above all, the presence of fimbriae (adhesins which attach organisms to the perineum and urothelium) on the bacterial fimbriae and on the cell surface make *E.coli* such a common pathogen (Table 9.5).

Risk factors for UTI

- Women
- Post-menopausal women
- New sexual activity, particularly in young women
- Indwelling urinary catheter or instrumentation of the urinary tract
- Urinary tract stones
- Urinary tract stasis (incomplete bladder emptying)
- Diabetes mellitus or immunosuppression.

Clinical features

The symptoms of *lower UTI* are frequency of micturition, dysuria, suprapubic pain and tenderness, haematuria and smelly urine. The clinical features of *acute pyelonephritis* are loin pain and tenderness, nausea, vomiting and fever. Localization of the site of infection on the basis of symptoms alone is unreliable. UTI can also present with few or no symptoms (particularly in the immunocompromised), or even abdominal pain, fever or haematuria in the absence of frequency or dysuria. In the elderly, new confusion may be the only symptom of UTI. In small children, who cannot complain of dysuria, symptoms are often 'atypical'. The possibility of UTI must always be considered in the fretful, febrile sick child who fails to thrive.

Natural history

Uncomplicated versus complicated infection *Uncomplicated infection* refers to UTI in an otherwise healthy non-pregnant woman with a functionally normal urinary tract and will rarely result in serious kidney damage. *Complicated infection* refers to infection in patients with abnormal urinary tracts (e.g. stones, obstruction) or systemic disease involving the kidney (e.g. diabetes mellitus, sickle cell disease/trait). They are more likely to fail treatment and develop complications which include renal papillary necrosis (p. 361) and the development of a renal or perinephric abscess with the risk of Gram-negative septicaemia. Most UTIs in men are also considered as complicated since they are often associated with urological abnormalities such as bladder outlet obstruction in elderly men.

Acute pyelonephritis This condition is associated with neutrophil infiltration of the renal parenchyma; small cortical abscesses and streaks of pus in the renal medulla are often present. There may be an acute deterioration in renal function but significant permanent kidney damage in adults with normal renal tracts is rare.

Reflux nephropathy Previously called chronic pyelonephritis or atrophic pyelonephritis, reflux nephropathy arises from childhood UTIs in combination with vesicoureteric reflux, leading to progressive renal scarring and presenting as hypertension or CKD in childhood and adult life. Vesicoureteric reflux refers to an incompetent valve between bladder and ureter, allowing reflux of urine up the ureter during bladder contraction and voiding. Reflux usually ceases around puberty but by that time the damage is done.

Recurrent UTI Recurrent UTI with the same or a different organism more than 2 weeks after stopping antibiotic treatment is considered to be *reinfection*, whereas *relapse* is diagnosed by recurrence of bacteriuria with the same organism within 7 days of completion of treatment. Relapse implies failure to eradicate the organism usually in association with anatomical renal tract abnormality, e.g. polycystic kidneys.

Investigations

Diagnosis

Uncomplicated UTIs in younger women (age ≤65 years old) can be diagnosed in patients without known urinary tract abnormalities, recent urinary tract instrumentation or systemic illness if they exhibit at least two of three cardinal symptoms – dysuria, urgency or frequency – along with absence of vaginal discharge. Neither urine dipstick testing for leukocyte esterase nor urine culture enhances diagnostic sensitivity.

Otherwise, diagnosis is based on culture of a clean-catch mid-stream specimen of urine (MSU) and the presence or absence of pyuria. Most Gram-negative organisms reduce nitrates to nitrites and produce a red colour in the reagent square. False-negative results are common. Dipsticks that detect significant pyuria depend on the release of esterases from leucocytes. Dipstick tests positive for both nitrite and leucocyte esterase are predictive of acute infection (sensitivity of 75% and specificity of 82%).

- Routine renal tract imaging of young women with UTI has a low diagnostic yield and is not indicated. Women with uncomplicated pyelonephritis who have persistent fever or clinical symptoms after 48–72 hours of appropriate antibiotic treatment require renal tract imaging to look for an abscess that requires drainage. Women with recurrent UTIs and all patients with complicated UTIs also require renal imaging. Contrast-enhanced CT scans give greater anatomical detail of the renal parenchyma and the perirenal areas than other imaging methods.

Management

Pre-treatment urine culture is essential. In patients with an indwelling urinary catheter, antibiotic treatment is indicated only in the presence of symptoms, and should be accompanied by replacement of the catheter.

Treatment of single isolated attack

- The most appropriate antibiotic choices are trimethoprim–sulfamethoxazole (160/800 mg twice daily for 3–7 days) or nitrofurantoin (100 mg twice daily for 5–7 days). Fluoroquinolones offered no advantage in cure rates; β-lactam antibiotics, such as amoxicillin–clavulanate, are less effective than the first-line recommendations. Most patients who delay antibiotic treatment to encourage spontaneous resolution eventually receive antibiotics and have longer times to resolution. Men with uncomplicated UTIs should be treated as above but for 7–14 days.
- Shorter 3–5 day courses with amoxicillin (250 mg three times daily), trimethoprim (200 mg twice daily) or an oral cephalosporin are also used and modified in light of the result of urine culture and sensitivity testing, and/or the clinical response.
- **Single-shot treatment** with 3 g of amoxicillin or 1.92 g of co-trimoxazole is used for patients with bladder symptoms of less than 36 hours' duration who have no previous history of UTI.
- **A high (2 L daily) fluid intake** should be encouraged during treatment and for some subsequent weeks. Urine culture should be repeated 5 days after treatment.
- **If the patient is acutely ill with high fever, loin pain and tenderness** (acute pyelonephritis), antibiotics are given intravenously, e.g. aztreonam, cefuroxime, ciprofloxacin or gentamicin, switching to a further 7 days'

treatment with oral therapy as symptoms improve. Intravenous fluids may be required to achieve a good urine output.

- **In patients presenting for the first time with high fever, loin pain and tenderness,** urgent renal ultrasound examination is required to exclude an obstructed pyonephrosis. If this is present it should be drained by percutaneous nephrostomy.

Recurrent infection In patients with a *relapse* of infection, a search should be made for an underlying cause, with treatment of the cause if possible, e.g. removal of stones. In addition, intensive (1 week intravenous) or prolonged (6 weeks oral) antibiotics are required. *Reinfection* where there is usually no underlying renal tract abnormality is managed initially with lifestyle advice (2 L daily fluid intake), voiding before bedtime and after intercourse, and avoidance of spermicidal jellies and constipation.

Colonization of the bladder by a pathogen is common after a urinary catheter has been in situ for more than a few days, partly due to organisms forming biofilms. So long as the bladder catheter is in place, antibiotics are likely to be ineffective and will encourage the development of resistant organisms. Only treat if the patient has symptoms or evidence of infection, and replace the catheter. When changing catheters, a single dose of antibiotic (e.g. gentamicin) is recommended.

Infection by *Candida* is a frequent complication of prolonged bladder catheterization. Treatment should be reserved for patients with evidence of invasive infection or those who are immunosuppressed. The catheter should be removed or replaced. In severe infections, continuous bladder irrigation with amphotericin is useful.

UTI in pregnancy

Approximately 6% of pregnant women have significant bacteriuria in pregnancy; if untreated, 20% of these will develop acute pyelonephritis with significant risk to both mother and fetus (e.g. septic shock, low birthweight and prematurity). Early detection of asymptomatic bacteriuria and antibiotic treatment is necessary.

Abacteriuric frequency or dysuria ('urethral syndrome')

This occurs in women and presents with dysuria and frequency but in the absence of bacteriuria. It may be associated with vaginitis in post-menopausal women, irritant chemicals (e.g. soaps) and sexual intercourse.

Bacterial prostatitis

Bacterial prostatitis is a relapsing infection which presents as perineal pain, recurrent epididymo-orchitis and prostatic tenderness, with pus in expressed prostatic secretion. Treatment is for 4–6 weeks with drugs that penetrate into the prostate, such as trimethoprim or ciprofloxacin. Long-term low-dose treatment may be required. Prostadynia (prostatic pain in the absence of active infection) may persist long after the infection. Amitriptyline and carbamazepine may alleviate the symptoms.

Tuberculosis of the urinary tract

Presentation is with symptoms of a UTI, i.e. dysuria, frequency or haematuria, and should be particularly considered in the Asian immigrant population of the UK and in countries with a high prevalence of tuberculosis. Classically, there is sterile pyuria (p. 362). Diagnosis depends on culture of mycobacteria from early-morning urine samples. Treatment is as for pulmonary tuberculosis (p. 543).

TUBULOINTERSTITIAL NEPHRITIS

Tubulointerstitial nephritis is primary injury to the renal tubules and interstitium that results in decreased renal function. It is a feature of bacterial pyelonephritis but in this context it rarely, if ever, leads to renal damage in the absence of reflux, obstruction or other complicating factors.

Acute tubulointerstitial nephritis

Most cases of acute tubulointerstitial nephritis (TIN) are due to an allergic drug reaction, most commonly drugs of the penicillin family and NSAIDs. Infections (e.g. streptococci) are a less common cause. Patients present with fever, eosinophilia and eosinophiluria, normal or only mildly increased urine protein excretion (<1 g/day) and AKI. Renal biopsy shows an intense interstitial cellular infiltrate and variable tubular necrosis. Management involves withdrawal of the offending drug, treatment of any underlying infection and treatment of AKI (p. 386). High-dose prednisolone therapy is often used, although its value has not been proven. The prognosis is generally good; patients should avoid further exposure to the offending drug.

Chronic tubulointerstitial nephritis

There are many causes of chronic TIN, including prolonged consumption of large amounts of analgesics, particularly NSAIDs ('analgesic nephropathy'), diabetes mellitus and toxins, e.g. lead. Presentation is usually with polyuria, proteinuria (usually <1 g/day) or uraemia. Polyuria and nocturia are the result of tubular damage in the medullary area of the kidney, leading to defects in the renal concentrating ability. Necrosis of the papillae, which may subsequently slough off and be passed in the urine, sometimes causes ureteric colic or acute ureteral obstruction. Management is largely supportive. In cases of analgesic nephropathy the drug should be stopped and replaced if necessary with paracetamol or dihydrocodeine.

HYPERTENSION AND THE KIDNEY

Hypertension can be the cause or the result of renal disease (renal hypertension), and it is often difficult to differentiate between the two on clinical grounds. Investigations should be performed on all patients, although renal imaging is usually unnecessary.

Essential hypertension

Hypertension leads to characteristic histological changes in the renal vessels and intrarenal vasculature over time. These include intimal thickening with reduplication of the elastic lamina, reduction in kidney size and an increase in the proportion of sclerotic glomeruli. The changes are usually accompanied by some deterioration in renal function, which is much more common in black Africans.

Accelerated or *malignant-phase hypertension* is marked by the development of fibrinoid necrosis in afferent glomerular arterioles and fibrin deposition in arteriolar walls. A rapid rise in blood pressure may trigger these arteriolar lesions, and a vicious circle is then established whereby fibrin deposition leads to renal damage, increased renin release and a further increase in blood pressure. There is progressive uraemia and, if untreated, fewer than 10% of patients survive 10 years.

Treatment of hypertension is described on page 380. The outlook is good if treatment is started before renal impairment has occurred.

Renal hypertension

Bilateral renal disease

Hypertension commonly complicates bilateral renal disease, such as in chronic glomerulonephritis, reflux nephropathy or analgesic nephropathy. Two main mechanisms are responsible:

- Activation of the renin–angiotensin–aldosterone system
- Retention of salt and water, leading to an increase in blood volume and hence blood pressure.

Good control of blood pressure will prevent further deterioration in renal function, with ACE inhibitors or angiotensin II blockers being the drugs of choice. These drugs confer an additional renoprotective effect for a given degree of blood pressure control when compared with other hypotensive drugs.

Renovascular disease

Narrowing of the renal arteries (renal artery stenosis, RAS) is usually due to atheroma and classically occurs in patients with evidence of generalized atheroma, e.g. peripheral vascular disease and coronary artery disease. In younger patients, particularly women, it is more commonly due to fibromuscular hyperplasia. Renal perfusion pressure is reduced and renal ischaemia results in a reduction in the pressure in afferent glomerular arterioles. The mechanism of hypertension with RAS is illustrated in Fig. 9.5.

Imaging for RAS is indicated in the following circumstances:

- Evidence of atheromatous vascular disease in patients with hypertension or progressive CKD
- A rise in the serum creatinine by more than 30% after introduction of an ACE inhibitor or angiotensin II receptor antagonist (an increase of 30% is acceptable and reflects reduction of glomerular perfusion)
- Abdominal bruits in a patient with hypertension or CKD
- Recurrent flash pulmonary oedema without cardiopulmonary disease
- Renal asymmetry of >1.5 cm in length on imaging.

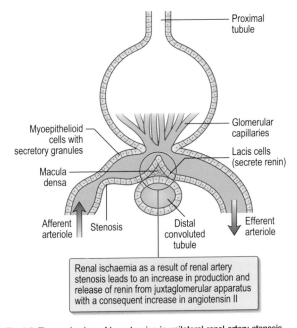

Fig. 9.5 The mechanism of hypertension in unilateral renal artery stenosis.
(Adapted from Davidson 1991 Principles and Practice of Medicine. Churchill Livingstone, Edinburgh.)

Options for renal artery imaging

The gold standard for diagnosing renal artery stenosis is renal arteriography. This requires cannulation of the femoral artery and less invasive imaging with MR or CT angiography or Doppler ultrasonography is often used in the first instance. The choice of test is based on institutional expertise and patient factors, e.g. CT with intravenous contrast is avoided in patients with poor renal function. If non-invasive imaging is inconclusive and clinical suspicion is high, conventional arteriography is necessary.

Management

Standard medical therapy for atherosclerotic vascular disease is indicated in all patients and includes lifestyle modification (increased exercise and smoking cessation), statins, antiplatelet therapy (p. 451) and antihypertensives for effective blood pressure control. Transluminal angioplasty (to dilate the stenotic region) and stent placement is used in patients with fibromuscular hyperplasia but does not offer any additional benefit (to medical treatment) in most patients with atheromatous stenosis.

RENAL CALCULI AND NEPHROCALCINOSIS

Renal (nephrolithiasis) and ureteral stones (urolithiasis) are very common world-wide, with a lifetime risk of about 10%, and in many patients it is a recurrent problem. The male:female ratio is 2:1. Prevalence of stone disease is much higher in the Middle East due to a higher oxalate- and lower calcium-containing diet (see below) and increased risk of dehydration in hot climates.

Aetiology

Most stones are composed of calcium oxalate and/or calcium phosphate: other types are uric acid, magnesium ammonium phosphate (struvite) and cystine stones. Stone formation occurs when normally soluble material, e.g. calcium, supersaturates the urine and begins the process of crystal formation. In normal urine, inhibitors of crystal formation also prevent stone formation.

Calcium stones

Hypercalciuria Increased urinary calcium excretion is the most common metabolic abnormality in calcium stone-formers. Causes of hypercalciuria are:

- Hypercalcaemia, of which the most common cause (p. 653), leading to stone formation, is primary hyperparathyroidism
- Excessive dietary intake of calcium
- Excessive resorption of calcium from bone, e.g. with prolonged immobilization
- Idiopathic hypercalciuria, in which there is increased absorption of calcium from the gut and in turn increased urinary excretion. Serum calcium levels are normal.

Primary renal disease, such as medullary sponge kidney and polycystic renal disease, is also associated with calcium stones. The alkaline urine seen in the renal tubular acidoses favours the precipitation of calcium phosphate.

Hyperoxaluria Increased oxalate excretion favours the formation of calcium oxalate, even if calcium excretion is normal. The main causes are:

- *Dietary hyperoxaluria:* a high dietary intake of oxalate-rich foods (e.g. spinach, rhubarb and tea) results in hyperoxaluria. Low dietary calcium intake can also result in hyperoxaluria via decreased intestinal binding of oxalate (by calcium) and the resulting increased oxalate absorption and urinary excretion.

- *Enteric hyperoxaluria:* chronic intestinal malabsorption of any cause leads to reduced levels of intestinal calcium for oxalate binding (see above). Dehydration secondary to fluid loss from the gut also plays a part in stone formation.

- *Primary hyperoxaluria:* this is a rare autosomal recessive enzyme deficiency resulting in high levels of endogenous oxalate production. There is widespread calcium oxalate crystal deposition in the kidneys, and later in other tissues (myocardium, tissues and bone). CKD develops in the late teens or early 20s.

Uric acid stones

These stones are associated with hyperuricaemia (p. 297) with or without clinical gout. Patients with ileostomies are also at risk of developing urate stones, as loss of bicarbonate from gastrointestinal secretions results in the production of an acid urine and reduced solubility of uric acid.

Infection-induced stones

UTI with organisms that produce urease (*Proteus, Klebsiella* and *Pseudomonas* spp.) is associated with stones containing ammonium, magnesium and calcium. Urease hydrolyses urea to ammonia and this raises the urine pH. An alkaline urine and high ammonia concentration favour stone formation. These stones are often large and fill the pelvicalyceal system, producing the typical radiopaque staghorn calculus.

Cystine stones

These stones occur with cystinuria, an autosomal recessive condition affecting cystine and dibasic amino acid transport (lysine, ornithine and arginine) in the epithelial cells of renal tubules and the gastrointestinal tract. Excessive urinary excretion of cystine, the least soluble of the amino acids, leads to the formation of crystals and calculi.

Clinical features

Most people with urinary tract calculi are asymptomatic; pain is the most common symptom (Table 9.6). Large staghorn renal calculi cause loin pain. *Ureteric*

Table 9.6 Clinical features of urinary tract calculi
Asymptomatic
Pain
Haematuria
Urinary tract infection Urinary tract obstruction

stones cause renal colic, a severe intermittent pain lasting for hours. The pain is felt anywhere between the loin and the groin and may radiate into the scrotum or labium or into the tip of the penis. Nausea, vomiting and sweating are common. Haematuria often occurs. There will be features of acute pyelonephritis or Gram-negative septicaemia if there is associated infection in an obstructed urinary system. *Bladder stones* present with urinary frequency and haematuria. *Urethral stones* may cause bladder outflow obstruction, resulting in anuria and painful bladder distension.

Differential diagnosis

Bleeding within the kidney, e.g. after renal biopsy, can produce clots that lodge temporarily in the ureter and produce ureteric colic. Pain may also occur from sloughed necrotic renal papillae. Pain from an ectopic pregnancy or leaking aortic aneurysm may be mistaken for renal colic.

Investigations

Investigations include a mid-stream specimen of urine for culture and measurement of serum urea, electrolytes, creatinine and calcium levels. A plain abdominal X-ray (KUB: kidney, ureters and bladder) may show a radiopaque stone in the line of the renal tract. Unenhanced helical (spiral) CT is the best diagnostic test available; a normal CT scan during an episode of pain excludes calculus disease as the cause of the pain. A detailed history may reveal possible aetiological factors for stone formation, e.g. vitamin D consumption (leading to hypercalcaemia), gouty arthritis, recurrent UTIs, intestinal resection. A further work-up to look for underlying metabolic risk factors is indicated in all patients other than the elderly with a single episode (Table 9.7).

Management

Initial treatment A strong analgesic, e.g. diclofenac 75 mg by intravenous infusion, is given to relieve the pain of renal colic. Patients are managed at home if there is no evidence of sepsis and they are able to take oral medications and fluids. Most small ureteric stones ($\leq$5 mm) will pass spontaneously. Indications for intervention include persistent pain, infection above the site of

Table 9.7 Investigations to identify the cause of stone formation

Urine
Chemical analysis of any stone passed
MSU for culture and sensitivity
24-hour urine collection for calcium, oxalate, uric acid Screen for cystinuria (purple colour of urine after addition of sodium nitroprusside)
Blood
Serum urea and electrolytes
Serum calcium
Serum urate Plasma bicarbonate (low in renal tubular acidosis)
Radiography
CT scan will normally have been performed at diagnosis
Imaging is also to look for a primary renal disease

CT, computed tomography; MSU, mid-stream urine specimen.

obstruction, and failure of the stone to pass down the ureter. The options for stone removal include the following:

- Extracorporeal shock wave lithotripsy (ESWL) will fragment most stones, which then pass spontaneously.
- Endoscopy (ureteroscopy) with a YAG laser is used for larger stones.
- Open surgery is rarely needed.

Prevention of recurrence Further treatment depends on the type of stone and any underlying condition identified during screening investigations (Table 9.7). For prevention of all stones, whatever the cause, a high intake of fluid (to produce a urine volume of 2–2.5 L/day) must be maintained, particularly during the summer months. This is the mainstay of treatment when no metabolic or renal abnormality has been identified ('idiopathic stone formers').

- *Idiopathic hypercalciuria.* Patients should be encouraged to consume a normal calcium diet and avoid foods containing large amounts of oxalate. A water softener may be helpful for patients who live in hard water areas. Thiazide diuretics, e.g. bendroflumethiazide 2.5 mg daily, reduce urinary calcium excretion and are used if hypercalciuria persists.
- *Mixed infective stones.* Meticulous control of bacteriuria, if necessary with long-term, low-dose, prophylactic antibiotics and a high fluid intake, helps to prevent recurrent stone formation.
- *Uric acid stones* are prevented by the long-term use of the xanthine oxidase inhibitor allopurinol, which allows the excretion of the more soluble

precursor compound hypoxanthine, in preference to uric acid. Oral sodium bicarbonate supplements to maintain an alkaline urine, and hence increased solubility of uric acid, are an alternative approach in those patients unable to tolerate allopurinol.

- *Cystine stones.* A very high fluid intake (5 L of water in 24 hours) is needed to maintain solubility of cystine in the urine. An alternative is D-penicillamine, which chelates cystine, forming a more soluble complex.

Nephrocalcinosis

Nephrocalcinosis is diffuse renal parenchymal calcification that is detectable radiologically. The causes are listed in Table 9.8. It is typically painless and hypertension and renal impairment commonly occur. Treatment is of the underlying cause.

URINARY TRACT OBSTRUCTION

The urinary tract may be obstructed at any point between the kidney and the urethral meatus, resulting in dilatation of the tract proximal to the obstruction. Dilatation of the renal pelvis is known as *hydronephrosis*. Eventually there is compression and thinning of the renal parenchyma, with a decrease in size of the kidney.

Aetiology

In adults the common causes are prostatic obstruction (hypertrophy or tumour), gynaecological cancer and calculi (Table 9.9).

Clinical features

- *Upper urinary tract obstruction* results in a dull ache in the flank or loin, which may be provoked by an increase in urine volume, e.g. high fluid intake or diuretics. Complete anuria is strongly suggestive of complete bilateral

Table 9.8 Common causes of nephrocalcinosis

Mainly medullary	Mainly cortical (rare)
Hypercalcaemia	Renal cortical necrosis
Renal tubular acidosis	
Primary hyperoxaluria	
Medullary sponge kidney	
Tuberculosis	

Table 9.9 Causes of urinary tract obstruction
Within the lumen
Calculus
Tumour of renal pelvis or ureter
Blood clot
Sloughed renal papillae (diabetes, NSAIDs, sickle cell disease or trait)
Within the wall
Congenital anomalies of the urinary tract (usually detected antenatally or in infancy)
Stricture: ureteric or urethral
Neuropathic bladder
Pressure from outside the wall
Prostatic hypertrophy/tumour
Pelvic tumours
Diverticulitis
Aortic aneurysm
Retroperitoneal fibrosis (periaortitis)
Accidental surgical ligation of the ureter
Retrocaval ureter (right-sided obstruction)
Pelviureteric compression (bands; aberrant vessels)
Phimosis

obstruction or complete obstruction of a single functioning kidney. Partial obstruction causes polyuria as a result of tubular damage and impairment of concentrating mechanisms.

- *Bladder outlet obstruction* results in hesitancy, poor stream, terminal dribbling and a sense of incomplete emptying. Retention with overflow is characterized by the frequent passage of small quantities of urine. Infection commonly occurs and may precipitate acute retention of urine.

Depending on the site of obstruction an enlarged bladder or hydronephrotic kidney may be felt on examination. Pelvic (for malignancy) and rectal examination (for prostate enlargement) is essential in determining the cause of obstruction.

Investigations

Imaging studies are performed to identify the site and nature of the obstruction and, together with serum creatinine, to assess function of the affected kidney.

- *Imaging:* ultrasonography is the initial investigation but helical/spiral CT scanning has a higher sensitivity for detecting calculi as well as details of the obstruction. Excretion urography identifies the site of obstruction and shows a characteristic appearance (a delayed nephrogram, which eventually becomes denser than the non-obstructed side).
- Radionuclide studies (p. 11) are unhelpful in acute obstruction but may help in longstanding obstruction, to differentiate true obstructive uropathy from retention of tracer in a low-pressure unobstructed pelvicalyceal system.
- Subsequent investigations may include retrograde and antegrade pyelography (p. 364), cystoscopy and pressure-flow studies during bladder filling and voiding.

Management

Surgery is the usual treatment for persistent urinary tract obstruction. Elimination of the obstruction may be associated with a massive post-operative diuresis, resulting partly from a solute diuresis from salt and urea retained during obstruction and partly from the renal concentrating defect. In some cases, definitive relief of obstruction is not possible and urinary diversion may be required. This may be simply an indwelling urethral catheter, a stent placed across the obstructing lesion or the formation of an ileal conduit.

ACUTE KIDNEY INJURY

Acute kidney injury (AKI), defined as an abrupt deterioration in renal function, usually over hours or days, which is usually (but not always) reversible over days or weeks, may cause sudden, life-threatening biochemical disturbances as a medical emergency. Oliguria is often a feature. The distinction between AKI and CKD or even acute-on-chronic kidney disease is not always obvious. AKI is usually recognized with a falling urine output, rising serum urea and creatinine, or both. It is important to consider situations when urea and creatinine are less accurate predictors of deteriorating renal function.

AKI may result from:

1. *Prerenal* causes (reduced kidney perfusion leads to a falling GFR)
2. *Renal* parenchymal disorders (injury to glomerulus, tubule or vessels)
3. Urinary tract obstruction (*postrenal*, functioning kidneys cannot excrete urine with back pressure affecting function)

The RIFLE criteria (*R*isk, *I*njury, *F*ailure, *L*oss, *E*nd-stage renal disease) (Table 9.10) help define AKI, by describing three levels of renal dysfunction (R, I, F) and two outcome measures (L, E) associated with a rise in serum creatinine or a decrease in urine output. These criteria indicate an increasing degree of renal damage and have a predictive value for mortality.

Table 9.10 RIFLE classification for acute kidney injury

Grade	Serum creatinine	Urine output criteria
Risk	↑ SCr to ≥1.5 × from baseline	<0.5 mL/kg/hour ≥6 hours
Injury	↑ SCr ≥2 × from baseline	<0.5 mL/kg/hour ≥12 hours
Failure	↑ SCr ≥3 × from baseline *or* SCr ≥350 μmol/L with an acute increase ≥40 μmol/L	<0.3 mL/kg/hour ≥24 hours
Loss	Persistent AKI > 4 weeks	
ESKD	Persistent renal failure >3 months	

SCr, serum creatinine; ESKD, end-stage kidney disease.
- *Baseline SCr is considered to be within 1 week.*
- *When baseline SCr is not known and in the absence of a history of chronic kidney disease, calculate a baseline SCr using the Modification of Diet in Renal Disease equation for assessment of kidney function, assuming a glomerular filtration rate of 75 mL/min/1.73 m².*
- *Only one criterion (SCr or urine output) has to be fulfilled to qualify for a stage.*
- *AKI should be both abrupt (within 1–7 days) and sustained (more than 24 hours).*

The Acute Kidney Injury Network (AKIN) has proposed a modification of the RIFLE criteria to include less severe AKI, a time constraint of 48 hours, and gives a correction for volume status before classification. 'R' in RIFLE is *stage 1* (a serum creatinine rise of ≥26.4 μmol/L, i.e. a 1.5-fold increase within 48 hours); *stage 2* is 'I', i.e. a two- to three-fold increase in serum creatinine; and 'F' is *stage 3*, i.e. an increase in serum creatinine of >300% (equal to ≥354 μmol/L). Urine output data are the same.

Epidemiology

Incidence varies widely, depending on the population studied and the definition of AKI used, e.g.:
- Community-acquired AKI on admission to hospital: approximately 5% in the UK (superimposed on CKD in half of these)
- Severe AKI (creatinine >500 μmol/L, often dialysis requiring): about 130–140 per million population per year
- Approximately 50% of patients with septic shock will have AKI.

Outcomes vary: uncomplicated AKI carries a good prognosis, with mortality rates <5–10%. In contrast, AKI complicating non-renal organ system failure (in the ITU setting) is associated with mortality rates of 50–70%, which have not changed for several decades. Sepsis-related AKI has a significantly worse prognosis than AKI in the absence of sepsis.

Approaching AKI

1. Prerenal AKI Falling renal blood flow leads to a falling GFR. This might either be due to changes in the circulation or intrarenal vasomotor changes that drop glomerular perfusion pressures. Common causes with a falling effective circulating volume include:

- Hypovolaemia of any cause, including dehydration or haemorrhage
- Hypotension without hypovolaemia, including cirrhosis or septic shock
- Low cardiac output, including cardiac failure or cardiogenic shock
- Combinations of the above.

Common intrarenal causes include:

- NSAIDs, ACE inhibitors, amphotericin B and calcineurin inhibitors, often in the context of added changes in renal blood flow

Autoregulation maintains glomerular filtration close to normal despite wide variations in renal perfusion pressure and volume status. Once autoregulation fails, GFR drops and AKI develops. Over time, reduced blood flow may lead to established parenchymal injury – but if renal perfusion is corrected early, AKI will resolve fully.

A few simple biochemical measures can help differentiate prerenal AKI from intrinsic renal disease (Table 9.11). Urine sodium will be low due to salt retention. The fractional excretion of sodium (FE_{Na}) is a more reliable measure of sodium retention.

Managing prerenal AKI largely depends on the underlying cause. Most cases of AKI have an element of hypovolaemia, so prompt fluid resuscitation is most

Table 9.11 Criteria for distinction between prerenal and intrinsic causes of renal failure

	Prerenal	Intrinsic
Urine specific gravity	>1.020	<1.010
Urine osmolality (mOsm/kg)	>500	<350
Urine sodium (mmol/L)	<20	>40
Fractional excretion of sodium (Na^+)	<1%	>1%

Fractional excretion of Na^+ = $\dfrac{urine\ [sodium] \div urine\ [creatinine]}{plasma\ [sodium]\ \ \ plasma\ [creatinine]} \times 100$

where [ ] is the concentration.

often indicated. Where uncertain as to the volume state of a patient, a fluid challenge of 250 mL crystalloid will often prove whether hypotension is fluid-responsive. Heart rate, blood pressure and urine output will all guide response to resuscitation. See also cardiogenic shock (p. 577) and septic shock (p. 581).

2. Postrenal AKI Here, uraemia results from obstruction of the urinary tract at any point from the calyces to the external urethral orifice – but, commonly, as bladder outflow obstruction (prostate disease in men) or bilateral ureteric obstruction (stones or tumours). Almost every case of unexplained AKI should result in an ultrasound to exclude obstruction, as once relieved (and if acute), renal function will return to baseline.

3. Renal parenchymal AKI This is most commonly (80–90%) due to *acute tubular necrosis* (ATN; see below and also Table 9.12). Almost any cause of prerenal AKI, if prolonged to the point at which renal autoregulation fails (see above), will lead to ischaemic ATN. If not ischaemic, then ATN usually results from direct tubular toxins. As a result, ATN is common in hospital practice. Other causes of parenchymal AKI include:

- Diseases affecting the intrarenal arteries and arterioles as well as glomerular capillaries, such as a vasculitis, accelerated hypertension, cholesterol

Table 9.12 Some causes of acute tubular necrosis

Haemorrhage
Burns
Diarrhoea and vomiting, fluid loss from fistulae
Acute pancreatitis
Diuretics
Myocardial infarction
Congestive cardiac failure
Endotoxic shock
Snake bite
Myoglobinaemia
Haemoglobinaemia (due to haemolysis, e.g. in falciparum malaria, 'blackwater fever')
Hepatorenal syndrome
Radiological contrast agents
Drugs, e.g. aminoglycosides, NSAIDs, ACE inhibitors, platinum derivatives
Abruptio placentae
Pre-eclampsia and eclampsia
ACE, angiotensin-converting enzyme; NSAIDs, non-steroidal anti-inflammatory drugs.

embolism, haemolytic uraemic syndrome, thrombotic thrombocytopenic purpura (TTP), pre-eclampsia and crescentic glomerulonephritis.

- Acute tubulointerstitial nephritis may also cause AKI. This also occurs when renal tubules are acutely obstructed by crystals: e.g. after rapid lysis of certain malignant tumours following chemotherapy (acute hyperuricaemic nephropathy).
- Acute bilateral suppurative pyelonephritis or pyelonephritis of a single kidney can cause acute uraemia.

Clinical and biochemical features

The early stages of AKI are often completely asymptomatic. It is not the accumulation of urea itself that causes symptoms, but a combination of many different metabolic abnormalities.

- *Alteration of urine volume*. Oliguria usually occurs in the early stages. Recovery of renal function typically occurs after 7–21 days and in the recovery phase, which may last some weeks, there is often passage of large amounts of dilute urine.
- *Biochemical abnormalities* include hyperkalaemia, metabolic acidosis (unless there is loss of hydrogen ions by vomiting or aspiration of gastric contents), hyponatraemia (due to water overload from continued drinking after the onset of oliguria or administration of 5% glucose), hypocalcaemia due to reduced renal production of 1,25-dihydroxycholecalciferol and hyperphosphataemia due to phosphate retention.
- *Symptoms* of uraemia are weakness, fatigue, anorexia, nausea and vomiting, followed by mental confusion, seizures and coma. There may be pruritus and bruising. Breathlessness occurs from a combination of anaemia and pulmonary oedema secondary to volume overload. Pericarditis occurs with severe untreated uraemia and may be complicated by a pericardial effusion and tamponade. Impaired platelet function causes bruising and exacerbates gastrointestinal bleeding. Infection occurs due to immune suppression.

Investigation of the uraemic emergency

The purpose of investigation, together with clinical examination, is three-fold:

1. To differentiate acute from chronic uraemia.
2. To document the degree of renal impairment and obtain baseline values so that the response to treatment can be monitored. This is accomplished by measurement of serum urea and creatinine.
3. To establish whether AKI is prerenal, renal or postrenal, and to determine the underlying cause so that specific treatment (e.g. intensive immunosuppression in Wegener's granulomatosis) may be instituted as early as possible and thus prevent progression to irreversible renal failure.

Investigations

- Blood count: anaemia and a very high erythrocyte sedimentation rate (ESR) may suggest myeloma or a vasculitis as the underlying cause.
- Urine and blood cultures to exclude infection.
- Urine dipstick testing and microscopy: glomerulonephritis is suggested by haematuria and proteinuria on dipstick testing and by the presence of red cell casts on urine microscopy (p. 361).
- Urinary electrolytes (see Table 9.11) may help to exclude a significant prerenal element to AKI.
- Serum calcium, phosphate and uric acid.
- Renal ultrasound excludes obstruction and gives an assessment of renal size; CT is useful for the diagnosis of retroperitoneal fibrosis and some other causes of urinary obstruction, and may also indicate cortical scarring.
- Histological investigations: renal biopsy should be performed in every patient with unexplained AKI and normal-sized kidneys.
- Optional investigations (depending on the case):
  - Serum protein electrophoresis for myeloma
  - Serum autoantibodies, ANCAs and complement
  - Antibodies to hepatitis B and C and HIV may suggest polyarteritis (hepatitis B virus), cryoglobulinaemia (hepatitis C virus) or HIV as the cause of AKI.

Management

The best form of management of AKI is prevention, e.g. by optimizing fluid balance in hospitalized patients (p. 330) and volume expansion (0.9% sodium chloride at 1 mL/kg/hour for 12 hours before the procedure and several hours afterwards) in patients with impaired kidney function (eGFR below 60 mL/min/ 1.73 m^2) undergoing radiological contrast studies. The principles of management of established AKI are summarized in Emergency Box 9.1. Hypovolaemia (prerenal) and obstruction (postrenal) must be excluded as contributing factors in all patients. Early specialist review is advisable – often unwell, patients with AKI should be monitored in a high-dependency setting. Good nursing, infection control and physiotherapy are vital. Fluid balance, as intake and output (particularly urine output), will be key to recovery. Daily weights, lying and standing blood pressure, medication review to withhold nephrotoxins, collateral history and past results will all form part of the management plan. Dialysis and haemofiltration are sometimes necessary; they do not hasten recovery from AKI but are performed as a bridge while patients are receiving treatment for the underlying cause or there is a natural improvement in kidney function. Indications for dialysis are listed in Table 9.13. Whether haemodialysis, haemofiltration or peritoneal dialysis (p. 399) is used depends on the facilities available and the clinical circumstances.

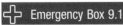

Emergency Box 9.1

Principles of management of a patient with acute kidney injury

Emergency resuscitation

To prevent death from hyperkalaemia (p. 342) or pulmonary oedema. Establish the aetiology and treat the underlying cause

- History, including family history, systemic disease, use of nephrotoxic drugs
- Examination includes assessment of haemodynamic status, pelvic and rectal examination
- Investigations (p. 391), which may include bladder catheterization or flush of existing catheter to exclude obstruction

Prevention of further renal damage

Early detection of infection and prompt treatment with antibiotics. Avoid hypovolaemia, nephrotoxic drugs, NSAIDs and ACE inhibitors.

Management of established renal failure

- Seek advice from a nephrologist
- Once fluid balance has been corrected, the daily fluid intake should equal fluid lost on the previous day plus insensible losses (approximately 500 mL)
- Diet – enteral nutrition is preferred over parenteral; sodium and potassium is restricted
- Nursing care, e.g. prevention of pressure sores
- Adjust doses of drugs that are excreted by the kidney, and monitor serum drug levels where appropriate (refer to a national formulary for guidance)
- Monitor daily: serum biochemistry, fluid input and output and body weight to assess fluid balance changes
- Frequent review regarding the need for dialysis

Careful fluid and electrolyte balance during recovery phase

Large volumes of dilute urine may be passed until the kidney recovers its concentrating ability.

ACE, angiotensin-converting enzyme; NSAIDs, non-steroidal anti-inflammatory drugs.

Prognosis

Prognosis depends on the underlying cause. The most common cause of death is sepsis as a result of impaired immune defence (from uraemia and malnutrition) and instrumentation (dialysis and urinary catheters and vascular lines). In patients who survive, renal function usually begins to recover within 1–3 weeks. AKI is irreversible in a few patients, probably because of cortical

Table 9.13 Indications for dialysis and/or haemofiltration in AKI

Progressive uraemia with encephalopathy or pericarditis

Severe biochemical derangement, especially if there is a rising trend in an oliguric patient and in hypercatabolic patients

Hyperkalaemia not controlled by conservative measures

Pulmonary oedema

Severe metabolic acidosis: pH < 7.1

For removal of drugs causing the AKI, e.g. gentamicin, lithium, severe aspirin overdose

AKI, acute kidney injury.

necrosis, which, unlike tubules which regenerate, heals with the formation of scar tissue.

CHRONIC KIDNEY DISEASE

CKD implies long-standing, and usually progressive, impairment in renal function. It is defined on the basis of persistent (>3 months) evidence of kidney damage (proteinuria, haematuria, or anatomical abnormality) and/or impaired GFR (Table 9.14). Patients at risk of CKD, e.g. with diabetes mellitus or hypertension, should be regularly screened to look for evidence of disease.

Aetiology

Causes of CKD vary depending on geographical area, racial group and age. Diabetes mellitus, hypertension and atherosclerotic renal vascular disease are the most common causes in European countries (Table 9.15). In parts of the Middle

Table 9.14 Classification of chronic kidney disease

Test	Measurement method	Definition
Impaired GFR	Formulae based on SCr	eGFR < 60 mL/min/1.73 m^2
Proteinuria	Early morning urine sample	ACR ≥ 30 mg/mmol or PCR ≥ 50 mg/mmol
Haematuria	Dipstick urinalysis	$>1+$ and urological causes excluded

ACR, albumin:creatinine ratio; (e)GFR, (estimated) glomerular filtration rate; PCR, protein:creatinine ratio; SCr, serum creatinine.

Table 9.15 Causes of chronic kidney disease

Congenital and inherited disease
Polycystic kidney disease (adult and infantile forms)
Tuberous sclerosis
Congenital obstructive uropathy
Other rare causes
Glomerular disease
Primary glomerulonephritides
Secondary glomerular disease, e.g. diabetes mellitus, amyloidosis, SLE
Vascular disease
Hypertensive nephrosclerosis (common in black Africans)
Reno-vascular disease
Small and medium-sized vessel vasculitis
Tubulointerstitial disease
See page 377
Urinary tract obstruction
Any causes of chronic obstruction (p. 374)
SLE, systemic lupus erythematosus.

East, schistosomiasis is a common cause due to a ureterovesical stricture causing urinary tract obstruction. Regardless of the underlying cause, fibrosis of the remaining tubules, glomeruli and small blood vessels results in progressive renal scarring and loss of renal function in some individuals.

Clinical features and investigations

The early stages of renal failure are often completely asymptomatic. With a declining GRF and an associated rise in serum urea and creatinine concentrations, there is an accumulation of symptoms and signs described below. The actual metabolites that are involved in the genesis of many of these clinical features is not known (Fig. 9.6). Investigations are similar to those in AKI (p. 386).

Anaemia Anaemia is primarily due to reduced erythropoietin production by the diseased kidney. Shortened red cell survival, increased blood loss (from the gut, during haemodialysis and as a result of repeated sampling) and dietary deficiency of haematinics (iron and folate) also contribute.

Bone disease The term 'renal osteodystrophy' embraces the various forms of bone disease that develop in CKD, i.e. osteomalacia, osteoporosis, secondary and tertiary hyperparathyroidism and osteosclerosis. Renal phosphate retention

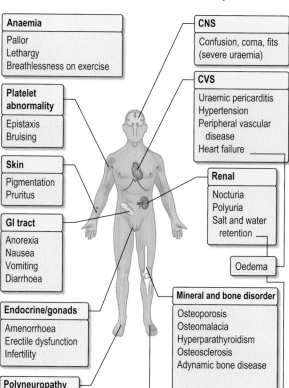

Anaemia

Pallor
Lethargy
Breathlessness on exercise

Platelet abnormality

Epistaxis
Bruising

Skin

Pigmentation
Pruritus

GI tract

Anorexia
Nausea
Vomiting
Diarrhoea

Endocrine/gonads

Amenorrhoea
Erectile dysfunction
Infertility

Polyneuropathy

CNS

Confusion, coma, fits
(severe uraemia)

CVS

Uraemic pericarditis
Hypertension
Peripheral vascular
  disease
Heart failure

Renal

Nocturia
Polyuria
Salt and water
  retention

Oedema

Mineral and bone disorder

Osteoporosis
Osteomalacia
Hyperparathyroidism
Osteosclerosis
Adynamic bone disease

Fig. 9.6 Symptoms and signs of chronic kidney disease. Oedema may be due to a combination of primary renal salt and water retention and heart failure. CNS, central nervous system; CVS, cardiovascular system; GI, gastrointestinal.

and impaired production of 1,25-dihydroxyvitamin D (the active hormonal form of vitamin D) lead to a fall in serum calcium concentration and hence to a compensatory increase in parathyroid hormone (PTH) secretion. A sustained excess of PTH results in skeletal decalcification with the classic radiological features described in Fig. 9.7. Osteosclerosis (hardening of bone) may be a result of hyperparathyroidism.

Neurological complications Neurological complications occur in almost all patients with severe CKD and are improved by dialysis. Polyneuropathy manifests as peripheral paraesthesiae and weakness. Autonomic dysfunction presents as postural hypotension and disturbed gastrointestinal motility. In advanced uraemia (serum urea >50–60 mmol/L) there is depressed cerebral

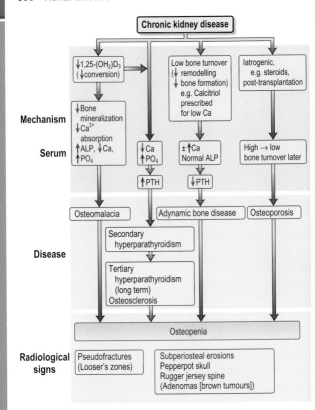

Fig. 9.7 Renal osteodystrophy. Pathogenesis and radiological features of renal bone disease. ALP, alkaline phosphatase; PTH, parathyroid hormone.

function, myoclonic twitching and fits. Median nerve compression in the carpal tunnel is common and is usually caused by β_2-microglobulin-related amyloidosis (a complication of dialysis).

Cardiovascular disease The highest mortality in CKD is from cardiovascular disease, particularly myocardial infarction, cardiac failure, sudden cardiac death and stroke. This occurs due to an increased frequency of hypertension, dyslipidaemia and vascular calcification. Renal disease also results in a form of cardiomyopathy with both systolic and diastolic dysfunction. Pericarditis and pericardial effusion occurs in severe uraemia.

Other complications These include an increased risk of peptic ulceration, acute pancreatitis, hyperuricaemia, erectile dysfunction and an increased incidence of malignancy.

Differentiating AKI from CKD

Distinction between AKI and CKD depends on the history, duration of symptoms and previous urinalysis or measurement of serum creatinine. A normochromic anaemia, small kidneys on ultrasonography and the presence of renal osteo-dystrophy favour a chronic process.

Management

The aims of treatment are:

- Specific therapy directed at the underlying cause of renal disease, e.g. immunosuppressive agents for vasculitis and tight metabolic control in diabetes
- Slow deterioration of kidney function (renoprotection)
- Reduce cardiovascular risk
- Treat the complications, e.g. anaemia
- Appropriate dose adjustment of prescribed drugs based on guidance in a national formulary.

Renoprotection

The goal of treatment should be to maintain the blood pressure at less than 120/80 mmHg and to maintain a urinary protein concentration of less than 0.3 g/24 hours. Good blood pressure control may slow the decline in renal function.

Patients with CKD and proteinuria >1 g/24 hours should receive:

- ACE inhibitor, increasing to maximum dose
- Angiotensin receptor antagonist if goals are not achieved
- Diuretic to prevent hyperkalaemia and help to control blood pressure
- Calcium channel blocker (verapamil or diltiazem) if goals not achieved.

Reduce cardiovascular risk

- Optimal control of blood pressure and reduction of proteinuria (as above)
- Statins to lower cholesterol to <4.5 mmol/L
- Cessation of smoking
- Optimize diabetic control, HbA_{1c} 53 mmol/mol (<7%)
- Normal protein diet (0.8–1 g/kg body weight/day).

Correction of complications

Hyperkalaemia Hyperkalaemia often responds to dietary restriction of potassium intake. Drugs which cause potassium retention should be stopped. Occasionally it is necessary to prescribe ion-exchange resins to remove potassium in the gastrointestinal tract. Emergency treatment of severe hyperkalaemia is described on page 342.

Calcium and phosphate Hyperphosphataemia is treated by dietary phosphate restriction and administration of oral phosphate-binding agents such as calcium carbonate (contraindicated with hypercalcaemia or hypercalciuria), sevelamer or lanthanum carbonate. The serum calcium should be maintained in the normal range through the use of synthetic vitamin D analogues such as 1_{α}-cholecalciferol or the vitamin D metabolite 1,25-dihydroxyvitamin D_3 (1,25-$(OH)_2D_3$).

Anaemia Iron deficiency is common in patients with CKD and should be treated. Recombinant human erythropoietin is an effective but expensive treatment for the anaemia of CKD. It is administered subcutaneously or intra-venously three times weekly. Target haemoglobin (Hb) is 11–12 g/dL and fail-ure to respond may be the result of haematinic deficiency, bleeding, malignancy or infection. The disadvantages of treatment are that erythropoietin may accelerate hypertension and, rarely, lead to encephalopathy with convulsions.

Acidosis Systemic acidosis accompanies the decline in renal function and may contribute to increased serum potassium levels as well as dyspnoea and lethargy. Treatment is with oral sodium bicarbonate (4.8 g or 57 mmol daily).

Infections Patients with CKD have an increased risk of infections which may be fatal. Influenza and pneumococcal vaccination should be administered.

Referral to a nephrologist

Most patients with CKD are managed in primary care and do not require referral to a nephrologist at the outset. Indications for specialist referral are based on the need for further investigation, complex treatment or because there is a high likelihood of progression to dialysis (Table 9.16).

Table 9.16 Indications for referral of a patient with CKD to a nephrologist

Patient group	Assessment
Severe CKD	GFR < 30 mL/min/1.73 m^2
Rapidly deteriorating kidney function	Fall in eGFR > 5 mL/min in 1 year or >10 mL/min/year in 5 years
Higher levels of proteinuria	ACR ≥ 70 mg/mmol or PCR ≥ 100 mg/mmol
Proteinuria and haematuria	Proteinuria with ≥ +1 blood on urine dipstick
Poorly controlled hypertension	Despite use of four antihypertensive drugs
Suspected rare or genetic cause of CKD	

ACR, albumin:creatinine ratio; CKD, chronic kidney disease; (e)GFR, (estimated) glomerular filtration rate; PCR, protein:creatinine ratio.

RENAL REPLACEMENT THERAPY

Dialysis

'Uraemic toxins' are efficiently removed from the blood by the process of diffusion across a semipermeable membrane towards the low concentrations present in dialysis fluid (Fig. 9.8). The gradient is maintained by replacing used dialysis fluid with fresh solution. In haemodialysis, blood in an extracorporeal circulation is exposed to dialysis fluid separated by an artificial semipermeable membrane. In peritoneal dialysis, the peritoneum is used as the semipermeable membrane and dialysis fluid is instilled into the peritoneal cavity.

Haemodialysis

Adequate dialysis requires a blood flow of at least 200 mL/min and is most reliably achieved by surgical construction of an arteriovenous fistula, usually in the forearm. This provides a permanent and easily accessible site for the insertion of needles. An adult of average size usually requires 4–5 hours of haemodialysis three times a week, which may be performed in hospital or at home. All patients are anticoagulated during treatment (usually with heparin) because contact of blood with foreign surfaces activates the clotting cascade. The most common acute complication of haemodialysis is hypotension, caused in part by excessive removal of extracellular fluid.

Peritoneal dialysis

A permanent tube (Tenckhoff catheter) is placed into the peritoneal cavity via a subcutaneous tunnel. The bags of dialysate are connected to the catheter using

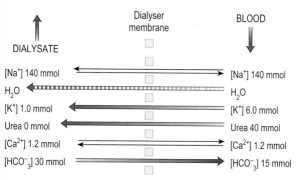

Fig. 9.8 The principle of haemodialysis.

a sterile, no-touch technique and the fluid run into the peritoneal cavity. Urea, creatinine, phosphate and other uraemic toxins pass into the dialysate down their concentration gradients and the dialysate is then collected. With continuous ambulatory peritoneal dialysis (CAPD) 1.5–3 L of dialysate are introduced and exchanged three to five times a day. Bacterial peritonitis, often with *S. epidermidis*, is the most common serious complication of peritoneal dialysis. Treatment is with appropriate antibiotics, often given intraperitoneally.

Haemofiltration

Haemofiltration involves the removal of plasma water and its dissolved constituents (e.g. Na^+, K^+, urea, phosphate) and replacing it with a solution of the desired biochemical composition. The procedure employs a highly permeable membrane, which allows large amounts of fluid and solute to be removed from the patient (Fig. 9.9). It is used mostly in the intensive care setting in the management of AKI.

Complications of all long-term dialysis

Cardiovascular disease (as a result of atheroma) and sepsis are the leading causes of death in long-term dialysis patients. Causes of fatal sepsis include peritonitis complicating peritoneal dialysis and *S. aureus* infection (including endocarditis) complicating the use of indwelling access devices for haemodialysis. Amyloidosis is the result of the accumulation and polymerization of β_2-microglobulin. This molecule (a component of human leucocyte antigen [HLA] proteins on most cell membranes) is normally excreted by the kidneys, but is not removed by dialysis membranes. Deposition results in the carpal tunnel syndrome and joint pains, particularly of the shoulders.

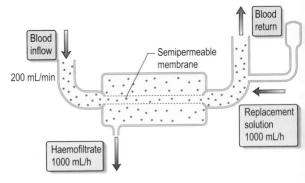

Fig. 9.9 Principles of haemofiltration.

Transplantation

Successful renal transplantation offers the potential for complete rehabilitation in, and is the treatment of choice for most patients with, end-stage renal failure. In the best centres, graft survival is 80% at 10 years. Kidneys are obtained from cadavers or, less frequently, a living donor, e.g. a close relative. The donor must be ABO compatible, and good HLA matching increases the chances of successful transplantation. The donor kidney is placed in the iliac fossa and anastomosed to the iliac vessels of the recipient; the donor ureter is placed into the recipient's bladder.

Long-term immunosuppressive treatment is necessary (unless the donor is an identical twin, i.e. genetically identical) to reduce the incidence of graft rejection. This treatment comprises corticosteroids, azathioprine or mycophenolate mofetil and ciclosporin or tacrolimus. Monoclonal and polyclonal antibodies such as antilymphocyte and anti-thymocyte globulin or basiliximab and daclizumab are potent immunosuppressives and are used in selected patients. The complications of renal transplantation and immunosuppression include opportunistic infection (e.g. with *Pneumocystis jiroveci*), hypertension, development of tumours (skin malignancies and lymphomas) and, occasionally, recurrence of the renal disease (e.g. Goodpasture's syndrome).

CYSTIC RENAL DISEASE

Solitary and multiple renal cysts

Renal cysts are common, particularly with advancing age. They are usually asymptomatic and discovered incidentally on ultrasonography performed for some other reason. Occasionally they may cause pain and/or haematuria.

Autosomal-dominant polycystic kidney disease

Autosomal-dominant polycystic kidney disease (ADPKD) is a common (1:1000) autosomal dominantly inherited condition in which multiple cysts develop throughout both kidneys. Cysts increase in size with advancing age and lead to renal enlargement and the progressive destruction of normal kidney tissue, with gradual loss of renal function. Most cases are due to a mutation in the *PKD1* gene (short arm of chromosome 16), which encodes for a protein, polycystin 1, an integral membrane protein which regulates tubular and vascular development in kidneys and other organs. A second gene, *PKD2*, on chromosome 4 accounts for the remaining cases.

Clinical features

The disease presents at any age after the second decade. Clinical features include:

- Acute loin pain due to cyst haemorrhage or infection, or urinary tract stone formation (uric acid calculi occur more commonly)
- Abdominal discomfort caused by renal enlargement
- Hypertension
- Progressive renal impairment. End-stage renal failure develops in about 50% of patients by 50–60 years of age.
- Liver cysts (usually clinically insignificant). Rarely cysts in the pancreas, spleen, ovary and other organs
- Subarachnoid haemorrhage – intracranial aneurysms are more common in ADPKD patients
- Mitral valve prolapse in 20%.

Diagnosis

Clinical examination commonly reveals large irregular kidneys, hypertension and possibly hepatomegaly. A definitive diagnosis is established by ultrasonography. In adults with a family history, criteria for diagnosis are at least two renal cysts in patients aged <30 years, two cysts in each kidney in patients aged 30–59 years and four cysts in each kidney in patient aged >60 years.

Management

No treatment has definitely been shown to slow disease progression or decrease cyst size. Blood pressure should be carefully controlled and disease progression monitored by serial measurements of serum creatinine. Many patients will eventually require renal replacement by dialysis and/or transplantation. Children and siblings of patients with the disease should be offered screening by renal ultrasonography in their 20s.

Medullary sponge kidney

Medullary sponge kidney is an uncommon condition characterized by dilatation of the collecting ducts in the papillae, sometimes with cystic change. In severe cases the medullary area has a sponge-like appearance. Small calculi form within the cysts and patients present with renal colic or haematuria. In 20% of patients there is hypercalciuria or renal tubular acidosis (p. 349). Renal function is usually well preserved. The diagnosis is made by excretion urography.

TUMOURS OF THE KIDNEY AND GENITOURINARY TRACT

Renal cell carcinoma

Renal cell carcinomas are the most common renal tumours in adults. Average age at presentation is 55 years, with a male:female ratio of 2:1. They arise from the proximal tubular epithelium and may be solitary, multiple and occasionally bilateral.

Clinical features

Haematuria, loin pain and a mass in the flank are the most common presenting features. Other features include malaise, weight loss and fever. Left-sided scrotal varicoceles occur if the renal tumour obstructs the gonadal vein where it enters the renal vein. Twenty-five per cent have metastases at presentation to bone, liver and the lung. Anaemia or polycythaemia and hypercalcaemia are other findings.

Investigations

- Ultrasonography will distinguish a simple benign cyst from a more complex cyst or solid tumour.
- CT scanning is more sensitive than ultrasound for detecting a renal mass and will show involvement of the renal vein or inferior vena cava. MRI is better than CT for tumour staging.

A presumptive diagnosis of renal carcinoma is made on imaging studies in patients with isolated solid renal masses and they will usually go straight to surgery (which provides tissue diagnosis and definitive treatment) without further investigation.

Management

Localized disease Radical nephrectomy is the preferred treatment. Partial nephrectomy is used if there is bilateral involvement or the contralateral kidney functions poorly. Ablative techniques (cryoablation or radiofrequency ablation) are used in patients with significant comorbid disease who would not tolerate surgery.

Metastatic or locally advanced disease Interleukin-2 and interferon produce a remission in 20% of cases. Targeted therapies which block the vascular endothelial growth factor (sunitinib, sorafenib, bevacizumab) or mTOR (temsirolimus) pathway are used in patients who cannot tolerate or do not respond to this treatment.

Prognosis

The 5-year survival rate is 60–70% with tumours confined to the renal parenchyma, but less than 5% in those with distant metastases.

Urothelial tumours

The calyces, renal pelvis, ureter, bladder and urethra are lined by transitional cell epithelium. Bladder tumours are the most common form of transitional cell malignancy. They occur most commonly after the age of 40 years and are four times more common in males. Predisposing factors for bladder cancer include:

- Cigarette smoking
- Exposure to industrial chemicals, e.g. β-naphthylamine, benzidine
- Exposure to drugs, e.g. phenacetin, cyclophosphamide
- Chronic inflammation, e.g. schistosomiasis.

Clinical features

Patients with bladder cancer usually present with painless haematuria (either visible or non-visible) or sometimes symptoms suggestive of a UTI (frequency, urgency, dysuria) in the absence of bacteriuria. Pain is usually due to locally advanced or metastatic disease but may sometimes occur from clot retention. Transitional cell cancers of the kidney and ureters present with haematuria and flank pain.

Investigations

Presentation is usually with haematuria and any patient over 40 years of age with haematuria should be assumed to have a urothelial tumour until proven otherwise (Fig. 9.3).

Management

Pelvic and ureteric tumours are treated with nephroureterectomy. Treatment of bladder tumours depends on the stage, but options include local diathermy or cystoscopic resection, bladder resection, radiotherapy and local and systemic chemotherapy.

DISEASES OF THE PROSTATE GLAND

The common diseases of the prostate gland are benign enlargement, carcinoma and prostatitis. Prostate-specific antigen (PSA) is a glycoprotein that is expressed by normal and neoplastic prostate tissue and secreted into the bloodstream. Serum concentrations can be increased in any of these conditions and also after perineal trauma and mechanical manipulation of the prostate (cystoscopy, prostate biopsy or surgery). Serum PSA concentration >4.0 ng/mL is abnormal and can be due to benign disease or cancer. However, prostate cancer is present in 50% of men with a serum PSA >10 ng/mL.

Benign enlargement of the prostate gland

Benign prostatic enlargement (hypertrophy, BPH) is common particularly after the age of 60 years. There is hyperplasia of both glandular and connective tissue elements of the gland. The aetiology is not known.

Clinical features

Frequency of micturition, nocturia, delay in initiation of micturition and postvoid dribbling are common symptoms. Acute urinary retention or retention with overflow incontinence also occurs. An enlarged smooth prostate may be felt on rectal examination.

Investigations

Serum electrolytes and renal ultrasonography are performed to exclude renal damage resulting from obstruction. Prostate cancer may present with similar symptoms. Serum PSA may be elevated in benign disease but an elevated value is usually an indication for specialist referral and prostate biopsy.

Management

Patients with mild symptoms are managed by 'watchful waiting'. Selective α_1-adrenoceptor antagonists, such as tamsulosin, relax smooth muscle in the bladder neck and prostate, producing an increase in urinary flow rate and an improvement in obstructive symptoms. The 5α-reductase inhibitor finasteride blocks conversion of testosterone to dihydrotestosterone (the androgen responsible for prostatic growth) and is an alternative to α-antagonists, particularly in men with a significantly enlarged prostate. Patients with acute retention of urine or retention with overflow require urethral catheterization or, if this is not possible, suprapubic catheter drainage. Further management is then with prostatectomy or a permanent catheter.

Prostatic carcinoma

Prostatic adenocarcinoma is common, accounting for 7% of all cancers in men. Malignant change within the prostate is increasingly common with increasing age, being present in 80% of men aged 80 years and over. In most cases these malignant foci remain dormant.

Clinical features

In developed countries, many patients now present as a result of screening for prostate cancer by measurement of serum PSA, although this is not widely recommended (see later). Presentation is also with symptoms of bladder outflow obstruction identical to those of BPH. Occasionally, presenting symptoms are due to metastases, particularly to bone. In some cases, malignancy is unsuspected until histological investigation is carried out on the resected specimen after prostatectomy. Rectal examination may reveal a hard irregular gland.

Investigation

The diagnosis is made using transrectal ultrasound of the prostate, elevated serum PSA (see above) and transrectal prostate biopsy. If metastases are present, serum PSA is usually markedly elevated (>16 ng/mL). Endorectal coil MRI is used to locally stage the tumour.

Management

Microscopic tumour is sometimes managed by watchful waiting. Treatment of disease confined to the gland is radical prostatectomy or radiotherapy, both resulting in 80–90% 5-year survival. The treatment of metastatic disease depends on removing androgenic drive to the tumour. This is achieved by bilateral orchidectomy, synthetic luteinizing hormone-releasing hormone analogues, e.g. goserelin, or antiandrogens, e.g. cyproterone acetate.

Screening

Screening for prostate cancer by annual measurement of serum PSA and digital rectal examination reduces the mortality from prostate cancer but the benefit is small and there is the potential for overdiagnosis and treatment-related complications. Most major medical organizations world-wide do not recommend screening for prostate cancer.

TESTICULAR TUMOUR

Testicular cancer is the most common cancer in young men. More than 96% of testicular tumours arise from germ cells. There are two main types: seminomas and teratomas. The aetiology is unknown and the risk of malignant change is greater in undescended testes.

Clinical features

Typically, the man or his partner finds a painless lump in the testicle. Presentation may also be with metastases in the lungs, causing cough and dyspnoea, or para-aortic lymph nodes, causing back pain.

Investigations

- Ultrasound scanning will help to differentiate between masses in the body of the testes and other intrascrotal swellings.
- Serum concentrations of the tumour markers α-fetoprotein (AFP) and/or the β- subunit of human chorionic gonadotrophin (β-hCG) are elevated in most men with teratomas. They are used to help make the diagnosis, to assess response to treatment and in following up patients. β-hCG is elevated in a minority of men with seminomas, and AFP is not elevated in men with pure seminomas.
- Tumour staging is assessed by chest X-ray and CT scanning of the chest, abdomen and pelvis.

Treatment

Orchidectomy is performed to permit histological evaluation of the primary tumour and to provide local tumour control. Seminomas with metastases below the diaphragm only are treated by radiotherapy. More widespread tumours are treated with chemotherapy. Teratomas with metastases are also treated with chemotherapy. Sperm banking should be offered prior to therapy to men who wish to preserve fertility.

URINARY INCONTINENCE

Normal bladder physiology

As the bladder fills with urine, two factors act to ensure continence until it is next emptied:

- Intravesical pressure remains low as a result of stretching of the bladder wall and the stability of the bladder muscle (detrusor), which does not contract involuntarily.
- The sphincter mechanisms of the bladder neck and urethral muscles.

At the onset of voiding, the sphincters relax (mediated by decreased sympathetic activity) and the detrusor muscle contracts (mediated by increased parasympathetic activity). Overall control and coordination of micturition is by higher brain centres, which include the cerebral cortex and the pons.

Stress incontinence

Stress incontinence occurs as a result of sphincter weakness, which may be iatrogenic in men (post-prostatectomy) or the result of childbirth in women. There is a small leak of urine when intra-abdominal pressure rises, e.g. with coughing, laughing or standing up. In young women, pelvic floor exercises may help.

In post-menopausal women the contributing factor of urethral atrophy may be helped by oestrogen creams.

Urge incontinence

In urge incontinence there is a strong desire to void and the patient may be unable to hold his or her urine. The usual cause is detrusor instability, which occurs most often in women, and the aetiology is not known. Mild cases may respond to bladder retraining (gradually increasing the time interval between voids). More severe cases are treated with anticholinergic agents, e.g. oxybutynin, which decrease detrusor excitability. Less commonly, urge incontinence is caused by bladder hypersensitivity from local pathology (e.g. UTI, bladder stones, tumours) and treatment is then of the underlying cause.

Overflow incontinence

Overflow incontinence is most often seen in men with prostatic hypertrophy causing outflow obstruction. There is leakage of small amounts of urine, and on abdominal examination the distended bladder is felt rising out of the pelvis. If the obstruction is not relieved with urethral or suprapubic catheterization, renal damage will develop.

Neurological causes

These are usually apparent from the history and examination, which reveal accompanying neurological deficits. Brainstem damage, e.g. trauma, may lead to incoordination of detrusor muscle activity and sphincter relaxation, so that the two contract together during voiding. This results in a high-pressure system with the risk of obstructive uropathy. The aim of treatment is to reduce outflow pressure, either with α-adrenergic blockers or by sphincterotomy. Autonomic neuropathy, e.g. in diabetic individuals, decreases detrusor excitability and results in a distended atonic bladder with a large residual urine which is liable to infection. Permanent catheterization may be necessary.

In elderly people, incontinence may be the result of a combination of factors: diuretic treatment, dementia (antisocial incontinence) and difficulty in getting to the toilet because of immobility.

COMMON PRESENTING SYMPTOMS OF HEART DISEASE

The common symptoms of heart disease are chest pain, breathlessness, palpitations, syncope, fatigue and peripheral oedema, but none are specific for cardiovascular disease. The severity of anginal pain, dyspnoea, palpitations or fatigue may be classified according to the New York Heart Association (NYHA) grading of 'cardiac status' (Table 10.1).

Chest pain

Chest pain or discomfort is a common presenting symptom of cardiovascular disease and must be differentiated from non-cardiac causes. The site of pain, its character, radiation and associated symptoms will often point to the cause (Table 10.2).

Dyspnoea

Causes are discussed on page 507. Left heart failure is the most common cardiac cause of exertional dyspnoea and may also cause orthopnoea and paroxysmal nocturnal dyspnoea.

Palpitations

Palpitations are an awareness of the heartbeat. The normal heartbeat is sensed when the patient is anxious, excited, exercising or lying on the left side. In other circumstances it usually indicates a cardiac arrhythmia, commonly ectopic beats or a paroxysmal tachycardia (p. 421).

Syncope

This is a temporary impairment of consciousness due to inadequate cerebral blood flow. There are many causes and the most common is a simple faint or vasovagal attack (Table 17.3; page 720). The cardiac causes of syncope are the result of either very fast (e.g. ventricular tachycardia) or very slow heart rates (e.g. complete heart block) which are unable to maintain an adequate cardiac output. Attacks occur suddenly and without warning. They last only 1 or 2 minutes, with complete recovery in seconds (compare with epilepsy, where complete recovery may be delayed for some hours). Obstruction to

Table 10.1 The New York Heart Association grading of 'cardiac status' (modified)

Grade 1	Uncompromised (no breathlessness)
Grade 2	Slightly compromised (on severe exertion)
Grade 3	Moderately compromised (on mild exertion)
Grade 4	Severely compromised (breathless at rest)

Table 10.2 Common causes of chest pain

Central	
Angina pectoris	Crushing pain on exercise, relieved by rest. May radiate to jaw or arms
ACS	Similar in character to angina but more severe, occurs at rest, lasts longer
Pericarditis	Sharp pain aggravated by movement, respiration and changes in posture
Aortic dissection	Severe tearing chest pain radiating through to the back
Massive PE	With dyspnoea, tachycardia and hypotension
Musculoskeletal	Tender to palpate over affected area
GORD	May be exacerbated by bending or lying down (at night). Pain may radiate into the neck
Lateral/peripheral	
Pulmonary infarct Pneumonia Pneumothorax	Pleuritic pain, i.e. sharp, well-localized, aggravated by inspiration, coughing and movement
Musculoskeletal	Sharp, well-localized pain with a tender area on palpation
Lung carcinoma	Constant dull pain
Herpes zoster	Burning unilateral pain corresponding to a dermatome that appears 2 to 3 days before the typical rash

ACS, acute coronary syndrome; GORD, gastro-oesophageal reflux disease; PE, pulmonary embolus.

ventricular outflow also causes syncope (e.g. aortic stenosis, hypertrophic cardiomyopathy), which typically occurs on exercise when the requirements for increased cardiac output cannot be met. Postural hypotension is a drop in systolic blood pressure (BP) of 20 mmHg or more on standing from a sitting or lying position.

Other symptoms

Tiredness and lethargy occur with heart failure and result from poor perfusion of brain and skeletal muscle, poor sleep, side effects of medication, particularly β-blockers, and electrolyte imbalance due to diuretic therapy. Heart failure also causes salt and water retention, leading to oedema, which in ambulant patients is most prominent over the ankles. In severe cases it may involve the genitalia and thighs.

INVESTIGATIONS IN CARDIAC DISEASE

The chest X-ray

A chest X-ray is usually taken in the postero-anterior (PA) direction at maximum inspiration (p. 509). A PA chest film can aid the identification of cardiomegaly, pericardial effusions, dissection or dilatation of the aorta, and calcification of the pericardium or heart valves. A cardiothoracic ratio (p. 510) of greater than 50% on a PA film is abnormal and normally indicates cardiac dilatation or pericardial effusion. Examination of the lung fields may show signs of left ventricular failure (Fig. 10.1), valvular heart disease (e.g. markedly enlarged left atrium in mitral valve disease) or pulmonary oligaemia (reduction of vascular markings) associated with pulmonary embolic disease.

THE ELECTROCARDIOGRAM

The electrocardiogram (ECG) is a recording from the body surface of the electrical activity of the heart. Each cardiac cell generates an action potential as it becomes depolarized and then repolarized during a normal cycle. Normally, depolarization of cardiac cells proceeds in an orderly fashion beginning in the sinus node (lying in the junction between superior vena cava and right atrium) and spreading sequentially through the atria, atrioventricular (AV) node (lying beneath the right atrial endocardium within the lower inter-atrial septum), and the His bundle in the interventricular septum, which divides into right and left bundle branches (Fig. 10.2). The right and left bundle branches continue down the right and left side of the interventricular septum and supply the Purkinje network which spreads through the subendocardial surface of the right ventricle and left ventricle, respectively. The main left bundle divides into an anterior superior division (the anterior hemi-bundle) and a posterior inferior division (the posterior hemi-bundle).

The standard ECG has 12 leads:

- Chest leads, V_1–V_6, look at the heart in a *horizontal plane* (Fig. 10.3).
- Limb leads look at the heart in a *vertical plane* (Fig. 10.4). Limb leads are unipolar (AVR, AVL and AVF) or bipolar (I, II, III).

The ECG machine is arranged so that when a depolarization wave spreads towards a lead the needle moves upwards on the trace (i.e. a positive deflection), and when it spreads away from the lead the needle moves downwards.

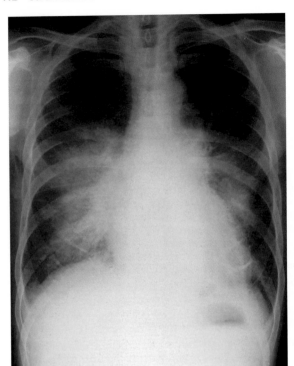

Fig. 10.1 Chest X-ray in acute left ventricular failure. This chest X-ray demonstrates cardiomegaly, hilar haziness, Kerley B lines, upper lobe venous blood engorgement and fluid in the right horizontal fissure. Hilar haziness and Kerley B lines (thin linear horizontal pulmonary opacities at the base of the lung periphery) indicate interstitial pulmonary oedema.

ECG waveform and definitions (Fig. 10.5)

Heart rate At normal paper speed (usually 25 mm/s) each 'big square' measures 5 mm wide and is equivalent to 0.2 s. The heart rate (if the rhythm is regular) is calculated by counting the number of big squares between two consecutive R waves and dividing into 300.

The P wave is the first deflection and is caused by atrial depolarization. When abnormal, it may be:

- Broad and notched (>0.12 s, i.e. three small squares) in left atrial enlargement ('P mitrale', e.g. mitral stenosis)
- Tall and peaked (>2.5 mm) in right atrial enlargement ('P pulmonale', e.g. pulmonary hypertension)

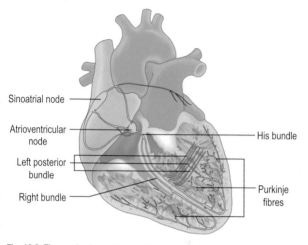

Fig. 10.2 The conducting system of the heart. In normal circumstances only the specialized conducting tissues of the heart undergo spontaneous depolarization (automaticity), which initiates an action potential. The sinus (SA) node discharges more rapidly than the other cells and is the normal pacemaker of the heart. The impulse generated by the SA node spreads first through the atria, producing atrial systole, and then through the atrioventricular (AV) node to the His-Purkinje system, producing ventricular systole.

- Replaced by flutter or fibrillation waves (p. 430)
- Absent in sinoatrial block (p. 423).

   The *QRS complex* represents ventricular activation or depolarization:

- A negative (downward) deflection preceding an R wave is called a Q wave. Normal Q waves are small and narrow; deep (>2 mm), wide (>1 mm) Q waves (except in AVR and V_1) indicate myocardial infarction (MI) (p. 453).
- A deflection upwards is called an R wave whether or not it is preceded by a Q wave.
- A negative deflection following an R wave is termed an S wave.

   Ventricular depolarization starts in the septum and spreads from left to right (Fig. 10.2). Subsequently, the main free walls of the ventricles are depolarized. Thus in the right ventricular leads (V_1 and V_2) the first deflection is upwards (R wave) as the septal depolarization wave spreads towards those leads. The second deflection is downwards (S wave) as the bigger left ventricle (in which depolarization is spreading away) outweighs the effect of the right ventricle (Fig. 10.3). The opposite pattern is seen in the left ventricular leads (V_5 and V_6), with an initial downwards deflection (small Q wave reflecting septal depolarization) followed by a large R wave caused by left ventricular depolarization.

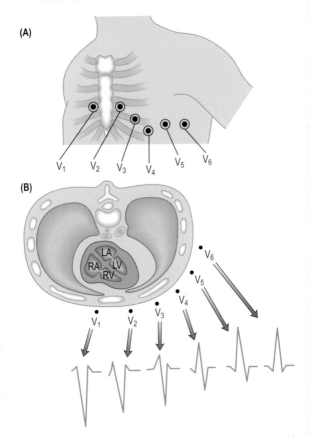

Fig. 10.3 ECG chest leads. (A) The V leads are attached to the chest wall overlying the intercostal spaces as shown: V_4 in the mid-clavicular line, V_5 in the anterior axillary line, V_6 in the mid-axillary line. (B) Leads V_1 and V_2 look at the right ventricle, V_3 and V_4 at the interventricular septum, and V_5 and V_6 at the left ventricle. The normal QRS complex in each lead is shown. The R wave in the chest (precordial) leads steadily increases in amplitude from lead V_1 to V_6 with a corresponding decrease in S wave depth, culminating in a predominantly positive complex in V_6. LA, left atrium; LV, left ventricle; RA, right atrium; RV, right ventricle.

Left ventricular hypertrophy with increased bulk of the left ventricular myocardium (e.g. with systemic hypertension) increases the voltage-induced depolarization of the free wall of the left ventricle. This gives rise to tall R waves (>25 mm) in the left ventricular leads (V_5, V_6) and/or deep S waves (>30 mm) in the right ventricular leads (V_1, V_2). The sum of the R wave in the left

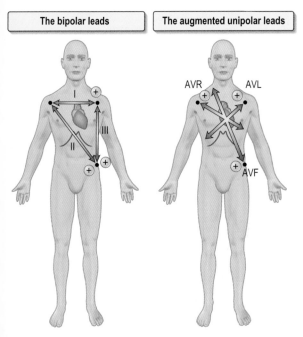

Fig. 10.4 ECG limb leads. Lead I is derived from electrodes on the right arm (negative pole) and left arm (positive pole), lead II is derived from electrodes on the right arm (negative pole) and left leg (positive pole) and lead III from electrodes on the left arm (negative pole) and the left leg (positive pole).

ventricular leads and the S wave in the right ventricular leads exceeds 40 mm. In addition to these changes, there may also be ST-segment depression and T-wave flattening or inversion in the left ventricular leads.

Right ventricular hypertrophy (e.g. in pulmonary hypertension) causes tall R waves in the right ventricular leads.

The QRS duration reflects the time that excitation takes to spread through the ventricle. A wide QRS complex (>0.10 s, 2.5 small squares) occurs if conduction is delayed, e.g. with right or left bundle branch block, or if conduction is through a pathway other than the right and left bundle branches, e.g. an impulse generated by an abnormal focus of activity in the ventricle (ventricular ectopic).

T waves result from ventricular repolarization. In general the direction of the T wave is the same as that of the QRS complex. Inverted T waves occur in many conditions and, although usually abnormal, they are a non-specific finding.

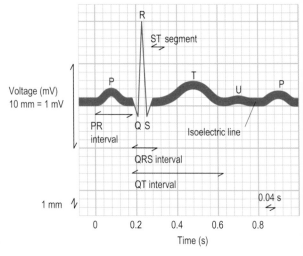

Fig. 10.5 The waves and elaboration of the normal ECG.

The *PR interval* is measured from the start of the P wave to the start of the QRS complex whether this is a Q wave or an R wave. It is the time taken for excitation to pass from the sinus node, through the atrium, atrioventricular node and His-Purkinje system to the ventricle. A prolonged PR interval (>0.2 s) indicates heart block (p. 423).

The *ST segment* is the period between the end of the QRS complex and the start of the T wave. ST elevation (>1 mm above the isoelectric line) occurs in the early stages of MI (p. 453) and with acute pericarditis (p. 458). ST segment depression (>0.5 mm below the isoelectric line) indicates myocardial ischaemia.

The *QT interval* extends from the start of the QRS complex to the end of the T wave. It is primarily a measure of the time taken for repolarization of the ventricular myocardium, which is dependent on heart rate (shorter at faster heart rates). The QT interval, corrected for heart rate ($QTc = QT/\sqrt{^2(R - R)}$), is normally ≤ 0.44 s in males and ≤ 0.46 s in females. Long QT syndrome (p. 433) is associated with an increased risk of torsades de pointes ventricular tachycardia and sudden death.

The *cardiac axis* refers to the overall direction of the wave of ventricular depolarization in the vertical plane measured from a zero reference point (Fig. 10.6). The normal range for the cardiac axis is between $-30°$ and $+90$. An axis more negative than $-30°$ is termed left axis deviation and an axis more positive than $+90°$ is termed right axis deviation. A simple method to calculate the axis is by inspection of the QRS complex in leads I, II and III. The axis

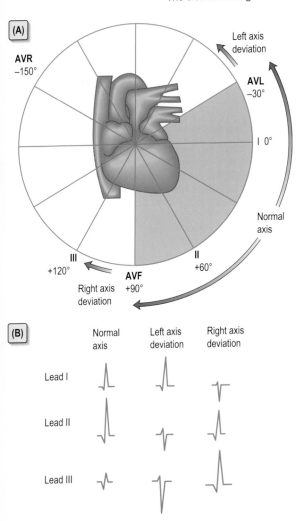

Fig. 10.6 Cardiac vectors. (A) The hexaxial reference system, illustrating the six leads in the frontal plane, e.g. lead I is 0°, lead II is +60°, lead III is 120°. (B) ECG leads showing the predominant positive and negative deflection with axis deviation.

is normal if leads I and II are positive; there is right axis deviation if lead I is negative and lead III positive, and left axis deviation if lead I is positive and leads II and III negative. Left axis deviation occurs due to a block of the anterior bundle of the main left bundle conducting system (Fig. 10.2), inferior MI and the Wolff–Parkinson–White syndrome. Right axis deviation may be normal and occurs in conditions in which there is right ventricular overload, dextrocardia, Wolff–Parkinson–White syndrome and left posterior hemiblock.

Exercise electrocardiography

Exercise electrocardiography assesses the cardiac response to exercise, but is used less often than previously because of its low sensitivity. The 12-lead ECG and BP are recorded whilst the patient walks or runs on a motorized treadmill using a standardized method (e.g. the Bruce protocol). Myocardial ischaemia provoked by exertion results in ST segment depression (>1 mm) in leads facing the affected area of ischaemic cardiac muscle. Exercise normally causes an increase in heart rate and BP. A sustained fall in BP usually indicates severe coronary artery disease. A slow recovery of the heart rate to basal levels has also been reported to be a predictor of mortality. Contraindications include unstable angina, severe hypertrophic cardiomyopathy, severe aortic stenosis and malignant hypertension. A positive test and indications for stopping the test are:

- Chest pain
- ST segment depression or elevation > 1 mm
- Fall in systolic BP > 20 mmHg
- Fall in heart rate despite an increase in workload
- BP > 240/110
- Significant arrhythmias or increased frequency of ventricular ectopics.

24-hour ambulatory taped electrocardiography

A 12-lead ECG is recorded continuously over a 24-hour period and is used to record transient changes such as a brief paroxysm of tachycardia, an occasional pause in rhythm or intermittent ST segment shifts. It is also called 'Holter' electrocardiography after its inventor. Event recording is used to record less frequent arrhythmias in which the patient triggers an ECG recording at the time of symptoms. They are both outpatient investigations.

Tilt testing

Tilt testing is performed to investigate suspected neurocardiogenic (vasovagal) syncope in which patients give a history of repeated episodes of syncope which occur without warning and are followed by a rapid recovery. The patient lies on a swivel motorized table in a flat position with safety straps applied across the chest and legs to hold them in position. BP, heart rate, symptoms and ECG are recorded after the table is tilted +60° to the vertical for 10–60 minutes, thus simulating going from a flat to an upright position. Reproduction of symptoms, bradycardia or hypotension indicates a positive test. The overall sensitivity, specificity and reproducibility are low.

Echocardiography

Echocardiography is an ultrasound examination of the heart (Fig. 10.7). Different modalities (e.g. M mode, two- and three-dimensional) are used to provide information about cardiac structure and function. The examination is performed in two ways:

- *Transthoracic echo* is the most common method and involves the placement of a handheld transducer on the chest wall. Ultrasound pulses are emitted through various body tissues, and reflected waves are detected by the transducer as an echo. The most common reasons for undertaking an echocardiogram are to assess ventricular function in patients with symptoms suggestive of heart failure, or to assess valvular disease. Left ventricular function is assessed by the ejection fraction (percentage of blood ejected from the left ventricle with each heartbeat) – normally > 55%.
- *Transoesophageal echo* uses miniaturized transducers incorporated into special endoscopes. It allows better visualization of some structures and pathology, e.g. aortic dissection, endocarditis.

Further refinements of the echocardiogram are Doppler and stress echocardiography. Doppler echocardiography uses the Doppler principle (in this case, the frequency of ultrasonic waves reflected from blood cells is related to their velocity and direction of flow) to identify and assess the severity of valve lesions, estimate cardiac output and assess coronary blood flow. Stress (exercise or pharmacological) echocardiography is used to assess myocardial wall motion as a surrogate for coronary artery perfusion. It is used in the detection of coronary artery disease, assessment of risk post-MI and perioperatively, and in patients in whom routine exercise ECG testing is non-diagnostic. For those who cannot exercise, pharmacological intervention with dobutamine is used to increase myocardial oxygen demand.

Cardiac nuclear imaging

Cardiac nuclear imaging is used to detect MI or to measure myocardial function, perfusion or viability, depending on the radiopharmaceutical used and the technique of imaging. A variety of radiotracers can be injected intravenously and these diffuse freely into myocardial tissue or attach to red blood cells.

Thallium-201 is taken up by cardiac myocytes. Ischaemic areas (produced by exercising the patient) with reduced tracer uptake are seen as 'cold spots' when imaged with a γ camera.

Technetium-99 m is used to label red blood cells and produce images of the left ventricle during systole and diastole.

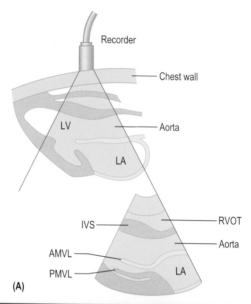

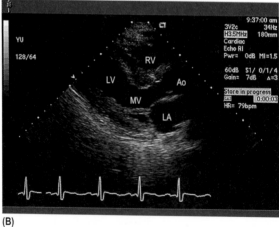

Fig. 10.7 Echocardiogram: an example of a two-dimensional long-axis view. (A) Diagram showing the anatomy of the area scanned and a diagrammatic representation of the echocardiogram. (B) Two-dimensional long-axis view. AMVL, anterior mitral valve leaflet; Ao, aorta; IVS, Inter-ventricular septum; LA, left atrium; LV, left ventricle; MV, mitral valve; PMVL, posterior mitral valve leaflet; RV, right ventricle; RVOT, right ventricular outflow tract.

Cardiac computed tomography

Computed tomography (CT) is useful for the assessment of the thoracic aorta and mediastinum, and multidetector thin slice scanners can assess calcium content of coronary arteries as an indicator of the presence and severity of coronary artery stenoses. CT coronary angiography has high sensitivity for the detection of coronary artery diseases. The current National Institute for Health and Care Excellence (NICE) chest pain guidelines recommend the use of CT calcium scoring in patients with chest pain and a 10–29% likelihood of coronary artery disease.

Cardiovascular magnetic resonance

Cardiovascular magnetic resonance (CMR) is a non-invasive imaging technique that does not involve harmful radiation. It is increasingly utilized in the investigation of cardiovascular disease to provide both anatomical and functional information. Contraindications are permanent pacemaker or defibrillator, intracerebral clips and significant claustrophobia. Coronary stents and prosthetic valves are not a contraindication.

Cardiac catheterization

A small catheter is passed through a peripheral vein (for study of right-sided heart structures) or artery (for study of left-sided heart structures) into the heart, permitting the securing of blood samples, measurement of intracardiac pressures and determination of cardiac anomalies. Specially designed catheters are then used to selectively engage the left and right coronary arteries, and contrast cine-angiograms are taken in order to define the coronary circulation and identify the presence and severity of any coronary artery disease. Coronary artery stenoses can be dilated (angioplasty) and metal stents can be placed to reduce the rate of restenosis – this is referred to as percutaneous coronary intervention (PCI). A further development is the introduction of stents coated with drugs (sirolimus or paclitaxel) to reduce cellular proliferation and restenosis rates still further. However, there is a risk of late-stent thrombosis.

CARDIAC ARRHYTHMIAS

An abnormality of cardiac rhythm is called a cardiac arrhythmia. Arrhythmia may cause sudden death, syncope, dizziness, palpitations or no symptoms at all. Twenty-four-hour ambulatory ECG monitoring and event recorders (p. 418) are often used to detect paroxysmal arrhythmias.

There are two main types of arrhythmia:

- *Bradycardia:* the heart rate is slow (<60 beats/min). Slower heart rates are more likely to cause symptomatic arrhythmias.
- *Tachycardia:* the heart rate is fast (>100 beats/min). Tachycardias are more likely to be symptomatic when the arrhythmia is fast and sustained. They are subdivided into *supraventricular tachycardias* (SVTs), which arise

from the atrium or the atrioventricular junction, and *ventricular tachycardias*, which arise from the ventricles.

Arrhythmias and conduction disturbances complicating acute MI are discussed on page 457.

General principles of management of arrhythmias

Patients with adverse symptoms and signs (low cardiac output, chest pain, hypotension, impaired consciousness or severe pulmonary oedema) require urgent treatment of their arrhythmia. Oxygen is given to all patients, intravenous access established and serum electrolyte abnormalities (potassium, magnesium, calcium) are corrected.

Sinus rhythms

The normal cardiac pacemaker is the sinus node (p. 411) with the rate of sinus node discharge under control of the autonomic nervous system with parasympathetic predominating (resulting in slowing of the spontaneous discharge rate).

Sinus arrhythmia

Fluctuations of autonomic tone result in phasic changes in the sinus discharge rate. During inspiration, parasympathetic tone falls and the heart rate quickens, and on expiration the heart rate falls. This variation is normal, particularly in children and young adults, and typically results in predictable irregularities of the pulse.

Bradycardia

Sinus bradycardia

Sinus bradycardia is normal during sleep and in well-trained athletes. Causes are:

- *Extrinsic to the heart:* drug therapy (β-blockers, digitalis and other antiarrhythmic drugs), hypothyroidism, hypothermia, cholestatic jaundice, raised intracranial pressure. Treatment of symptomatic bradycardia is that of the underlying cause.
- *Intrinsic to the heart:* acute ischaemia and infarction of the sinus node (as a complication of MI) and chronic degenerative changes such as fibrosis of the atrium and sinus node (sick sinus syndrome) occurring in elderly people. Patients with persistent symptomatic bradycardia are treated with a permanent cardiac pacemaker. First-line treatment in the acute situation with adverse signs is atropine (500 µg intravenously repeated to a maximum of 3 mg, but contraindicated in myasthenia gravis and paralytic ileus). Temporary pacing (transcutaneous, or transvenous if expertise available) is an alternative.

- *Sick sinus syndrome*. Bradycardia is caused by intermittent failure of sinus node depolarization (sinus arrest) or failure of the sinus impulse to propagate through the perinodal tissue to the atria (sinoatrial block). The slow heart rate predisposes to ectopic pacemaker activity and tachyarrhythmias are common (tachy–brady syndrome). The ECG shows severe sinus bradycardia or intermittent long pauses between consecutive P waves (>2 s, dropped P waves). Permanent pacemaker insertion is indicated in symptomatic patients. Antiarrhythmic drugs are used to treat tachycardias. Thromboembolism is common in sinus node dysfunction and patients are anticoagulated unless there is a contraindication.
- Neurally mediated, e.g. carotid sinus syndrome and vasovagal attacks, resulting in bradycardia and syncope.

Heart block

The common causes of heart block are coronary artery disease, cardiomyopathy and, particularly in elderly people, fibrosis of the conducting tissue. Block in either the AV node or the His bundle results in AV block, whereas block lower in the conduction system (Fig. 10.2) produces right or left bundle branch block.

Atrioventricular block

There are three forms:

First-degree AV block This is the result of delayed atrioventricular conduction and is reflected by a prolonged PR interval (>0.22 s) on the ECG. No change in heart rate occurs and treatment is unnecessary.

Second-degree AV block This occurs when some atrial impulses fail to reach the ventricles.

There are several forms (Fig. 10.8):

- *Mobitz type I* (Wenckebach) *block* is generally caused by AV node block and results in progressive PR interval prolongation until a P wave fails to conduct, i.e. absent QRS after the P wave. The PR interval then returns to normal and the cycle repeats itself.
- *Mobitz type II block* is due to a block at an infra-nodal level so the QRS is widened and QRS complexes are dropped without PR prolongation. The ratio of non-conducted P waves to QRS complexes is usually specified. For example, a 2:1 Mobitz type II block refers to two P waves for every QRS complex.

Progression from second-degree AV block to complete heart block occurs more frequently following acute anterior MI and in Mobitz type II block, and treatment is with a cardiac pacemaker. Patients with Wenckebach AV block or those with second-degree block following acute inferior infarction are usually monitored.

Third-degree AV block Complete heart block occurs when there is complete dissociation between atrial and ventricular activity; P waves and QRS complexes occur independently of one another and ventricular contractions

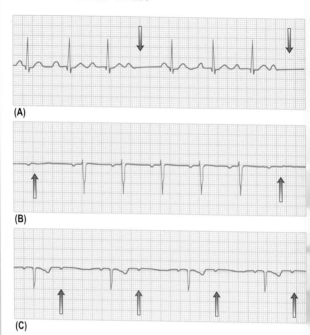

Fig. 10.8 Three varieties of second-degree atrioventricular (AV) block.
(A) Wenckebach (Mobitz type I) AV block. The PR interval gradually prolongs until the P wave does not conduct to the ventricles (arrows). (B) Mobitz type II AV block. The P waves that do not conduct to the ventricles (arrows) are not preceded by gradual PR interval prolongation. (C) Two P waves to each QRS complex. The PR interval prior to the dropped P wave is always the same. It is not possible to define this type of AV block as type I or type II Mobitz block and it is, therefore, a third variety of second-degree AV block (arrows show P waves), not conducted to the ventricles.

are maintained by a spontaneous escape rhythm originating below the site of the block in the:

- *His bundle* (Fig. 10.2) – which gives rise to a narrow complex QRS (<0.12 s) at a rate of 50–60 beats/min and is relatively reliable. Recent onset block due to transient causes, e.g. ischaemia, may respond to intravenous atropine (p. 422) without the need for pacing. Chronic narrow-complex AV block usually requires permanent pacing.
- *His–Purkinje system* (i.e. distally) – gives rise to a broad QRS complex (>0.12 s), is slow (<40 beats/min), unreliable and often associated with dizziness and blackouts (Stokes–Adams attacks). Permanent pacemaker insertion is indicated.

Bundle branch block

Complete block of a bundle branch (see Fig. 10.2) is associated with a wide QRS complex (≥ 0.12 s) with an abnormal pattern and is usually asymptomatic. The shape of the QRS depends on whether the right or the left bundle is blocked (Fig. 10.9):

- Right bundle branch block (RBBB) – there is sequential spread of an impulse (i.e. first the left ventricle and then the right) resulting in a secondary R wave (RSR') in V_1 and a slurred S wave in V_5 and V_6. RBBB occurs in normal healthy individuals, pulmonary embolus, right ventricular hypertrophy, ischaemic heart disease and congenital heart disease, e.g. atrial and ventricular septal defect and Fallot's tetralogy.
- Left bundle branch block (LBBB – the opposite occurs with an RSR' pattern in the left ventricular leads (I, AVL, V_4–V_6) and deep slurred S waves in V_1 and V_2. LBBB indicates underlying cardiac pathology and occurs in aortic stenosis, hypertension, severe coronary artery disease and following cardiac surgery.

Supraventricular tachycardias

SVTs arise from the atrium or the atrioventricular junction. Conduction is via the His-Purkinje system and the QRS shape during tachycardia is usually similar to that seen in the same patient during baseline rhythm.

Sinus tachycardia

Sinus tachycardia is a physiological response during exercise and excitement. It also occurs with fever, pain, anaemia, heart failure, thyrotoxicosis, acute pulmonary embolism, hypovolaemia and drugs (e.g. catecholamines and atropine). Treatment is aimed at correction of the underlying cause. If necessary, β-blockers may be used to slow the sinus rate, e.g. in hyperthyroidism.

Atrioventricular junctional tachycardias

Tachycardia arises as a result of re-entry circuits in which there are two separate pathways for impulse conduction. They are usually referred to as paroxysmal SVTs and are often seen in young patients with no evidence of structural heart disease.

Atrioventricular nodal re-entry tachycardia

AVNRT is the most common type of SVT and is twice as common in women as in men. It is due to the presence of a 'ring' of conducting pathway in the AV node, of which the 'limbs' have differing conduction times and refractory periods. This allows a re-entry circuit and an impulse to produce a circus movement tachycardia. On the ECG, the P waves are either not visible or are seen immediately before or after the QRS complex (Fig. 10.10). The QRS complex is usually of normal shape because the ventricles are activated in the normal way. Occasionally the QRS complex is wide, because of a rate-related bundle branch

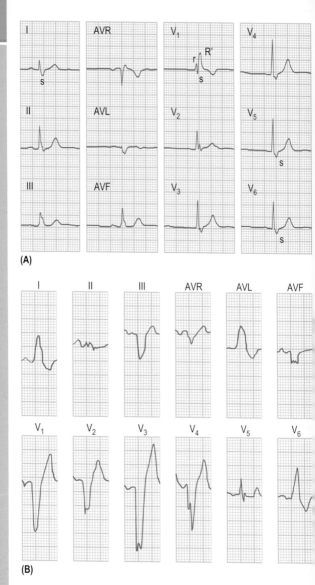

Fig. 10.9 Bundle branch block. A 12-lead ECG showing (A) right bundle branch block. Note an RSR pattern with the tall R in lead V_1–V_2 and the broad S waves in leads I and V_5 and V_6. (B) Left bundle branch block. The QRS duration is greater than 0.12 s. Note the broad notched R waves with ST depression in leads I, AVL and V_6, and the broad QRS waves in V_1–V_3.

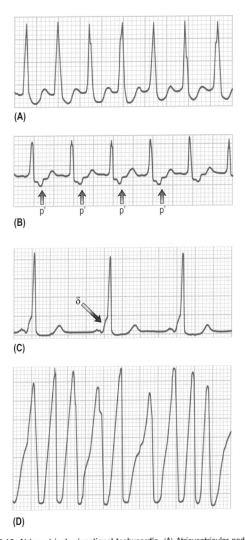

Fig. 10.10 Atrioventricular junctional tachycardia. (A) Atrioventricular nodal re-entry tachycardia. The QRS complexes are narrow and the P waves cannot be seen. (B) Atrioventricular re-entry tachycardia (Wolff–Parkinson–White [WPW] syndrome). The tachycardia P waves (arrows) are clearly seen after narrow QRS complexes. (C) An electrocardiogram taken in a patient with WPW syndrome during sinus rhythm. Note the short PR interval and the δ wave (arrow). (D) Atrial fibrillation in the WPW syndrome. Note tachycardia with broad QRS complexes with fast and irregular ventricular rate.

Table 10.3 Clinical indicators for the identification of sustained ventricular tachycardia (12-lead ECG) in a patient presenting with wide complex tachycardia

Ventricular tachycardia is more likely than supraventricular tachycardia with:
History of ischaemic heart disease
QRS interval > 140 ms
Atrioventricular dissociation – P waves have no relationship to the QRS complexes
Capture complexes – intermittent normal QRS complex
RS interval > 100 ms
Bifid, upright QRS complex with a taller first peak in V_1
Deep S wave in V_6
Concordant QRS direction in leads V_1–V_6, i.e. all positive or all negative complexes

block, and it may be difficult to distinguish from ventricular tachycardia (Table 10.3).

Atrioventricular reciprocating tachycardia

AVRT is due to the presence of an accessory pathway that connects the atria and ventricles and is capable of antegrade or retrograde conduction, or both. In contrast to AVNRT, each part of the circuit is activated sequentially in, so atrial activation occurs after ventricular activation and the P wave is usually clearly seen between the QRS and T wave. Wolff–Parkinson–White syndrome is the best-known type of AVRT in which there is an accessory pathway (bundle of Kent) between atria and ventricles. The resting ECG in Wolff–Parkinson–White syndrome shows evidence of the pathway's existence if the path allows some of the atrial depolarization to pass quickly to the ventricle before it gets through the AV node. The early depolarization of part of the ventricle leads to a shortened PR interval and a slurred start to the QRS (delta wave). The QRS is narrow (Fig. 10.10). These patients are also prone to atrial and occasionally ventricular fibrillation.

Symptoms

The usual history is of rapid regular palpitations, usually with abrupt onset and sudden termination. Other symptoms are dizziness, dyspnoea, central chest pain and syncope. Exertion, coffee, tea or alcohol may aggravate the arrhythmia.

Acute management

The aim of treatment is to restore and maintain sinus rhythm:

- *Unstable patient* – emergency cardioversion is required in patients whose arrhythmia is accompanied by adverse symptoms and signs.

- *Haemodynamically stable patient:*
  - Increase vagal stimulation of the sinus node by the Valsalva manoeuvre (ask the patient to blow into a 20-mL syringe with enough force to push back the plunger) or right carotid sinus massage (contraindicated in the presence of a carotid bruit).
  - Adenosine (p. 491) is a very short-acting AV nodal-blocking drug that will terminate most junctional tachycardias. Other treatments are intravenous verapamil (p. 501) or β-blockers, e.g. metoprolol. Verapamil is contraindicated with β-blockers, if the QRS is wide and therefore differentiation from VT difficult or if there is atrial fibrillation (AF) and an accessory pathway.

Long-term management

Radiofrequency ablation of the accessory pathway via a cardiac catheter is successful in about 95% of cases. Flecainide, verapamil, sotalol and amiodarone are the drugs most commonly used.

Atrial tachyarrhythmias

AF, flutter, tachycardia and ectopic beats all arise from the atrial myocardium. In some cases, automaticity is acquired by damaged atrial cells. They share common aetiologies (Table 10.4). Baseline investigations in a patient with an atrial arrhythmia include an ECG, thyroid function tests and transthoracic echocardiogram.

Table 10.4 Causes of atrial arrhythmias
General
Hypertension, age, obesity
Cardiac
Ischaemic heart disease, rheumatic heart disease, valvular heart disease Cardiomyopathy Lone atrial fibrillation (no cause identified) Wolff–Parkinson–White syndrome Pericarditis, myocarditis Atrial septal defect, cardiac surgery
Pulmonary
Pneumonia, pulmonary embolus, carcinoma of the bronchus, chronic obstructive pulmonary disease
Metabolic
Acute and chronic alcohol use, electrolyte imbalance,
Endocrine
Diabetes mellitus, thyrotoxicosis

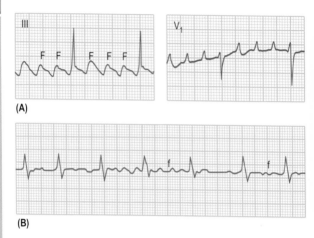

Fig. 10.11 Atrial flutter and atrial fibrillation. (A) Atrial flutter: the flutter waves are marked with an F, only half of which are transmitted to the ventricles. (B) Atrial fibrillation: there are no P waves; the ventricular response is fast and irregular.

Atrial fibrillation

AF is the most common arrhythmia and occurs in 15% of patients over 75 years of age. It also occurs, particularly in a paroxysmal form (stopping spontaneously within 7 days), in younger patients. Atrial activity is chaotic and mechanically ineffective. The AV node conducts a proportion of the atrial impulses to produce an irregular ventricular response – giving rise to an irregularly irregular pulse. In some patients, it is an incidental finding; in others, symptoms range from palpitations and fatigue to acute heart failure. AF is associated with a five-fold increased risk of stroke, primarily as a result of embolism of a thrombus that has formed in the atrium. There are no clear P waves on the ECG (Fig. 10.11), only a fine oscillation of the baseline (so-called fibrillation or f waves).

Management

When AF is caused by an acute precipitating event, the underlying cause should be treated:

- *Haemodynamically unstable patient* (p. 422) – immediate heparinization and attempted *cardioversion with a synchronized DC shock* (p. 490).
  If cardioversion fails or AF recurs, intravenous amiodarone is given (p. 491) *before a further attempt at cardioversion. A second dose of amiodarone can be given.*
- *Stable patient* – two strategies are available for the long-term management of AF: rate control or rhythm control (i.e. conversion to, and maintaining

sinus rhythm). Randomized studies in heart failure and in older patients have shown that neither strategy has net benefits compared with the other.

- *Rate control* aims to reduce heart rate at rest and during exercise, but the patient remains in AF. β-blockers (p. 495) or calcium antagonists (verapamil, diltiazem, p. 501) are the preferred treatment except in predominantly sedentary people where digoxin (p. 493) is used.
- *Rhythm control* is generally appropriate in patients who are < 65 years of age, highly symptomatic, patients with heart failure and individuals with recent onset AF (<48 h). Conversion to sinus rhythm is achieved by electrical DC cardioversion (p. 490) and then administration of β-blockers to suppress the arrhythmia. Other agents used depend on the presence (use amiodarone) or absence (sotalol, flecainide, propafenone) of underlying heart disease. Catheter ablation techniques such as pulmonary vein isolation are used in patients who do not respond to antiarrhythmic drugs.
  Patients with infrequent symptomatic paroxysms of AF (less than one per month) that are haemodynamically well tolerated and whom have little underlying heart disease are treated on an as-needed basis ('pill in the pocket') by oral flecainide (p. 493) or propafenone.

Assessment for anticoagulation

AF is associated with an increased risk of thromboembolism, and anticoagulation with warfarin or with dabigatran 150 mg twice daily should be given for at least 3 weeks before (with the exception of those who require emergency cardioversion or new-onset AF < 48 h duration) and 4 weeks after cardioversion. Longer-term anticoagulation is indicated in underlying rheumatic mitral stenosis or in the presence of a mechanical heart valve. Otherwise, a scoring system known as CHADS$_2$ (Congestive heart failure, Hypertension, Age ≥75, Diabetes mellitus and previous Stroke or transient ischaemic attack [TIA]) is used to determine the need for anticoagulation. Each factor scores 1 except previous stroke or TIA, which scores 2. A total score of 2 implies that oral anticoagulation is needed. When the score is <2 the CHADS$_2$VASc scoring system is applied, which adds Vascular disease (aorta, coronary or peripheral arteries), Age 65–74 and female Sex category. Each factor scores 1, except previous age >75 and stroke or TIA, which score 2. A CHADS$_2$VASc score of 2 requires oral anticoagulation and a score of 1 merits consideration for oral anticoagulation or aspirin. A score of 0 should not require any antithrombotic prophylaxis.

When oral anticoagulation is required, either warfarin (international normalized ratio [INR] 2.0–3.0) or one of the novel oral anticoagulants (NOACs) can be used. These newer agents fall into two classes: direct thrombin inhibitors (e.g. dabigatran) and oral direct factor Xa inhibitors (e.g. rivaroxaban and apixaban). NOACs specifically block a single step in the coagulation cascade in contrast to warfarin, which blocks several vitamin K-dependent factors (II, VII, IX and X). Unlike warfarin, the NOACs have rapid onset of action, shorter half-life, fewer food and drug interactions and do not require INR testing. Trial data have shown them to be equally effective and safer as compared to warfarin. However, these agents require dose reduction or avoidance in patients with renal impairment, elderly patients or those with low body weight.

Atrial flutter

Atrial flutter is often associated with AF. The atrial rate is typically 300 beats/min and the AV node usually conducts every second flutter beat, giving a ventricular rate of 150 beats/min. The ECG (Fig. 10.11A) characteristically shows 'sawtooth' flutter waves (F waves), which are most clearly seen when AV conduction is transiently impaired by carotid sinus massage or drugs. The treatment of atrial flutter is similar to AF, except that most cases of flutter can be cured by radiofrequency catheter ablation of the re-entry circuit.

Ventricular tachyarrhythmias

Ventricular ectopic premature beats (extrasystoles)

These are asymptomatic or patients complain of extra beats, missed beats or heavy beats. The ectopic electrical activity is not conducted to the ventricles through the normal conducting tissue and thus the QRS complex on the ECG is widened, with a bizarre configuration (Fig. 10.12). Treatment is with β-blockers if symptomatic.

Sustained ventricular tachycardia

Ventricular tachycardia (VT) and ventricular fibrillation (VF) are usually associated with underlying heart disease. The ECG in sustained VT (>30 s) shows a rapid ventricular rhythm with broad abnormal QRS complexes. Supraventricular tachycardia with bundle branch block also produces a broad complex tachycardia, which can sometimes be differentiated from VT on ECG criteria (Table 10.3). However, the majority of broad complex tachycardias are VT and if in doubt treat as such. Urgent DC cardioversion is necessary if the patient

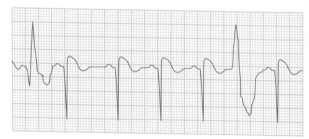

Fig. 10.12 A rhythm strip demonstrating two ventricular ectopic beats of different morphology (multimorphological).

is haemodynamically compromised (p. 422). If there is no haemodynamic compromise, treatment of VT is usually with intravenous β-blockers (esmolol) or amiodarone (p. 491). Recurrence is prevented with β-blockers or an implantable cardioverter–defibrillator (ICD). This is a small device implanted behind the rectus abdominis and connected to the heart; it recognizes VT or VF and automatically delivers a defibrillation shock to the heart.

Non-sustained ventricular tachycardia

This is defined as VT ≥ 5 consecutive beats but lasting < 30 s. It is common in patients with heart disease (and in a few individuals with normal hearts). The treatments indicated are β-blockers in symptomatic patients or an ICD in patients with poor left ventricular function (ejection fraction < 30%) in whom it improves survival.

Ventricular fibrillation

VF is a very rapid and irregular ventricular activation (Fig. 10.13) with no mechanical effect and hence no cardiac output. The patient is pulseless and becomes rapidly unconscious, and respiration ceases (cardiac arrest). Treatment is immediate defibrillation (Emergency Box 10.1). Survivors of VF are, in the absence of an identifiable reversible cause (e.g. during the first 2 days of acute MI, severe metabolic disturbance), at high risk of sudden death and treatment is with an ICD.

Long QT syndrome

Ventricular repolarization (QT interval) is greatly prolonged (p. 416). The causes include congenital (mutations in sodium and potassium-channel genes), electrolyte disturbances (hypokalaemia, hypocalcaemia, hypomagnesaemia) and a variety of drugs (e.g. tricyclic antidepressants, phenothiazines and macrolide antibiotics). Symptoms are palpitations and syncope, as a result of a polymorphic VT (torsade de pointes, rapid irregular sharp QRS complexes that

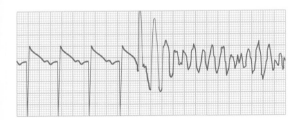

Fig. 10.13 A rhythm strip demonstrating four beats of sinus rhythm followed by a ventricular ectopic beat that initiates ventricular fibrillation. The ST segment is elevated owing to acute myocardial infarction.

✚ Emergency Box 10.1

Basic life support (BLS)

- Assess if patient is responsive – gently shake shoulders and ask loudly 'Are you alright?'
- If there is no response, move onto AIRWAY. Call for help and ask for AED.

Airway

- Turn the victim on his/her back on a firm surface.
- Open the airway using head tilt and chin lift – place your hand on victim's forehead and tilt the head back and with fingertips underneath the point of the chin, lift the chin to open the airway.

Breathing

- Keeping the airway open, look (chest movement), listen (breath sounds) and feel (victim's expired air on your cheek) for normal breathing. Assess for no more than 10 seconds.
- If victim is not breathing normally, start chest compressions (see below).
- After 30 chest compressions, give two rescue breaths: use head tilt and chin lift, pinch the nose closed, take a breath and create a seal with your lips around his mouth, exhale over 1 minute. Watch for the rise and fall of the patient's chest, indicating adequate ventilation.

Circulation

- Circulation is assessed by palpation of the carotid pulse at the same time as assessing for respiratory effort.
- Circulation is achieved by external chest compression.
- Place the heel of one hand in the centre of the victim's chest. Place the heel of your other hand on top of the first hand. Interlock the fingers of your hands and with straight arms press down on the sternum 5–6 cm. After each compression, release all the pressure on the chest.
- Continue with chest compressions and rescue breaths in a ratio of 30:2 with 100–120 compressions per minute.
- Attach AED pads. AED assesses rhythm and delivers shock if indicated. Immediately resume CPR.

Advanced life support (ALS)

- Institute as soon as help arrives; continue cardiac massage throughout except during actual defibrillation.
- Give 100% O_2 via Ambu-bag, intubate as soon as possible and initiate positive-pressure ventilation.
- Establish intravenous access and connect ECG leads.
- Drugs administered by the peripheral route should be followed by a flush of 20 mL of 0.9% saline.
- If intravenous access not possible, give drugs by the intraosseous route (tibia and humerus).

Advanced life-support algorithm*

Unresponsive?

↓

Open airway
Look for signs of life

→ Call resuscitation team

↓

CPR 30:2
Until defibrillator/monitor attached

↓

Assess rhythm

Shockable
(VF/pulseless VT)

Non-shockable
(PEA/asystole)

1 shock
150–200J biphasic for 1st shock, 150–300J for subsequent shocks

↓

Immediately resume:
CPR 30:2 for 2 min

During CPR
- Correct reversible causes*
- Check electrode position and contact
- Attempt/verify:
  IV access
  airway and oxygen
- Give adrenaline 1 mg i.v. immediately in PEA/asystole
- Give adrenaline 1 mg and amiodarone 300 mg after 3rd shock in VF
- Give adrenaline every 3–5 min in all cases

Immediately resume:
CPR 30:2 for 2 min

*Reversible causes
- Hypoxia
- Hypovolaemia
- Hyper/hypokalaemia/ metabolic
- Hypothermia
- Tension pneumothorax
- Tamponade, cardiac
- Toxins
- Thrombosis (coronary or pulmonary)

AED, Automated External Defibrillator; CPR, cardiopulmonary resuscitation; EMD, electromechanical dissociation; VF/VT, ventricular fibrillation/ventricular tachycardia; PEA, Pulseless Electrical Activity.

*Reproduced with permission from the Resuscitation Council; http://www.resus.org.uk

continuously change from an upright to an inverted position on the ECG), that usually terminates spontaneously but may degenerate into VF. In acquired cases, treatment is that of the underlying cause and intravenous isoprenaline.

Cardiac arrest

In cardiac arrest there is no effective cardiac output. The patient is unconscious and apnoeic with absent arterial pulses (best felt in the carotid artery in the neck). Irreversible brain damage occurs within 3 minutes if an adequate circulation is not established. Management is described in Emergency Box 10.1. Resuscitation is stopped when there is return of spontaneous circulation and a pulse, or further attempts at resuscitation are deemed futile. Post-resuscitation care centres on maintaining arterial oxygen saturation (94–98%), blood glucose values <10 mmol/L and therapeutic hypothermia.

Prognosis In many patients resuscitation is unsuccessful, particularly in those who collapse out of hospital and are brought into hospital in an arrested state. In patients who are successfully resuscitated, the prognosis is often poor because they have severe underlying heart diseases. The exceptions are those who are successfully resuscitated from a VF arrest in the early stages of MI, when the prognosis is much the same as for other patients with an infarct.

Studies suggest that therapeutic hypothermia (32–34°C for 12–24 hours) might improve neurological outcomes in unconscious adult patients with spontaneous circulation after an out-of-hospital cardiac arrest due to ventricular fibrillation.

HEART FAILURE

Heart failure is a complex syndrome that can result from any structural or functional cardiac disorder that impairs the ability of the heart to function as a pump and maintain sufficient cardiac output to meet the demands of the body. It is a common condition, with an estimated annual incidence of 10% in patients over 65 years. The long-term outcome is poor and approximately 50% of patients are dead within 5 years.

Aetiology

Ischaemic heart disease is the most common cause in the developed world and hypertension is the most common cause in Africa (Table 10.5). Any factor that increases myocardial work (arrhythmias, anaemia, hyperthyroidism, pregnancy, obesity) may aggravate existing heart failure or initiate failure.

Pathophysiology

When the heart fails, compensatory mechanisms attempt to maintain cardiac output and peripheral perfusion. However, as heart failure progresses, the mechanisms are overwhelmed and become pathophysiological. These mechanisms involve the following factors.

Table 10.5 Causes of heart failure

Main causes
Ischaemic heart disease
Cardiomyopathy (dilated)
Hypertension
Other causes
Cardiomyopathy (hypertrophic, restrictive)
Valvular heart disease (mitral, aortic, tricuspid)
Congenital heart disease (atrial septal defect, ventricular septal defect)
Alcohol and chemotherapy, e.g. imatinib, doxorubicin
Hyperdynamic circulation (anaemia, thyrotoxicosis, Paget's disease)
Right heart failure (RV infarct, pulmonary hypertension, pulmonary embolism, cor pulmonale, COPD)
Severe bradycardia or tachycardia
Pericardial disease (constrictive pericarditis, pericardial effusion)
Infections (Chagas' disease)
COPD, chronic obstructive pulmonary disease; RV, right ventricle.

Activation of the sympathetic nervous system

Activation of the sympathetic nervous system improves ventricular function by increasing heart rate and myocardial contractility. Constriction of venous capacitance vessels redistributes flow centrally, and the increased venous return to the heart (preload) further augments ventricular function via the Starling mechanism (Fig. 10.14). Sympathetic stimulation, however, also leads to arteriolar constriction; this increases the afterload, which eventually reduces cardiac output.

Renin–angiotensin system

The fall in cardiac output and increased sympathetic tone lead to diminished renal perfusion, activation of the renin–angiotensin system and hence increased fluid retention. Salt and water retention further increases venous pressure and maintains stroke volume by the Starling mechanism (see Fig. 10.14). As salt and water retention increases, however, peripheral and pulmonary congestion causes oedema and contributes to dyspnoea. Angiotensin II also causes arteriolar constriction, thus increasing the afterload and the work of the heart.

Natriuretic peptides

Natriuretic peptides are released from the atria (atrial natriuretic peptide [ANP]), ventricles (brain natriuretic peptide [BNP] – so-called because it was first

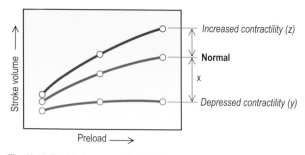

Fig. 10.14 The Starling curve. Starling's law states that the stroke volume is directly proportional to the diastolic filling (i.e. the preload or ventricular end-diastolic pressure). As the preload is increased, the stroke volume rises (normal). Increasing contractility (e.g. increased with sympathetic stimulation) shifts the curve upwards and to the left (z). If the ventricle is overstretched, the stroke volume will fall (x). In heart failure (y) the ventricular function curve is relatively flat, so that increasing the preload has only a small effect on cardiac output.

discovered in the brain) and vascular endothelium (C-type peptide). They have diuretic, natriuretic and hypotensive properties. The effect of their action may represent a beneficial, albeit inadequate, compensatory response leading to reduced cardiac load (preload and afterload). The N terminal fragment released from pro-BNP (NTproBNP) and BNP itself correlate with the severity of heart failure and they are therefore predictors of cardiovascular events and mortality. There is increasing interest in monitoring levels to help guide heart failure therapy.

Ventricular dilatation

Myocardial failure leads to a reduction of the volume of blood ejected with each heartbeat, and thus an increase in the volume of blood remaining after systole. The increased diastolic volume stretches the myocardial fibres and, as Starling's law would suggest, myocardial contraction is restored. Once heart failure is established, however, the compensatory effects of cardiac dilatation become limited by the flattened contour of Starling's curve. Eventually the increased venous pressure contributes to the development of pulmonary and peripheral oedema. In addition, as ventricular diameter increases, greater tension is required in the myocardium to expel a given volume of blood, and oxygen requirements increase.

Ventricular remodelling

This is a process of hypertrophy, loss of myocytes and increased interstitial fibrosis which all contribute to progressive and irreversible pump (contractile) failure. The process is multifactorial and includes apoptosis of myocytes and changes in cardiac contractile gene expression (e.g. myosin).

Clinical features

Most patients with heart failure present insidiously.

The clinical syndromes are:

- *Left ventricular systolic dysfunction (LVSD)* (or heart failure and a reduced ejection fraction) – commonly caused by ischaemic heart disease, but can also occur with valvular heart disease and hypertension.
- *Right ventricular systolic dysfunction (RVSD)* – occurs secondary to LVSD, with primary and secondary pulmonary hypertension, right ventricular infarction and adult congenital heart disease.
- *Diastolic heart failure* (or heart failure with normal ejection fraction) – a syndrome consisting of symptoms and signs of heart failure but with a normal or near-normal left ventricular ejection fraction (above 45–50%) and evidence of diastolic dysfunction on echocardiography (e.g. abnormal left ventricular relaxation and filling, usually with left ventricular hypertrophy). This leads to impairment of diastolic ventricular filling and hence decreased cardiac output. Diastolic heart failure is more common in elderly hypertensive patients but may occur with primary cardiomyopathies.

Symptoms

Symptoms include exertional dyspnoea, orthopnoea, paroxysmal nocturnal dyspnoea and fatigue.

Signs

There is one or more of the following: tachycardia, elevated jugular venous pulse (JVP), cardiomegaly with a displaced apex beat, third and fourth heart sounds, bi-basal lung crackles, pleural effusion, ankle oedema (plus sacral oedema in bed-bound patients), ascites and tender hepatomegaly.

The NYHA classification of heart failure (Table 10.6) is useful in the assessment of severity and the response to therapy.

Table 10.6 New York Heart Association classification of heart failure

Class 1	No limitation. Normal physical exercise does not cause fatigue, dyspnoea or palpitations
Class II	Mild limitation. Comfortable at rest but normal physical activity produces fatigue, dyspnoea or palpitations
Class III	Marked limitation. Comfortable at rest but less gentle physical activity produces marked symptoms of heart failure
Class IV	Symptoms of heart failure occur at rest and are exacerbated by any physical activity

Investigations

The aim of investigation in a patient with symptoms and signs of heart failure is to objectively show evidence of cardiac dysfunction (usually by echocardiography) and to establish the cause (Fig. 10.15):

- *Chest X-ray* shows cardiac enlargement and features of left ventricular failure (p. 412), but can be normal.
- *ECG* may show evidence of underlying causes, e.g. arrhythmias, ischaemia, left ventricular hypertrophy in hypertension.
- *Blood tests.* Full blood count (to look for anaemia which may exacerbate heart failure), liver biochemistry (may be altered due to hepatic congestion), blood glucose (for diabetes), urea and electrolytes (as a baseline before starting diuretics and angiotensin-converting enzyme inhibitors [ACEIs]), and thyroid function tests (in the elderly and those with atrial fibrillation).

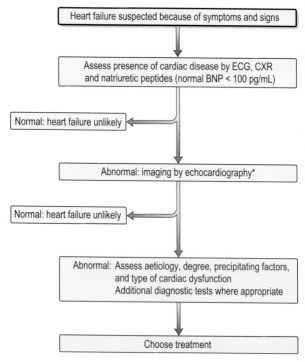

Fig. 10.15 Algorithm for the diagnosis of heart failure. BNP, brain natriuretic peptide; CXR, chest X-ray; ECG, electrocardiogram. Based on the European Society of Cardiology and NICE guidelines. *Prior to BNP testing in patients with previous myocardial infarction.

Normal plasma concentrations of BNP (<100 pg/mL) or NTproBNP (p. 437) exclude heart failure.

- *Echocardiography* is performed in all patients with new-onset heart failure. It allows an assessment of ventricular systolic and diastolic function, shows regional wall motion abnormalities and may reveal the aetiology of heart failure. An ejection fraction of <0.45 is usually accepted as evidence for systolic dysfunction.
- *Other investigations.* Cardiac catheterization, thallium perfusion imaging, positron emission tomography (PET) scanning, cardiac magnetic resonance imaging (MRI) or dobutamine stress echocardiography (p. 419) may be of benefit in selected patients to identify those with *hibernating myocardium* (a region of impaired myocardial contractility due to persistently impaired coronary blood flow) in whom revascularization will improve left ventricular function and long-term prognosis.

Treatment of chronic heart failure

Treatment is aimed at relieving symptoms, minimising cardiac dysfunction, retarding disease progression and improving quality and length of survival (Table 10.7).

Drug treatment

Vasodilator therapy

- *ACEIs* (p. 497), e.g. perindopril, lisinopril and rampiril, inhibit the production of angiotensin II, a potent vasoconstrictor, and increase concentrations of the vasodilator bradykinin. They enhance renal salt and water excretion and increase cardiac output by reducing afterload. They improve symptoms, limit the development of progressive heart failure and prolong survival, and should be given to all patients with heart failure. The major side effect is first-dose hypotension. ACEI treatment should be introduced gradually with a low initial dose and gradual titration every 2 days to full dose with regular BP monitoring and a check on serum potassium and renal function; creatinine levels normally rise by about 10–15% during ACEI therapy.
- *Angiotensin II type 1 receptor antagonists* (ARAs, p. 498) (e.g. losartan, irbesartan, candesartan and valsartan) block binding of angiotensin II to the type 1 receptor (AT1) and are indicated as second-line therapy in patients intolerant of ACEIs. Unlike ACEIs, they do not affect bradykinin metabolism and do not produce a cough. Both ACEIs and ARAs are contraindicated in patients with bilateral renal artery stenosis.
- *Vasodilators.* Isosorbide mononitrate (vasodilator reduces preload) in combination with hydralazine (arteriolar vasodilator reduces afterload) improves symptoms and survival and is used in patients intolerant of ACEIs and ARAs. Ivabradine is also used.

Table 10.7 Summary of the management of chronic heart failure

General measures*

Education of patients and family

Physical activity: reduce during exacerbations to reduce work of the heart. Encourage low-level (e.g. 20- to 30-minute walks three to five times weekly) with compensated heart failure

Diet and social: weight reduction if necessary, no added salt diet, avoid alcohol (negative inotropic effects), stop smoking (p. 512)

Vaccinate against pneumococcal disease and influenza

Correct aggravating factors, e.g. arrhythmias, anaemia, hypertension and pulmonary infections

Driving: unrestricted, except symptomatic heart failure disqualifies driving large lorries and buses

Sexual activity: tell patients on nitrates not to take phosphodiesterase type 5 inhibitors

Pharmacological treatment

ACEI (or ARA)*

β-Blocker*

Diuretic

Spironolactone/eplerenone

Digoxin

Vasodilators

Inotropic agents

Non-pharmacological treatment (in selected cases)

Revascularization (coronary artery bypass graft)

Cardiac resynchronization therapy (biventricular pacing)

Implantable cardioverter–defibrillator

Replacement of diseased valves

Repair of congenital heart disease

Cardiac transplantation

Left ventricular assist device and artificial heart (bridge to transplantation)

ACEI, angiotensin-converting enzyme inhibitor; ARA, angiotensin II receptor antagonist.
*In all patients. ACEI (ARA) and β-blockers improve prognosis.

β-Blockers Bisoprolol, carvedilol and nebivolol (p. 495) improve symptoms and reduce cardiovascular mortality in patients with chronic stable heart failure. This effect is thought to arise through blockade of the chronically activated sympathetic system. They are started at a low dose and gradually titrated upwards.

Diuretics (see Table 8.4 and p. 351) are used in patients with fluid overload. They act by promoting renal sodium excretion, with enhanced water excretion as a secondary effect. The resulting loss of fluid reduces ventricular filling pressures (preload) and thus decreases pulmonary and systemic congestion.

- *Loop diuretics*, e.g. furosemide (20–40 mg daily, maximum 250–500 mg daily) and bumetanide, are potent diuretics used in moderate/severe heart failure. When given intravenously, they also induce venodilatation, a beneficial action independent of their diuretic effect.
- *Thiazide diuretics*, e.g. bendroflumethiazide (2.5 mg daily, maximum 10 mg daily), are mild diuretics that inhibit sodium reabsorption in the distal renal tubule. The exception is metolazone (2.5 mg daily, maximum 10 mg daily), which causes a profound diuresis and is only used in severe and resistant heart failure.
- *Aldosterone antagonists.* Spironolactone and eplerenone are relatively weak diuretics with a potassium-sparing action. Spironolactone (25 mg daily) in combination with conventional treatment improves survival in patients with moderate/severe heart failure and should be given to all these patients. However, gynaecomastia or breast pain is a common side effect. Eplerenone reduces mortality in patients with acute MI and heart failure.

Digoxin is indicated in patients with heart failure and atrial fibrillation. It is also used as add-on therapy in patients in sinus rhythm who remain symptomatic despite standard treatment (vasodilators, β-blockers, diuretics).

Inotropes (p. 579) are occasionally used in patients not responding to oral medication.

Non-pharmacological treatment

Revascularization Coronary artery disease is the most common cause of heart failure. Revascularization with angioplasty and stenting or surgery can result in improvement in regional abnormalities in wall motion in up to one-third of patients and may thus have a role to play in some individuals.

Cardiac resynchronization therapy (also known as biventricular pacing) aims to improve the coordination of the atria and both ventricles. It is indicated for patients with left ventricular systolic dysfunction who have moderate or severe symptoms of heart failure and a widened QRS on ECG.

Implantable cardioverter–defibrillator (ICD) is indicated for patients with symptomatic ventricular arrhythmias or left ventricular ejection fraction < 30% on optimal medical therapy. Sudden death from ventricular tachyarrhythmias is reduced.

Cardiac transplantation is the treatment of choice for younger patients with severe intractable heart failure and a life expectancy of < 6 months. The expected 1-year survival following transplantation is over 90%, with 75% alive at 5 years. Death is usually the result of operative mortality, organ rejection and overwhelming infection secondary to immunosuppressive treatment. After this time the greatest threat to health is accelerated coronary atherosclerosis, the cause of which is unknown.

Prognosis

There is usually a gradual deterioration necessitating increased doses of diuretics, and sometimes admission to hospital. The prognosis is poor in those with severe heart failure (i.e. breathless at rest or on minimal exertion), with a 1-year survival rate of 50%.

Acute heart failure

Acute heart failure is a medical emergency, with left or right heart failure developing over minutes or hours. Aetiology is similar to chronic heart failure and initial investigations are similar (ECG, chest X-ray, blood tests, transthoracic echocardiogram) with additional blood tests of serum troponin (for myocardial necrosis) and D-dimer (for evidence of pulmonary embolism).

Clinical features

Several clinical syndromes are defined:

- Acute decompensation of chronic heart failure
- Hypertensive heart failure – high BP, preserved left ventricular function, pulmonary oedema on chest X-ray
- Acute pulmonary oedema – acutely breathless, tachycardia, profuse sweating (sympathetic overactivity), wheezes and crackles throughout the chest, hypoxia, pulmonary oedema on chest X-ray
- Cardiogenic shock – hypotension, tachycardia, oliguria, cold extremities
- High output cardiac failure – e.g. septic shock, warm peripheries, pulmonary congestion, BP may be low
- Right heart failure – low cardiac output, elevated jugular venous pressure, hepatomegaly, hypotension.

Management

In many cases the patient is so unwell that treatment (Emergency Box 10.2) must begin before the investigations are completed. Patients are managed in a high dependency unit. All require prophylactic anticoagulation, e.g. enoxaparin (p. 247). Some patients will require central venous cannulation, arterial lines and pulmonary artery cannulation for monitoring and to direct therapy. Initial therapy includes oxygen, diuretics (furosemide 50 mg i.v.) and vasodilator therapy (glyceryl trinitrate intravenous infusion 50 mg in 50 mL 0.9% saline at 2–10 mL/h) providing systolic BP is > 85 mmHg. Inotropic support can be added in patients who do not respond to initial therapy (p. 579). Mechanical assist devices can be used in patients who fail to respond to standard medical therapy but in whom there is transient myocardial dysfunction with likelihood of recovery.

Emergency Box 10.2

Management of acute heart failure with systolic dysfunction

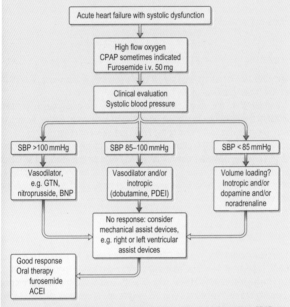

ACEI, angiotensin-converting enzyme inhibitor; BNP, brain natriuretic peptide; CPAP, continuous positive airway pressure (p. 584); GTN, glyceryl trinitrate; PDEI, phosphodies-terase inhibitor; SBP, systolic blood pressure.

ISCHAEMIC HEART DISEASE

Myocardial ischaemia results from an imbalance between the supply of oxygen to cardiac muscle and myocardial demand. The most common cause is coronary artery atheroma (coronary artery disease), which results in a fixed obstruction to coronary blood flow. Less common causes of myocardial ischaemia are coronary artery thrombosis, spasm or, rarely, arteritis (e.g. polyarteritis). Increased demand for oxygen due to an increase in cardiac output occurs in thyrotoxicosis or myocardial hypertrophy (e.g. from aortic stenosis or hypertension).

Coronary artery disease (CAD) is the single largest cause of death in many parts of the world, including the UK. However, in the last decade the mortality rate in the UK has fallen. Atheroma consists of atherosclerotic plaques (an accumulation of lipid, macrophages and smooth muscle cells in the intima of arteries) which narrow the lumen of the artery. The risk factors, listed below, contribute to the development of atheroma through vascular endothelial dysfunction, biochemical abnormalities, immunological factors and inflammation. Some of these risk factors cannot be changed, i.e. they are irreversible, and others can be modified.

Irreversible risk factors for coronary artery disease

Age CAD rate increases with age. It rarely presents in the young, except in familial hyperlipidaemia (p. 693).

Gender Men are more often affected than pre-menopausal women, although the incidence in women after the menopause is similar to that in men, possible due to the loss of the protective effect of oestrogen.

Family history CAD is often present in several members of the same family. It is unclear, however, whether family history is an independent risk factor as so many other factors are familial. A positive family history refers to those in whom a first-degree relative has developed ischaemic heart disease before the age of 50 years.

Potentially changeable risk factors

Hyperlipidaemia The risk of CAD is directly related to serum cholesterol levels, but there is an inverse relationship with high-density lipoproteins (HDLs). High triglyceride levels are also independently linked with coronary atheroma. Lowering serum cholesterol slows the progression of coronary atherosclerosis and causes regression of the disease.

Cigarette smoking increases the risk of CAD, more so in men. The risk from smoking declines to almost normal after 10 years of abstention.

Hypertension (systolic and diastolic) is linked to an increased incidence of CAD.

Metabolic factors Diabetes mellitus, an abnormal glucose tolerance, raised fasting glucose, lack of exercise and obesity have all been linked to an increased incidence of atheroma.

Diets high in fats (particularly saturated fat intake) and low in antioxidant intake (fruit and vegetables) are associated with CAD.

Other risk factors Lack of exercise, psychosocial factors (work stress, lack of social support, depression), elevated serum C-reactive protein (CRP) levels (as an inflammatory marker), high alcohol intake and coagulation factors (high levels of fibrinogen, factor VII and homocysteine) are also associated with CAD, while moderate alcohol consumption (one to two drinks per day) is associated with a reduced risk of CAD.

Estimation of cardiovascular risk

Atherosclerotic disease manifest in one vascular bed is often advanced in other territories. Patients with intermittent claudication have a two- to four-fold increased risk of CAD, stroke or heart failure. Following MI, there is a three- to six-fold increase in the risk of heart failure and stroke. Patients with symptomatic cardiovascular disease therefore require intense lifestyle and drug therapy to improve their modifiable risk factors, i.e. secondary prevention. The cardiovascular disease risk for asymptomatic apparently healthy people can be estimated using prediction charts which take into account a number of risk factors, e.g. diabetes mellitus, BP and lipid profile. In the UK, NICE guidelines recommend that primary care should use the QRISK2 risk assessment tool to target high-risk people (10-year risk of cardiovascular disease $\geq 10\%$) for primary preventative measures.

Angina

Angina pectoris is a descriptive term for chest pain arising from the heart as a result of myocardial ischaemia.

Clinical features

Angina is usually described as a central, crushing, retrosternal chest pain, coming on with exertion and relieved by rest within a few minutes. It is often exacerbated by cold weather, anger and excitement, and it frequently radiates to the arms and neck. Variants of classic angina include:

- *Decubitus angina* – occurs on lying down.
- *Nocturnal angina* – occurs at night and may waken the patient from sleep.
- *Variant (Prinzmetal's) angina* – caused by coronary artery spasm and results in angina that occurs without provocation, usually at rest.
- *Unstable angina* – increases rapidly in severity, occurs at rest, or is of recent onset (less than 1 month) (see Acute coronary syndromes).
- *Cardiac syndrome* X – patients with symptoms of angina, a positive exercise test and normal coronary arteries on angiogram. It is thought to result from functional abnormalities of the coronary microcirculation. The prognostic and therapeutic implications are not known.

  Physical examination in patients with angina is often normal, but must include a search for risk factors (e.g. hypertension and xanthelasma occurring in hyperlipidaemia) and underlying causes (e.g. aortic stenosis).

Diagnosis

The diagnosis of angina is largely based on the clinical history. Occasionally, chest wall pain or oesophageal reflux causes diagnostic confusion.

Investigations

- Resting ECG may show ST segment depression and T-wave flattening or inversion during an attack. The ECG is usually normal between attacks.
- Exercise ECG testing is positive (p. 418) in most people with CAD, but a normal test does not exclude the diagnosis. ST segment depression (>1 mm) at a low workload (within 6 minutes of starting the Bruce protocol) or a paradoxical fall in BP with exercise usually indicates severe CAD and is an indication for coronary angiography.
- Other testing protocols (pharmacological stress testing with myocardial perfusion imaging or stress echocardiography [p. 419]) are used in patients who cannot exercise or have baseline ECG abnormalities that can interfere with interpretation of the exercise ECG test. They may also be helpful in patients with an equivocal exercise test.
- Coronary angiography (p. 421) is occasionally used in patients with chest pain where the diagnosis of angina is uncertain. More commonly it is used to delineate the exact coronary anatomy before coronary intervention (p. 449) or surgery is considered. CT coronary angiography and CMR are also being increasingly used to provide information about coronary anatomy.

Management

This is two-fold:

- Identify and treat risk factors for CAD and offer secondary prevention
- Symptomatic treatment of angina.

Secondary prevention Patients with angina are at a high risk of experiencing subsequent cardiovascular events, including MI, sudden death and stroke. Modification of risk factors has a beneficial effect on subsequent morbidity and mortality, and includes smoking cessation, control of hypertension, maintaining ideal body weight, regular exercise and glycaemic control in diabetes mellitus. In addition, aspirin and statins reduce subsequent risk:

- Aspirin (75 mg daily, p. 246) inhibits platelet cyclo-oxygenase and formation of the aggregating agent thromboxane A_2, and reduces the risk of coronary events in patients with CAD. Clopidogrel (75 mg daily, p. 246) is an alternative when aspirin is not tolerated, or is contraindicated.
- Lipid-lowering agents reduce mortality and incidence of MI in patients with CAD and should be used in patients to achieve a cholesterol level of less than 5.0 mmol/L. Guidelines on introduction of lipid-lowering therapy are illustrated on page 694. A statin (p. 701) is used unless the triglycerides are above 3.5 mmol/L, in which case a fibrate is indicated.

Symptomatic treatment Acute attacks are treated with sublingual glyceryl trinitrate tablet or spray (p. 499). Patients should be encouraged to use this before exertion, rather than waiting for the pain to develop. The main side effect is a severe bursting headache, which is relieved by inactivating the tablet either by swallowing or spitting it out.

Most patients will require regular prophylactic therapy. Nitrates, β-blockers or calcium antagonists are most commonly used (p. 501), with treatment being tailored to the individual patient. Some patients will require combination therapy and revascularization for those not controlled on medical therapy:

- *β-Adrenergic blocking drugs* (p. 495), e.g. atenolol and metoprolol, reduce heart rate and the force of ventricular contraction, both of which reduce myocardial oxygen demand.

- *Calcium antagonists* (p. 501), e.g. diltiazem, amlodipine, block calcium influx into the cell and the utilization of calcium within the cell. They relax the coronary arteries and reduce the force of left ventricular contraction, thereby reducing oxygen demand. The side effects (postural dizziness, headache, ankle oedema) are the result of systemic vasodilatation. High-dose nifedipine increases mortality and should not be used in this situation.

- *Nitrates* (p. 499) reduce venous and intracardiac diastolic pressure, reduce impedance to the emptying of the left ventricle, and dilate coronary arteries. They are available in a variety of slow-release preparations, including infiltrated skin plasters, buccal pellets and long-acting oral nitrate preparations, e.g. isosorbide mononitrate, isosorbide dinitrate. The major side effect is headache, which tends to diminish with continued use.

- *Other treatments* are usually reserved for patients where there are contraindications or inadequate response to the above agents. *Nicorandil* combines nitrate-like activity with potassium-channel blockade; it has both arterial and venous vasodilating properties. *Ranolazine* interacts with sodium channels and can improve exercise tolerance but causes QT prolongation. *Ivabradine* inhibits the cardiac pacemaker I_f current and lowers the heart rate. It is used in patients who have a contraindication or intolerance of β-blockers.

When angina persists or worsens in spite of general measures and optimal medical treatment, patients should be considered for coronary artery bypass grafting (CABG) or percutaneous coronary intervention.

Percutaneous coronary intervention (PCI) Localized atheromatous lesions are dilated at cardiac catheterization using small inflatable balloons. Stent placement reduces the risk of restenosis. Studies support an initial strategy of optimal medical management in patients with stable angina symptoms, but revascularization should be considered in patients who remain symptomatic despite two anti-anginals. This technique is most useful for isolated, proximal, non-calcified atheromatous plaques. Complications include death, acute MI, the need for urgent CABG and restenosis. Dual antiplatelet therapy with aspirin and clopidogrel is routinely given (p. 246) for 6–12 months. The addition of the antiplatelet glycoprotein IIb/IIIa antagonists (tirofiban, eptifibatide, abciximab) has further reduced periprocedural complications. Drug-eluting stents which release antiproliferative agents (sirolimus, paclitaxel) reduce restenosis rates still further but there is a risk of late stent thrombosis. Bare metal stents may be preferred in patients requiring anticoagulation and early surgery.

Coronary artery bypass grafting The left or right internal mammary artery is used to bypass stenoses in the left anterior descending or right coronary artery, respectively. Less commonly, the saphenous vein from the leg is anastomosed between the proximal aorta and coronary artery distal to the obstruction. Surgery successfully relieves angina in about 90% of cases and, when performed for left main stem obstruction or three-vessel disease, an improved lifespan and quality of life can be expected. Operative mortality rate is less than 1%. In most patients the angina eventually recurs because of accelerated atherosclerosis in the graft (particularly vein grafts), which can be treated by stenting. CABG is recommended for patients with triple vessel coronary artery disease and impaired left ventricular function (left ventricular ejection fraction [LVEF] 35–49%). Left stem disease with a stenosis of $\geq 50\%$ is also an indication for revascularization.

Acute coronary syndromes

Acute coronary syndromes (ACSs) encompass a spectrum of unstable coronary artery disease. The mechanism common to all ACSs is rupture or erosion of the fibrous cap of a coronary artery atheromatous plaque with subsequent formation of a platelet-rich clot and vasoconstriction produced by platelet release of serotonin and thromboxane A_2. Patients with ACS include those whose clinical presentations cover the following diagnoses:

- Unstable angina
- Non-ST-elevation MI (NSTEMI)
- ST-elevation MI (STEMI).

Unstable angina differs from NSTEMI in that in the latter the occluding thrombus is sufficient to cause myocardial damage and an elevation in serum markers of myocardial injury (troponin and creatine kinase). In patients presenting with symptoms suggestive of ACS, serum troponin should be measured on arrival at hospital and at 12 hours after the onset of symptoms; a normal serum troponin at 12 hours suggests unstable angina rather than MI. In both unstable angina and NSTEMI the ECG may be normal or show evidence of ischaemia with T-wave inversion and/or ST segment depression. Both unstable angina and NSTEMI may be complicated by MI with ST segment elevation (STEMI) if treatment is inadequate. In STEMI there is complete occlusion of the coronary artery by thrombus with usually more severe symptoms, typical ECG changes of MI (Fig. 10.16) and elevated troponin and creatine kinase (pp. 453–457).

Clinical features

The diagnosis of ACS is made in a patient with worsening pain on minimal exertion, chest pain at rest, or chest pain unrelieved in the usual time by nitrates or rest. In some patients, chest pain is absent and presentation is with collapse, arrhythmia or new-onset heart failure. Other causes of chest pain must be considered in all patients, e.g. aortic dissection, musculoskeletal pain, gastro-oesophageal reflux disease.

Treatment of NSTEMI and unstable angina

Emergency Box 10.3 summarizes the initial investigation and management of patients presenting with suspected ACS.

- *Antiplatelet therapy.* In the absence of contraindications, aspirin (300 mg initially, then 75 mg daily, p. 246) is indicated in all patients. It reduces the risk of subsequent vascular events and deaths and is continued indefinitely. Clopidogrel (300 mg initially, then 75 mg daily for 12 months, p. 246) or prasugrel (60 mg initially then 10 mg o.d.) or ticagrelor (180 mg initially then 90 mg b.d.). Platelet glycoprotein IIb/IIIa receptor inhibitors (e.g. abciximab, tirofiban) are added for high-risk patients.
- *Antithrombins.* Heparin interferes with thrombus formation at the site of plaque rupture and reduces the risk of ischaemic events and death. Low molecular weight heparin, e.g. enoxaparin (1 mg/kg s.c. twice daily [p. 247]), has better efficacy than unfractionated heparin. Treatment should be for at least 48 hours. The synthetic pentasaccharide, fondaparinux, inhibits factor Xa of the coagulation cascade. It has a lower risk of bleeding than heparin and may become the antithrombin of choice in ACS. Bivalirudin reversibly binds to and inhibits clot-bound thrombin.
- *Anti-ischaemia agents.* Nitrates (p. 495) are given sublingually or by intravenous infusion with continuing pain for 24–48 hours. β-blockers (p. 495), e.g. metoprolol, are the first-line oral anti-anginal of choice given their secondary preventative effects in CAD.
- *Plaque stabilization.* Statins (p. 701) and an ACEI (p. 497) are continued long term and reduce future cardiovascular events.

Oral medication is continued indefinitely after hospital discharge, with the exception of clopidogrel, which is stopped after 12 months.

Risk stratification

There are several risk stratification scoring systems (e.g. Thrombolysis in Myocardial Infarction [TIMI] and the Global Registry of Acute Coronary Events [GRACE]) that can predict subsequent risk of STEMI and death in patients with unstable angina/NSTEMI and provide a basis for therapeutic decision-making. The TIMI score is shown in Table 10.8. The GRACE score includes age, heart rate, systolic BP and serum creatinine. Early coronary angiography with a view to surgery or PCI is recommended in patients at intermediate/high risk. Coronary stenting may stabilize the disrupted coronary plaque and reduces angiographic restenosis rates compared to angioplasty alone. Low-risk patients should have a cardiac stress test (p. 448), usually an exercise ECG, if they remain pain-free with no evidence of ischaemia, heart failure or arrhythmias.

Emergency Box 10.3

Immediate management of acute coronary syndrome (ACS)

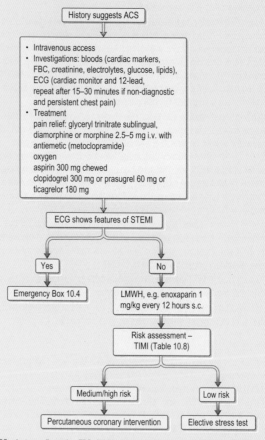

ECG, electrocardiography; FBC, full blood count; LMWH, low-molecular-weight heparin; STEMI, ST segment elevation myocardial infarction; TIMI, thrombolysis in myocardial infarction.

Table 10.8 The Thrombolysis in Myocardial Infarction (TIMI) risk score in acute coronary syndrome

Risk factor	Score*
Age > 65 years	1
More than three coronary artery disease risk factors – hypertension, hyperlipidaemia, family history, diabetes, smoking	1
Known CAD (stenosis of ≥ 50% on angiography)	1
Aspirin use in the last 7 days	1
At least two episodes of rest pain in the last 24 hours	1
ST deviation on admission ECG (horizontal ST depression or transient ST elevation > 1 mm)	1
Elevated cardiac markers (creatine kinase-myocardial bound or troponin)	1

CAD, coronary artery disease; ECG, electrocardiogram.
*Low risk = score 0–2. Intermediate risk = score 3–4. High risk = score 5–7.

ST segment elevation myocardial infarction (STEMI)

MI is the most common cause of death in developed countries. It is almost always the result of rupture of an atherosclerotic plaque, with the development of thrombosis and total occlusion of the artery.

Clinical features

Central chest pain similar to that occurring in angina is the most common presenting symptom. Unlike angina, it usually occurs at rest, is more severe and lasts for some hours. The pain may radiate to the left arm, neck or jaw and is often associated with sweating, breathlessness, nausea, vomiting and restlessness. There may be no physical signs unless complications develop (p. 457), although the patient often appears pale, sweaty and grey. About 20% of patients have no pain, and such 'silent' infarctions either go unnoticed or present with hypotension, arrhythmias or pulmonary oedema. This occurs most commonly in elderly patients or those with diabetes or hypertension.

Investigations

The diagnosis is made on the basis of the clinical history and early ECG appearances. Serial changes (over 3 days) in the ECG and serum levels of cardiac markers confirm the diagnosis and allow an assessment of infarct size (on the magnitude of the enzyme and protein rise, and extent of ECG changes). A normal ECG in the early stages does not exclude the diagnosis.

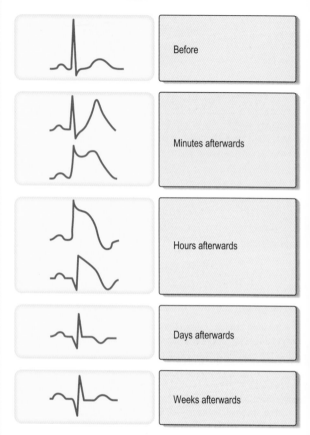

	Before
	Minutes afterwards
	Hours afterwards
	Days afterwards
	Weeks afterwards

Fig. 10.16 Electrocardiographic evolution of myocardial infarction. After the first few minutes, the T waves become tall, pointed and upright and there is ST segment elevation. After the first few hours, the T waves invert, the R wave voltage is decreased and Q waves develop. After a few days, the ST segment returns to normal. After weeks or months, the T wave may return to upright but the Q wave remains.

The ECG shows a characteristic pattern. Within hours there is ST segment elevation (>1 mm in two or more contiguous leads) followed by T-wave flattening or inversion (Fig. 10.16). Pathological Q waves are broad (>1 mm) and deep (>2 mm, or >25% of the amplitude of the following R wave) negative deflections that start the QRS complex. They develop because the infarcted muscle is electrically silent so that the recording leads 'look through' the infarcted area. This means that the electrical activity being recorded (on the opposite ventricular wall) is moving away from the electrode and is therefore negative. New LBBB is also an indicator of acute MI.

Typically, ECG changes are confined to the leads that 'face' the infarct. Leads II, III and AVF are involved in inferior infarcts; I, AVL and V_5–V_6 in lateral infarcts; and V_2–V_4 in anterior infarcts. As there are no posterior leads, a posterior wall infarct is diagnosed by the appearance of reciprocal changes in V_1 and V_2 (i.e. the development of tall initial R waves, ST segment depression and tall upright T waves). New or presumed new LBBB is also compatible with a diagnosis of MI.

Cardiac markers Necrotic cardiac muscle releases several enzymes and proteins into the systemic circulation:

- Troponin T and troponin I are regulatory proteins, highly specific and sensitive for cardiac muscle damage. They are released within hours of event onset, persist for several days, and are more sensitive and cardiac specific than CK-MB (the MB isoform of creatine kinase, which is found mainly in heart muscle).

Other investigations These include a chest X-ray, full blood count, serum urea and electrolytes, blood glucose and lipids (lipids taken within the first 12 hours reflect preinfarction levels, but after this time they are altered for up to 6 weeks).

Management

The aims of treatment are relief of pain, limitation of infarct size and treatment of complications. The immediate and subsequent management is summarized in Emergency Boxes 10.3 and 10.4. Treatment is urgent: prolonged times between symptom onset and treatment to recanalize the artery are associated with impaired ST-segment resolution, larger infarct sizes and higher mortality ('time is muscle').

Limitation of infarct size

Immediate primary angioplasty is the optimal treatment for recanalization of the infarct-related arteries (p. 421). When compared with thrombolysis (see below), PCI reduced mortality, re-infarction, recurrent ischaemia, stroke and the need for CABG. However, it is only a therapeutic option when rapid access to a catheterization laboratory is possible, the cardiologist is experienced in interventional cardiology and a full support team is immediately available. PCI is also used as 'rescue' therapy in patients who have received thrombolysis and who seem on clinical grounds not to have reperfused (ongoing chest pain and < 50% resolution of ST elevation 45–60 minutes after start of thrombolysis).

Fibrinolytic agents (thrombolysis) enhance the breakdown of occlusive thromboses by the activation of plasminogen to form plasmin. They are indicated where primary PCI is not available and there are no contraindications to thrombolysis (p. 251). Maximum benefit is derived from thrombolytic agents if they are given early ('time is muscle' – minutes count) and

➕ Emergency Box 10.4

Management of ST elevation myocardial infarction (STEMI)

Immediate management

- Immediate investigations and treatment (see Emergency Box 10.3).
- Reperfusion therapy: preferred therapy for patients presenting within 90 minutes of onset is primary angioplasty with dual antiplatelet therapy. If presenting after 90 minutes and within 12 hours (preferably 6 hours), treat with thrombolysis, e.g. double-bolus reteplase or single-bolus tenecteplase.
- Metoprolol (5 mg slow i.v. injection) if heart rate > 100 beats/min. Repeat every 15 minutes, titrated against heart rate and BP. Do not give if hypotension, heart failure, bradycardia, asthma.
- Insulin infusion if blood glucose > 11 mmol/L; aim for blood glucose of 7–10 mmol/L.
- Treat complications (p. 457).

Subsequent management of uncomplicated infarction

- Repeat ECG, serum cardiac markers and electrolytes at 24 and 48 hours after admission.
- Initiate secondary prevention therapy: aspirin, clopidogrel, statin, metoprolol, ACEI and modification of CAD risk factors (as for ACS).
- Transfer from CCU to medical ward after 48 hours.
- Mobilize gradually and discharge from hospital after 5 days.
- Submaximal exercise ECG test prior to discharge if primary angioplasty not performed.
- Refer to cardiac rehabilitation programme.
- No driving for 1 month; special assessment is required for heavy goods or public service licence holder before driving. Usually return to work in 2 months.

ACS, acute coronary syndrome; BP, blood pressure; CAD, coronary artery disease; CCU, coronary care unit; ECG, electrocardiography.

in some centres pre-hospital thrombolysis is used. There is little benefit of thrombolysis more than 12 hours after the onset of symptoms. Of the four thrombolytic agents available, reteplase and tenecteplase are preferred in the pre-hospital setting because they can be administered as a bolus intravenous injection. Streptokinase and alteplase are given by intravenous infusion. Streptokinase is the cheapest thrombolytic agent available but may induce the development of antistreptokinase antibodies and reduce the effectiveness of subsequent treatment. It should not be used beyond 4 days after first administration.

Mortality is increased in diabetic patients with MI, largely due to the high incidence of heart failure. This is due in part to metabolic changes which occur in the early stages of MI, and is reduced by rigorous control of blood glucose with insulin infusion, and monitoring with 2-hourly BM Stix. This regimen is also indicated in patients not known to be diabetic who have an admission blood glucose of > 11 mmol/L. β-Blockers reduce infarct size and the incidence of sudden death. Metoprolol (5–10 mg i.v.) should be given, particularly if the heart rate is greater than 100 beats/min and there is persistent pain.

Subsequent management ACEIs (or angiotensin receptor blocker if intolerant) reduce mortality and prevent the development of heart failure and should be started on the first day after MI. Treatment with ACEIs, aspirin, statin and β-blockers is continued indefinitely (see ACS for doses). Aldosterone antagonist, e.g. eplerenone 25 mg/day (p. 352), is given to patients with clinical evidence of heart failure and reduced ejection fraction on echocardiogram. Gradual mobilization takes place on the second day and if the patient is fully ambulant and pain-free, a submaximal exercise tolerance test is performed (70% of age-predicted maximal heart rate) before hospital discharge on day 5 or 6 in uncomplicated cases. Patients with test results suggesting ischaemia are referred for coronary angiography.

Complications (Table 10.9)

Disturbances of rate, rhythm and conduction (p. 421)

- *Atrial arrhythmias.* Sinus tachycardia is common; treatment is that of the underlying cause, particularly pain, anxiety and heart failure. Sinus

Table 10.9 Complications of myocardial infarction

Heart failure
Rupture of free wall of infarcted ventricle (usually fatal)
Rupture of the interventricular septum (ventricular septal defect)
Mitral regurgitation
Arrhythmias
Heart block
Pericarditis
Thromboembolism
Dressler's syndrome*
Ventricular aneurysm*
*May develop weeks or months after myocardial infarction.

bradycardia is especially associated with acute inferior wall MI. Treatment is initially with intravenous atropine (p. 422). Atrial fibrillation occurs in about 10% of cases and is usually a transient rhythm disturbance. Treatment with digoxin or β-blockers is indicated if the fast rate is exacerbating ischaemia or causing heart failure.

- *Ventricular arrhythmias.* Ventricular ectopic beats are common and may precede the development of VT or VF. Antiarrhythmic drug treatment has not been shown to affect progression to these more serious arrhythmias. VT may degenerate into VF (p. 433) or may itself produce shock or heart failure. Treatment of VT is with intravenous amiodarone (p. 491) or direct current cardioversion if there is hypotension. VF may be primary (occurring in the first 24–48 hours) or secondary (occurring late after infarction and associated with large infarcts and heart failure). Cardiac arrest requires defibrillation. Recurrences may be prevented with intravenous amiodarone. Late VT/VF is associated with a poor prognosis and a high incidence of sudden death, and is an indication for an implantable cardioverter-defibrillator (ICD).

- *Heart block occurring with inferior infarction* is common and usually resolves spontaneously. Some patients respond to intravenous atropine, but a temporary pacemaker may be necessary if the rhythm is very slow or producing symptoms.

- *Complete heart block occurring with anterior wall infarction* indicates the involvement of both bundle branches by extensive myocardial necrosis, and hence a very poor prognosis. The ventricular rhythm in this case is unreliable and a temporary pacing wire is necessary. Heart block is often permanent and a permanent pacing wire may be necessary.

Heart failure in a mild form occurs in up to 40% of patients following MI. Extensive infarction may cause acute heart failure (p. 444), which may also occur following rupture of the ventricular septum or mitral valve papillary muscle. Both conditions present with worsening heart failure, a systolic thrill and a loud pansystolic murmur. Mortality is high, and urgent surgical correction is often needed. Hypotension with a raised JVP is usually a complication of right ventricular infarction, which may occur with inferior wall infarcts. Initial treatment is with volume expansion, and pericardial effusion (which produces similar signs) should be ruled out on an echocardiogram.

Embolism Patients with severe left ventricular dysfunction, persistent AF or mural thrombus on echocardiography are at risk of embolism from left ventricular or left atrial clot and should be anticoagulated with warfarin to achieve a target INR of 2–3.

Pericarditis is characterized by sharp chest pain and a pericardial rub. Treatment is with non-steroidal anti-inflammatory drugs (NSAIDs) until spontaneous resolution occurs within 1–2 days. Late pericarditis (2–12 weeks after) with fever and a pericardial effusion (Dressler's syndrome) is rare and corticosteroids may be necessary in some patients.

Post-ACS drug therapy and assessment

A range of pharmaceuticals are advantageous in reducing mortality over the years following MI. Therefore post-MI most patients should be taking most of the following medications:

- Aspirin (75 mg o.d.)
- A second anti-platelet agent (e.g. clopidogrel)
- An oral β-blocker to maintain heart rate <60 beats/min
- ACEIs or angiotensin receptor blockers, particularly if left ventricular ejection fraction is below 40%
- High-intensity statins with target low-density lipoprotein (LDL) cholesterol < 1.8 mmol/L
- Aldosterone antagonist – post-MI with clinical evidence of heart failure and left ventricular ejection fraction ≤ 40% if the serum creatinine is < 221 μmol/L (men) or < 177 μmol/L (women) and the serum potassium < 5.0 mEq/L.

RHEUMATIC FEVER

Rheumatic fever is an inflammatory disease that usually has its first onset between 5 and 15 years of age as a result of infection with group A streptococci. It is a complication of less than 1% of streptococcal pharyngitis, developing 2–3 weeks after the onset of sore throat. It is thought to develop because of an autoimmune reaction triggered by the streptococci rather than direct infection of the heart.

Epidemiology

The incidence in developed countries has decreased dramatically since the 1920s as a result of improved sanitation, a change in the virulence of the organism and the use of antibiotics. The disease is more common in women than in men.

Clinical features

The disease presents suddenly, with fever, joint pains and loss of appetite. The major clinical features are as follows:

- Changing heart murmurs, mitral and aortic regurgitation, heart failure and chest pain, caused by carditis affecting all three layers of the heart
- Polyarthritis – fleeting and affecting the large joints, e.g. knees, ankles and elbows
- Skin manifestations – erythema marginatum (transient pink coalescent rings develop on the trunk) and small non-tender subcutaneous nodules which occur over tendons, joints and bony prominences
- Sydenham's chorea ('St Vitus' dance') indicates involvement of the central nervous system and presents with 'fidgety' and spasmodic, unintentional movements.

Investigations

Blood count shows a leucocytosis and a raised erythrocyte sedimentation rate (ESR).

The diagnosis is based on the revised Duckett Jones criteria, which depend on the combination of certain clinical features and evidence of recent streptococcal infection.

Treatment

Treatment is with complete bed rest and high-dose aspirin. Penicillin is given to eradicate residual streptococcal infection, and then long term to all patients with persistent cardiac damage.

Chronic rheumatic heart disease

More than 50% of those who suffer acute rheumatic fever with carditis will develop chronic rheumatic valvular disease 10–20 years later, predominantly affecting the mitral and aortic valves (pp. 461–467).

VALVULAR HEART DISEASE

Cardiac valves may be incompetent (regurgitant), stenotic or both. The most common problems are acquired left-sided valvular lesions: aortic stenosis, mitral stenosis, mitral regurgitation and aortic regurgitation. Abnormal valves produce turbulent blood flow, which is heard as a murmur on auscultation; a few murmurs are also felt as a thrill on palpation. Murmurs may sometimes be heard with normal hearts ('innocent murmurs'), often reflecting a hyperdynamic circulation, e.g. in pregnancy, anaemia and thyrotoxicosis. Benign murmurs are soft, short, systolic, may vary with posture, and are not associated with signs of organic heart disease.

Diagnosis of valve dysfunction is made clinically and by echocardiography. The severity is assessed by Doppler echocardiography, which measures the direction and velocity of blood flow and allows a calculation to be made of the pressure across a stenotic valve. Transoesophageal echocardiography, cardiac magnetic resonance or invasive cardiac catheterization are usually only necessary to assess complex situations, such as coexisting valvular and ischaemic heart disease, or suspected dysfunction of a prosthetic valve. Treatment of valve dysfunction is both medical and surgical: this may be valve replacement, valve repair (some incompetent valves) or valvotomy (the fused cusps of a stenotic valve are separated along the commissures). The timing of surgery is critical and must not be delayed until there is irreversible ventricular dysfunction or pulmonary hypertension.

Prosthetic heart valves

Prosthetic heart valves are either mechanical or tissue (bioprosthetic). Tissue prostheses are derived from human (homograft), or from porcine or bovine (xenograft) origin. Tissue valves tend to degenerate after about 10 years but patients do not need long-term anticoagulation. These valves are often used in elderly patients. Mechanical valves last much longer but are thrombogenic and patients need lifelong anticoagulation. There are several types of mechanical valve: a ball-and-cage design (Starr–Edwards), tilting disc (Björk–Shiley) or a double tilting disc (St Jude). All damaged and prosthetic valves carry a risk of infection.

The individual valve lesions are considered separately below, but disease may affect more than one valve (particularly in rheumatic heart disease and infective endocarditis), when a combination of clinical features is produced.

Mitral stenosis

Aetiology

Most cases of mitral stenosis are a result of previous rheumatic heart disease, although a reliable history of rheumatic fever is not always obtained.

Pathophysiology

Thickening and immobility of the valve leaflets leads to obstruction of blood flow from the left atrium to left ventricle. As a result there is an increase in left atrial pressure, pulmonary hypertension and right heart dysfunction. Atrial fibrillation is common due to the elevation of left atrial pressure and dilatation. Thrombus may form in the dilated atrium and give rise to systemic emboli (e.g. to the brain, resulting in a stroke). Chronically elevated left atrial pressure leads to an increase in pulmonary capillary pressure and pulmonary oedema. Pulmonary arterial vasoconstriction leads to pulmonary hypertension and eventually right ventricular hypertrophy, dilatation and failure.

Symptoms

Exertional dyspnoea which becomes progressively more severe is usually the first symptom. A cough productive of blood-tinged sputum is common, and frank haemoptysis may occasionally occur. The onset of atrial fibrillation may produce an abrupt deterioration and precipitate pulmonary oedema. Pulmonary hypertension eventually leads to right heart failure with fatigue and lower limb oedema.

Signs

- Mitral facies or malar flush occurs with severe stenosis. This is a cyanotic or dusky-pink discoloration on the upper cheeks.
- The pulse is low volume and may become irregular if atrial fibrillation develops.
- The apex beat is 'tapping' in quality as a result of a combination of a palpable first heart sound and left ventricular backward displacement produced by an enlarging right ventricle.

- Auscultation at the apex reveals a loud first heart sound, an opening snap (when the mitral valve opens) in early diastole, followed by a rumbling mid-diastolic murmur. If the patient is in sinus rhythm the murmur becomes louder when atrial systole occurs (presystolic accentuation), as a result of increased flow across the narrowed valve.

The presence of a loud second heart sound, parasternal heave, elevated JVP, ascites and peripheral oedema indicate that pulmonary hypertension producing right ventricular overload has developed.

Investigations

Investigations are performed to confirm the diagnosis, to estimate the severity of valve stenosis and to look for pulmonary hypertension.

Chest X-ray shows an enlarged left atrium, pulmonary venous hypertension and sometimes a calcified mitral valve. Pulmonary oedema is present in severe disease.

ECG usually shows atrial fibrillation. In patients in sinus rhythm, left atrial hypertrophy results in a bifid P wave ('P mitrale'). With progressive disease there are features of right ventricular hypertrophy.

Echocardiography confirms the diagnosis and assesses severity. A valve area of <2 cm^2 indicates moderate mitral stenosis while an area <1 cm^2 indicates severe stenosis.

Management

General Treatment is often not required for mild mitral stenosis. Complications are treated medically, e.g. β-blockers/digoxin for atrial fibrillation, diuretics for heart failure and anticoagulation in patients with atrial fibrillation to prevent clot formation and embolization.

Specific Mechanical relief of the mitral stenosis is indicated if symptoms are more than mild or if pulmonary hypertension develops. In many cases, percutaneous balloon valvotomy (access to the mitral valve is obtained via a catheter passed through the femoral vein, right atrium and interatrial septum, and a balloon inflated across the valve to split the commissures) provides relief of symptoms. In other cases, open valvotomy (splitting of the valve leaflets) or mitral valve replacement is necessary. The latter is performed if there is associated mitral regurgitation, a badly calcified valve or thrombus in the left atrium despite anticoagulation.

Mitral regurgitation

Aetiology

Prolapsing mitral valve is the most common cause in the developed world but rheumatic heart disease continues to be a common cause in the developing world (Table 10.10).

Table 10.10 Causes of mitral regurgitation

Rheumatic heart disease
Mitral valve prolapse
Infective endocarditis*
Ruptured chordae tendineae*
Rupture of the papillary muscle* complicating myocardial infarction
Papillary muscle dysfunction
Dilating left ventricle disease causing 'functional' mitral regurgitation
Hypertrophic cardiomyopathy
Rarely: systemic lupus erythematosus, Marfan's syndrome
Ehlers–Danlos syndrome

These disorders may produce acute regurgitation.

Pathophysiology

The circulatory changes depend on the speed of onset and severity of regurgitation. Long-standing regurgitation produces little increase in the left atrial pressure because flow is accommodated by an enlarged left atrium. With acute mitral regurgitation there is a rise in left atrial pressure, resulting in an increase in pulmonary venous pressure and pulmonary oedema. The left ventricle dilates, but more so with chronic regurgitation.

Symptoms

Acute regurgitation presents as pulmonary oedema. Chronic regurgitation causes progressive exertional dyspnoea, fatigue and lethargy (resulting from reduced cardiac output). In the later stages the symptoms of right heart failure also occur and eventually lead to congestive cardiac failure. Thromboembolism is less common than with mitral stenosis, although infective endocarditis is much more common.

Signs

The apex beat is displaced laterally, with a diffuse thrusting character. The first heart sound is soft. There is a pansystolic murmur (palpated as a thrill), loudest at the apex and radiating widely over the precordium and into the axilla. A third heart sound is often present, caused by rapid filling of the dilated left ventricle in early diastole.

Investigations

- Chest X-ray and ECG changes are not sensitive or specific for the diagnosis of mitral regurgitation. On both, evidence of enlargement of the left atrium, the left ventricle or both, is seen late in the course of the disease.

- Echocardiography can establish the aetiology and haemodynamic consequences of mitral regurgitation. Doppler and colour flow Doppler is used to measure the severity of mitral regurgitation. Cardiac magnetic resonance or cardiac catheterization is rarely needed for further evaluation.

Management

Mild mitral regurgitation in the absence of symptoms can be managed conservatively by following the patient with serial echocardiograms every 1–5 years. Medical management involves diuretics and ACEIs. Surgical intervention is recommended in patients with symptomatic severe mitral regurgitation, left ventricular ejection fraction >30% and end-diastolic dimension of under 55 mm; and in asymptomatic patients with left ventricular dysfunction (end-systolic dimension >45 mm and/or ejection fraction of under 60%). Patients with asymptomatic severe mitral regurgitation and preserved left ventricular function should be considered for surgery in the presence of atrial fibrillation and/or pulmonary hypertension. Emergency valve replacement is necessary with acute severe mitral regurgitation.

Prolapsing ('floppy') mitral valve

This is a common condition that occurs mainly in young women. One or more of the mitral valve leaflets prolapses back into the left atrium during ventricular systole, producing mitral regurgitation in a few cases.

Aetiology

The cause is unknown, but it is associated with Marfan's syndrome, hyperthyroidism and rheumatic or ischaemic heart disease.

Clinical features

Most patients are asymptomatic. Atypical chest pain is the most common symptom. Some patients complain of palpitations caused by atrial and ventricular arrhythmias. The typical finding on examination is a mid-systolic click, which may be followed by a murmur. Occasionally, there are features of mitral regurgitation.

Investigation

Echocardiography is diagnostic and shows the prolapsing valve cusps.

Management

Chest pain and palpitations are treated with β-blockers. Anticoagulation to prevent thromboembolism is indicated if there is significant mitral regurgitation and atrial fibrillation.

Aortic stenosis

Aetiology

There are three main causes of aortic valve stenosis:

- Degeneration and calcification of a normal valve – presenting in the elderly
- Calcification of a congenital bicuspid valve – presenting in middle age
- Rheumatic heart disease.

Pathophysiology

Obstruction to left ventricular emptying results in left ventricular hypertrophy. In turn this results in increased myocardial oxygen demand, relative ischaemia of the myocardium and consequent angina and arrhythmias. Left ventricular systolic function is typically preserved in aortic stenosis (cf. aortic regurgitation).

Symptoms

There are usually no symptoms until the stenosis is moderately severe (aortic orifice reduced to a third of its normal size). The classic symptoms are angina, exertional syncope and dyspnoea. Ventricular arrhythmias may cause sudden death.

Signs

The carotid pulse is slow rising (plateau pulse) and the apex beat thrusting. There is a harsh systolic ejection murmur (palpated as a thrill) at the right upper sternal border and radiating to the neck. The second heart sound may become soft or inaudible when the valve becomes immobile.

Investigations

- Chest X-ray shows a normal heart size, prominence of the ascending aorta (post-stenotic dilatation) and there may be valvular calcification.
- ECG shows evidence of left ventricular hypertrophy and a left ventricular strain pattern when the disease is severe (depressed ST segment and T-wave inversion in the leads orientated to the left ventricle, i.e. I, AVL, V_5 and V_6).
- Echocardiography is diagnostic in most cases. Doppler examination of the valve allows an assessment of the pressure gradient across the valve during systole.
- Cardiac catheterization is used to exclude coronary artery disease prior to recommending surgery.

Management

Aortic valve replacement is indicated in symptomatic patients, as the onset of symptoms is associated with 75% mortality at 3 years. Some would recommend valve replacement for asymptomatic patients with a critically stenotic valve (valve area ≤ 0.6 cm^2 or the valve gradient exceeds 50 mmHg on echocardiography) or with a left ventricular ejection fraction of $<50\%$. Balloon aortic valvotomy is sometimes used in childhood or adolescence but aortic valve replacement will usually be needed a few years later. If patients are unsuitable for open valve replacement, transcatheter aortic valve implantation (TAVI) with a balloon expandable stent valve may be considered.

Aortic regurgitation

Aetiology

Aortic regurgitation results from either disease of the valve cusps or dilatation of the aortic root and valve ring. The most common causes are rheumatic fever and infective endocarditis complicating an already damaged valve (Table 10.11).

Pathophysiology

Chronic regurgitation volume loads the left ventricle and results in hypertrophy and dilatation. The stroke volume is increased, which results in an increased pulse pressure and the myriad of clinical signs described below. Eventually, contraction of the ventricle deteriorates, resulting in left ventricular failure. The adaptations to the volume load entering the left ventricle do not occur with acute regurgitation and patients may present with pulmonary oedema and a reduced stroke volume (hence many of the signs of chronic regurgitation are absent).

Table 10.11 Causes and associations of aortic regurgitation

Acute aortic regurgitation	Chronic aortic regurgitation
Infective endocarditis	Chronic rheumatic heart disease
Acute rheumatic fever	Bicuspid aortic valve
Dissection of the aorta	Aortic endocarditis
Ruptured sinus of Valsalva aneurysm	Arthritides:
Failure of prosthetic heart valve	• Reiter's syndrome
	• Ankylosing spondylitis
	• Rheumatoid arthritis
	Severe hypertension
	Marfan's syndrome
	Syphilis
	Osteogenesis imperfecta

Symptoms

In chronic regurgitation, patients remain asymptomatic for many years before developing dyspnoea, orthopnoea and fatigue as a result of left ventricular failure.

Signs

- A 'collapsing' (water-hammer) pulse with wide pulse pressure is pathognomonic.
- The apex beat is displaced laterally and is thrusting in quality.
- A blowing early diastolic murmur is heard at the left sternal edge in the fourth intercostal space. It is accentuated when the patient sits forward with the breath held in expiration. Increased stroke volume produces turbulent flow across the aortic valve, heard as a mid-systolic murmur.
- A mid-diastolic murmur (Austin Flint murmur) may be heard over the cardiac apex and is thought to be produced as a result of the aortic jet impinging on the mitral valve, producing premature closure of the valve and physiological stenosis.

Investigations

- Chest X-ray shows a large heart and occasionally dilatation of the ascending aorta.
- ECG shows evidence of left ventricular hypertrophy (see aortic stenosis).
- Echocardiography with Doppler examination of the aortic valve helps estimate the severity of regurgitation.
- Cardiac catheterization is needed to assess for coronary artery disease in patients undergoing surgery.

Management

Mild symptoms may respond to the reduction of afterload with vasodilators and diuretics. ACEIs are useful in patients with left ventricular dysfunction. The timing of surgery and aortic valve replacement is critical and must not be delayed until there is irreversible left ventricular dysfunction.

Tricuspid and pulmonary valve disease

Tricuspid and pulmonary valve disease is uncommon. Tricuspid stenosis is almost always the result of rheumatic fever and is frequently associated with mitral and aortic valve disease, which tends to dominate the clinical picture.

Tricuspid regurgitation is usually functional and secondary to dilatation of the right ventricle (and hence tricuspid valve ring) in severe right ventricular failure. Much less commonly it is caused by rheumatic heart disease, infective endocarditis or carcinoid syndrome (p. 100). On examination there is a pansystolic murmur heard at the lower left sternal edge, the jugular venous pressure is elevated, with giant 'v' waves (produced by the regurgitant jet through the tricuspid valve in systole), and the liver is enlarged and pulsates in systole. There may be severe peripheral oedema and ascites. In functional tricuspid regurgitation these signs improve with diuretic therapy.

Pulmonary regurgitation results from pulmonary hypertension and dilatation of the valve ring. Occasionally it is the result of endocarditis (usually in intravenous drug abusers). Auscultation reveals an early diastolic murmur heard at the upper left sternal edge (Graham Steell murmur), similar to that of aortic regurgitation. Usually there are no symptoms and treatment is rarely required. Pulmonary stenosis is usually a congenital lesion but may present in adult life with fatigue, syncope and right ventricular failure.

Infective endocarditis

Infective endocarditis is an infection of the endocardium or vascular endothelium of the heart. It may occur as a fulminating or acute infection, but more commonly runs an insidious course and is known as subacute (bacterial) endocarditis (SBE).

Infection occurs in the following:

- On valves which have a congenital or acquired defect (usually on the left side of the heart). Right-sided endocarditis is more common in intravenous drug addicts.
- On normal valves with virulent organisms such as *Streptococcus pneumoniae* or *Staphylococcus aureus*.
- On prosthetic valves, when infection may be 'early' (within 60 days of valve surgery and acquired in perioperative period) or 'late' (following bacteraemia). Infected prosthetic valves often need to be replaced.
- In association with a ventricular septal defect or persistent ductus arteriosus.

Aetiology

Streptococcus viridans, *Staphylococcus aureus* and enterococci are common causes (Table 10.12). Blood cultures remain negative in 5–10% of patients, especially in the context of prior antibiotic therapy. Culture-negative endocarditis is particularly likely with organisms which are difficult to isolate in culture: *Coxiella burnetii* (the cause of Q fever), *Chlamydia* spp., *Bartonella* spp. (organisms that cause trench fever and cat scratch disease) and *Legionella*.

Pathology

A mass of fibrin, platelets and infectious organisms form vegetations along the edges of the valve. Virulent organisms destroy the valve, producing regurgitation and worsening heart failure.

Table 10.12 Modified Duke criteria for the diagnosis of infective endocarditis

Major criteria

Positive blood cultures for infective endocarditis

Typical microorganism for infective endocarditis from two separate blood cultures in the absence of a primary focus: e.g. *Streptococcus viridans*, *Streptococcus bovis*, community-acquired *Staphylococcus aureus* or enterococci

Persistently positive blood cultures, defined as recovery of a microorganism consistent with infective endocarditis from blood cultures drawn more than 12 hours apart *or* all of three or the majority of four or more separate blood cultures, with first and last drawn at least 1 hour apart

Single positive blood culture for *Coxiella burnetii* or antiphase IgG antibody titre > 1:800

Evidence for endocardial involvement

TTE (TOE in prosthetic valve) showing oscillating intracardiac mass on a valve or supporting structures, in the path of regurgitant jet or on implanted material, in the absence of an alternative anatomic explanation, *or*

Abscess

New partial dehiscence of prosthetic valve

New valvular regurgitation

Minor criteria

Predisposition, e.g. prosthetic valve, intravenous drug use

Fever – 38°C

Vascular phenomena (e.g. major arterial emboli, septic pulmonary infarcts)

Immunological phenomena (e.g. Osler's nodes, glomerulonephritis)

Echocardiogram – findings consistent with infective endocarditis but not meeting major criteria

Microbiological evidence – positive blood culture but not meeting major criteria

TTE, transthoracic echocardiogram; TOE, transoesophageal echocardiogram.

Clinical features

Symptoms and signs result from:

- Systemic features of infection, such as malaise, fever, night sweats, weight loss and anaemia. Slight splenomegaly is common. Clubbing is rare and occurs late.
- Valve destruction, leading to heart failure and new or changing heart murmurs (in 90% of cases).

- Vascular phenomena due to embolization of vegetations and metastatic abscess formation in the brain, spleen and kidney. Embolization from right-sided endocarditis causes pulmonary infarction and pneumonia.
- Immune complex deposition in blood vessels producing a vasculitis and petechial haemorrhages in the skin, under the nails (splinter haemorrhages) and in the retinae (Roth's spots). Osler's nodes (tender subcutaneous nodules in the fingers) and Janeway lesions (painless erythematous macules on the palms) are uncommon. Immune complex deposition in the joints causes arthralgia and, in the kidney, acute glomerulonephritis. Microscopic haematuria occurs in 70% of cases but acute kidney injury is uncommon.

    Endocarditis should always be excluded in any patient with a heart murmur and fever.

Investigation

- Blood cultures must be taken before antibiotics are started. Three sets (i.e. six bottles) taken over 24 hours will identify the organism in 75% of cases. Special culture techniques are occasionally necessary if blood cultures are negative.
- Transthoracic echocardiography (TTE) identifies vegetations and underlying valvular dysfunction. Small vegetations may be missed and a normal echocardiogram does not exclude endocarditis. Transoesophageal echocardiography (TOE) is more sensitive (but not 100%) particularly in cases of suspected prosthetic valve endocarditis.
- Serological tests may be helpful if unusual organisms are suspected, e.g. *Coxiella, Bartonella, Legionella*.
- Chest X-ray may show heart failure or evidence of septic emboli in right-sided endocarditis.
- ECG may show MI (emboli to the coronary circulation) or conduction defects (due to extension of the infection to the valve annulus and adjacent septum).
- Blood count shows a normochromic, normocytic anaemia with a raised ESR and often a leucocytosis.
- Urine Stix testing shows haematuria in most cases.
- Serum immunoglobulins are increased and complement levels decreased as a result of immune complex formation.

Diagnostic criteria

The Duke classification for diagnosis of endocarditis relies upon major and minor criteria (see Table 10.12). A definite diagnosis of endocarditis requires one of the following:

- Direct evidence of infective endocarditis by histology or culture of organism, e.g. from a vegetation
- Two major criteria

- One major and any three minor criteria
- Five minor criteria.

Possible endocarditis is diagnosed if there is one major and one minor criterion or three minor.

Management

Drug therapy Treatment is with bactericidal antibiotics, given intravenously for the first 2 weeks and by mouth for a further 2–4 weeks. While awaiting the results of blood cultures, a combination of intravenous benzylpenicillin and gentamicin is given unless staphylococcal endocarditis is suspected, when vancomycin should be substituted for penicillin. Subsequent treatment depends on the results of blood cultures and the antibiotic sensitivity of the organism. Antibiotic doses are adjusted to ensure adequate bactericidal activity (microbiological assays of minimum bactericidal concentrations).

Surgery

Surgery to replace the valve should be considered when there is severe heart failure, early infection of prosthetic material, worsening renal failure and extensive damage to the valve.

PULMONARY HEART DISEASE

Pulmonary hypertension

The lung circulation offers a low resistance to flow compared to the systemic circulation and the normal mean pulmonary artery pressure (PAP) at rest is 10–14 mmHg (compared to mean systemic arterial pressure of about 90 mmHg). Pulmonary hypertension is characterized by an elevated PAP (>25 mmHg at rest) and secondary right ventricular failure.

Aetiology

Pulmonary hypertension occurs due to an increase in pulmonary vascular resistance or an increase in pulmonary blood flow. Specific causes are listed in Table 10.13.

Clinical features

Exertional dyspnoea, lethargy and fatigue are the initial symptoms due to an inability to increase cardiac output with exercise. As right ventricular failure develops there is peripheral oedema and abdominal pain from hepatic congestion. On examination there is a loud pulmonary second sound, and a right parasternal heave (caused by right ventricular hypertrophy). In advanced disease there are features of right heart failure (cor pulmonale): elevated jugular venous pressure with a prominent V wave if tricuspid regurgitation is present,

Table 10.13 Causes of pulmonary hypertension

Pulmonary arterial hypertension:

Idiopathic (no cause identified)
Autoimmune rheumatic diseases, e.g. systemic sclerosis, systemic lupus erythematosus, rheumatoid arthritis
Congenital heart disease with systemic-to-pulmonary communication (atrial septal defect, ventricular septal defect)
Portal hypertension (portopulmonary hypertension)
Drugs: long-term use of cocaine and amphetamines, dexfenfluramine
HIV infection
Hereditary
Schistosomiasis
Chronic haemolytic anaemia
Pulmonary veno-occlusive disease

Pulmonary hypertension secondary to:

Left heart disease: valvular, systolic dysfunction, diastolic dysfunction
Lung disease and/or hypoxia, e.g. chronic obstructive pulmonary disease, obstructive sleep apnoea, lung fibrosis
Thromboembolic occlusion of proximal or distal pulmonary vasculature
Multifactorial mechanisms: myeloproliferative disorders, sarcoidosis, glycogen storage disease

hepatomegaly, a pulsatile liver, peripheral oedema, ascites and a pleural effusion. There are also features of the underlying disease.

Investigations

The aim of investigation is to confirm the presence of pulmonary hypertension and demonstrate the cause:

- Chest X-ray shows enlarged proximal pulmonary arteries which taper distally. It may also reveal the underlying cause (e.g. emphysema, calcified mitral valve).
- ECG shows right ventricular hypertrophy and P pulmonale (p. 412).
- Echocardiography shows right ventricular dilatation and/or hypertrophy and may also reveal the cause of pulmonary hypertension, e.g. intracardiac shunt. It is possible to measure the peak PAP with Doppler echocardiography.
- Right heart catheterization may be indicated to confirm the diagnosis (elevated PAP), to determine the pulmonary wedge pressure (PWP), to calculate the cardiac output and to assess for pulmonary vascular resistance and reactivity.

Management

The initial treatment is oxygen, warfarin (due to a higher risk of intrapulmonary thrombosis), diuretics for oedema and oral calcium-channel blockers as pulmonary vasodilators, together with treatment of the underlying cause. In more advanced disease, treatment is aimed at decreasing pulmonary vascular resistance and includes oral endothelin receptor antagonists (bosentan, sitaxentan), prostanoid analogues (inhaled iloprost, treprostinil, beraprost), intravenous epoprostenol and oral sildenafil or tadalafil. In primary pulmonary hypertension there is a progressive downhill course and many patients ultimately require heart and lung transplantation.

Pulmonary embolism

Pulmonary embolism (PE) is a common and potentially lethal condition. Unfortunately, the diagnosis is often missed because the presenting symptoms are vague or non-specific. Emboli usually arise from thrombi in the iliofemoral veins (deep venous thrombosis, p. 488). The risk factors for thromboembolism are listed on p. 241. Rarely, PE results from clot formation in the right heart.

Pathology

A massive embolism obstructs the right ventricular outflow tract and therefore suddenly increases pulmonary vascular resistance, causing acute right heart failure. A small embolus impacts in a terminal, peripheral pulmonary vessel and may be clinically silent unless it causes pulmonary infarction. Lung tissue is ventilated but not perfused, resulting in impaired gas exchange. It is important to consider PE in the differential diagnosis of chest pain with elevated troponin. The rise in troponin reflects right ventricular ischaemia and is associated with adverse outcomes.

Clinical features

- Small/medium PEs present with breathlessness, pleuritic chest pain, and haemoptysis if there is pulmonary infarction. On examination the patient may be tachypnoeic and have a pleural rub and an exudative (occasionally bloodstained) pleural effusion can develop.
- Massive PE presents as a medical emergency: the patient has severe central chest pain and suddenly becomes shocked, pale and sweaty, with marked tachypnoea and tachycardia. Syncope and death may follow rapidly. On examination the patient is shocked, with central cyanosis. There is elevation of the jugular venous pressure, a right ventricular heave, accentuation of the second heart sound and a gallop rhythm (acute right heart failure).
- Multiple recurrent PEs present with symptoms and signs of pulmonary hypertension (pp. 471–472), developing over weeks to months.

Investigations

A clinical pre-test probability score of PE is used prior to investigation (Table 10.14), which helps to decide on the most appropriate first-line diagnostic test and interpretation of the results (Emergency Box 10.5):

- Chest X-ray, ECG and blood gases may all be normal with small/medium emboli and any abnormalities with massive emboli are non-specific. The chest X-ray and ECG are useful to exclude other conditions that may present similarly. The chest X-ray may show decreased vascular markings and a raised hemidiaphragm (caused by loss of lung volume). With pulmonary infarction, a late feature is the development of a wedge-shaped opacity adjacent to the pleural edge, sometimes with a pleural effusion. The most

Table 10.14 Revised Geneva score for the clinical prediction of a pulmonary embolism

	Score
Risk factors	
Age > 65 years	+1
Previous deep venous thrombosis or pulmonary embolism	+3
Surgery or fracture within 1 month	+2
Active malignancy	+2
Symptoms	
Unilateral leg pain	+3
Haemoptysis	+2
Clinical signs	
Heart rate (beats/min)	
75–94	+3
≥95	+5
Pain on leg deep vein palpation and unilateral oedema	+4
Clinical probability	**Total score**
Low	0–3
Intermediate	4–10
High	≥11

NB: diagnosis of pulmonary embolism (PE) is not excluded on this basis alone; about 8% of patients with a low clinical score will have a PE.
(After Righini M, Le Gal G, Aujesky D, et al. (2008) Lancet 371: 1343–1352, with permission from Elsevier.)

✚ Emergency Box 10.5

Management of suspected and confirmed pulmonary embolism (PE)

Investigation and diagnosis

Investigation and diagnosis

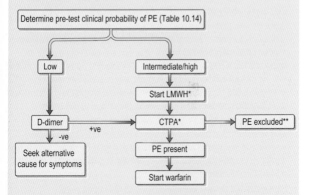

- D dimer, arterial blood gas, ECG, CXR, CTPA or echo
- High flow oxygen if hypoxaemic
- Thrombolysis (p. 251) for massive embolism with persistent hypotension
- Analgesia: morphine (5–10 mg i.v.) relieves pain and anxiety
- Prevention of further thrombi: LMWH and oral warfarin (p. 248). NOACs (p. 250) are also used in patients with VTE (dabigatran, rivaroxaban and apixaban).
- Intravenous fluids (to raise the filling pressure) for patients presenting with moderate/severe embolism.

CTPA, CT pulmonary angiogram; CXR, chest X-ray; ECG, electrocardiogram; LMWH, low-molecular-weight heparin; NOACs, novel oral anticoagulants; VTE, venous thromboembolis.

*Patients with massive PE and persistent hypotension should be treated with thrombolysis. In these cases, bedside echocardiography is an alternative diagnostic test to CTPA if CT is not immediately available or the patient is too unstable for transfer to the radiology department.

**Rarely, CTPA is inconclusive and high pre-test clinical probability patients may need further imaging, e.g. repeat CTPA (if poor quality initially), Doppler ultrasound of legs (to look for a source thrombus) or $\dot{V}/\dot{Q}$ scan.

common ECG finding is sinus tachycardia or there may be new-onset atrial fibrillation. The features of acute right heart strain may be seen: tall peaked P waves in lead II, right axis deviation and right bundle branch block. Arterial blood gases show hypoxaemia and hypocapnia with massive emboli.

- Plasma D-dimers are a subset of fibrinogen degradation products released into the circulation when a clot begins to dissolve. D-dimers are, however, elevated in many other conditions (e.g. cancer, pregnancy, post-operatively) and a positive result is not diagnostic of thromboembolic disease. The value of D-dimer testing is in patients with a low pre-test clinical probability score (Table 10.14 and Emergency Box 10.5).
- Spiral CT with *intravenous* contrast (CT pulmonary angiography, CTPA) images the pulmonary vessels directly and is highly sensitive for the detection of large proximal pulmonary emboli. It is increasingly being used as the diagnostic test of choice for patients with suspected PE. Subsegmental emboli may be missed and occasionally patients may need further imaging (Emergency Box 10.5). One of the benefits over $\dot{V}/\dot{Q}$ scan is the ability to detect an alternative pathology that may explain the clinical presentation.
- Radionuclide lung scan ($\dot{V}/\dot{Q}$ scan) demonstrates areas of ventilated lung with perfusion defects (ventilation-perfusion defects). Pulmonary embolism is excluded in patients with a normal scan. However, there is high incidence of non-diagnostic scans, especially in patients with coexistent chronic lung disease, who will then need further imaging.
- Ultrasound will detect clots in the pelvic or iliofemoral veins.
- MRI gives similar results and is used if CT is contraindicated.
- Echocardiography is diagnostic in massive PE and can be performed at the bedside. It demonstrates proximal thrombus and right ventricular dilatation.

Management

Management of PE is summarized in Emergency Box 10.5. Patients are classed as *high risk* and *not high risk* based on the presence of shock or hypotension *High-risk* patients should proceed to CTPA. A negative test should lead to investigations for other causes of haemodynamic instability. Echocardiography may be useful if patients are too unstable for CTPA. In *not high-risk* patients, the clinical probability of pulmonary embolus should be determined using a scoring system such as the revised Geneva rules (Table 10.14) and D-dimer assay. The only definite indication for thrombolysis in acute massive embolism is persistent arterial hypotension. Surgical embolectomy is occasionally undertaken if thrombolysis is contraindicated or ineffective. In contrast, patients who are cardiovascularly stable and who have no coexistent serious medical pathology can be treated at home once the diagnosis is confirmed. Anticoagulation is continued for 6 weeks to 6 months (p. 248), depending on the likelihood of recurrence of thromboembolism, and lifelong treatment is indicated for recurrent emboli. Insertion of a vena caval filter is used to prevent further emboli when emboli recur despite adequate anticoagulation or in high-risk individuals where anticoagulation is contraindicated.

Pulmonary embolism in pregnancy

Pulmonary embolism occurs more frequently in pregnancy and is the leading cause of maternal death in the developed world. Compression ultrasonography of the legs is the initial investigation. CTPA is required if ultrasound is normal and delivers a lower dose of radiation to the fetus than $\dot{V}/\dot{Q}$ scanning. Warfarin is teratogenic and confirmed PE is treated with low-molecular-weight heparin (LMWH).

MYOCARDIAL DISEASE

Myocarditis

Myocarditis is an inflammation of the myocardium. The most common cause in the UK is viral, particularly Coxsackie virus infection, but it may also occur with diphtheria, rheumatic fever, radiation injury and some drugs. Myocarditis in association with human immunodeficiency virus (HIV) infection is seen at post-mortem in up to 20% of cases but causes clinical problems in less than 10% of cases.

Clinical features

Patients present with an acute illness characterized by fever and varying degrees of biventricular failure. Cardiac arrhythmias and pericarditis may also occur.

Investigations

- Chest X-ray may show cardiac enlargement.
- ECG shows non-specific T-wave and ST changes and arrhythmias.
- The diagnosis is supported by demonstration of an increase in serum viral titres. Cardiac biopsy is not usually performed as the findings rarely influence management. Cardiac enzymes are elevated.

Management

Treatment is with bed rest and treatment of heart failure. The prognosis is generally good.

CARDIOMYOPATHY

Cardiomyopathies comprise a group of diseases of the myocardium that affect the mechanical (hypertrophic, arrhythmogenic right ventricular, dilated and restrictive cardiomyopathy) or electrical function (conduction system disease and ion channelopathies, e.g. long QT syndrome) of the heart. Diagnosis of myocardial disease is usually by imaging (echocardiogram and CMR).

Hypertrophic cardiomyopathy

Hypertrophic cardiomyopathy (HCM) is characterized by marked ventricular hypertrophy in the absence of abnormal loading conditions such as hypertension and valvular disease. There is usually disproportionate involvement of the interventricular septum. The hypertrophic non-compliant ventricles impair diastolic filling, so that stroke volume is reduced. Most cases are familial, autosomal dominant and caused by mutations in genes encoding sarcomeric proteins, e.g. troponin T and β-myosin. It is the most common cause of sudden cardiac death in young people.

Clinical features

Patients may be symptom-free (and detected through family screening) or have breathlessness, angina or syncope. Complications include sudden death, atrial and ventricular arrhythmias, thromboembolism, infective endocarditis and heart failure. The carotid pulse is jerky because of rapid ejection and sudden obstruction to the ventricular outflow during systole. An ejection systolic murmur occurs because of left ventricular outflow obstruction, and the pansystolic murmur of functional mitral regurgitation may also be heard.

Investigations

- ECG is almost always abnormal. A pattern of left ventricular hypertrophy with no discernible cause is diagnostic.
- Cardiac imaging shows ventricular hypertrophy (on echo and magnetic resonance [MR]) and fibrosis (on MR).
- Genetic analysis may confirm the diagnosis and provide prognostic information.

Management

Amiodarone reduces the risk of arrhythmias and sudden death. Individuals at highest risk are fitted with an ICD. Chest pain and dyspnoea are treated with β-blockers and verapamil. Vasodilators should be avoided because they may aggravate left ventricular outflow obstruction or cause refractory hypotension. In selected cases, outflow tract gradients are reduced by surgical resection or alcohol ablation of the septum, or by dual-chamber pacing.

Dilated cardiomyopathy

Dilated cardiomyopathy (DCM) is characterized by a dilated left ventricle which contracts poorly. Inheritance is autosomal dominant in the familial disease.

Clinical features

Shortness of breath is usually the first complaint; less often, patients present with embolism (from mural thrombus) or arrhythmia. Subsequently, there is progressive heart failure with the symptoms and signs of biventricular failure.

Investigations

- Chest X-ray may show cardiac enlargement.
- ECG is often abnormal. The changes are non-specific and include arrhythmias and T-wave flattening.
- Cardiac imaging shows dilated ventricles with global hypokinesis. Cardiac MR may show other aetiologies of left ventricular dysfunction, e.g. previous MI.

Other tests such as coronary angiography, viral and autoimmune screen and endomyocardial biopsy may be needed to exclude other diseases (Table 10.15) that present with the clinical features of DCM.

Management

Heart failure and atrial fibrillation are treated in the conventional way (pp. 436, 430). Cardiac resynchronization therapy and ICDs are used in patients with NYHA III/IV grading. Severe cardiomyopathy is treated with cardiac transplantation.

Primary restrictive cardiomyopathy

The rigid myocardium restricts diastolic ventricular filling and the clinical features resemble those of constrictive pericarditis (pp. 481–482). In the UK the most common cause is amyloidosis. The ECG, chest X-ray and echocardiogram are often abnormal, but the findings are non-specific. Diagnosis is by cardiac catheterization, which shows characteristic pressure changes. An endomyocardial biopsy may be taken during the catheter procedure, thus providing histological diagnosis. There is no specific treatment and the prognosis is poor, with most patients dying less than a year after diagnosis. Cardiac transplantation is performed in selected cases.

Table 10.15 Heart muscle disease presenting with features of dilated cardiomyopathy

Ischaemia
Hypertension
Congenital heart disease
Peripartum cardiomyopathy
Infections, e.g. cytomegalovirus, HIV
Alcohol excess
Muscular dystrophy
Amyloidosis
Haemochromatosis

Arrhythmogenic right ventricular cardiomyopathy

There is progressive fibro-adipose replacement of the wall of the right ventricle. The typical presentation is ventricular tachycardia or sudden death in a young man.

PERICARDIAL DISEASE

The normal pericardium is a fibroelastic sac containing a thin layer of fluid (50 mL) that surrounds the heart and roots of the great vessels.

Acute pericarditis

Aetiology

In the UK, acute inflammation of the pericardium is most commonly secondary to viral infection (Coxsackie B, echovirus, HIV infection) or MI. Other causes include uraemia, autoimmune rheumatic diseases, trauma, infection (bacterial, tuberculosis, fungal) and malignancy (breast, lung, leukaemia and lymphoma).

Clinical features

There is sharp retrosternal chest pain which is characteristically relieved by leaning forward. Pain may be worse on inspiration and radiate to the neck and shoulders. The cardinal clinical sign is a pericardial friction rub, which may be transient.

Diagnosis

The ECG is diagnostic. There is concave upwards (saddle-shaped) ST segment elevation across all leads and return towards baseline as inflammation subsides. ST segment elevation is convex upwards in MI and limited to the leads that face the infarct.

Management

Treatment is of the underlying disorder plus NSAIDs. Systemic corticosteroids are used in resistant cases. NSAIDs should not be used in the few days following MI as they are associated with a higher rate of myocardial rupture. Complications of acute pericarditis are pericardial effusion and chronic pericarditis (>6–12 months).

Pericardial effusion and tamponade

Pericardial effusion is an accumulation of fluid in the pericardial sac which may result from any of the causes of pericarditis. Hypothyroidism also causes a pericardial effusion which rarely compromises ventricular function. Pericardial tamponade is a medical emergency and occurs when a large amount of pericardial fluid (which has often accumulated rapidly) restricts diastolic ventricular filling and causes a marked reduction in cardiac output.

Clinical features

The effusion obscures the apex beat and the heart sounds are soft. The signs of pericardial tamponade are hypotension, tachycardia and an elevated jugular venous pressure, which paradoxically rises with inspiration (Kussmaul's sign). There is invariably pulsus paradoxus (a fall in BP of more than 10 mmHg on inspiration). This is the result of increased venous return to the right side of the heart during inspiration. The increased right ventricular volume thus occupies more space within the rigid pericardium and impairs left ventricular filling.

Investigations

- Chest X-ray shows a large globular heart.
- ECG shows low-voltage complexes with sinus tachycardia.
- Echocardiography is diagnostic, showing an echo-free space around the heart.
- Invasive tests to establish the cause of the effusion may only be necessary with a persistent effusion, if a purulent, tuberculous or malignant effusion is suspected, or if the effusion is not known to be secondary to an underlying illness. Pericardiocentesis (aspiration of fluid under echocardiographic guidance) and pericardial biopsy for culture, cytology/histology and polymerase chain reaction (PCR) (for tuberculosis) give a greater diagnostic yield with large effusions.

Management

Most pericardial effusions resolve spontaneously. Tamponade requires emergency pericardiocentesis. Pericardial fluid is drained percutaneously by introducing a needle into the pericardial sac. If the effusion recurs, despite treatment of the underlying cause, excision of a pericardial segment allows fluid to be absorbed through the pleural and mediastinal lymphatics.

Constrictive pericarditis

In the UK, most cases of constrictive pericarditis are idiopathic in origin or result from intrapericardial haemorrhage during heart surgery.

Clinical features

The heart becomes encased within a rigid fibrotic pericardial sac which prevents adequate diastolic filling of the ventricles. The clinical features resemble those of right-sided heart failure, with jugular venous distension, dependent oedema, hepatomegaly and ascites. Kussmaul's sign (JVP rises paradoxically with inspiration) is usually present and there may be pulsus paradoxus, atrial fibrillation and, on auscultation, a pericardial knock caused by rapid ventricular filling. Clinically, constrictive pericarditis cannot be distinguished from restrictive cardiomyopathy (p. 479).

Investigations

A chest X-ray shows a normal heart size and pericardial calcification (best seen on the lateral film). Diagnosis is made by CT or MRI, which shows pericardial thickening and calcification.

Management

Treatment is by surgical excision of the pericardium.

SYSTEMIC HYPERTENSION

The level of BP is said to be abnormal when it is associated with a clear increase in morbidity and mortality from heart disease, stroke and renal failure. This level varies with age, sex, race and country. The definition of hypertension is over 140/90 mmHg, based on at least two readings on separate occasions. The validity of a single BP measurement is unclear (BP rises acutely in certain situations, e.g. visiting the doctor). In the UK, NICE recommends that ambulatory BP monitoring (ABPM) is offered to patients with a clinic BP of $\geq 140/90$ mmHg to confirm the diagnosis of hypertension. Home BP monitoring (HBPM) can also be used.

Aetiology

Essential hypertension   Most patients with hypertension (80–90%) have no known underlying cause, i.e. 'primary' or 'essential' hypertension. Essential hypertension has a multifactorial aetiology:

- Genetic component
- Low birthweight
- Obesity
- Excess alcohol intake
- High salt intake
- The metabolic syndrome (p. 165).

Secondary hypertension   Secondary hypertension is the result of a specific and potentially treatable cause:

- Renal disease accounts for over 80% of cases of secondary hypertension. The common causes are diabetic nephropathy, chronic glomerulonephritis, adult polycystic kidneys, chronic tubulointerstitial nephritis and renovascular disease.
- Endocrine disease (p. 645): Conn's syndrome, adrenal hyperplasia, phaeochromocytoma, Cushing's syndrome and acromegaly.

- Coarctation of the aorta is a congenital narrowing of the aorta at, or just distal to, the insertion of the ductus arteriosus, i.e. distal to the left subclavian artery. There is hypertension due to decreased renal perfusion, delayed (radiofemoral delay) pulses in the legs, a mid-late systolic murmur and 'rib notching' (collateral arteries erode the undersurface of ribs) on X-ray.
- Pre-eclampsia occurring in the third trimester of pregnancy.
- Drugs, including oestrogen-containing oral contraceptives, other steroids, NSAIDs and vasopressin.

Clinical features

Hypertension is generally asymptomatic. Secondary causes of hypertension may be suggested by specific features, such as attacks of sweating and tachycardia in phaeochromocytoma. Malignant or accelerated hypertension describes a rapid rise in BP with severe hypertension (diastolic BP > 120 mmHg). The characteristic histological change is fibrinoid necrosis of the vessel wall and untreated it will result in end-organ damage in the kidneys (haematuria, proteinuria, progressive kidney disease), brain (cerebral oedema and haemorrhage), retina (flame-shaped haemorrhages, cotton wool spots, hard exudates and papilloedema) and cardiovascular system (acute heart failure and aortic dissection).

Examination In most patients the only finding is high BP, but in other patients, signs relating to the cause (e.g. abdominal bruit in renal artery stenosis, delayed femoral pulses in coarctation of the aorta) or the end-organ effects of hypertension may be present: e.g. loud second heart sound, left ventricular heave, fourth heart sound in hypertensive heart disease, and retinal abnormalities. The latter are graded according to severity:

- Grade 1 – increased tortuosity and reflectiveness of the retinal arteries (silver wiring)
- Grade 2 – grade 1 plus arteriovenous nipping
- Grade 3 – grade 2 plus flame-shaped haemorrhages and soft 'cotton wool' exudates
- Grade 4 – grade 3 plus papilloedema.

Risk assessment and investigations

Patients with hypertension should have their cardiovascular risk assessed using an appropriate calculator – NICE recommends QRISK2-2014 (http://www.qrisk.org/index.php). Investigations are carried out to identify end-organ damage and those patients with secondary causes of hypertension. Routine investigation should include:

- Serum urea and electrolytes, which may show evidence of renal impairment, in which case more specific renal investigations (e.g. renal ultrasound, renal angiography) are indicated. Hypokalaemia occurs in Conn's syndrome.

- Urinalysis for protein and blood, which may indicate renal disease (either the cause or the effect of hypertension).
- Blood glucose.
- Serum lipids.
- ECG, which may show evidence of left ventricular hypertrophy or myocardial ischaemia.

Patients under 40 years old with no risk factors or those where an underlying cause is suspected (e.g. from clinical examination or abnormal baseline investigations) should undergo further investigation for secondary causes of hypertension.

Management

Treatment is begun immediately in patients with malignant or severe hypertension (BP ≥ 180/110 mmHg). In other patients, treatment is started if repeated measurements confirm sustained hypertension (Table 10.16). For most patients, target BP during treatment is 140/90 mmHg. For patients with diabetes, chronic kidney disease or cardiovascular disease, a lower target of 130/80 mmHg is recommended.

Non-pharmacological measures in the treatment of hypertension include:

- Weight reduction (aim for body mass index [BMI] < 25 kg/m^2)
- Low-fat and low saturated fat diet

Table 10.16 Indications for treatment based on sustained blood pressure recordings

Severity	BP (mmHg)	Intervention
Stage 1 hypertension	Clinic BP ≥ 140/90 and daytime average ABPM or HBPM ≥ 135/85	Offer treatment to everyone under 80 years old with at least one of the following risk factors: • Target organ damage • Cardiovascular disease • Renal disease • Diabetes • 10-year cardiovascular risk ≥ 20%
Stage 2 hypertension	Clinic BP ≥ 160/100 and daytime average ABPM or HBPM ≥ 150/95	All patients should be offered treatment
Severe hypertension	>180/110	Treat immediately

ABPM, ambulatory blood pressure monitoring; BP, blood pressure; HBPM, home blood pressure monitoring.

- Low-salt diet (<6 g sodium chloride per day)
- Limited alcohol consumption (<21 units and <14 units per week for men and women, respectively)
- Dynamic exercise (at least 30 minutes brisk walk per day)
- Increased fruit and vegetable consumption
- Reduce cardiovascular risk by stopping smoking and increasing oily fish consumption.

In most hypertensive patients, statins (p. 701) are also given to reduce the overall cardiovascular risk burden. Glycaemic control should be optimized in diabetics (HbA$_{1c}$ < 53 mmol/mol). For each class of antihypertensive there will be indications and contraindications in specific patient groups. A single antihypertensive drug is used initially, but combination treatment will be needed in many patients to control BP. In patients without compelling reasons for a particular drug class, a treatment algorithm such as the one advocated by NICE (Fig. 10.17) is used to advise on the sequencing of drugs and logical drug combinations. This algorithm is based on the observation that younger people and Caucasians tend to have higher renin levels compared to older people or the black population. Thus the 'A' drugs which reduce BP at least in part by suppression of the renin–angiotensin system are more effective as initial blood-pressure-lowering therapy in younger Caucasian patients.

Group A: ACE inhibitors (p. 497), e.g. captopril, enalapril, lisinopril and ramipril, block the conversion of angiotensin I to angiotensin II, which is a potent vasoconstrictor, and block degradation of bradykinin, which is a vasodilator. Side effects include first-dose hypotension and cough, proteinuria, rashes and leucopenia in high doses. ACEIs are contraindicated in renal artery stenosis because inhibition of the renin–angiotensin system in this instance may lead to loss of renal blood flow and infarction of the kidney.

Group B: Angiotensin II receptor antagonists (p. 498), e.g. losartan, valsartan, irbesartan and candesartan, selectively block receptors for angiotensin II. They share some of the actions of ACEIs and are useful in patients who cannot tolerate ACEIs because of cough.

Group C: Calcium antagonists (p. 501), e.g. amlodipine and nifedipine, act predominantly by dilatation of peripheral arterioles. Side effects include bradycardia and cardiac conduction defects (verapamil and diltiazem), headaches, flushing and fluid retention.

Group D: Diuretics increase renal sodium and water excretion and directly dilate arterioles (p. 351). Loop diuretics, e.g. furosemide, and thiazide diuretics, e.g. bendroflumethiazide (bendrofluazide), are equally effective in lowering BP, although thiazides are usually preferred, as the duration of action is longer, the diuresis is not so severe and they are cheaper. Thiazide diuretics cause hypercholesterolaemia, hypokalaemia, hyponatraemia, hyperuricaemia (may precipitate gout) and impairment of glucose tolerance.

β-**Adrenergic blocking agents** (p. 495) are no longer a preferred initial therapy for hypertension. They are used in younger patients, particularly those

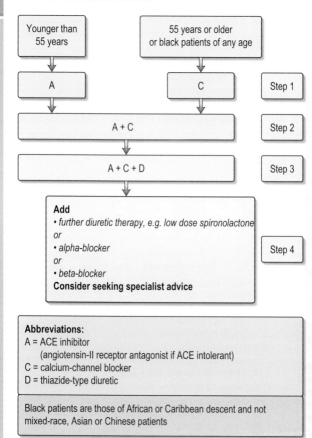

Fig. 10.17 Choosing drugs for patients newly diagnosed with hypertension.
National Institute for Health and Clinical Excellence (2016). NICE pathway: treatment steps for hypertension. http://pathways.nice.org.uk/pathways/hypertension. Pathway last updated 26/4/16.

with an intolerance or contraindication to ACEIs and angiotensin-II receptor antagonists; women of child-bearing potential; or patients with evidence of increased sympathetic drive. β-Blockers reduce renin production and sympathetic nervous system activity. Complications include bradycardia, bronchospasm, cold extremities, fatigue and weakness.

Other agents α-Blocking agents (e.g. doxazosin), hydralazine, an aldosterone antagonist (spironolactone) and centrally acting agents (e.g. clonidine, moxonidine) may be indicated in specific circumstances.

Management of severe hypertension

Patients with malignant (p. 483) or severe hypertension (diastolic BP > 140 mmHg) should be admitted to hospital for treatment. The aim should be to reduce the diastolic BP slowly (over 24–48 hours) to about 100–110 mmHg and this is usually achieved with oral antihypertensives, e.g. atenolol or amlodipine. Sublingual and intravenous antihypertensives are not recommended because they may produce a precipitous fall in BP, leading to cerebral infarction. When rapid control of BP is required (e.g. aortic dissection), the agent of choice is intravenous sodium nitroprusside (starting dose 0.3 μg/kg/min, i.e. 100 mg nitroprusside in 250 mL saline at 2–5 mL/h) or labetalol.

ARTERIAL AND VENOUS DISEASE

Aortic aneurysms

An aneurysm is a permanent localized dilatation of an artery. They may be asymptomatic or cause symptoms by pressure effects or vessel rupture, occasionally with fistula formation, or they may be a source of emboli. Aortic aneurysms (vessel diameter > 3 cm) are usually abdominal and most result from a degenerative process and present in elderly men. Some are the result of connective tissue disease.

Abdominal Abdominal aortic aneurysms can be asymptomatic (e.g. found as a pulsating mass on abdominal examination). In the UK, ultrasound screening should be offered to men aged 65–74 years. Aneurysms may also cause symptoms due to pressure effects (epigastric or back pain) or rupture. The latter is a surgical emergency presenting with epigastric pain radiating to the back, and hypovolaemic shock. Diagnosis is by ultrasonography or CT scan. Surgical replacement of the aneurysmal segment with a prosthetic graft is indicated for a symptomatic aneurysm or large asymptomatic aneurysms (>5.5 cm). In patients who are poor surgical risks, endovascular repair with insertion of an aortic stent is being increasingly employed.

Thoracic Cystic medial necrosis and atherosclerosis are the usual causes of thoracic aneurysms. Cardiovascular syphilis is no longer a common cause. Thoracic aneurysms may be asymptomatic, cause pressure on local structures (causing back pain, dysphagia and cough) or result in aortic regurgitation if the aortic root is involved.

Dissecting aortic aneurysm Aortic dissection results from a tear in the intima: blood under high pressure creates a false lumen in the diseased media. Typically there is an abrupt onset of severe, tearing central chest pain, radiating through to the back. Involvement of branch arteries may produce neurological signs, absent pulses and unequal BP in the arms. The chest X-ray shows a widened mediastinum and the diagnosis is confirmed by CT scanning and transoesophageal echocardiography or MRI. Management involves urgent control of BP (p. 487) and surgical repair for proximal aortic dissection.

Raynaud's disease and phenomenon

Raynaud's phenomenon consists of intermittent spasm in the arteries supplying the fingers and toes. It is usually precipitated by cold and relieved by heat. There is initial pallor (resulting from vasoconstriction) followed by cyanosis and, finally, redness from hyperaemia. Raynaud's disease (no underlying disorder) occurs most commonly in young women and must be differentiated from secondary causes of Raynaud's phenomenon, e.g. autoimmune rheumatic disease and β-blocker therapy. Treatment is by keeping the hands and feet warm, stopping smoking and stopping β-blockers. Medical treatment includes oral nifedipine and occasionally prostacyclin infusions. Lumbar sympathectomy may help lower limb symptoms.

Venous disease

Superficial thrombophlebitis This usually occurs in the leg. The vein is painful, tender and hard, with overlying redness. Treatment is with simple analgesia, e.g. NSAIDs. Anticoagulation with fondaparinux can limit the extension of superficial thrombosis. Thromboembolic events are uncommon.

   Deep venous thrombosis Thrombosis can occur in any vein, but those of the pelvis and leg are the most common sites. The risk factors for deep venous thrombosis (DVT) are listed on page 241.

Clinical features

DVT is often asymptomatic but the leg may be warm and swollen, with calf tenderness and superficial venous distension. The differential diagnosis includes ruptured Baker's cyst (p. 278), oedema from other causes and cellulitis.

Investigations

Measurement of serum D-dimer is the initial investigation in patients with a low clinical probability score (Table 10.17) and no further investigation is indicated if D-dimers are normal. In all other patients, venous compression ultrasonography, which is a reliable test for iliofemoral thrombosis, is indicated. It is not reliable for calf vein thrombosis, and repeat scanning 1 week later with interim heparin treatment is indicated if the initial scan is negative and there is high index of clinical suspicion.

Management

This is discussed on page 242.

Table 10.17 Wells score for the clinical probability of a deep venous thrombosis (DVT)

History	Score if present
Lower limb trauma or surgery or immobilization in a plaster cast	+1
Bedridden for more than 3 days or surgery within the last 4 weeks	+1
Malignancy (including treatment up to 6 months previously)	+1
Tenderness along deep venous system	+1
Clinical findings	
Entire limb swollen	+1
Calf swelling more than 3 cm compared to asymptomatic side, measured at 10 cm below tibial tuberosity	+1
Pitting oedema (greater in symptomatic leg)	+1
Dilated collateral superficial veins (non-varicose)	+1
Possible alternative diagnosis	
Alternative diagnosis (e.g. musculoskeletal injury, haematoma, chronic oedema, cellulitis of the leg, arthritis of the leg, Baker's cyst) as likely or greater than that of DVT	−2

Total score	≤0	1–2	≥3
Risk of DVT	3% (low)	17% (moderate)	75% (high)

The main aim of therapy is to prevent pulmonary embolism. Anticoagulation is initially with LMWH and subsequently with warfarin, usually continued for 3 months in above-knee DVTs. Anticoagulation of below-knee DVTs is recommended for 6 weeks, as 30% of patients will have proximal extension of the clot. Thrombolytic therapy is occasionally used for patients with a large iliofemoral thrombosis.

The main complications of DVT are pulmonary embolus, post-thrombotic syndrome (permanent pain, swelling, oedema and sometimes venous eczema may result from destruction of the deep-vein valves) and recurrence of thrombosis. Elastic support stockings are used for the post-thrombotic syndrome.

Prevention

Hospital-acquired venous thromboembolism is largely preventable. All patients should be assessed on admission to hospital and those at risk should be considered for pharmacological prophylaxis (fondaparinux, LMWH or unfractionated heparin if renal impairment) unless they have a risk factor for bleeding.

THERAPEUTICS FOR THE CARDIOVASCULAR SYSTEM

Electrical cardioversion

Cardioversion is the delivery of energy that is synchronized to the QRS complex, whereas defibrillation is non-synchronized delivery of energy, i.e. the shock is delivered randomly during the cardiac cycle (Table 10.18). In the patient who has had a cardiac arrest and is not responding to repeated defibrillation, a difficult decision is when to stop resuscitation and defibrillation efforts. This depends on the patient, the circumstances of the arrest and how long the patient has had a non-perfusing cardiac rhythm. In general, if a patient arrests in hospital and resuscitation has not resulted in a perfusing cardiac rhythm after 30 minutes, then further attempts are unlikely to be successful. The prognosis is poorer in patients who arrest outside hospital. There are exceptions: resuscitation is continued for longer in a hypothermic patient.

Indications

- Elective cardioversion:
  - atrial tachyarrhythmias.
- Emergency cardioversion:
  - atrial tachyarrhythmias causing haemodynamic compromise, e.g. hypotension, pulmonary oedema, myocardial ischaemia, impaired conscious level
  - VT
  - VF.

Contraindications

- Digitalis toxicity (relative contraindication) – induction of ventricular arrhythmias by cardioversion is more likely
- Atrial fibrillation with onset more than 24 hours previously (due to risk of embolism) unless patient has high-risk symptoms and signs (p. 430).

Table 10.18 Energy levels for biphasic defibrillators

Arrhythmia	Initial shock energy (J)
Broad-complex tachycardia	120–150
Atrial flutter and narrow-complex tachycardia	70–120
Atrial fibrillation	120–150
Ventricular arrhythmias	150–200

DRUGS FOR ARRHYTHMIAS

Adenosine

Mechanism of action

Adenosine is a purine nucleotide. It acts on adenosine receptors and enhances the flow of potassium out of myocardial cells; it produces hyperpolarization of the cell membrane and stabilizes the cell membrane. It has potent effects on the sinus (SA) node, causing complete heart block for a fraction of a second after i.v. administration and producing sinus bradycardia.

Indications

The main indication is reversion to sinus rhythm of atrioventricular junctional tachycardia.

Preparations and dose

3 mg/mL.

Intravenous injection By rapid i.v. injection into a central or large peripheral vein, 6 mg over 2 seconds with cardiac monitoring and resuscitation equipment available; if necessary, followed by 12 mg after 1–2 minutes, and then 12 mg after a further 1–2 minutes; increments should not be given if high-level AV block develops at any dose.

Side effects

Unwanted effects are common; however, they are usually transient. Patients should be warned before drug administration of side effects usually lasting less than 1 minute:

- Bradycardia and AV block
- Facial flushing, headache, chest pain or tightness
- Bronchospasm, sense of impending doom.

Cautions/contraindications

Contraindicated in asthma, second- or third-degree AV block and sick sinus syndrome (unless pacemaker fitted).

Amiodarone hydrochloride

Mechanism of action

Class III (Vaughan Williams' classification) drug action, which prolongs the duration of the action potential, thus increasing the absolute refractory period. Inhibits the potassium channels involved in repolarization.

Indications

Intravenous injection of amiodarone is used in cardiopulmonary resuscitation for ventricular fibrillation or pulseless tachycardia unresponsive to other interventions. Oral and i.v. amiodarone is used in the treatment of arrhythmias (supraventricular and ventricular tachycardia, atrial fibrillation and flutter), particularly when other drugs are ineffective or contraindicated. In the non-emergency setting it should only be initiated under specialist supervision. Unlike many other antiarrhythmic drugs, amiodarone causes little or no myocardial depression.

Preparations and dose

Tablets: 100 mg, 200 mg. Injection: 30 mg/mL or concentrate 50 mg/mL.

Oral Oral administration is 200 mg three times daily for 1 week reduced to 200 mg twice daily for a further week; the maintenance dose is usually 200 mg daily or the minimum required to control the arrhythmia.

Intravenous Intravenous administration is via central line catheter (in an emergency, e.g. ventricular tachycardia, can be given via a large peripheral line, but is a vesicant drug and therefore requires caution), initially 5 mg/kg in 250 mL glucose 5% (drug incompatible with sodium chloride) over 20–120 minutes with ECG monitoring. This may be repeated if necessary to a maximum of 1.2 g in 24 hours in 500 mL. As soon as an adequate response has been obtained, oral therapy should be initiated and the i.v. therapy phased out.

Side effects

Amiodarone therapy can be proarrhythmogenic in patients with significant structural heart disease. Amiodarone contains iodine and can cause both hypothyroidism and hyperthyroidism. Thyroid function tests including T_3 should be measured before treatment and then every 6 months of treatment. Liver toxicity can also occur, so liver biochemistry should be measured before and then every 6 months of treatment. Other side effects are reversible corneal microdeposits (drivers may be dazzled by headlights at night), phototoxic skin reactions (advise use of sunblock creams), slate-grey skin pigmentation, pneumonitis and peripheral neuropathy.

Cautions/contraindications

It is contraindicated in sinus bradycardia or sinoatrial heart block, unless pacemaker fitted, iodine sensitivity and thyroid dysfunction.

Many drugs interact with amiodarone, including warfarin and digoxin (check *British National Formulary* for full list). It has a very long half-life (extending to several weeks) and many months may be required to achieve steady-state concentrations; this is also important when drug interactions are considered.

Flecainide

Mechanism of action

Class Ic (Vaughan Williams' classification) antiarrhythmic drug. It is a membrane-depressant drug that reduces the rate of entry of sodium into the cell (sodium channel blocker). This may slow conduction, delay recovery or reduce the spontaneous discharge rate of myocardial cells.

Indications

AV nodal reciprocating tachycardia, arrhythmias associated with accessory conducting pathways (e.g. Wolff–Parkinson–White syndrome), paroxysmal atrial fibrillation. Occasionally it is used in ventricular tachyarrhythmias resistant to other treatments.

Preparations and dose

IVT – 50 mg twice daily, increased to maximum 300 mg daily.
'On demand' treatment for AF – 200 mg or 300 mg if weight greater than 70 kg, at the onset of paroxysm.

Side effects

Side effects include dizziness, visual disturbances, dyspnoea, palpitations, proarrhythmic effects, headache, fatigue and nausea in 5–10% of patients. Rarely, bronchospasm, heart block, bone marrow suppression and increased ventricular rate in AF/flutter are seen.

Cautions/contraindications

Class Ic agents increase mortality in post-MI patients with ventricular ectopy and should therefore be reserved for patients who **do not** have significant coronary artery disease, left ventricular dysfunction, or other forms of significant structural heart disease. Interactions with other drugs, including β-blockers and calcium-channel blockers, can occur (check *British National Formulary* for full list).

β-Blockers

See page 495.

Digoxin

Mechanism of action

This drug blocks AV conduction and reduces heart rate by enhancing vagal nerve activity and inhibiting sympathetic activity. It is positively inotropic (enhancing strength of cardiac contraction) by inhibition of Na^+/K^+-ATPase and secondary activation of the Na^+/Ca^{2+} membrane exchange pump, thereby increasing intracellular calcium levels.

Indications

Digoxin is used in heart failure with atrial fibrillation or patients in sinus rhythm who remain symptomatic despite ACEI, β-blocker and diuretic uses. It is also used for rate control in sedentary patients with atrial fibrillation/flutter.

Preparations and dose

Tablets: 62.5, 125 and 250 μg. Injection: 250 μg/mL.

Check renal function and electrolytes before starting therapy; reduce dose in the elderly and in renal impairment.

Oral Rapid digitalization for atrial fibrillation/flutter 0.75–1.5 mg in divided doses over 24 hours and then maintenance of 125–250 μg once daily according to heart rate and renal function. For heart failure (sinus rhythm) 62.5–125 μg once daily is given.

Intravenous infusion Intravenous infusion for emergency loading dose for atrial fibrillation or flutter 0.75–1 mg (diluted in glucose 5% or sodium chloride 0.9% to a concentration of not more than 62.5 μg/mL) over at least 2 hours and then maintenance dose the next day by mouth.

Side effects

Side effects include nausea, vomiting, diarrhoea, conduction disturbances, blurred or yellow vision and ventricular arrhythmias. Side effects are common because of the narrow therapeutic index (the margin between effectiveness and toxicity). Hypokalaemia and renal impairment (reduce dose) increase the risk of toxicity. In suspected toxicity, measure plasma potassium concentration first and correct if hypokalaemia is evident. Plasma digoxin concentrations should be measured if toxicity is suspected; concentrations of > 2 mmol/L usually suggest toxicity. In severe toxicity, give anti-digoxin antibodies.

Contraindications

Digoxin is contraindicated in arrhythmias associated with accessory conduction pathways, e.g. Wolff–Parkinson–White syndrome, because the accessory pathway is not affected. Blocking the normal pathway can increase the speed of conduction in the abnormal pathway and lead to ventricular arrhythmias. Caution should be demonstrated in left ventricular outflow tract obstruction. Diltiazem, verapamil, spironolactone and amiodarone inhibit renal excretion of digoxin; avoid with amiodarone and measure plasma levels with other drugs (see *British National Formulary* for full interaction list). Tetracycline, erythromycin and possibly other macrolides enhance the effect of digoxin. Rifampicin reduces serum concentrations.

DRUGS FOR HEART FAILURE

Diuretics

See Table 7.4 and pages 351–353.

β-Blockers

Mechanism of action

The β-adrenoceptors in the heart, peripheral vasculature, bronchi, pancreas and liver are blocked. They decrease heart rate, reduce the force of cardiac contraction and lower BP. These effects reduce myocardial oxygen demand and give more time for coronary perfusion. β-Blockers improve functional status and reduce cardiovascular morbidity and mortality in patients with heart failure.

Indications

The main indicators are angina, MI, arrhythmias, stable heart failure, hypertension, alleviation of symptoms of anxiety, prophylaxis of migraine, prevention of variceal bleeding and symptomatic treatment of hyperthyroidism (no effect on thyroid function tests).

Preparations and dose

Most β-blockers are equally effective, but there are differences between them which may affect the choice in particular diseases or individual patients, e.g. atenolol and metoprolol are used in angina; sotalol in the management of supraventricular and ventricular arrhythmias; propranolol in the treatment of hyperthyroidism, prevention of variceal bleeding and prophylaxis of migraine (usually); bisoprolol and carvedilol in the management of heart failure (usually specialist initiated) and nebivolol in the treatment of stable mild–moderate heart failure in patients over 70 years old.

Propranolol

Tablets: 10 mg, 40 mg, 80 mg, 160 mg. Oral solution: 5 mg/mL. Injection 1 mg/mL.
Oral
- Portal hypertension: initially 40 mg twice daily, increased according to heart rate; maximum 160 mg twice daily
- Angina: initially 40 mg two to three times daily; maintenance dose 120–240 mg daily
- Arrhythmias: anxiety, hyperthyroidism, migraine prophylaxis, essential tremor, 10–40 mg three times daily
- Hypertension: initially 80 mg twice daily, increased at weekly intervals as required; maintenance 160–320 mg daily.

Intravenous Arrhythmias and thyrotoxic crisis: 1 mg over 1 minute; if necessary, repeat at 2-minute intervals; maximum 10 mg.

Atenolol

Tablets: 25 mg, 50 mg, 100 mg.
Oral
- Angina: 25–100 mg daily in one or two doses
- After MI: 25–100 mg daily
- Hypertension: 25–50 mg daily.

Intravenous For arrhythmias: 2.5 mg at a rate of 1 mg/min, repeated at 5-minute intervals to a maximum of 10 mg, or by infusion 150 µg/kg over 20 minutes, repeated every 12 hours if required.

Bisoprolol

Tablets: 1.25 mg, 2.5 mg, 3.75 mg, 5 mg, 7.5 mg, 10 mg.
- Hypertension and angina, usually 5–10 mg once daily; maximum 20 mg daily
- Heart failure, initially 1.25 mg daily titrated up at weekly intervals over 8–10 weeks to maximum 10 mg daily.

Metoprolol

Tablets: 50 mg, 100 mg. Injection: 1 mg/mL.
Oral
- After MI: 100 mg twice daily
- Angina, arrhythmias, anxiety, thyrotoxicosis, migraine prophylaxis, essential tremor: 50–100 mg two to three times daily
- Hypertension: 50–100 mg twice daily.

Intravenous For arrhythmias: up to 5 mg at a rate of 1–2 mg/min, repeated after 5 minutes to a maximum of 10–15 mg.

Sotalol Tablets: 40 mg, 80 mg, 160 mg, Injection: 10 mg/mL.

Sotalol use is limited to the treatment of ventricular arrhythmias or the prevention of supraventricular arrhythmias.

Oral 80 mg daily in one to two divided doses, increased gradually at intervals of 2–3 days to usual dose of 160–320 mg daily.

Intravenous Over 10 minutes: 20–120 mg with ECG monitoring repeated at 6-hourly intervals if necessary.

Side effects

Side effects include bradycardia, exacerbation of intermittent claudication, lethargy, nightmares, hallucinations, deterioration of glucose tolerance and interference with metabolic and autonomic responses to hypoglycaemia in diabetics.

Contraindications

These comprise asthma, severe peripheral arterial disease, second- or third-degree heart block, marked bradycardia, hypotension, phaeochromocytoma (apart from specific use with α-blockers).

DRUGS AFFECTING THE RENIN–ANGIOTENSIN SYSTEM

Renin produced by the kidney in response to glomerular hypoperfusion catalyses cleavage of angiotensinogen (produced by the liver) to angiotensin (AT), which in turn is cleaved by angiotensin-converting enzyme (ACE) to angiotensin II, which acts on two receptors. The AT_1 receptor mediates the vasoconstrictor effects of AT. The actions of the AT_2 receptor are less well defined.

Angiotensin-converting enzyme inhibitors

Mechanism of action

These drugs inhibit the conversion of angiotensin I to angiotensin II and reduce angiotensin II-mediated vasoconstriction.

Indications

ACEIs improve symptoms and significantly improve survival in all grades of heart failure. They are also recommended in patients at risk of developing heart failure (e.g. ischaemic heart disease). Other indications are hypertension and diabetic nephropathy.

Preparations and dose

Perindopril

Tablets: 2 mg, 4 mg, 8 mg.

- Hypertension, initially 4 mg once daily (use 2 mg if in addition to diuretic, in the elderly, in renal impairment) subsequently adjusted according to response to maximum 8 mg daily
- Heart failure: initially 2 mg once daily, increased after at least 2 weeks to maintenance usually 4 mg daily
- Ischaemic heart disease, diabetic nephropathy: 4 mg daily increased after 2 weeks to 8 mg daily.

Lisinopril

Tablets: 2.5 mg, 5 mg, 10 mg, 20 mg.

- Hypertension: initially 10 mg once daily (2.5–5 mg if in addition to diuretic, in the elderly, in renal impairment), usual maintenance 20 mg daily, maximum 80 mg daily

- Heart failure: initially 2.5 mg once daily, increased by 10 mg every 2 weeks if tolerated to maintenance 35 mg daily
- Ischaemic heart disease, diabetic nephropathy: 5–10 mg daily. Immediately post-STEMI start at 2.5 mg if systolic BP 100–120 mmHg and gradually increase to maintenance dose of 5–10 mg. Do not give if systolic BP < 100 mmHg.

Ramipril

Tablets: 1.25 mg, 2.5 mg, 5 mg, 10 mg.

- Hypertension: initially 1.25 mg daily, increased weekly to maintenance 2.5–5 mg daily, maximum 10 mg once daily
- Heart failure: initially 1.25 mg daily, increased if necessary to maximum 10 mg daily
- Ischaemic heart disease, diabetic nephropathy: 2.5 mg twice daily, maintenance 2.5–5 mg daily.

Side effects

After the first dose, side effects can include hypotension (use small initial doses in heart failure and patients taking diuretics, dry cough, hyperkalaemia, sudden deterioration in renal function in patients with renal artery stenosis and in patients taking NSAIDs (check urea and electrolytes 1–2 weeks after starting treatment), loss of taste, rashes and hypersensitivity reactions.

Cautions/contraindications

These include bilateral renal artery stenosis, pregnancy, angio-oedema, severe renal failure, severe or symptomatic mitral or aortic stenosis and hypertrophic obstructive cardiomyopathy (risk of hypotension).

Angiotensin II receptor antagonists

Mechanism of action

These are antagonists of the type 1 subtype of the angiotensin II receptor (AT_1 receptor).

Indications

Indications include hypertension, heart failure or diabetic nephropathy in patients intolerant to ACE inhibitors because of cough.

Preparations and dose

Candesartan

Tablets: 2 mg, 4 mg, 8 mg, 16 mg, 32 mg.

- Hypertension: initially 8 mg daily, increased as necessary to 32 mg daily
- Heart failure: initially 4 mg once daily increased at intervals of at least 2 weeks to target dose of 32 mg.

Valsartan

Capsules: 40 mg, 80 mg, 160 mg.

- Hypertension: 80 mg once daily (40 mg in caution groups) and increased if necessary after 4 weeks to 160 mg daily
- Ischaemic heart disease: 20 mg twice daily increased gradually to 160 mg twice daily.

Side effects

These include postural hypotension, rash, abnormalities in liver biochemistry and hyperkalaemia.

Caution/contraindications

Lower doses should be given in liver and renal impairment, patients taking high-dose diuretics and the elderly (over 75 years). Caution should be applied in renal artery stenosis, aortic or mitral valve stenosis and in obstructive hypertrophic cardiomyopathy.

NITRATES, CALCIUM-CHANNEL BLOCKERS AND POTASSIUM-CHANNEL ACTIVATORS

Nitrates, calcium-channel blockers and potassium-channel activators have a vasodilating effect, leading to a reduction in venous return, which reduces left ventricular work and dilatation of the coronary circulation.

Nitrates

Mechanism of action

An increase in cyclic guanosine monophosphate (cGMP) in vascular smooth muscle cells causes a decrease in intracellular calcium levels and smooth muscle relaxation with dilatation of veins and arteries, including the coronary circulation. Nitrates reduce venous return, which reduces left ventricular work.

Indications

These drugs are used as a prophylaxis for and in the treatment of angina, as an adjunct in congestive heart failure and intravenously in the treatment of acute heart failure and acute coronary syndrome.

Preparations and dose

Glyceryl trinitrate – short acting

Sublingual tablets: 300 μg, 500 μg, 600 μg (expire after 8 weeks once bottle opened). Spray: 400 μg/dose.

- Angina: one or two tablets or sprays under the tongue (sublingual use avoids hepatic first-pass metabolism) repeated as required. More effective if taken before exertion known to precipitate angina. Tablets (unlike spray) can be spat out if side effects occur (headache, hypotension).

Glyceryl trinitrate – transdermal

Patches releasing approx: 5 mg, 10 mg, 15 mg/24 h.

- Angina: apply patch to chest or outer arm and replace at different site every 24 hours. If tolerance (with reduced therapeutic effect) is suspected, the patch should be left off for 4–8 consecutive hours – usually at night as this is the least symptomatic period.

Glyceryl trinitrate – long-acting tablets

Buccal tablets: 2 mg, 3 mg, 5 mg.

- Angina: 1–5 mg three times daily
- Heart failure: 5 mg (increased to 10 mg in severe cases) three times daily.

Glyceryl trinitrate injection

5 mg/mL, diluted to 100 µg/mL, i.e. 5 mg in 50 mL, in glucose 5% or sodium chloride 0.9% administered via a syringe pump.

- 0.6–0.9 mg/h i.v., then increase dose cautiously until response is achieved, keeping systolic BP > 100 mmHg. Usual range 2–10 mg/h.

Isosorbide mononitrate

Tablets: 10 mg, 20 mg, 40 mg.

- 10–40 mg twice daily, 8 hours apart rather than 12 to prevent nitrate tolerance.

Isosorbide mononitrate (modified release)

Tablets: 25 mg, 50 mg, 60 mg.

- 25–60 mg once daily. Reserve for patients where twice-daily dosing (above) has proved unacceptable. Build up dose gradually to avoid headaches. Up to 120 mg daily may be required.

Side effects

These are mainly due to vasodilating properties and are minimized by initiating therapy with a low dose. They include flushing, headache, postural hypotension, and methaemoglobinaemia with excessive dosage.

Cautions/contraindications

Nitrates are contraindicated in hypotension and hypovolaemia, hypertrophic obstructive cardiomyopathy, aortic stenosis, mitral stenosis, cardiac tamponade and constrictive pericarditis. Nitrates potentiate the effect of other vasodilators and hypotensive drugs. Sildenafil is contraindicated in patients taking nitrates.

Calcium-channel blockers

This group of drugs includes different modified-release preparations of calcium-channel blockers that have different bioavailabilities, and so the brand should be stated on the prescription.

Mechanism of action

These drugs block calcium channels and modify calcium uptake into myocardium and vascular smooth muscle cells. The dihydropyridine calcium-channel blockers (e.g. amlodipine, nifedipine, nimodipine) are potent vasodilators with little effect on cardiac contractility or conduction. In contrast, verapamil, and to a lesser extent diltiazem, are weak vasodilators but depress cardiac conduction and contractility.

Indications

Indicators for use are hypertension and prophylaxis for angina. Verapamil is used in the treatment of some arrhythmias. Nimodipine is for the prevention of ischaemic neurological deficits following aneurysmal subarachnoid haemorrhage.

Preparations and dose

Amlodipine

Tablets: 5 mg, 10 mg.

- 5–10 mg once daily.

Verapamil

Tablets: 40 mg, 80 mg, 120 mg, 160 mg. Oral solution: 40 mg/5 mL. Modified-release (slow-release, SR) tablets: 120 mg, 240 mg; injection: 2.5 mg/mL.

- Angina: 80–120 mg three times daily. SR 240 mg once or twice daily
- Hypertension: 240–480 mg daily in two to three divided doses. SR 120–240 mg once or twice daily
- Supraventricular arrhythmias: oral 40–120 mg three times daily, i.v. 5–10 mg over 10 minutes, further 5 mg after 5–10 minutes if required.

Nifedipine modified release

Adalat LA tablets: 20 mg, 30 mg, 60 mg.

- Angina: initially 30 mg once daily, increased if necessary to 90 mg once daily
- Hypertension: initially 20 mg once daily, increased if necessary.

Diltiazem

Tablets: 60 mg.

- Angina: 60 mg three times daily.

Diltiazem slow release

Capsules for twice daily use: 90 mg, 120 mg, 180 mg. Capsules for once daily use: 120 mg, 180 mg, 240 mg, 300 mg.

- Hypertension: 120 mg twice daily
- Angina: 90 mg twice daily, increased to 180 mg twice daily if required
- Angina and hypertension: 240 mg once daily, increased to 300 mg once daily.

Side effects

These are mainly due to vasodilator properties: flushing, dizziness, tachycardia, hypotension, ankle swelling and headache. Side effects are minimized by starting with a low dose and increasing slowly. Constipation occurs with verapamil. Worsening heart failure can be seen with verapamil and diltiazem.

Cautions/contraindications

The major contraindication is aortic stenosis. Verapamil and diltiazem diminish cardiac contractility and slow cardiac conduction; thus they are relatively contraindicated in patients taking β-blockers, left ventricular failure, sick sinus syndrome and heart failure. Verapamil is contraindicated for treatment of arrhythmias complicating Wolff–Parkinson–White syndrome. Short-acting calcium antagonists increase mortality and are contraindicated immediately after MI.

Potassium-channel activators

Mechanism of action

The mechanism of action here is a hybrid of nitrates (p. 499) and calcium-channel blockers. Potassium-channel activators cause an increase in potassium flow into the cell, which indirectly leads to calcium-channel blockade and arterial dilatation.

Indications

Use is indicated in cases of refractory angina in patients who are uncontrolled on standard regimens of aspirin, β-blockers, nitrates, calcium antagonists and statins.

Preparations and dose

Nicorandil

Tablets: 10 mg, 20 mg.

- 5–30 mg twice daily.

Side effects

These include headache (often temporary), flushing, nausea, vomiting, dizziness, hypotension, tachycardia.

Cautions/contraindications

Nicorandil use is contraindicated in left ventricular failure and cardiogenic shock. Sildenafil is contraindicated in patients taking nicorandil.

11 Respiratory disease

BASIC STRUCTURE OF THE RESPIRATORY SYSTEM

The main function of the lungs is to provide continuous gas exchange between inspired air (supplying oxygen) and blood in the pulmonary circulation (removing carbon dioxide). The lungs are each enclosed within a double membrane; visceral pleura covers the surface of the lung and is continuous at the hilum with the parietal pleura, which lines the inside of the thoracic cavity. The interpleural space between these layers normally contains only a tiny amount of lubricating fluid. The right lung is divided into three lobes, whereas the left lung has two. The trachea divides at the carina (lying under the junction of manubrium sterni and second right costal cartilage) into right and left main bronchi. Within the lungs the bronchi branch again, forming secondary and tertiary bronchi, then smaller bronchioles, and finally terminal bronchioles ending at the alveoli.

The airways are lined by epithelium containing ciliated columnar cells and mucous (goblet) cells – fewer of the latter in the smaller airways. Mucus traps macrophages, inhaled particles and bacteria, and is moved by the cilia in a cephalad direction, thus clearing the lungs (the mucociliary escalator). Gas exchange occurs in the alveolus where capillary blood flow and inspired air are separated only by a thin wall composed mainly of type 1 pneumocytes and capillary endothelial cells and the capillary and alveolar basement membranes are fused as one.

FUNCTION OF THE RESPIRATORY SYSTEM

The lung has a dual blood supply: pulmonary (venous blood) and systemic (arterial blood). The pulmonary circulation delivers deoxygenated blood to the lungs from the right side of the heart via the pulmonary artery. Oxygen from inhaled air passes through the alveoli into the bloodstream and oxygenated blood is returned to the left heart via the pulmonary veins. The bronchial (systemic) system carries arterial blood from the descending aorta to oxygenate lung tissue primarily along the larger conducting airways. In contrast, carbon dioxide passes from the capillaries which surround the alveoli, into the alveolar spaces, and is breathed out.

Inspiratory airflow is achieved by creating a sub-atmospheric pressure in the alveoli by increasing the volume of the thoracic cavity under the action of the inspiratory muscles: descent of the diaphragm (innervated by the phrenic nerve, C3–C5) and contraction of the intercostal muscles with movement of the ribs upwards and outwards. The accessory muscles of respiration are also recruited (sternomastoids and scalenes) during exercise or respiratory distress. Expiration is a passive process, relying on the elastic recoil of the lung and chest wall. During exercise, ventilation is increased and expiration becomes active, with contraction of the muscles of the abdominal wall and the internal intercostals.

SYMPTOMS OF RESPIRATORY DISEASE

Common symptoms of respiratory disease are cough, sputum production, haemoptysis, breathlessness, wheeze and chest pain (p. 409).

Cough is the most common manifestation of lower respiratory tract disease. It is initiated by mechanical (e.g. touch and displacement) or chemical (e.g. noxious fumes) stimulation of specialized cough receptors on the epithelium of the upper and lower respiratory tract. Impulses are carried by afferent nerves to a 'cough centre' in the medulla. This generates efferent signals (via phrenic nerve and efferent branches of the vagus) to expiratory musculature to generate a cough.

Cough lasting only a few weeks is most commonly due to an acute respiratory tract infection. Asthma, gastro-oesophageal reflux disease and postnasal drip are the most common causes of a persistent cough (Table 11.1). A postnasal drip is due to rhinitis, acute nasopharyngitis or sinusitis and symptoms, other than cough, are nasal discharge, a sensation of liquid dripping back into the throat and frequent throat clearing. Cough may be the only symptom of asthma when it is typically worse at night, on waking and after exercise. A chronic cough, sometimes accompanied by sputum production, is common in smokers. However, a worsening cough may be the presenting symptom of bronchial carcinoma and needs investigation.

Sputum Cigarette smoking is the commonest cause of excess mucus production. Mucoid sputum is clear and white but can contain black specks resulting from the inhalation of carbon. Yellow or green sputum is due to the presence of cellular material, including bronchial epithelial cells, or neutrophil or eosinophil granulocytes. Yellow sputum is not necessarily due to infection, as eosinophils in the sputum, as seen in asthma, can give the same

---

Table 11.1 Causes of persistent cough

*Postnasal drip

*Asthma

*Gastro-oesophageal reflux disease

Post-viral cough

Lung airway disease: COPD, bronchiectasis, tumour, foreign body

Lung parenchymal disease: interstitial lung disease, lung abscess

Drugs: ACE inhibitors

*Commonest causes and responsible for 99% of cases who are non-smokers, not taking ACE inhibitors and with a normal chest X-ray.

COPD, chronic obstructive pulmonary disease; ACE, angiotensin-converting enzyme.

appearance. The production of large quantities of yellow or green sputum is characteristic of bronchiectasis.

Haemoptysis (coughing blood) always requires investigation. Common causes are bronchiectasis, bronchial carcinoma, pulmonary embolism, bronchitis and lung infections including pneumonia (rust-coloured sputum), abscess and tuberculosis. Pulmonary oedema is associated with the production of pink frothy sputum. Rarer causes are benign tumours, bleeding disorders, granulomatosis with polyangitis (p. 549) and Goodpasture's syndrome (p. 552). A chest X-ray should be performed in all patients, and subsequent investigations (e.g. bronchoscopy, computed tomography (CT) of the thorax, ventilation–perfusion scan) decided from the history and examination.

Massive haemoptysis (>200 mL in 24 hours) is most often due to pulmonary TB, bronchiectasis, lung abscess or malignancy (primary or secondary). It may be life-threatening due to asphyxiation and is an indication for hospital admission. Initial management includes administration of oxygen, placement of a large-bore intravenous catheter, blood samples (full blood count, clotting screen, urea and electrolytes), arterial blood gases and chest X-ray. There should be early referral to a respiratory physician and thoracic surgeon.

Breathlessness Dyspnoea is the subjective sensation of shortness of breath. Orthopnoea is breathlessness that occurs when lying flat and is the result of abdominal contents pushing the diaphragm into the thorax. Paroxysmal nocturnal dyspnoea is a manifestation of left heart failure: the patient wakes up gasping for breath and finds some relief by sitting upright. The mechanism is similar to orthopnoea, but because sensory awareness is depressed during sleep, severe interstitial pulmonary oedema can accumulate.

The cause of breathlessness (Table 11.2) is often apparent from the clinical history and examination, particularly with sudden and acute breathlessness. In acute breathlessness, appropriate initial investigations include a chest X-ray, pulse oximetry and sometimes arterial blood gases. ECG, full blood count, serum electrolytes, blood glucose, serum troponin (suspected cardiac cause) and D-dimers (suspected pulmonary embolism) may be indicated depending on the clinical circumstances. Pulmonary embolism can be a difficult diagnosis to make and chest X-ray, blood gases and ECG may be normal (p. 473). Simple lung function tests, pulse oximetry, a full blood count and a chest X-ray are the initial investigations for most patients with chronic breathlessness. Echocardiography is indicated if a cardiac cause is suspected.

Psychogenic breathlessness is usually described as 'inability to take a deep breath' and rarely disturbs sleep: it may be better with exercise.

Wheezing is the result of airflow limitation and due to localized (e.g. cancer, foreign body) or generalized (e.g. asthma and chronic obstructive pulmonary disease [COPD]) obstruction of the airways. Asthma is a common cause of wheezing and is likely when patients present with episodic wheezing, cough and dyspnoea which responds favourably to inhaled bronchodilators. Wheeze should be distinguished from stridor, which is a harsh inspiratory wheezing sound caused by obstruction of the trachea or major bronchi, e.g. by tumour.

Table 11.2 Causes of breathlessness

Acute (onset over minutes/ hours)	Chronic (onset over days/ months)
Acute asthma	Asthma
Exacerbation COPD	COPD
Pneumothorax	Diffuse parenchymal lung disease
Pulmonary embolism	Pleural effusion
Pneumonia	Cancer of the bronchus/trachea
Hypersensitivity pneumonitis	Heart failure
Upper airway obstruction: Inhaled foreign body Anaphylaxis	Severe anaemia
Left heart failure	
Cardiac tamponade	
Panic with hyperventilation	

COPD, chronic obstructive pulmonary disease.

Chest pain (p. 409) due to respiratory disease is often a localized sharp pain made worse by deep breathing or coughing (referred to as pleuritic pain) and is most commonly caused by infection or by pleural irritation from a pulmonary embolism.

INVESTIGATION OF RESPIRATORY DISEASE

Sputum

Sputum is commonly sent for microbiology (Gram stain and culture in pneumonia, auramine stain in suspected tuberculosis) and cytology for malignant cells, but may be falsely negative. A 5% saline nebulizer will encourage productive coughing if sputum is difficult to obtain. Yellow/green sputum indicates inflammation (infection or allergy). Haemoptysis is discussed above.

Respiratory function tests

Respiratory function tests include simple outpatient investigations to assess airflow limitation and lung volumes. Normal values vary for age, sex and height, and between individuals.

Peak expiratory flow rate

Peak expiratory flow rate (PEFR) records the maximum expiratory flow rate during a forced expiration after full inspiration and is measured with a peak flow meter. It is useful in monitoring the response to treatment of asthma and many patients will monitor their own PEFR at home.

The spirometer

The spirometer is used to measure forced expiratory volume (FEV) and forced vital capacity (FVC). The patient exhales as fast and as long as possible from a full inspiration; the volume expired in the first second is the FEV_1 and the total volume expired is the FVC. The FEV_1/FVC ratio is a measure of airflow limitation and is normally about 75%:

- Airflow limitation: FEV_1/FVC $< 75\%$
- Restrictive lung disease: FEV_1/FVC $> 75\%$.

More sophisticated techniques allow the measurement of total lung capacity (TLC) and residual volume (RV). These are increased in obstructive lung disease such as asthma or COPD, because of air trapping, and reduced in lung fibrosis. Transfer factor (T_{CO}) measures the transfer of a low concentration of added carbon monoxide in the inspired air to haemoglobin. The transfer coefficient (K_{CO}) is the value corrected for differences in lung volume. Gas transfer is reduced early on in emphysema and lung fibrosis.

Arterial blood gas sampling This is used to measure partial pressures of oxygen and carbon dioxide within arterial blood (p. 583), the values of which are used in the assessment of the breathless patient and the management of respiratory failure and acute asthma. Arterial oxygen saturation (S_aO_2) can be continuously measured non-invasively using an oximeter with either ear or finger probes. Normal ranges are from 94–98%. However, carbon dioxide levels are not measured and hypoventilation with carbon dioxide retention would go undetected.

Walking distance

A 6-minute period is also used to assess lung function.

Imaging

Chest X-ray

Routine films are taken postero-anteriorly (PA), i.e. the film is placed in front of the patient with the X-ray source behind. AP films are taken only in patients who are unable to stand; the cardiac outline appears bigger and the scapulae cannot be moved out of the way. Fig. 11.1 shows a normal chest X-ray and suggests a systematic approach to read a film. The solitary pulmonary nodule detected on chest X-ray is a common clinical problem (Table 11.3). Risk factors for malignancy in this situation are older age, smoker, occupational exposure to carcinogens, increasing size of lesion ($80\% > 3$ cm), irregular border, eccentric calcification of the lesion and increasing size compared to an old X-ray. CT scan is usually necessary for further evaluation.

Computed tomography (CT scan)

The initial imaging tool for the lung parenchyma is the chest X-ray. However, a CT scan can detect lung disease in symptomatic patients with a normal chest X-ray.

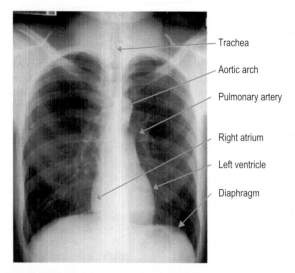

Trachea

Aortic arch

Pulmonary artery

Right atrium

Left ventricle

Diaphragm

Fig. 11.1 A normal chest X-ray and suggested checklist for review of a film.

Checklist

- Patient name and date of film
- View – PA or AP?
- Film centring – equal distance between each clavicular head and spinal processes?
- Trachea – deviated from midline?
- Soft tissues: neck, shoulders, breast
- Bony outline: ribs, clavicles, spine
- Diaphragms – right diaphragm usually 2–3 cm higher than left
- Cardiothoracic ratio – maximum transverse diameter of the heart normally less than 50% maximum transverse diameter of the thorax measured from inside of ribs on PA film
- Mediastinum – widened? (>6 cm on upright film or >25% of thoracic width at aortic knob)
- Hilar region – lymphadenopathy?, enlarged pulmonary arteries and veins?
- Lungs – opacities, consolidation, fluid, nodules?

It can be used as a guide to the type and site of lung or pleural biopsy, and is used in the staging of bronchial carcinoma. Multi-slice (high-resolution) CT scanning (sampling lung parenchyma with scans of 1–2 mm thickness at intervals of 10–20 mm) is particularly useful in the detection and evaluation of diffuse parenchymal lung disease and in diagnosis of bronchiectasis. CT angiography (helical CT using intravenous contrast) is used in the diagnosis of pulmonary emboli.

Table 11.3 Causes of a solitary pulmonary nodule

Benign	Malignant
Infectious granuloma, e.g. tuberculosis	Bronchial carcinoma
Other infections, e.g. localized pneumonia, abscess, hydatid cyst	Single metastasis
Benign neoplasms	Lymphoma
Arteriovenous malformation	Pulmonary carcinoid
Bronchogenic cyst	
Pulmonary infarct	
Inflammatory, rheumatoid nodule, granulomatosis with polyangiitis	

Magnetic resonance imaging (MRI)

MRI is used in the staging of lung cancer to assess tumour invasion in the mediastinum, lung apex and chest wall. It also provides accurate images of the heart and aorta. MRI is less useful than CT scanning in the assessment of the lung parenchyma.

Positron emission tomography (PET)

PET scanning is used in the investigation of pulmonary nodules to differentiate benign from malignant, and in the staging of lung cancer.

Scintigraphic imaging

Ventilation–perfusion ($\dot{V}/\dot{Q}$) scanning is used in the diagnosis of pulmonary emboli. Xenon-133 gas is inhaled (the ventilation scan) and microaggregates of albumin labelled with technetium-99 m are injected intravenously (the perfusion scan). Pulmonary emboli are detected as 'cold areas' on the perfusion scan relative to the ventilation scan. However, many lung diseases affect pulmonary blood flow as well as ventilation and the $\dot{V}/\dot{Q}$ scan is only diagnostic when it is reported as normal (excluding PE) or high probability (diagnostic of pulmonary emboli).

Pleural aspiration and biopsy

Pleural aspiration is used for both diagnostic and therapeutic reasons (to drain large effusions for symptom relief, to instill therapeutic agents such as sclerosants). A diagnostic fluid sample is obtained with a fine bore needle and a 50 mL syringe to investigate the cause of a pleural effusion (p. 558). Complications of pleural aspiration include pneumothorax, damage to the neurovascular bundle which lies in the subcostal groove, infection and seeding of malignant cells along the tract with a malignant effusion. Pulmonary oedema may occur when large quantities of fluid (>1 L) are removed rapidly for therapeutic purposes.

Bronchoscopy

A flexible bronchoscope is passed through the nose. The airways as far as the subsegmental bronchi are inspected under intravenous midazolam sedation, topical lidocaine anaesthesia and pre-medication with an antimuscarinic agent such as atropine (to reduce bronchial secretions). Biopsies and brushings are taken of macroscopic abnormalities and washings for appropriate microbiological staining and culture and cytological examination for malignant cells. Diffuse parenchymal lung disease is investigated by transbronchial biopsy. Complications of bronchoscopy ± biopsy include respiratory depression, pneumothorax, respiratory obstruction, cardiac arrhythmias and haemorrhage.

Mediastinoscopy

Mediastinoscopy is used in the diagnosis of mediastinal masses and in staging nodal disease in carcinoma of the bronchus. An incision is made just above the sternum and a mediastinoscope inserted by blunt dissection.

Video-assisted thoracoscopic (VATS) lung biopsy

This technique is less invasive than open thoracotomy for obtaining a lung biopsy. It is used in the investigation of diffuse and localized lung disease.

SMOKING

Cigarette smoking has declined in recent years in the Western world, but is on the increase in many developing countries. Tobacco smoke contains over 40 different carcinogens and is associated with an increased risk of cancer in the gastrointestinal tract (oral cavity, oesophagus, stomach and pancreas), respiratory (larynx and bronchus) and urogenital system (bladder, kidney, cervix). Cigarette smoking is a risk factor for ischaemic heart disease and peripheral vascular disease and is the major cause of COPD (p. 516). Environmental tobacco smoke ('passive' smoking) also increases the risk of lung cancer and COPD. Persuading an individual to stop smoking is an essential part of the management of many respiratory diseases and has a preventative role in the 'well' person. Population-targeted approaches such as advertising and banning smoking in public places has reduced smoking prevalence. Individually targeted smoking cessation strategies are best delivered by a smoking cessation clinic and are non-pharmacological (behavioural therapy, self-help programmes, group counselling) and pharmacological treatments:

- Nicotine replacement therapy as gum, lozenges, patches, tablets, nasal spray
- Bupropion tablets – mode of action in smoking cessation is not clear
- Varenicline tablets – partial agonist at the nicotinic acid acetylcholine receptor.

The pharmacological therapies all require the smoker to commit to a target stop date.

DISEASES OF THE UPPER RESPIRATORY TRACT

The common cold (acute coryza)

The common cold is usually caused by infection with one of the rhinoviruses. Spread is by droplets and close personal contact. After an incubation period of 12 hours to 5 days there is malaise, slight pyrexia, a sore throat and a watery nasal discharge, which becomes mucopurulent after a few days. Treatment is symptomatic. The differential diagnosis is mainly from rhinitis (see below).

Sinusitis (see p. 707)

Rhinitis

Rhinitis is defined clinically as sneezing attacks, nasal discharge or blockage occurring for more than 1 hour on most days:

- For a limited period of the year *(seasonal or intermittent rhinitis)*
- Throughout the whole year *(perennial or persistent rhinitis)*.

Seasonal rhinitis is often called 'hay fever' and occurs during the summer months. It is caused by allergy to grass and tree pollen and a variety of mould spores (e.g. *Aspergillus fumigatus*) which grow on cultivated plants. In addition to the nasal symptoms, there may be itching of the eyes and soft palate.

Perennial rhinitis may be allergic (the allergens are similar to those for asthma) or non-allergic (triggered by cold air, smoke and perfume). Patients rarely have symptoms affecting the eyes or soft palate. Some develop nasal polyps which may cause nasal obstruction, loss of smell and taste, and mouth breathing.

Diagnosis

The diagnosis of rhinitis is clinical. Skin-prick testing or measurement of specific serum immunoglobulin E (IgE) antibody against the particular antigen (RAST test) in conjunction with a detailed clinical history will identify causal antigens.

Management

This involves avoidance of allergens, if practical, antihistamines, e.g. cetirizine or loratadine tablets, decongestants and topical steroids, e.g. beclometasone spray twice daily. A 2-week course of low-dose oral prednisolone (5–10 mg daily) is used when other treatments fail.

Acute pharyngitis

Viruses, particularly from the adenovirus group, are the most common cause of acute pharyngitis. Symptoms are a sore throat and fever which are self-limiting and only require symptomatic treatment. More persistent and severe pharyngitis may imply bacterial infection, often secondary invaders, of which the most common organisms are haemolytic streptococcus, *Haemophilus influenzae* and *Staphylococcus aureus*. This is treated with penicillin V 500 mg four times a day for 10 days (erythromycin if allergic).

Acute laryngotracheobronchitis (croup)

This is usually the result of infection with one of the parainfluenza viruses or measles virus. Symptoms are most severe in children under 3 years of age. Inflammatory oedema involving the larynx causes a hoarse voice, barking cough (croup) and stridor (p. 507). Tracheitis produces a burning retrosternal pain. Treatment is with oxygen therapy, oral or intramuscular corticosteroids and nebulized adrenaline. Endotracheal intubation is occasionally necessary and, rarely, tracheostomy.

Influenza

The influenza virus exists in two main forms, A and B. The surface of the virion is coated with haemagglutinin (H) and an enzyme, neuraminidase (N), which are necessary for attachment to the host respiratory epithelium. Human immunity develops against the H and N antigens. Influenza A has the capacity to undergo antigenic 'shift', and major changes in the H and N antigens are associated with pandemic infections which may cause millions of deaths worldwide. The H5N1 strain is passed from birds to humans (avian flu) and the H1N1 strain is endemic in pigs and birds. A new strain of swine-origin H1N1 is responsible for the latest pandemic, declared in June 2009. Minor antigenic 'drifts' are associated with less severe epidemics.

Clinical features

The incubation period is 1–3 days. There is then an abrupt onset of fever, generalized aching in the limbs, severe headache, sore throat and dry cough, all of which may last several weeks. Influenza and the common cold (p. 513) can have similar symptoms. In general, flu symptoms are worse than a common cold: fever, generalized aching and dry cough are more common with flu, and a runny and stuffy nose are more common with a cold.

Diagnosis

Laboratory diagnosis is not always necessary, but serology shows a four-fold rise in antibody titre over a 2-week period, or the virus can be demonstrated in throat or nasal secretion.

Management

Treatment is symptomatic (paracetamol, bed rest, maintenance of fluid intake), together with antibiotics to prevent secondary infection for individuals with chronic bronchitis, heart or renal disease. Neuraminidase inhibitors, e.g. zanamivir and oseltamivir, help to shorten the duration of symptoms in patients with influenza, if given within 48 hours of the first symptom. The cost–benefit of zanamivir and oseltamivir remains unproven but these are currently recommended in the UK for patients with suspected influenza over the age of 65 and 'at-risk' adults, as part of a strategy to reduce admissions to hospital when influenza is circulating in the community.

Complications

Pneumonia is the most common complication. This is either viral or the result of secondary infection with bacteria, of which *S. aureus* is the most serious, with a mortality rate of up to 20%.

Prophylaxis

Influenza vaccine is prepared from current strains. It is effective in 70% of people and lasts for about a year. It is recommended in individuals over 65 years of age or people under 65 years of age who are more likely to acquire the infection or suffer from a severe illness (see *British National Formulary* for a detailed list).

Inhalation of foreign bodies

Children inhale foreign bodies – frequently peanuts – more often than do adults. In adults, inhalation is usually associated with a depressed conscious level, such as after an alcoholic binge. A large object may totally occlude the airways and rapidly result in death. Smaller objects impact more peripherally (usually in the right main bronchus, because it is more vertical than the left) and cause choking or persistent wheeze, presentation at a later stage with persistent suppurative pneumonia or lung abscess. In an emergency the foreign body is dislodged from the airway using the Heimlich manoeuvre: the subject is gripped from behind with the arms around the upper abdomen, a sharp forceful squeeze pushes the diaphragm into the thorax and the rapid airflow generated may be sufficient to force the foreign body out of the trachea or bronchus. In the non-emergency situation, bronchoscopy is used to remove the foreign body.

DISEASES OF THE LOWER RESPIRATORY TRACT

Acute bronchitis

Acute bronchitis is usually viral but may be complicated by bacterial infection, particularly in smokers and in patients with chronic airflow limitation. Symptoms are cough, retrosternal discomfort, chest tightness and wheezing, which usually resolve spontaneously over 4–8 days.

Chronic obstructive pulmonary disease (COPD)

COPD is characterized by poorly reversible airflow limitation that is usually progressive and associated with a persistent inflammatory response of the lungs. COPD is now the preferred term for patients previously diagnosed as having chronic bronchitis or emphysema.

Epidemiology and aetiology

Cigarette smoking is the major cause of COPD and is related to the daily average of cigarettes smoked and years spent smoking. Most smokers will eventually develop abnormal lung function if they continue to smoke. Chronic exposure to pollutants at work (mining, building and chemical industries), outdoor air pollution, and inhalation of smoke from biomass fuels used in heating and cooking in poorly ventilated areas play a role, particularly in developing countries. α_1-Antitrypsin deficiency (p. 179) causes early-onset COPD but otherwise patients are rarely symptomatic before middle age. The cost of COPD is considerable due to direct (hospital admissions, outpatient visits, drug costs) and indirect costs (loss of working days).

Pathophysiology

In chronic bronchitis, there is airway narrowing, and hence airflow limitation, as a result of hypertrophy and hyperplasia of mucus-secreting glands of the bronchial tree, bronchial wall inflammation and mucosal oedema. The epithelial cell layer may ulcerate and, when the ulcers heal, squamous epithelium may replace columnar epithelium (squamous metaplasia). Emphysema is defined pathologically as dilatation and destruction of the lung tissue distal to the terminal bronchioles. Emphysematous changes lead to loss of elastic recoil, which normally keeps airways open during expiration; this is associated with expiratory airflow limitation and air trapping. Although it has been suggested that these definitions separate patients into two different clinical groups (the 'pink puffers' with predominant emphysema and the 'blue bloaters' with predominant chronic bronchitis), most have both emphysema and chronic bronchitis, irrespective of the clinical signs.

Pathogenesis

- *Cigarette smoke* causes mucous gland hypertrophy in the larger airways and leads to an increase in neutrophils, macrophages and lymphocyes in the airways and walls of the bronchi and bronchioles. These cells release inflammatory mediators (elastases, proteases, interleukin-1 [IL-1] and IL-8 and tumour necrosis factor-α [TNF-α]) that attract inflammatory cells (and further amplify the process), induce structural changes and break down connective tissue (protease–antiprotease imbalance) in the lung parenchyma, resulting in emphysema. α_1-Antitrypsin is a major protease inhibitor which can be inactivated by cigarette smoke.

- *Respiratory infections* are a precipitating cause of acute exacerbations of COPD, but it is not known if they contribute to the progressive airflow limitation that characterizes COPD.
- α_1-*Antitrypsin deficiency* (p. 179) is a cause of early-onset emphysema.

Clinical features

Symptoms and signs help to distinguish COPD from asthma (Table 11.4). The characteristic symptoms of COPD are cough with the production of sputum, wheeze and breathlessness following many years of a smoker's cough. Frequent infective exacerbations occur, giving purulent sputum. On examination the patient with severe disease is breathless at rest, with prolonged expiration, chest expansion is poor and the lungs are hyperinflated (loss of normal cardiac and liver dullness, 'barrel-shaped chest, protruding abdomen). Pursed lips on expiration help to prevent alveolar and airway collapse. Use of the accessory muscles of respiration (scalene and sternocleidomastoid) reflect the increased work of breathing (Fig. 11.2). There may be a wheeze or quiet breath sounds. In 'pink puffers', breathlessness is the predominant problem; they are not cyanosed. 'Blue bloaters' hypoventilate; they are cyanosed, may be oedematous and have features of CO_2 retention (warm peripheries with a bounding pulse, flapping tremor of the outstretched hands and confusion in severe cases).

Table 11.4 Differentiating features of COPD and asthma

	COPD	Asthma
Smoker or ex-smoker	Most	Possibly
Symptoms under age 35	Rare	Common
Atopic features (rhinitis, eczema)	Uncommon	Common
Cellular infiltrate	Macrophages, neutrophils, CD8+ T cells	Eosinophils, CD4+ T cells
Cough and sputum	Daily/common	Intermittent
Breathlessness	Persistent and progressive	Variable
Night time symptoms	Uncommon	Common
Significant diurnal or day-to-day variability of symptoms	Uncommon	Common
Bronchodilator response (FEV_1 and PEFR)	<15%	>20%
Corticosteroid response	Variable	Good

FEV_1, forced expiratory volume in first second; PEFR, peak expiratory flow rate.

Thin with loss of muscle mass

Pursed-lip breathing

Increased work of breathing:

- leaning forward
- accessory muscles of respiration
- tracheal tug
- nasal flare
- paradoxical abdominal movement
- indrawing of intercostal muscles

Hyperinflated chest – 'barrel chest'

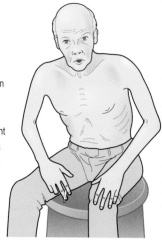

Fig. 11.2 Some clinical signs in a patient with chronic obstructive pulmonary disease.

In addition to pulmonary manifestations, patients with COPD develop systemic problems, including skeletal muscle dysfunction (loss of muscle bulk and skeletal muscle strength), nutritional abnormalities, weight loss and depression. Skeletal muscle dysfunction is due to a combination of factors (ageing, malnutrition, systemic inflammation, inactivity, hypoxia) and affects both respiratory and limb muscles. It contributes to reduced exercise tolerance independently of the reduced lung function.

Complications

- Respiratory failure (p. 582)
- Cor pulmonale, i.e. heart disease secondary to disease of the lung (p. 471).

Investigations

The diagnosis is made on the basis of history (breathlessness and sputum production in a chronic smoker), physical examination and confirmation of airflow limitation with lung function testing:

- *Lung function tests* show progressive airflow limitation (Table 11.5). The FEV_1: FVC ratio is reduced and the PEFR is low. Some patients have partially reversible airflow limitation with an increase in FEV_1 (but usually < 15%) following inhalation of a β_2-agonist. Serial peak flow measurements may be

Table 11.5 Classification of severity (GOLD criteria)

Stage of COPD	Function	Symptoms
Stage I, mild	FEV$_1$/FVC < 70% FEV$_1$ ≥ 80% predicted	Chronic cough, none/mild breathlessness
Stage II, moderate	FEV$_1$/FVC < 70% 50% ≤ FEV$_1$ < 80% predicted	Breathlessness on exertion
Stage III, severe	FEV$_1$/FVC < 70% 30% ≤ FEV$_1$ < 50% predicted	Breathless on minimal exertion. May be weight loss and depression
Stage IV, very severe	FEV$_1$/FVC < 70% FEV$_1$ < 30% predicted *or* FEV$_1$ < 50% predicted plus respiratory failure	Breathless at rest

(Modified from the Global Strategy for the Diagnosis, Management and Prevention of COPD, www.goldcopd.com.)

necessary to exclude asthma (Table 11.4). Additional testing of lung function is necessary if there is diagnostic uncertainty. Lung volumes are normal or increased, and the loss of alveoli with emphysema results in a decreased gas transfer coefficient of carbon monoxide.

- *Chest X-ray* may be normal or show evidence of hyperinflated lungs indicated by low, flattened diaphragms and a long narrow heart shadow. There are reduced peripheral lung markings and bullae (complete destruction of lung tissue producing an airspace greater than 1 cm).
- *High-resolution CT scans* are used, particularly to show emphysematous bullae.
- *Haemoglobin and PCV* may be high as a result of persistent hypoxaemia and secondary polycythaemia (p. 221).
- *Arterial blood gases* may be normal or show hypoxia ± hypercapnia in advanced cases.
- *α_1-Antitrypsin* serum levels and genotype are measured in early-onset disease (<40 years) or family history.
- *ECG* and *echocardiography* is used to assess cardiac status if clinical features of cor pulmonale (p. 417).

Management

COPD care should be delivered by a multidisciplinary team that includes a GP and respiratory physicians, respiratory nurse specialists, physiotherapy, occupational therapy, dietetics and palliative care in end-stage COPD.

Cessation of smoking   It is essential to persuade the patient to stop smoking. This may slow the rate of deterioration.

Bronchodilators   A stepwise approach to drug therapy is used similar to that used in asthma (p. 526). Inhaled long-acting once-daily antimuscarinic agents such as tiotropium or aclidinium, are used as initial maintenance therapy with a rescue short-acting β_2-agonist (p. 564) to prevent or reduce acute symptoms. A long-acting β_2-agonist is added in patients with persistent dyspnoea. Dry powder inhalers are simpler to use than metered dose inhalers but technique still needs to be checked. Nebulized therapy may be useful for patients with disabling breathlessness despite inhalers.

Phosphodiesterase type 4 inhibitors   Roflumilast is a phosphodiesterase inhibitor with anti-inflammatory properties. It is used as an adjunct to bronchodilators for the maintenance treatment of COPD patients.

Corticosteroids   Assessment of reversibility is made with a 2-week course of oral prednisolone (30 mg daily), with measurement of lung function before and after the treatment period. If there is objective evidence of benefit ($>15\%$ improvement in FEV_1), oral steroids are gradually reduced and replaced with inhaled corticosteroids. Combinations of corticosteroids with long-acting $\beta2$-agonists may protect against lung function decline but do not improve overall mortality.

Prevention of infection   Acute exacerbations of COPD are commonly due to bacterial or viral infection. Patients should receive pneumococcal vaccine and annual influenza vaccination and receive prompt antibiotic treatment for acute exacerbations.

Oxygen   Long-term domiciliary oxygen therapy is provided by oxygen concentrators and has a survival benefit in selected groups of patients:

- $P_aO_2 < 7.3$ kPa when breathing room air
- $P_aO_2 < 8.0$ kPa with secondary polycythaemia, nocturnal hypoxaemia, peripheral oedema or evidence of pulmonary hypertension.

Assessment for home oxygen should include blood gas measurements made 3 weeks apart in a stable patient receiving bronchodilator treatment. It is prescribed to patients who no longer smoke (supported by a carboxyhaemoglobin concentration $< 3\%$). Oxygen is given for 19 hours per day (every day) at a flow rate of 1–3 L/min via nasal prongs to increase arterial oxygen saturation to $>90\%$.

Additional treatments   include mucolytics to reduce sputum viscosity, venesection for polycythaemia, diuretics for oedema, exercise training to improve sense of well-being and breathlessness, and high-calorie dietary supplements in those with low BMI. Surgery is beneficial for a minority of patients: bullectomy for patients with large emphysematous bullae and lung volume reduction surgery for selected patients with severe COPD ($FEV_1 < 1$ L).

Acute exacerbation of COPD

Diagnosis is made on the basis of increased breathlessness or an increase in sputum volume or purulence. The major complication is respiratory failure.

Exacerbations are usually the result of a superimposed viral or bacterial respiratory tract infection and are investigated and treated in a similar manner to asthma (p. 533) but with some essential modifications (see below). Some patients with mild exacerbations may be managed at home by a dedicated multidisciplinary team (including nurses, physiotherapists and occupational therapists). Management of patients admitted to hospital:

- Controlled oxygen is given with the aim of maintaining $S_a0_2 > 88$–92% and $P_a0_2 > 8$ kPa without increasing $P_a co_2$. These patients often depend on a degree of hypoxaemia to maintain respiratory drive and, therefore, if oxygen is necessary, low concentrations (24%) are given via a Venturi mask (fixed oxygen concentration mask), so as not to reduce respiratory drive and precipitate worsening hypercapnia and respiratory acidosis. The oxygen concentration is increased in increments (28% and then 35%) if clinical examination and arterial blood gases (repeated at 30–60-minute intervals) do not show hypoventilation, carbon dioxide retention and worsening acidosis.

- Patients with life-threatening respiratory failure require ventilatory assistance. Bilevel positive airway pressure (BiPAP, p. 584) avoids the need for intubation and mechanical ventilation in some patients. It is indicated in patients with signs of worsening respiratory distress (respiratory rate > 30/min) and respiratory acidosis (blood pH $\leq$ 7.35, $P_a co_2 > 6$ kPa) who have failed to respond to optimal medical treatment and controlled oxygen.

- Bronchodilators (salbutamol and ipratropium bromide) are given 4–6 hourly together with oral prednisolone 40 mg. In the presence of type 2 respiratory failure, nebulizers should be air driven and controlled oxygen given by nasal cannulae simultaneously.

- Antibiotics, e.g. cefaclor or co-amoxiclav, are given if there is a history of more purulent sputum production or with chest X-ray changes. Patients should be encouraged to cough up sputum, initially with the help of a physiotherapist. Antibiotic treatment is modified depending on sputum culture results.

- Aminophylline use is controversial because of its modest benefits and high incidence of side effects. It is used for patients with moderate to severe exacerbations who are not responding to standard treatment as above.

- Low-molecular-weight heparin is given to prevent thromboembolism.

- Respiratory stimulants such as doxapram are no longer routinely used due to the increasing availability of non-invasive ventilatory support.

- Exacerbations of COPD are occasionally the result of pneumothorax, heart failure or pulmonary embolism, and these must be excluded.

Long term prognosis

This is assessed by the BODE predictive index (**b**ody mass index, degree of airflow **o**bstruction – FEV$_1$, **d**yspnoea, **e**xercise capacity). In the most severe category, a patient with BMI < 21, FEV$_1$ $< 35\%$ predicted, shortness of breath on dressing, and walking distance <149 m in 6 minutes has a mortality rate of 80% at 4 years.

Obstructive sleep apnoea (OSA)

There is repeated apnoea (cessation of breathing for 10 seconds or more) as a result of obstruction of the upper airway during sleep. It affects about 2% of the population and is most common in overweight middle-aged men. It can also occur in children, particularly those with enlarged tonsils.

Aetiology

Apnoea occurs if the upper airway at the back of the throat is sucked closed when the patient breathes in. This occurs during sleep because the muscles that hold the airway open are hypotonic. Airway closure continues until the patient is woken up by the struggle to breathe against a blocked throat. These awakenings are so brief that the patient remains unaware of them but may be woken hundreds of times at night, leading to sleep deprivation and daytime sleepiness. Contributing factors include alcohol ingestion before sleep, obesity and COPD. It is more common in patients with hypothyroidism and acromegaly.

Clinical features

Loud snoring and excessive daytime sleepiness (leading to impairment of work performance and driving) occur in the majority of patients. Apnoeas may be witnessed by bed partners. Other symptoms are irritability, personality change, morning headaches, impotence and nocturnal choking. Patients with OSA have an increased risk of hypertension, heart failure, myocardial infarction and stroke.

Diagnosis

The Epworth Sleepiness Scale is a simple tool that helps discriminate OSA from simple snoring. The patient is asked how likely, or not, they would be to fall asleep in eight specified situations – watching television, and sitting and talking to someone are two examples. A high score equates with significant excess sleepiness. Frequent falls in arterial oxygen saturation during sleep (measured by oximetry at home) may confirm the diagnosis. If this is normal or equivocal, inpatient sleep studies are indicated. This usually involves oximetry supplemented by video-recording in a room specifically adapted for sleep studies. The diagnosis of sleep apnoea/hypopnoea is confirmed if there are more than 10–15 apnoeas or hypopnoeas in any 1 hour of sleep.

Management

- Weight loss, removal of markedly enlarged tonsils and correction of facial deformities may help.

- CPAP (continuous positive airway pressure, p. 584) to the airway via a tight-fitting nasal mask – nasal CPAP – during sleep keeps the pharyngeal walls open and is an effective treatment.

Bronchiectasis

Bronchiectasis is abnormal and permanent dilatation of the central and medium-sized airways. This in turn leads to impaired clearance of bronchial secretions with secondary bacterial infection and bronchial inflammation. It may be localized to a lobe or generalized throughout the bronchial tree.

Aetiology

Cystic fibrosis and post-infectious (bronchial damage following pneumonia, whooping cough, TB) are the common causes. Many cases are idiopathic. Rarer causes are immunodeficiency (acquired immunodeficiency syndrome [AIDS] and immunoglobulin deficiency), congenital ciliary defect (e.g. Kartagener's syndrome: immotile cilia, situs invertus, chronic sinusitis) and airway obstruction (e.g. inhaled foreign body). Bronchiectasis associated with COPD is becoming increasingly recognized.

Clinical features

There is usually a history of a chronic productive cough and recurrent chest infections. In severe disease there is production of copious amounts of thick, foul-smelling green sputum. Other symptoms are haemoptysis (which may be massive and life-threatening), breathlessness and wheeze. On examination there is clubbing and coarse crackles over the affected area, usually the lung bases.

Investigations

- Chest X-ray may be normal or show dilated bronchi with thickened bronchial walls, and sometimes multiple cysts containing fluid.
- High-resolution CT scanning (p. 509) is the gold standard for diagnosis. It shows airway dilatation, bronchial wall thickening and bronchial wall cysts that are not shown on a standard chest X-ray.
- Sputum culture is essential during an infective exacerbation. The common organisms are *S. aureus*, *Pseudomonas aeruginosa* and *H. influenzae*.
- Further investigations, e.g. serum immunoglobulins, sweat test (p. 525), in patients where an underlying cause is suspected.

Management

Patients should be advised on smoking cessation (p. 512) and physiotherapy techniques to improve sputum clearance. They should receive annual influenza vaccination, pneumococcal vaccination and prompt antibiotic treatment for exacerbations:

- Respiratory physiotherapy promotes mucociliary clearance and sputum production. Techniques include the active cycle of breathing technique (ACBT), postural drainage, chest percussion and the use of devices that provide positive expiratory pressure with or without airway oscillation (e.g. the 'flutter' or 'acapella').
- Antibiotics are given to patients presenting with increased cough, sputum production or purulence. In mild cases, intermittent chemotherapy with cefaclor 500 mg three times daily may be the only therapy needed. Flucloxacillin is the best treatment if *S. aureus* is isolated on sputum culture. If the sputum remains yellow or green despite regular physiotherapy and antibiotics it is probable that there is infection with *P. aeruginosa*. Specific antibiotics, e.g. ceftazidime, are required and are administered by aerosol or parenterally. Oral ciprofloxacin is an alternative. Long-term azithromycin has an immunomodulatory effect and been demonstrated to reduce exacerbation frequency.
- Bronchodilators (β_2-agonists and/or anticholinergics) may provide symptomatic relief even without an objective improvement in FEV_1.
- Inhaled or oral steroids can decrease the rate of progression.
- Surgery is reserved for the very small minority with localized disease. Severe disease sometimes requires lung or heart–lung transplantation.

Complications

These are listed in Table 11.6.

Cystic fibrosis

Cystic fibrosis (CF) is an autosomal recessive condition occurring in 1:2415 live births in the UK. It is much less common in Afro-Caribbean and Asian people. It is caused by mutations in a single gene on chromosome 7 that encodes the CF transmembrane conductance regulator (CFTR) protein, a chloride channel and regulatory protein found in epithelial cell membranes in the lungs, pancreas, gastrointestinal and reproductive tract. The most common mutation is ΔF_{508} (deletion, phenylalanine at position 508). Deranged transport of chloride

Table 11.6 Complications of bronchiectasis

Haemoptysis – may be massive
Pneumonia
Empyema
Aspergillus and non-tuberculous mycobacteria
Metastatic cerebral abscess
Pneumothorax
Respiratory failure

and/or other CFTR-affected ions, such as sodium and bicarbonate, leads to an alteration in the viscosity and tenacity of mucus produced at these epithelial surfaces and to increased salt content in sweat gland secretions.

Clinical features

Although the lungs of babies born with CF are structurally normal at birth, frequent respiratory infections are an early presenting feature. The resultant inflammatory response damages the airway, leading to progressive bronchiectasis, airflow limitation and eventually respiratory failure. Finger clubbing is present in most patients, particularly with more advanced disease. Sinusitis and nasal polyps occur in most patients. In the newborn, thick tenacious intestinal secretions cause small bowel obstruction (meconium ileus). Meconium ileus equivalent syndrome presents in later life with small bowel obstruction. There may be steatorrhoea and diabetes mellitus as a result of pancreatic insufficiency. Liver disease occurs in around 20% of patients. Males are infertile because of failure of development of the vas deferens. Chronic ill-health in children leads to impaired growth and delayed puberty. Many patients are undernourished.

Investigations

Most new CF diagnoses are currently made at newborn screening. The test involves measuring immunoreactive trypsinogen at the time of the neonatal heel prick test. If the concentration is raised, formal testing is performed. Evaluation for CF is indicated in patients with suggestive symptoms or signs, or a sibling with the disease:

- Sweat sodium measurement is the initial investigation. A value ≥ 60 mmol/L is diagnostic. Lower values, but above the normal range, still require DNA analysis
- Blood DNA analysis of the gene defect
- Radiology showing features of CF.

Genetic screening for the carrier state, together with counselling, should be offered to persons or couples with a family history of CF.

Management

Patients with CF should be managed in a specialist centre by a multidisciplinary group of experienced healthcare professionals. Management of bronchiectasis and exocrine pancreatic insufficiency is described on pages 523 and 194. Lung damage associated with persistent infection with *P. aeruginosa* is a major cause of morbidity and mortality in patients with CF. Nebulized antipseudomonal antibiotic therapy, e.g. tobramycin, improves lung function, slows the rate of respiratory decline and decreases the risk of infective exacerbations and hospitalization in these patients. Regular sputum culture for *Pseudomonas* allows early detection and treatment. Other organisms such as *Burkholderia cepacia*, methicillin-resistant *S. aureus* (MRSA) and *Stenotrophomonas malto-phila* have been associated with worsening respiratory outcomes, and eradication regimes for these bacteria are being used. Non-tuberculous mycobacterial disease, in particular *Mycobacterium* abscessus can be associated with a rapid decline and active infection may preclude transplantation. Close contact promotes cross-infection, so siblings and fellow sufferers with CF may pass the organism from one to another.

Inhalation of recombinant DNAase (dornase alfa) improves FEV_1 and may influence survival. Nebulized hypertonic saline draws water to the cell surface, while inhaled mannitol increases mucociliary clearance. Ivacaftor is the first drug available for CF that improves CFTR function (available for patients with the G551D mutation). Some patients with severe respiratory disease have received lung or heart–lung transplantations.

Prognosis

Ninety per cent of children now survive into their teens and the median survival for those born after 1990 is about 40 years. Most mortality is the result of pulmonary disease.

ASTHMA

Asthma is a common chronic inflammatory condition of the lung airways, the cause of which is incompletely understood. It has three characteristics: airflow limitation, airway hyperresponsiveness to a range of stimuli and inflammation of the bronchi. Airflow limitation is usually reversible, either spontaneously or with treatment; in chronic asthma it may be irreversible as a result of airway wall remodelling and mucus impaction.

Epidemiology

The prevalence of asthma is increasing, particularly in the second decade of life, when 10–15% of the population is affected. Asthma is more common in developed countries (particularly the UK, Australia and New Zealand) than in Far Eastern countries and Eastern Europe.

Classification

Asthma can be subdivided into various different subtypes.

Many people with childhood onset persistent asthma are allergic to inhaled allergens and may have persisting reactions to common triggers such as dust mite, animal danders, pollens and fungi. Late onset asthma in adults may be triggered by chemicals in the workplace.

Asthma may also start in middle age with no definite external cause identified.

There are various other subtypes (or endotypes) including brittle asthma and steroid resistant asthma.

Aetiology

Two major factors are involved in the development of asthma:

- *Atopy* is the term used in individuals who readily develop IgE antibodies against common environmental antigens such as the house-dust mite, grass pollen and fungal spores from *Aspergillus fumigatus*. Genetic and environmental factors affect serum IgE levels. Included in the genetic influence is the interleukin-4 (IL-4) gene cluster on chromosome 5 which controls the production of the cytokines IL-3, IL-4, IL-5 and IL-13, which in turn affect mast and eosinophil cell development and longevity, and IgE production. Environmental factors include childhood exposure to allergens and maternal smoking, and intestinal bacterial and childhood infections. Growing up in a relatively clean environment may predispose towards an IgE response to allergens.

- *Increased responsiveness of the airways of the lung* to stimuli such as inhaled histamine and methacholine (bronchial provocation tests, see below).

Genetic and envirinmental factors may also be implicated. Factors which can precipitate asthma are discussed on page 528.

Pathogenesis

The primary abnormality in asthma is narrowing of the airway, which is due to smooth muscle contraction, thickening of the airway wall by cellular infiltration and inflammation, and the presence of secretions within the airway lumen. The pathogenesis of asthma is complex and not fully understood. It involves a number of cells, mediators, nerves and vascular leakage which can be activated by several mechanisms, of which exposure to allergens is the most relevant.

Inflammation Mast cells, eosinophils, T lymphocytes and dentritic cells are increased in the bronchial wall, mucous membranes and secretions of asthmatics. Dentritic cells may play a role in the initial uptake and presentation of allergens to lymphocytes, predominantly of the T-helper 2 (Th2) phenotype. These lymphocytes, when stimulated by the appropriate antigen, release a restricted panel of cytokines (IL-3, IL-4, IL-5, IL-9 and IL-13, GM-CSF), which play a part in the migration and activation of mast cells and eosinophils. In addition, production of IL-4 and IL-13 helps maintain the proallergic Th2 phenotype, favouring switching of antibody production by B lymphocytes to IgE. These IgE molecules attach to mast cells via high-affinity receptors, which in turn release a number of powerful mediators acting on smooth muscle and small blood vessels, such as histamine, tryptase, prostaglandin D_2 and leukotriene C_4, which cause the immediate asthmatic reaction. Activation of eosinophils, by IgE binding, leads to release of a variety of mediators, such as eosinophilic cationic protein, which are predominantly toxic to airway cells.

Remodelling Airway smooth muscle undergoes hypertrophy and hyperplasia, leading to a larger fraction of the wall being occupied by smooth muscle tissue. The airway wall is further thickened by deposition of repair collagens and matrix proteins below the basement membrane. The airway epithelium is damaged, with loss of the ciliated columnar cells into the lumen. The epithelium undergoes metaplasia with an increase in the number of mucus-secreting goblet cells.

Precipitating factors

The major allergen is the house-dust mite and its faeces. Non-specific factors causing wheezing include viral infections, cold air, exercise, irritant dusts, vapours and fumes (cigarette smoke, perfume, exhaust fumes), emotion and drugs (non-steroidal anti-inflammatory drugs (NSAIDs), aspirin and β-blockers).

Over 250 materials encountered at the workplace give rise to occupational asthma, which typically improves on days away from work and during holidays. Common occupations associated with asthma are veterinary medicine and animal handling (allergens from mouse, rat and rabbit urine and fur), bakery (wheat, rye) and laundry work (biological enzymes).

A rare cause of asthma is the airborne spores of *A. fumigatus*, a soil mould. There are fleeting shadows on the chest X-ray and peripheral blood eosinophilia (allergic bronchopulmonary aspergillosis), not to be confused with the severe aspergillus pneumonia occurring in the immunocompromised.

Clinical features

The principal symptoms of asthma are wheezing attacks, shortness of breath, chest tightness and cough (may be the only symptom). Symptoms tend to be intermittent, worse at night and in the early morning and provoked by triggers as above. Some patients have just one or two attacks a year, whereas others have chronic symptoms. On examination, during an attack, there is reduced chest expansion, prolonged expiratory time and bilateral expiratory polyphonic wheezes.

Investigations

The diagnosis of asthma is made on the history and evidence of airflow obstruction (by spirometry or PEF) when symptomatic. There is no single satisfactory diagnostic test for all asthmatic patients:

- Demonstration of variable (at least 15%) airflow limitation by measurement of PEFR or FEV_1:
  - Measurement of PEFR by the patient on waking, during the day and before bed – most asthmatic individuals will show obvious diurnal variation, with lowest values occurring in the early morning (the 'morning dip', Fig. 11.3).
  - An increase after inhalation of a bronchodilator, e.g. salbutamol.
  - A decrease after 6 minutes of exercise, e.g. running.

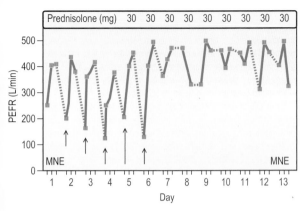

Fig. 11.3 Diurnal variability in peak expiratory flow rate (PEFR) in asthma, showing the effect of steroids. The arrows indicate the morning 'dips'. M, morning; N, noon; E, evening.

- Histamine or methacholine challenge in difficult cases. Bronchial hyperreactivity is demonstrated by asking the patient to inhale gradually increasing doses of histamine or methacholine and demonstrating a fall in FEV_1. The test should not be performed on individuals who have poor lung function ($FEV_1 < 1.5$ L) or a history of 'brittle' asthma.

- Skin-prick tests should be performed in all cases of asthma to help identify allergic causes. A weal develops 15 minutes after allergen injection in the epidermis of the forearm. Measurement of allergen-specific IgE in the serum is also sometimes used.

- Chest X-ray is performed during an acute attack (see later) or to identify the pulmonary shadows associated with allergic bronchopulmonary aspergillosis.

- A trial of corticosteroids should be undertaken in all patients who present with severe airflow limitation. A substantial improvement in FEV_1 ($>15\%$) confirms the presence of a reversible element and indicates that the administration of inhaled steroids will prove beneficial to the patient.

Management

The effective management of asthma centres on patient and family education, anti-smoking advice (p. 512), the avoidance of precipitating factors and specific drug treatment. Self-management programmes have been incorporated into patient care and involve individualized self-treatment plans based on self-monitoring of PEFR and symptoms and a written action plan showing patients how to act early in exacerbations. Patients should be offered influenza immunization.

Avoidance of precipitating factors Patients should be discouraged from smoking and advised to avoid allergens, e.g. pets, which have been identified as extrinsic causes. Occupational asthma should be identified early because removal of the patient from exposure may cure the asthma and continued exposure may become self-perpetuating even when exposure ceases. β-Blockers in any form are absolutely contraindicated in patients with asthma. Individuals intolerant of aspirin should avoid all NSAIDs.

Drug treatment Most drugs are delivered directly into the lungs as aerosols (metered-dose inhaler ± spacer, p. 563) or dry powder inhalers, which means that lower doses can be used and systemic side effects are reduced compared to oral treatment. Asthma is managed with a stepwise approach that depends partly on repeated measurements of PEFR by the patient (Fig. 11.4). The aim is that the patient starts treatment at the step most appropriate to the initial severity, and when control of symptoms is achieved, treatment is gradually reduced to the previous step over a period of 1–3 months. The aim of treatment is to have control of the disease, i.e. no day or night symptoms, no exacerbations, no need for relieving bronchodilators and normal lung function (FEV_1 or PEF > 80% predicted):

- β_2-Adrenoceptor agonists (p. 564), e.g. salbutamol, terbutaline and the longer-acting, salmeterol and formoterol, relax bronchial smooth muscle and cause bronchial dilatation.
- Antimuscarinic bronchodilators (p. 565), e.g. ipratropium bromide or oxitropium bromide, cause bronchodilatation and may be additive to adrenoceptor stimulants.
- Corticosteroids are powerful anti-inflammatory agents. Inhaled steroids (p. 568), e.g. beclometasone dipropionate, budesonide and fluticasone propionate, are used as maintenance treatment in all but very mild asthmatic individuals. Side effects of inhaled steroids are oral candidiasis, hoarseness and, rarely, cataract formation. Oral steroids are occasionally necessary in those patients not controlled on inhaled steroids. Side effects are listed on page 665.
- Anti-inflammatory agents, e.g. sodium cromoglicate, prevent activation of inflammatory cells and may be useful in mild asthma. They are not as effective as inhaled steroids, but are free of side effects, and thus may have some advantages in children.
- Cysteinyl leukotriene receptor antagonists (LTRAs), e.g. montelukast and zafirlukast, are given orally. Leukotrienes are inflammatory mediators released by mast cells which cause bronchoconstriction and increased production of mucus. LTRAs are particularly useful in patients who still have symptoms despite taking high-dose inhaled or oral corticosteroids, and in patients with asthma induced by aspirin.
- Steroid-sparing agents. Methotrexate, ciclosporin, anti-IgE monoclonal antibody (omalizumab), intravenous immunoglobulin and etanecerpt are used occasionally.

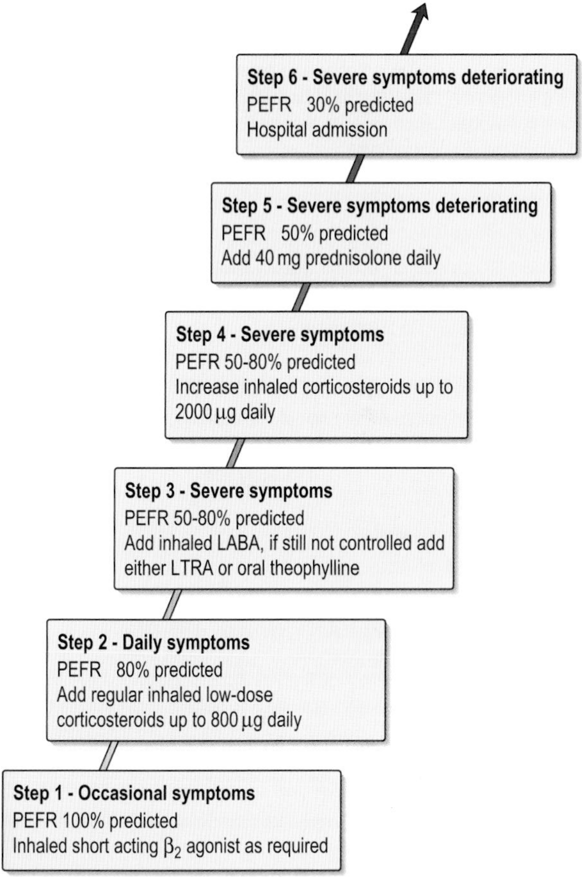

Step 6 - Severe symptoms deteriorating
PEFR 30% predicted
Hospital admission

Step 5 - Severe symptoms deteriorating
PEFR 50% predicted
Add 40 mg prednisolone daily

Step 4 - Severe symptoms
PEFR 50-80% predicted
Increase inhaled corticosteroids up to
2000 µg daily

Step 3 - Severe symptoms
PEFR 50-80% predicted
Add inhaled LABA, if still not controlled add
either LTRA or oral theophylline

Step 2 - Daily symptoms
PEFR 80% predicted
Add regular inhaled low-dose
corticosteroids up to 800 µg daily

Step 1 - Occasional symptoms
PEFR 100% predicted
Inhaled short acting β_2 agonist as required

- Patient measures PEFR at home to guide treatment.
- Short-acting inhaled β agonist taken at any step as needed for symptom relief.
- A rescue of oral steroids (used for shortest time possible) may be needed at any step.
- Decrease treatment after 1–3 months' stability

LTRA - leukotriene receptor antagonist
LABA - inhaled long-acting β_2 agonist
PEFR - peak expiratory flow rate

Fig. 11.4 The stepwise management of asthma in adults.

Acute severe asthma

This is severe progressive asthmatic symptoms over a number of hours or days. It is a medical emergency that must be recognized and treated immediately at home with subsequent transfer to hospital (Emergency Box 11.1). In the UK, 1400 patients die from asthma each year and 90% of these deaths are preventable by correct management.

Clinical features

Patients with acute severe asthma typically have:
- Inability to complete a sentence in one breath
- Respiratory rate ≥ 25 breaths/min
- Heart rate ≥ 110 beats/min
- PEFR 33–50% of predicted normal or patient's best.

Life-threatening features are any one of the following in a patient with acute severe asthma:
- Silent chest, cyanosis or feeble respiratory effort
- Exhaustion, altered conscious level
- Bradycardia or hypotension
- PEFR $< 33\%$ of predicted or best
- $P_a o_2 < 8$ kPa.

    Near fatal asthma is $P_a co_2 > 6$ kPa, and a low or falling arterial pH.

    The management of acute severe asthma is shown in Emergency Box 11.1. Patients with moderate asthma (defined as increasing symptoms, PEFR 50–75%, no features of acute severe asthma) who present to hospital are treated with a nebulized β-agonist. Provided they improve and are then stable for at least 1 hour, they may be discharged with oral prednisolone 40 mg daily for 1 week.

PNEUMONIA

Pneumonia is defined as an inflammation of the substance of the lungs and is usually caused by bacteria. Pneumonia can be classified anatomically, e.g. lobar (affecting the whole of one lobe) and bronchopneumonia (affecting the lobules and bronchi), according to the setting where the infection was contracted (community versus hospital acquired) or on the basis of aetiology (Table 11.7). *Streptococcus pneumoniae* (pneumococcus) is the commonest single cause. Mycobacterium tuberculosis is a cause of pneumonia and is considered separately, as both mode of presentation and treatment are different from the other pneumonias. In about 25% of patients, no organism is isolated. Pneumonia may also result from chemical causes (e.g. aspiration of vomit) and radiotherapy.

Management of acute severe asthma in hospital

Initial treatment
- Oxygen therapy to maintain oxygen saturation (SpO_2) 94–98%.
- Nebulized salbutamol 5 mg or terbutaline 10 mg with oxygen as the driving gas.
- Hydrocortisone 200 mg intravenously.
- Antibiotics if evidence of infection: focal shadowing on the chest X-ray, purulent sputum*.
- Fluids, aim for 2.5–3 L/day, intravenously if necessary.

Investigations
- Chest X-ray to exclude pneumothorax or pneumonia.
- Pulse oximetry (continuous).
- Arterial blood gases if SpO_2 < 92%. May need repeat depending on response.
- PEFR before and after initial treatment.
- Urea and electrolytes – steroids and salbutamol may result in hypokalaemia.

If improved – continue
Oxygen therapy
Prednisolone oral, 40–50 mg for 7 days
Nebulized β_2-agonist 4-hourly.

After 24 hours
Add in high-dose inhaled corticosteroid
Change nebulized to inhaled β_2-agonist.

Discharge from hospital when:
- Free of SOB or wheeze
- PEFR > 75% predicted & diurnal variability <25%
- Stable on discharge treatment for 24 h.
Before discharge: check inhaler technique, determine reason for exacerbation and issue a written asthma plan discussed with patient.

Life-threatening features present or poor response to treatment
Oxygen therapy
Hydrocortisone 200 mg i.v. 4-hourly
Nebulized β_2-agonist every 10–20 min
Add nebulized ipratropium bromide 0.5 mg 4-6-hourly
Magnesium sulphate 1.2–2 g i.v. over 20 min.
If no improvement give:
Salbutamol 3–20 µg/min (5 mg salbutamol in 500 mL 0.9% saline or 5% dextrose, infuse at 0.3–2 mL/min)
Inform ITU of possible admission for intubation and mechanical ventilation.

*There is little evidence that antibiotics are helpful in managing patients with asthma. During acute exacerbations, yellow or green sputum containing eosinophils and bronchial epithelial cells may be coughed up. This is usually due to viral rather than bacterial infection and antibiotics are not always required.

Table 11.7 The aetiology of pneumonia in the UK

Infecting agent	Clinical circumstances
Streptococcus pneumoniae	Community pneumonia patients usually previously fit
Mycoplasma pneumoniae	As above
Influenza A virus (usually with a bacterial component)	As above
Haemophilus influenzae	Pre-existing lung disease: COPD
Chlamydia pneumoniae	Community-acquired pneumonia
Chlamydia psittaci	Contact with birds (though not inevitable)
Staphylococcus aureus	Children, intravenous drug abusers, associated with influenza virus infections
Legionella pneumophila	Institutional outbreaks (hospitals and hotels), sporadic, endemic
Coxiella burnetii	Abattoir and animal-hide workers
Pseudomonas aeruginosa	Cystic fibrosis
Enteric Gram-negative bacilli	In acutely ill or debilitated patients
Pneumocystis jiroveci Actinomyces israelii Nocardia asteroides Cytomegalovirus Aspergillus fumigatus	Immunosuppressed (AIDS, lymphomas, leukaemias, use of cytotoxic drugs and corticosteroids)

NB: Causes vary in different countries. Streptococcus pneumoniae accounts for 35–80% of cases in the UK.

Clinical features

Symptoms and signs vary according to the infecting agent and to the immune state of the patient. Most commonly there is pyrexia, combined with respiratory symptoms such as cough, sputum production, pleurisy and dyspnoea. Signs of consolidation and a pleural rub may be present. There may be a pleural effusion. Elderly patients often have fewer symptoms than younger patients or may present with a confusional state. The severity of community-acquired pneumonia is assessed by clinical and laboratory criteria (Table 11.8). Precipitating factors for pneumonia are underlying lung disease, smoking, alcohol abuse, immunosuppression and other chronic illnesses. The clinical history should enquire about contact with birds (possible psittacosis), and farm animals (Coxiella burnetii, causative organism of Q fever), recent stays in large hotels

Table 11.8 Diagnosis of severe community-acquired pneumonia using CURB-65 and other criteria

Score 1 (maximum score = 6) for each of:

- **C**onfusion – new disorientation in person, place or time
- **U**rea >7 mmol/L
- **R**espiratory rate ≥ 30/min
- **B**lood pressure
  Systolic <90
  Diastolic ≤ 60 mmHg
- **A**ge > 65 years

Score 0–1 – Treat as outpatient
Score 2 – Admit to hospital
Score ≥ 3 (severe pneumonia) – often require ITU care

Other markers of severe pneumonia

- Chest X-ray – more than one lobe involved
- $P_aO_2 < 8$ kPa
- Low albumin (<35 g/L)
- White cell count (<4 × 10⁹/L or >20 × 10⁹/L)
- Blood culture – positive

or institutions (*Legionella pneumophila*), chronic alcohol abuse (*Mycobacterium tuberculosis*, anaerobic organisms), intravenous drug abuse (*S. aureus, M. tuberculosis*) and contact with other patients with pneumonia.

Investigations

Many otherwise fit patients with mild (see Table 11.8) community-acquired pneumonia are treated as outpatients and the only investigation needed is a chest X-ray. Patients admitted to hospital require investigations to identify the cause and severity of the pneumonia:

- *Chest X-ray* confirms the area of consolidation, but these changes may lag behind the clinical course (Fig. 11.5). The chest X-ray is repeated at 6 weeks after the acute illness and any persisting abnormalities suggest a bronchial abnormality usually a carcinoma. The chest X-ray is repeated more frequently if the acute illness is not responding to treatment.
- *Sputum* for Gram stain, culture and sensitivity tests.
- *Blood tests*. A white cell count above 15 × 10⁹/L suggests bacterial infection. There may be lymphopenia with *Legionella* pneumonia. Marked red cell agglutination on the blood film suggests the presence of cold agglutinins (immunoglobulins that agglutinate red cells at 4°C), which

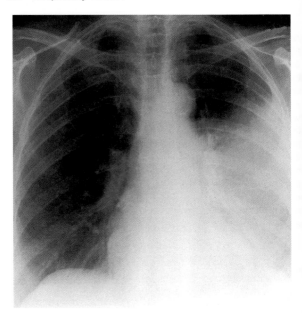

Fig. 11.5 Chest X-ray showing lobar pneumonia. There is an ill-defined area of opacity in the left lower zone without loss of volume (i.e. no shift of structures such as the mediastinum or trachea). The opacity is caused by the filling of alveolar spaces with fluid instead of air.

are raised in 50% of patients with *Mycoplasma* pneumonia. Liver biochemistry may be non-specifically abnormal and serum electrolytes may show a raised urea and hyponatraemia. Blood cultures are also taken.

- *Serology.* Some organisms, e.g. mycoplasma, causing pneumonia can be diagnosed by detection of a raised IgM antibody by immunofluorescent tests or by a four-fold rise in antibody titre from blood taken early in the clinical course and 10–14 days later.
- *Arterial blood gases.* $P_a\text{O}_2 < 8$ kPa or rising $P_a\text{CO}_2$ indicates severe pneumonia.
- *Urine* is sent for legionella and pneumococcal antigen testing in patients with indicators of severe pneumonia (Table 11.8).

Differential diagnosis

This includes pulmonary embolism, pulmonary oedema, pulmonary haemorrhage, bronchial carcinoma, hypersensitivity pneumonitis and some types of diffuse parenchymal lung disease with acute onset.

Management

Antibiotic treatment of community-acquired pneumonia is summarized in Fig. 11.6. In addition, pleuritic pain requires analgesia, and humidified oxygen is given if there is hypoxaemia. Fluids are encouraged, to avoid dehydration. Physiotherapy is needed to help and encourage the patient to cough. Patients with severe pneumonia should be assessed for management on the intensive care unit (ICU). Hospital-acquired (nosocomial) pneumonia occurs in patients who are beyond 2 days of their initial admission to hospital or who have been in a healthcare setting within the last 3 months (including nursing/residential homes). It is often due to infection with Gram-negative organisms and treatment is with co-amoxiclav 625 mg three times daily or in more severe cases a second-generation cephalosporin, e.g. cefuroxime, and an aminoglycoside (e.g. gentamicin). Metronidazole is added in patients at risk of anaerobic infection, e.g. prolonged ICU stay or aspiration in a comatose patient. Antibiotic treatment in all cases is adjusted on the basis of the results of sputum microscopy and culture.

Complications

Complications of pneumonia include lung abscess and empyema (p. 539).

Specific forms of pneumonia

Mycoplasma pneumoniae commonly presents in young adults with generalized features such as headaches and malaise, which may precede chest symptoms by 1–5 days. Physical signs in the chest may be scanty, and chest X-ray appearances frequently do not correlate with the clinical state of the patient. Treatment is with macrolides, e.g. clarithromycin 500 mg twice daily (or erythromycin or azithromycin) for 7–10 days. Extrapulmonary complications (myocarditis, erythema multiforme, haemolytic anaemia and meningoencephalitis) will occasionally dominate the clinical picture.

Haemophilus influenzae is commonly the cause of pneumonia in patients with COPD. There are no other features to differentiate it from other causes of bacterial pneumonia. Treatment is with oral amoxicillin 500 mg three times daily.

Chlamydia *Chlamydia pneumoniae* accounts for 4–13% of cases of community-acquired pneumonia. Patients with *C. psittaci* pneumonia may give a history of contact with infected birds, particularly parrots. Symptoms include malaise, fever, cough and muscular pains, which may be low grade and protracted over many months. Occasionally the presentation mimics meningitis, with a high fever, prostration, photophobia and neck stiffness. Diagnosis of *Chlamydia* infection is made by demonstrating a rising serum titre of complement-fixing antibody. *C. pneumoniae* is distinguished from *C. psittaci* infection by type-specific immunofluorescence tests. Treatment of *Chlamydia* infection is with macrolides or tetracycline.

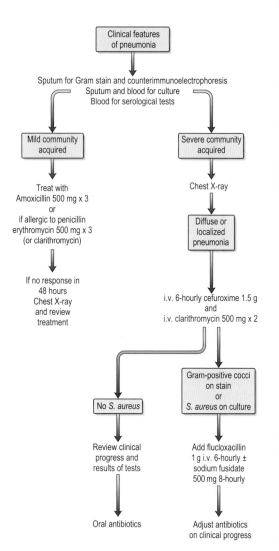

Fig. 11.6 Algorithm for the management of community-acquired pneumonia.

- Severity of pneumonia is assessed using criteria listed in Table 11.8
- Fluoroquinolones, e.g. ciprofloxacin, are recommended for those intolerant of penicillins or macrolides
- Choice of antibiotics may be narrowed once microbiological results are available
- Intravenous antibiotics are switched to oral when the patient has been apyrexial for 24 hours and there is no contraindication to oral treatment
- Antibiotic treatment is usually for a total of 7–10 days.

Staphylococcus aureus usually causes pneumonia only after a preceding influenza viral illness or in staphylococcal septicaemia (occurs in intravenous drug users or in patients with central venous catheters). It results in patchy areas of consolidation which can break down to form abscesses that appear as cysts on the chest X-ray. Pneumothorax, effusions and empyemas are frequent, and septicaemia may develop with metastatic abscesses in other organs. All patients with this form of pneumonia are extremely ill and the mortality rate is in excess of 25%. Treatment is with intravenous flucloxacillin.

Legionella pneumophila is acquired by the inhalation of aerosols or microaspiration of infected water containing *Legionella*. Infection is linked to contamination of water distribution systems in hotels, hospitals and workplaces and may also occur sporadically and in the immunosuppressed. Pneumonia tends to be more severe than with most other pathogens associated with community-acquired pneumonia.

A strong presumptive diagnosis of *L. pneumophila* infection is possible in the majority of patients if they have three of the four following features:

- A prodromal virus-like illness
- A dry cough, confusion or diarrhoea
- Lymphopenia without marked leucocytosis
- Hyponatraemia.

Diagnosis is by specific antigen detection in the urine or by direct fluorescent antibody staining of the organism in the pleural fluid, sputum or bronchial washings. Treatment is with clarithromycin, ciprofloxacin or rifampicin for 14–21 days.

Pseudomonas aeruginosa is seen in the immunocompromised and in patients with CF, in whom its presence is associated with a worsening of the clinical condition and increasing mortality. Treatment includes intravenous ceftazidime, ciprofloxacin, tobramycin or ticarcillin. Inhaled tobramycin is used in CF patients (p. 525).

Pneumocystis jiroveci is the most common opportunistic infection in patients with untreated AIDS. The clinical features and treatment of this and other opportunistic infection are described on page 51.

Aspiration pneumonia Aspiration of gastric contents into the lungs can produce a severe destructive pneumonia as a result of the corrosive effect of gastric acid – Mendelson's syndrome. Aspiration usually occurs into the posterior segment of the right lower lobe because of the bronchial anatomy. It is associated with periods of impaired consciousness, structural abnormalities, such as tracheo-oesophageal fistulae or oesophageal strictures, and bulbar palsy. Infection is often due to anaerobes, and treatment must include metronidazole.

Complications of pneumonia: lung abscess and empyema

A lung abscess results from localized suppuration of the lung associated with cavity formation, often with a fluid level on the chest X-ray. Empyema means the presence of pus in the pleural cavity, usually from rupture of a lung abscess into the pleural cavity, or from bacterial spread from a severe pneumonia.

A lung abscess develops in the following circumstances:

- Complicating aspiration pneumonia or bacterial pneumonia caused by *S. aureus* or *Klebsiella pneumoniae*
- Secondary to bronchial obstruction by tumour or foreign body
- From septic emboli from a focus elsewhere (usually *S. aureus*)
- Secondary to infarction.

Clinical features

Lung abscess presents with persisting or worsening pneumonia, often with the production of copious amounts of foul-smelling sputum. With empyema the patient is usually very ill, with a high fever and neutrophil leucocytosis. There may be malaise, weight loss and clubbing of the digits.

Investigations

Bacteriological investigation is best conducted on specimens obtained by transtracheal aspiration, bronchoscopy or percutaneous transthoracic aspiration. Bronchoscopy is helpful to exclude carcinomas and foreign bodies.

Management

Antibiotics are given to cover both aerobic and anaerobic organisms. Intravenous cefuroxime, and metronidazole are given for 5 days, followed by oral cefaclor and metronidazole for several weeks. Empyemas should be treated by prompt tube drainage or rib resection and drainage of the empyema cavity. Abscesses occasionally require surgery.

TUBERCULOSIS

Epidemiology

Tuberculosis (TB) is the most common cause of death world-wide from a single infectious disease and is on the increase in most parts of the world. The reasons for this are primarily inadequate programmes for disease control, multiple drug resistance, immunosuppression associated with human immunodeficiency virus (HIV) infection (when the disease may present atypically) and a rapid rise in the world population of young adults, the group with the highest mortality from tuberculosis. In the UK the incidence of tuberculosis is highest in Asian and West Indian immigrants, children of these immigrants, the homeless and those with HIV infection. Rates in the otherwise healthy indigenous white population have fallen to very low levels.

Pathology

The initial infection with *M. tuberculosis* is known as primary tuberculosis and usually occurs in the upper region of the lung producing a subpleural lesion called the Ghon focus (Fig. 11.7). The primary lesion may also occur in the gastrointestinal tract, particularly the ileocaecal region. The primary focus is characterized by exudation and infiltration with neutrophil granulocytes. These are replaced by macrophages which engulf the bacilli and result in the typical granulomatous lesions, which consist of central areas of caseation surrounded by epithelioid cells and Langhans' giant cells (both derived from the macrophage). The primary focus is almost always accompanied by caseous lesions in the regional lymph nodes (mediastinal and cervical) – together these constitute the Ghon complex. In most people the primary infection and the lymph nodes heal completely and become calcified. However, they may harbour tubercle bacilli which may become reactivated if there is depression of the host defence system. Occasionally there is dissemination of the primary infection, producing miliary tuberculosis.

Reactivation results in typical post-primary tuberculosis. Post-primary tuberculosis refers to all forms of tuberculosis that develop after the first few weeks of the primary infection when immunity to the mycobacteria has developed. Reinfection after successful treatment for TB is uncommon except in immunocompromised patients such as HIV-infected individuals.

Clinical features

Primary TB is usually symptomless; occasionally there may be erythema nodosum (p. 816), a small pleural effusion or pulmonary collapse caused by compression of a lobar bronchus by enlarged nodes (Fig. 11.7). Miliary TB is the result of acute dissemination of tubercle bacilli via the bloodstream. Patients, especially the elderly, may present with non-specific ill-health, fever of unknown origin, weight loss and a few other localizing symptoms. Occasionally the disease presents as tuberculous meningitis, and in the later stages there may be enlargement of the liver and spleen. Choroidal tubercles (yellowy/white raised lesions about one-quarter the diameter of the optic disc) are occasionally seen in the eye. Most commonly clinical tuberculosis represents delayed reactivation. Symptoms begin insidiously, with malaise, anorexia, weight loss, fever and cough. Sputum is mucoid purulent or bloodstained, but night sweats are uncommon. There are often no physical signs, although occasionally signs of a pneumonia or pleural effusion may be present.

Tuberculous disease (as above) must be differentiated from latent tuberculous infection. Infection implies the presence of small numbers of tubercle bacilli in the body; the tuberculin test is positive (as with disease), but the chest X-ray is normal and the patient asymptomatic.

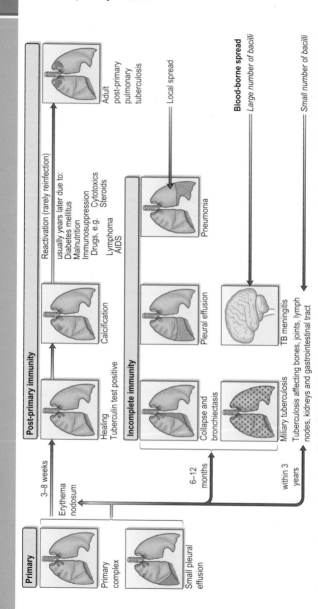

Investigations

In order to minimize the risk of transmission to other people, patients who are suspected of having pulmonary TB should be isolated in a ward side-room until sputum specimens are negative. This is to minimize the risk of transmission to other patients in a confirmed case. Because of the rising incidence of drug-resistant TB, the diagnosis is confirmed bacteriologically whenever possible and to obtain drug sensitivities.

Chest X-ray typically shows patchy or nodular shadows in the upper zones, with loss of volume, and fibrosis with or without cavitation. With miliary tuberculosis the chest X-ray may be normal or show miliary shadows 1–2 mm in diameter throughout the lung.

Sputum is stained with an auramine-phenol fluorescent test or the less sensitive Ziehl–Neelsen (ZN) stain for acid- and alcohol-fast bacilli. Culture of sputum is more sensitive than microscopy and allows antibiotic sensitivity testing. Where pulmonary tuberculosis is suspected, serial sputum samples on at least three occasions (ideally immediately upon waking) should be collected. Solid culture mediums take 4–8 weeks for organism recovery and are gradually being replaced by liquid culture mediums (Bactec) which shorten the recovery time by 2–3 weeks. Sensitivity testing takes a further 3–4 weeks.

- Bronchoscopy with washings of the affected lobes is useful if no sputum is available.
- The diagnosis of extrapulmonary TB depends on a high index of clinical suspicion. Recovery of the organism from specimens is still necessary wherever possible. This may involve lymph node biopsy, bone biopsy, urine testing or aspiration of pericardial fluid.
- Lumbar puncture and cerebrospinal fluid (CSF) examination for evidence of tuberculous infection is indicated in all cases of miliary TB. This is due to the high rate of blood-borne spread to meninges, and positive CSF will alter the length of treatment.
- Skin testing for TB (Mantoux test) is rarely of any value in the diagnosis or exclusion of active TB. It is neither sensitive nor specific.
- Whole blood interferon-γ assay detects interferon produced by T cells after incubation with TB antigens in individuals who have been sensitized to TB.
- HIV testing should be considered if risk assessment shows the patient to be from an area or background with increased risk of HIV co-infection. TB is an AIDS-defining illness.

Management

Tuberculosis should be treated by experienced physicians working closely with TB nurse specialists or TB health visitors. The latter are helpful in monitoring patients' compliance with treatment and the accuracy and continuity of prescribing. It is a statutory requirement in the UK that all cases of TB must be notified to the local Public Health Authority so that contact tracing and screening can be arranged.

Patients who are ill, sputum-smear positive (patients with three negative smears are considered non-infectious), highly infectious patients (particularly multidrug-resistant TB), and those unlikely to be compliant with treatment should be initially treated in hospital.

A 6-month regimen comprising rifampicin, isoniazid, pyrazinamide and ethambutol for the initial 2 months followed by rifampicin and isoniazid for a further 4 months, is standard treatment. Four drugs should be continued for longer than 2 months if susceptibility testing is still outstanding. Pyridoxine 10 mg daily is given to reduce the risk of isoniazid-induced peripheral neuropathy. Treatment time is extended in TB meningitis (to 12 months) and bone TB (to 9 months). Streptomycin is now rarely used in the UK, but it may be added if the organism is resistant to isoniazid. Significant side effects are uncommon and are listed in Table 11.9. A transient asymptomatic rise in the serum aminotransferase level may occur with rifampicin, but treatment is only stopped if hepatitis develops. The major causes of treatment failure are incorrect prescribing by the doctor and inadequate compliance by the patient. Vagrants, alcoholics, homeless and the mentally ill are most likely to be non-compliant with therapy. In order to improve compliance, special clinics are used to supervise treatment regimens where the ingestion of every drug dose is witnessed (directly observed therapy, DOTS). Incentives to attend include free meals and cash payments.

Table 11.9 Side effects of the main antituberculous drugs

Rifampicin	Stains body secretions and urine pink
	Induces liver enzymes – concomitant drug treatment may be less effective
	Elevation of liver transferases and hepatitis
	Thrombocytopenia (rarely)
Isoniazid	Polyneuropathy (rarely), prevented by co-administration of pyridoxine
	Allergic reactions – skin rash and fever Hepatitis
Pyrazinamide	Hepatitis – rarely
	Hyperuricaemia and gout
	Rash and arthralgia
Ethambutol	Optic neuritis – testing of visual acuity (Snellen chart) and red-green colour perception performed before treatment. Patients asked to report visual changes (defects, colour blindness, acuity) during treatment

Multidrug-resistant (MDR, resistance to isoniazid and rifampicin) and extensively drug-resistant TB (EDR, resistance to first-line and some second-line treatment) is a world-wide major problem. It occurs mainly in HIV-infected patients who can then transmit the infection to healthcare workers and other patients. Treatment of MDR and EDR is difficult and uses combination treatment (including capreomycin, clarithromycin, azithromycin and ciprofloxacin) to which the organism is sensitive for up to 2 years.

Prevention and chemoprophylaxis

Close contacts of a case are screened for evidence of disease with a chest X-ray and a Mantoux test (positive if area of induration $\geq$ 10 mm 72 hours after intradermal injection of purified protein derivative of *Mycobacterium* TB) or whole-blood interferon-γ assay. Antituberculous treatment is given if the chest X-ray shows evidence of disease or if the Mantoux test is negative initially but becomes positive on repeat testing 6 weeks later. In adults, an initial positive tuberculin test with a normal chest X-ray is not usually taken as indication of disease.

Vaccination with BCG (bacille Calmette–Guérin) reduces the risk of developing tuberculosis: it is a bovine strain of *M. tuberculosis* which has lost its virulence after growth in the laboratory for many years. Immunization produces cellular immunity and a positive Mantoux test. In the UK, BCG vaccination is offered to infants living in areas with a high immigrant population, to previously unvaccinated new immigrants from high-prevalence countries for TB, to persons at occupational risk of TB (healthcare workers, veterinary staff, staff of prisons) and to contacts of known cases. BCG vaccination is given to all persons in developing countries where TB is more prevalent.

Targeted tuberculin testing for latent TB infection is an essential component of TB control and identifies people at high risk for developing clinical disease. High-risk groups for developing TB include recent immigrants from high-prevalence countries, injection drug users and HIV-positive patients. Patients with tuberculous infection identified by tuberculin testing are usually treated with one drug for 6 months (chemoprophylaxis) to prevent progression to disease.

Patients with chest X-ray changes compatible with previous tuberculosis and who are about to undergo treatment with an immunosuppressive agent should also receive chemoprophylaxis with isoniazid.

DIFFUSE DISEASES OF THE LUNG PARENCHYMA

Diffuse parenchymal lung diseases (DPLDs), also referred to as interstitial lung disease, comprise a heterogenous group of lung diseases with bilateral diffuse lung injury and inflammation that can progress to lung fibrosis (Fig. 11.8). The process involves not only the interstitial space but also the alveoli, bronchioles and blood vessels. The diseases have common clinical, radiological and pulmonary function features. Presentation is with shortness

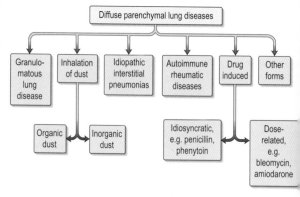

Fig. 11.8 Causes of diffuse parenchymal lung diseases.

of breath on exertion, a persistent non-productive cough, an abnormal chest X-ray (bilateral diffuse pulmonary infiltrates), or with pulmonary symptoms associated with another disease such as a connective tissue disease. Pulmonary infection, malignancy and pulmonary oedema may mimic interstitial lung disease.

Granulomatous lung disease

A granuloma is a mass or nodule of chronic inflammatory tissue formed by the response of macrophages and histiocytes to a slowly soluble antigen or irritant. It is characterized by the presence of epithelioid multinucleate giant cells. Sarcoidosis is the most common cause of lung granulomas.

Sarcoidosis

Sarcoidosis is a multisystem granulomatous disorder of unknown cause typically affecting young and middle-aged adults. It usually presents with bilateral hilar lymphadenopathy (BHL) and/or pulmonary infiltrations, and skin or eye lesions. In about half of cases, the disease is detected incidentally on a routine chest X-ray in an asymptomatic individual.

Epidemiology

Sarcoidosis has a female preponderance, is most common in northern Europe and is uncommon in Japan. The course of the disease is more severe in African blacks than in whites.

Immunopathology

- Typical non-caseating (compare with TB) sarcoid granuloma consists of a focal accumulation of epithelioid cells, macrophages and lymphocytes, mainly T cells.

- Depressed cell-mediated reactivity to antigens, such as tuberculin and *Candida albicans*, and an overall lymphopenia with low circulating T cells, as a result of sequestration of lymphocytes within the lung and slightly increased B cells.
- Increased number of cells (particularly CD4 helper) in bronchoalveolar lavage.
- Transbronchial biopsies show infiltration of alveolar walls and interstitial spaces with mononuclear cells before granuloma formation.

Clinical features

Sarcoidosis can affect any organ, particularly the lung, skin and eyes (Table 11.10). Lung disease presents with a non-productive cough, breathlessness and sometimes a wheeze. Pulmonary infiltration may predominate, and, in a minority of patients there is progressive fibrosis resulting in increasing effort dyspnoea, cor pulmonale and death. Chest examination is normal or there are fine crackles, particularly anteriorly. Finger clubbing is rare and, when present, alternative diagnoses should be considered, e.g. other causes of pulmonary fibrosis, tuberculosis, malignancy. Löfgren's syndrome consists of the triad of erythema nodosum (p. 816), arthralgia and BHL on chest X-ray (see later); it carries an excellent prognosis. Asymptomatic disease may be identified when a chest X-ray is performed for other reasons. Fatigue is a major problem in many patients.

Table 11.10 Clinical features of sarcoidosis

System	Symptoms and signs
Chest	Cough, breathlessness, wheeze, fine crackles on examination
Skin	Erythema nodosum, waxy maculopapular lesions, lupus pernio (red/blue infiltration of the nose), infiltration of scars by granulomas
Eye	Anterior and posterior uveitis, conjunctival nodules, lacrimal gland enlargement, uveoparotid fever (Heerfordt's syndrome: uveitis, parotid gland enlargement and facial nerve palsy)
Bone	Arthralgias, bone cysts
Metabolic	Hypercalcaemia (sarcoid macrophages produce 1,25-dihydroxyvitamin D)
Liver	Granulomatous hepatitis, hepatosplenomegaly
Neurological	Meningeal inflammation, seizures, mass lesions, hypothalamic–pituitary infiltration, diffuse sensorimotor neuropathy, mononeuropathy
Cardiac	Rarely: ventricular arrhythmias, conduction defects, cardiomyopathy with cardiac failure

Investigations

Diagnosis depends on a compatible clinical picture, exclusion of diseases with a similar presentation (see Differential diagnosis) and biopsy for histological diagnosis if possible. Common biopsy sites are enlarged lymph nodes, skin lesions and transbronchial biopsy at bronchoscopy.

- Chest X-ray allows the disease to be staged. High-resolution chest CT scan provides a better assessment of pulmonary involvement and identifies abnormal nodes for biopsy.
- Pulmonary function tests assess disease severity and the response to treatment. There is a restrictive lung defect in patients with pulmonary infiltration, with a decrease in total lung capacity, FEV_1, FVC and gas transfer.
- Blood tests – a full blood count, liver biochemistry, serum creatinine and calcium – are performed to look for abnormalities and evidence of organ involvement. Serum angiotensin-converting enzyme (ACE) is raised in >75% patients but it has limited sensitivity and specificity and does not provide additional information to other tests in disease monitoring.
- Tuberculin test is negative in 80% of patients. It is of interest but of no diagnostic value.

Differential diagnosis

The differential diagnosis of BHL includes:

- Lymphoma
- Pulmonary tuberculosis
- Bronchial carcinoma with secondary spread.

The combination of symmetrical BHL and erythema nodosum only occurs in sarcoidosis. Non-caseating granulomas also occur in lymphoma, fungal infection, tuberculosis (also caseating) and in response to foreign bodies and occupational exposure to beryllium.

Management

Hilar lymphadenopathy with no other evidence of lung involvement on chest X-ray or lung function testing does not require treatment. The disease remits spontaneously within 2 years in over two-thirds of patients.

Infiltration or abnormal lung function tests that persist for 6 months after diagnosis are treated with 30 mg prednisolone for 6 weeks, reducing to 15 mg on alternate days for 6–12 months. Other definite indications for steroid treatment are hypercalcaemia, neurological or myocardial involvement and ocular involvement (topical steroids are used in some cases). Steroid-sparing agents (methotrexate, azathioprine, cyclophosphamide) are sometimes used in patients needing long-term steroids for disease control.

Prognosis

In patients of African origin the mortality rate may be up to 10%, but it is less than 5% in Caucasians. Death is mainly as a result of respiratory failure or renal damage from hypercalciuria.

Granulomatous lung disease with vasculitis

There are two main groups:

- Pulmonary vasculitis associated with primary autoimmune rheumatic diseases including rheumatoid arthritis, systemic lupus erythematosus and systemic sclerosis (see Ch. 7).
- The vasculitides associated with the presence of antineutrophil cytoplasmic antibodies (ANCAs) including eosinophilic granulomatosis with polyangiitis (Churg–Strauss syndrome) (p. 312), microscopic polyangiitis (p. 312) and granulomatosis with polyangiitis (GPA).

GPA is a vasculitis of unknown aetiology characterized by lesions involving the upper respiratory tract, the lungs and the kidneys. The disease often starts with rhinorrhoea, with subsequent nasal mucosal ulceration, cough, haemoptysis and pleuritic pain. Chest X-ray shows nodular masses or pneumonic infiltrates with cavitation which often show a migratory pattern. ANCAs (p. 276) are found in the serum in over 90% of cases with active disease, and measurement is useful both diagnostically and as a guide to disease activity in the treated patient. Typical histological changes are best shown in the kidney, where there is a necrotizing microvascular glomerulonephritis. Treatment is with cyclophosphamide; rituximab is also being used.

Idiopathic interstitial pneumonias

This group accounts for about 40% of cases of diffuse parenchymal lung disease and, as the name suggests, no underlying causes can be identified. Idiopathic pulmonary fibrosis (previously called cryptogenic fibrosing alveolitis) is the commonest type. Other types are non-specific interstitial pneumonitis, cryptogenic organizing pneumonia, acute interstitial pneumonia, desquamative interstitial pneumonia and respiratory bronchiolitis.

Idiopathic pulmonary fibrosis (IPF)

There is patchy fibrosis of the interstitium and minimal or absent inflammation, acute fibroblastic proliferation and collagen deposition. It usually presents in the late sixties and is more common in males.

Clinical features

Presentation is with progressive breathlessness and a non-productive cough. Eventually there is respiratory failure, pulmonary hypertension and cor pulmonale. Finger clubbing occurs in two-thirds of cases, and fine inspiratory basal crackles are heard on auscultation. Rarely, an acute form known as the Hamman–Rich syndrome occurs.

Investigations

The aim of investigation is to confirm the presence of pulmonary fibrosis and exclude identifiable (and potentially reversible) causes.

- Chest X-ray appearances are initially of a ground-glass appearance, progressing to fibrosis and honeycomb lung. These changes are most prominent in the lower lung zones.
- High-resolution CT scan is the most sensitive imaging technique, and shows bilateral irregular linear opacities and honeycombing.
- Respiratory function tests show a restrictive defect (p. 509) with reduced lung volumes and impaired gas transfer.
- Blood gases show hypoxaemia with a normal $P_a\text{co}_2$.
- Autoantibodies, such as antinuclear factor and rheumatoid factor, are performed to exclude connective tissue disease.
- Histological confirmation is necessary in some patients. Transbronchial lung biopsy is rarely diagnostic but can exclude other conditions that present similarly, e.g. sarcoidosis. A video-assisted thoracoscopic lung biopsy is performed to obtain a larger specimen and a clear histological diagnosis.

Differential diagnosis

This is from other causes of diffuse parenchymal lung disease (Fig. 11.8). A detailed history, including occupational exposure (past and present) and drug history, is required to exclude other causes of pulmonary fibrosis.

Treatment

Corticosteroids are no longer routinely used and attention is now focused on targeting the underlying aberrant fibroblastic proliferation and tissue remodelling. Pirfenidone, a novel antifibrotic tablet, has been shown to slow the rate of FVC decline. Careful attention should be paid to treating gastro-oesophageal reflux disease (GORD), as this is thought to contribute to repetitive alveolar epithelial damage. Even with treatment, IPF is a life-limiting disease and transplant assessment should be considered. All patients should have their need for supportive care assessed with respect to oxygen therapy, pulmonary rehabilitation and palliative care input.

Prognosis

The median survival without lung transplantation is approximately 5 years.

Hypersensitivity pneumonitis

This condition was previously called extrinsic allergic alveolitis and is characterized by a widespread diffuse inflammatory reaction in the alveoli and small

Table 11.11 Hypersensitivity pneumonitis – some causes

Disease	Situation	Antigens
Farmer's lung	Forking mouldy hay or other vegetable material	*Micropolyspora faeni*
Bird fancier's lung	Handling pigeons, cleaning lofts or budgerigar cages	Proteins present in feathers and excreta
Malt worker's lung	Turning germinating barley	*Aspergillus clavatus*
Humidifier fever	Contaminated humidifying systems in air conditioners or humidifiers	A variety of bacteria or amoebae
Mushroom workers	Turning mushroom compost	Thermophilic actinomycetes
Cheese washer's lung	Mouldy cheese	*Penicillium casei* *Aspergillus clavatus*
Wine maker's lung	Mould on grapes	Botrytis

airways of the lung as a response to inhalation of organic dusts (Table 11.11). By far the most common condition is farmer's lung, which affects up to 1 in 10 of the farming community in poor wet areas around the world.

Clinical features

There is fever, malaise, cough and shortness of breath several hours after exposure to the causative antigen. Physical examination reveals tachypnoea, and coarse end-inspiratory crackles and inspiratory squeaks due to bronchiolitis. Continuing exposure leads to a chronic illness with weight loss, effort dyspnoea, cough and the features of pulmonary fibrosis.

Investigations

- Chest X-ray shows fluffy nodular shadowing with the subsequent development of streaky shadows, particularly in the upper zones.
- High-resolution CT shows reticular and nodular changes with ground-glass opacity.
- Full blood count shows a raised white cell count in acute cases.
- Lung function tests show a restrictive defect with a decrease in gas transfer.
- Precipitating antibodies to causative antigens are present in the serum (these are evidence of exposure and not disease).
- Bronchoalveolar lavage shows increased T lymphocytes and granulocytes.

Management

Prevention is the aim, with avoidance of exposure to the antigen if possible. Prednisolone in large doses (30–60 mg daily) may be required to cause regression of the disease in the early stages.

Other types of diffuse lung disease

Intrapulmonary haemorrhage can produce diffuse infiltrates on the chest X-ray. In Goodpasture's syndrome, antibodies are directed against the basement membrane of both kidney and lung. There is cough, haemoptysis and tiredness followed by acute glomerulonephritis. Treatment is usually with corticosteroids. Diffuse alveolar haemorrhage is similar but tends to occur in children, the kidneys are less frequently involved and there are no anti-basement membrane antibodies. Other rarer causes of DPLD are Langerhan's cell histiocytosis and pulmonary alveolar proteinosis.

OCCUPATIONAL LUNG DISEASE

Exposure to dusts, gases, vapours and fumes at work can lead to the following types of lung disease:

- Acute bronchitis and pulmonary oedema from irritants such as sulphur dioxide, chlorine, ammonia or oxides of nitrogen
- Pulmonary fibrosis from inhalation of inorganic dust, e.g. coal, silica, asbestos, iron and tin
- Occupational asthma – this is the commonest industrial lung disease in the developed world
- Hypersensitivity pneumonitis
- Bronchial carcinoma due to asbestos, polycyclic hydrocarbons and radon in mines.

Coal worker's pneumoconiosis

Small coal particles escape the normal clearance mechanisms of the airways (trapped in the nose, removed by the mucociliary clearance system, destroyed by alveolar macrophages) to reach the acinus and initiate an inflammatory reaction and subsequent fibrosis. Improved working conditions and reduction in the coal industry has led to a considerable reduction in the number of cases of pneumoconiosis. Simple pneumoconiosis produces small pulmonary nodules on the chest X-ray; there is considerable debate as to whether this has any effect on respiratory function and symptoms. However, with continued exposure there may be progression to progressive massive fibrosis (PMF) characterized by large (1–10 cm) fibrotic masses, predominantly in the upper lobes. Unlike simple pneumoconiosis, the disease may progress after exposure to coal dust has ceased. Symptoms are breathlessness and cough productive of black sputum. Eventually respiratory failure may supervene. There is no specific treatment and further exposure must be prevented. Patients with PMF and some with simple pneumoconiosis (depending on the severity of radiological changes) are eligible for disability benefit in the UK.

Asbestosis

Asbestos is a mixture of fibrous silicates which have the common properties of resistance to heat, acid and alkali: hence, their widespread use at one time. Chrysotile or white asbestos constitutes 90% of the world production and is less fibrogenic than the other forms – crocidolite (blue asbestos) and amosite (brown asbestos). Most people with asbestos-related lung disease have a clear history of occupational exposure such as fitting or working with asbestos insulation (builders, plumbers and electricians), shipyard workers or ship engineering workers. The diseases caused by asbestos (Table 11.12)

Table 11.12 The effects of asbestos on the lung

Disease	Pathology and clinical features
Asbestos bodies	No symptoms or change in lung function
	Serve only as a marker of exposure
Pleural plaques	Fibrotic plaques on parietal and diaphragmatic pleura
	Usually produce no symptoms
Pleural effusion	Pleural biopsy often needed to differentiate from malignant effusion
	Pleuritic pain and dyspnoea
Diffuse pleural thickening*	Thickening of parietal and visceral pleura. Effort dyspnoea and restrictive ventilatory defect
Mesothelioma*	Tumour arising from mesothelial cells of pleura, peritoneum and pericardium
	Often presents with dull diffuse progressive chest pain and a pleural effusion
	Treatment is with chemotherapy or debulking procedures. Prognosis is poor
Asbestosis*	Breathlessness, finger clubbing, bilateral inspiratory crackles
	Pulmonary function tests show a restrictive ventilatory defect
Lung cancer, often adenocarcinoma*	Presentation and treatment is that of lung cancer (see below)

*The diseases indicated are all eligible for compensation under the Social Security Act of 1975 (UK).

are all characterized by a long latency period (20–40 years) between exposure and disease. Diagnosis of asbestos-related lung disease is made on the basis of the history of exposure and typical chest X-ray appearances. High-resolution CT scanning, lung function testing and pleural biopsy are sometimes needed.

CARCINOMA OF THE LUNG

Epidemiology

Bronchial carcinoma accounts for 95% of primary lung tumours. The rest are benign tumours and rarer types of cancers, e.g. alveolar cell carcinoma. Bronchial carcinoma is the most common malignant tumour in the Western world, and in the UK is the third most common cause of death after heart disease and cerebrovascular disease. Although the rising mortality of this disease has levelled off in men, it continues to rise in women and the ratio in men-to-women is now 1.2:1.

Aetiology

Smoking is by far the most common aetiological factor, although there is a higher incidence in urban areas than in rural areas even when allowances are made for smoking. Other aetiological factors are passive smoking, exposure to asbestos and, possibly, also contact with arsenic, chromium, iron oxides and the products of coal combustion.

Pathology

This is broadly divided into small cell and non-small cell cancer (Table 11.13).

Clinical features

Local effects of tumour within a bronchus Cough, chest pain, haemoptysis and breathlessness are typical symptoms. Because evidence suggests that cough is neglected by patients and healthcare professionals, campaigns in the UK have highlighted the 'three week cough' as a symptom that merits a chest X-ray.

 Spread within the chest Tumour may directly involve the pleura and ribs, causing pain and bone fractures. Spread to involve the brachial plexus causes pain in the shoulder and inner arm (Pancoast's tumour), spread to the sympathetic ganglion causes Horner's syndrome (p. 733), and spread to the left recurrent laryngeal nerve causes hoarseness and a bovine cough. In addition, the tumour may directly involve the oesophagus, heart or superior vena cava (causing upper limb oedema, facial congestion and distended neck veins).

 Metastatic disease Metastases are most commonly to bone (presenting with pain and sometimes spinal cord compression) and brain (change in personality, epilepsy, focal neurological signs). The liver, adrenal glands and skin are also frequent sites for metastases.

Table 11.13 Types of bronchial carcinoma (indicates per cent lung carcinomas)

Cell type	Characteristics
Non-small cell	
Squamous (40%)	Most present as obstructive lesion leading to infection
	Occasionally cavitates
	Local spread common
	Widespread metastases occur late
Large cell (25%)	Poorly differentiated tumour
	Metastasize early
Adenocarcinoma (10%)	Most common lung cancer associated with asbestos exposure
	Proportionately more common in non-smokers
	Usually occurs peripherally
	Local and distant metastases
Small cell (20–30%)	Arises from endocrine cells (Kulchitsky cells)
	Secretes polypeptide hormones (Table 11.14)
	Early development of widespread metastases
	Responds to chemotherapy. Poor prognosis

Non-metastatic manifestations These are rare apart from finger clubbing (Table 11.14). There may be non-specific features such as malaise, lethargy and weight loss. Approximately 10% of small cell tumours produce ectopic hormones giving rise to paraneoplastic syndromes.

There are often no physical signs, although lymphadenopathy, signs of a pleural effusion, lobar collapse or unresolved pneumonia may be present.

Investigations

The aim of investigation is to confirm the diagnosis, determine the histology and assess tumour spread as a guide to treatment.

Confirm the diagnosis The chest X-ray will usually be abnormal by the time a lung cancer is causing symptoms. Tumours usually appear as a round shadow, the edge of which often has a fluffy or spiked appearance. There may be evidence of cavitation, lobar collapse, a pleural effusion or secondary pneumonia. Spread through the lymphatic channels gives rise to lymphangitis carcinomatosis, appearing as streaky shadowing throughout the lung. A minority of tumours are confined to the central airways and mediastinum without an

Table 11.14 Non-metastatic extrapulmonary manifestations of bronchial carcinoma

Endocrine	Ectopic secretion of: 　ACTH, causing Cushing's syndrome 　ADH, causing dilutional hyponatraemia 　PTH-like substance, causing hypercalcaemia 　HCG or related hormones resulting in gynaecomastia
Neurological	Cerebellar degeneration
	Myopathy, polyneuropathies
	Myasthenic syndrome (Eaton–Lambert syndrome)
Vascular/ haematological (rare)	Thrombophlebitis migrans
	Non-bacterial thrombotic endocarditis
	Disseminated intravascular coagulation
	Anaemia
Skeletal	Clubbing
	Hypertrophic pulmonary osteoarthropathy (clubbing, painful wrists and ankles)
Cutaneous (rare)	Dermatomyositis
	Acanthosis nigricans (pigmented overgrowth of skin in axillae or groin)
	Herpes zoster

ACTH, adrenocorticotrophic hormone; ADH, antidiuretic hormone; HCG, human chorionic gonadotrophin; PTH, parathyroid hormone.

obvious change on chest X-ray and in patients with suspicious symptoms: e.g. a smoker with haemoptysis, bronchoscopy or CT scanning is necessary to make the diagnosis.

Determine the histology Sputum is examined by a cytologist for malignant cells. Bronchoscopy is used to obtain biopsies for histological investigation and washings for cytology. Transthoracic fine needle aspiration biopsy under radiographic or CT screening is useful for obtaining tissue diagnosis from peripheral lesions.

Assess spread of the tumour At bronchoscopy, involvement of the first 2 cm of either the main bronchus or of the recurrent laryngeal nerve (vocal cord paresis) indicates inoperability. Patients being considered for surgery should have a CT of the thorax to include the liver and adrenal glands to assess the mediastinum and the extent of tumour spread. PET scanning is the investigation of choice for confirmation or exclusion of intrathoracic lymph node metastases and is used when available to assess suitability for surgery.

Determine patient suitability for major operation Physical examination and respiratory function tests.

Treatment

Treatment of lung cancer involves several different modalities and is best planned by a multidisciplinary team.

Non-small cell lung cancer

- Surgery can be curative in non-small cell cancer. Neo-adjuvant chemotherapy may downstage tumours to render them operable. Adjuvant post-operative chemotherapy and radiotherapy improves survival.
- Radiotherapy in high doses can produce good results in patients with localized squamous carcinoma if surgery is declined. Complications are radiation pneumonitis and fibrosis. Palliative radiotherapy is useful for bone pain, haemoptysis and superior vena cava obstruction (p. 257).
- Chemotherapy is given in advanced disease and improves median survival from 6–10 months.

Small cell lung cancer

Limited disease (confined to a single anatomical or radiation field) is treated with combined chemo- and radiotherapy, with 25% survival at 5 years.

Extensive disease is treated with chemotherapy, with a median survival of 9–13 months and 2-year survival of 20%.

Symptomatic treatments

Local treatments such as endoscopic laser therapy, endobronchial irradiation and transbronchial stenting are used to treat distressing symptoms arising from airway narrowing. Malignant pleural effusions should be aspirated to dryness and a sclerosing agent (e.g. tetracycline, bleomycin) instilled into the pleural space. In the terminal stages, the quality of life must be maintained as far as possible. In addition to general nursing, counselling and medical care, patients may need oral or intravenous opiates for pain (given with laxatives to prevent constipation), and prednisolone may improve the appetite.

Differential diagnosis

In most cases the diagnosis is straightforward. The differential diagnosis is usually from other solitary nodules on the chest X-ray (Table 11.3).

Metastatic tumours in the lung

Metastases in the lung are common, usually presenting as round shadows 1.5–3 cm in diameter. The most common primary sites are the kidney, prostate, breast, bone, gastrointestinal tract, cervix or ovary.

DISEASES OF THE CHEST WALL AND PLEURA

Rib fractures

Rib fractures are caused by trauma, coughing, osteoporosis or secondary to metastatic bone disease. Pain limits chest expansion and coughing, which can lead to pneumonia. Lateral and oblique X-rays may show fractures not visible on a PA chest X-ray. Treatment is with oral analgesia, local infiltration or an intercostal nerve block. Fracture of a rib in more than one place can lead to a flail segment with paradoxical movement of part of the chest wall on inspiration and inefficient ventilation; intermittent positive pressure ventilation may be necessary.

Kyphosis and scoliosis of the spine

Kyphosis describes bowing of the thoracic spine ('humpback') and is congenital or secondary to osteoporosis and vertebral fractures. Scoliosis describes a curved spine ('S' shaped) and is congential or secondary to neuromuscular disease, e.g. spina bifida. Kyphoscoliosis is a combination of kyphosis and scoliosis. If severe, these spinal abnormalities may diminish lung capacity. Treatment is to correct the spinal deformity if possible. Positive airway pressure ventilation through a tightly fitting nasal mask is necessary for respiratory failure.

Pleurisy

Inflammation of the pleura without an effusion results in localized sharp pain made worse on deep inspiration, coughing and bending or twisting movements. Common causes are pneumonia, pulmonary infarct and carcinoma. Epidemic myalgia (Bornholm disease) is due to infection with Coxsackie B virus. It is characterized by an upper respiratory tract infection followed by pleuritic pain and abdominal pain with tender muscles. The chest X-ray remains normal and the illness clears in 1 week.

Pleural effusion

A pleural effusion is an excessive accumulation of fluid in the pleural space. It can be detected clinically when there is 500 mL or more present, and by plain chest X-ray when there is more than 300 mL. Massive effusions are most commonly malignant in origin. A pleural effusion may be asymptomatic (if small) or cause breathlessness. The typical physical signs and chest X-ray appearances are shown in Fig. 11.9.

Aetiology

Pleural effusions are transudates or exudates (Table 11.15). Transudates occur when the balance of hydrostatic forces in the chest favour the accumulation of

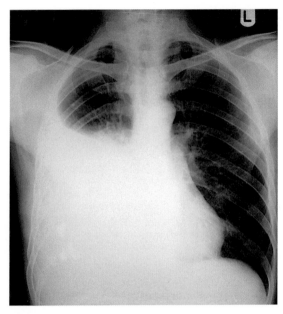

Fig. 11.9 The chest radiographic appearances of a pleural effusion. With a large effusion there is a dense homogenous shadow occupying part of the hemithorax and a meniscus visible on an erect chest X-ray.

Physical signs on the affected side:

- Reduced chest wall movement
- Dull ('stony dull') to percussion
- Absent breath sounds
- Reduced vocal resonance
- Mediastinum shifted away.

pleural fluid; occasionally, they occur because of movement of fluid from the peritoneum or retroperitoneal space. Exudates occur with damaged or altered pleura (resulting in loss of tissue fluid and protein) or from impaired lymphatic drainage of the pleural space. Differentiation of transudate from exudate is the key to subsequent management; treatment for a transudative effusion is that of the underlying disease, while treatment of an exudate often requires specific pleural intervention. More rarely, effusions consist of blood (haemothorax), pus (empyema, p. 539) or lymph (chylothorax). Chylous effusions are caused by leakage of lymph from the thoracic duct as a result of trauma or infiltration by carcinoma.

Table 11.15 Causes of a pleural effusion

Transudate	Exudate
Pleural fluid protein <30 g/L*	Pleural fluid protein >30 g/L*
Common	
Heart failure	Infection (empyema/parapneumonic effusion/tuberculosis)
Hypoalbuminaemia, e.g. nephrotic syndrome, cirrhosis	Malignancy (primary and secondary)
Constrictive pericarditis	Pulmonary embolus with infarction
Hypothyroidism	Connective tissue disease
Ovarian fibroma producing right-sided effusion (Meig's syndrome)	Rare causes (post-myocardial infarction syndrome, acute pancreatitis, mesothelioma, sarcoidosis, chylothorax, drugs, e.g. methotrexate, amiodarone)

*If pleural fluid protein is 25–35 g/L or serum protein level is abnormal, apply Light's criteria (for which simultaneous sampling of venous blood for protein and lactate dehydrogenase [LDH] is required):
- pleural fluid protein/serum protein > 0.5
- pleural fluid LDH/serum LDH > 0.6
- pleural fluid LDH > two-thirds of the upper limit of normal serum LDH.

One or more of above suggest an exudate.

Investigations

Diagnostic pleural fluid aspiration is the initial investigation, unless the clinical picture clearly suggests a transudate, e.g. left ventricular failure. Small effusions or where initial 'blind' aspiration is unsuccessful require image guidance – usually ultrasound. Large effusions causing breathlessness are initially managed with large-volume thoracocentesis (e.g. 1 L) for diagnostic and therapeutic purposes. Appearance of the pleural fluid is noted (purulent in empyema, turbid in infected effusion, milky in chylothorax) and the sample sent for protein, lactate dehydrogenase (LDH), glucose, pH (<7.3 suggests infection), cytology (differential white cell count and malignant cells) and microbiology (Gram stain and culture after inoculating into blood culture bottles, acid-fast bacilli stain and culture) if infection is suspected. Cytology may be negative in a malignant effusion. Occasionally, amylase is measured in suspected pancreatitis-associated effusion and a lipid profile in suspected chylothorax.

Contrast-enhanced thoracic CT scan is performed if diagnostic aspiration does not provide a diagnosis. It is most useful when pleural fluid is still present, as this improves the contrast between pleural abnormality and fluid. CT scanning allows identification of pleural nodularity and image-guided needle biopsy of any focal area of abnormality.

Pleural biopsy for tissue diagnosis (TB smear, culture and histology) is obtained by CT-guided biopsy, blind biopsy (via an Abram's needle) or a video-assisted thoracoscopic approach that allows multiple biopsies to be taken under direct visualization.

Management

This depends on the underlying cause. Exudates are usually drained, and transudates are managed by treatment of the underlying cause. Malignant effusions usually reaccumulate after drainage. They can be treated by aspiration to dryness, followed by instillation into the pleural space of a sclerosing agent such as talc, tetracycline or bleomycin.

Pneumothorax

Pneumothorax is air in the pleural space leading to partial or complete collapse of the lung and occurs spontaneously or secondary to chest trauma. A 'tension pneumothorax' is rare unless the patient is on a mechanical ventilator or nasal non-invasive ventilation. In this situation the pleural tear acts as a one-way valve through which air passes during inspiration but is unable to exit on expiration. There is a unilateral increase in intrapleural pressure, with increasing respiratory distress and eventually shock and cardiorespiratory arrest. Treatment is immediate decompression by needle thoracocentesis (second intercostal space, mid-clavicular line) and then intercostal tube drainage.

Aetiology

Spontaneous pneumothorax typically occurs in young men (typically tall and thin) and is the result of rupture of a pleural bleb which is thought to be due to a congenital defect in the connective tissue of the alveolar wall. Secondary pneumothorax is associated with underlying lung disease, usually COPD.

Clinical features

There is a sudden onset of pleuritic chest pain and breathlessness. With a large pneumothorax there are reduced breath sounds and hyperresonant percussion on examination.

Investigations

A standard PA chest X-ray (Fig. 11.10) will usually confirm the diagnosis. In patients with severe bullous lung disease, CT scanning will differentiate emphysematous bullae from pneumothoraces and save the patient a potentially dangerous needle aspiration. CT will also detect pneumothoraces too small to be visible on chest X-ray.

Management

Management of a spontaneous primary pneumothorax is shown in Fig. 11.11. The management of patients with secondary pneumothoraces differs in four respects:

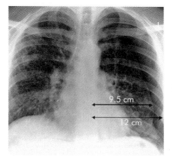

Volume of pneumothorax
$(12^3 - 9.5^3)/12^3 = 50\%$

Fig. 11.10 The chest radiographic appearances of a pneumothorax.

- The visceral-pleura line (marked by the right-hand top arrowhead)
- Loss of pulmonary markings over the left lung
- Mediastinum is shifted away from the pneumothorax and diaphragm on the same side is pushed downwards with large pneumothoraces.

The size of a pneumothorax is estimated by measuring the distance from the lateral edge of the lung to the inner wall of the ribs. A distance >2 cm implies that the pneumothorax is at least 50%, and hence large in size.

(From Henry M, Arnold T, Harvey J on behalf of the BTS Pleural Disease Group. BTS guidelines for the management of spontaneous pneumothorax. Thorax 2003; 58 [Suppl ii]: ii39–52 with permission of the BMJ Publishing Group & British Thoracic Society.)

- Patients remain in hospital
- Attempt aspiration only in minimally breathless patients, <50 years old with small pneumothoraces
- Chest drain insertion indicated in all other patients
- Oxygen given via a fixed-performance mask to patients with COPD (p. 521).

Indications for surgical referral in patients with pneumothorax include persistent air leaks, recurrent pneumothorax and after a first pneumothorax in professions at risk (pilots, divers). Cessation of smoking reduces the recurrence rate. All patients are advised not to fly for 2 weeks after successful treatment of a pneumothorax.

DISORDERS OF THE DIAPHRAGM

Unilateral diaphragmatic paralysis is usually asymptomatic and discovered incidentally on patients having imaging for some other reason. The commonest cause is involvement of the phrenic nerve (C2–C4) in the thorax by a bronchial carcinoma. Chest X-ray shows an elevated hemidiaphragm on the affected side and the diagnosis is made on fluoroscopy (the diaphragm moves paradoxically upward during inspiration). Bilateral diaphragmatic weakness causes orthopnoea, paradoxical (inward) movement of the abdominal wall on inspiration and a large fall in FVC on lying down. Causes include trauma or generalized muscular or neurological

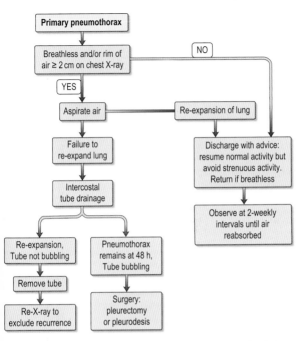

Fig. 11.11 Treatment of a primary spontaneous pneumothorax. All patients admitted to hospital should receive high-flow oxygen (10 L/min) to increase absorption of air from the pleural cavity.

(From Henry M, Arnold T, Harvey J on behalf of the BTS Pleural Disease Group. BTS guidelines for the management of spontaneous pneumothorax. Thorax 2003; 58 [Suppl ii]: ii39–52 with permission of the BMJ Publishing Group & British Thoracic Society.)

conditions (motor neurone disease, muscular dystrophy, Guillain–Barré syndrome). Treatment is either diaphragmatic pacing or night-time assisted ventilation.

THERAPEUTICS

Most drugs described in this section are used in the management of asthma and COPD. Drug inhalation delivers the drug directly to the airways; the dose is smaller than that for the drugs given by mouth, and side effects are reduced. Metered-dose inhalers (MDIs) are the method of first choice for drug delivery. An MDI with a spacer device removes the need to coordinate actuation of an MDI and inhalation, and may improve drug delivery for patients who have difficulty using a pressurized MDI. The MDI increases airway drug deposition and reduces oropharyngeal deposition. Local adverse effects from inhaled corticosteroids, e.g. oropharyngeal candidiasis, are reduced and a spacer device should be co-prescribed with inhaled corticosteroids for children, patients on high doses and those with poor inhaler technique. Breath-activated inhalers or dry powder inhalers are also available. A nebulizer converts a solution of a drug into an aerosol for inhalation and delivers a higher dose of drug than is usual with standard inhalers. Nebulizers are used in the management of acute severe asthma, chronic persistent asthma and brittle asthma.

Bronchodilators

Short-acting selective β_2-adrenoceptor stimulants

Mechanism of action

They interact with β-receptors on the surface of a variety of cells, which leads to bronchial smooth muscle relaxation, decreased release of mediators from mast cells, inhibited neutrophil and eosinophil functional responses and increased mucociliary transport.

Indications

Inhalers are used on an as-required basis for relief of symptoms in mild asthma and on an as-required or regular basis in COPD. Oral preparations are used by patients who cannot manage the inhaler route, and the intravenous route is used for acute severe asthma. In asthma patients using an inhaler on a daily basis, regular inhaled preventative corticosteroid treatment is given (Fig. 11.4).

Preparations and dose

Salbutamol *By inhaler (MDI): 100 μg/puff. Breath-actuated inhaler: 100 μg/ puff. Tablets: 2 mg, 4 mg. Oral solution: 2 mg/5 mL. Nebules: 2.5 mg/2.5 mL, 5 mg/2.5 mL. For infusion: 5 mg/5 mL.*

Inhaled MDI or breath-actuated inhaler: one to two puffs inhaled when required up to three to four times daily.

Oral 4 mg three to four times daily. Elderly and sensitive patients 2 mg initially.

Nebules 2.5–5 mg inhalation of nebulized solution, repeated according to clinical need.

IV infusion Add 5 mg in 5 mL to a 500 mL bag of sodium chloride 0.9% or glucose 5%, to give a 10 μg/mL solution. Infuse at a rate of 5 μg per minute and adjust according to response. Usual maintenance: 3–20 μg/min.

Terbutaline *Inhaler: 250 μg/puff. Dry powder inhaler: 500 μg/inhalation. Injection: 500 μg/mL.*

Inhaled

- One to two puffs of inhaler when required up to three to four times daily
- One inhalation of dry powder inhaler when required up to four times daily.

IV 250–500 μg up to four times daily. Give i.v. over 1–2 minutes or dilute 1.5–2.5 mg in 500 mL glucose 5% and give as a continuous infusion at a rate of 1.5–5 μg/min for 8–10 hours.

Side effects

Fine tremor, tachycardia, palpitations, headache, disturbances of sleep. Hypokalaemia with high doses (monitor plasma potassium in severe asthma).

Cautions/contraindications

Caution in untreated/poorly controlled hyperthyroidism, arrhythmias.

Long-acting selective inhaled β_2-adrenoceptor stimulants (LABA)

Mechanism of action

See short-acting selective β_2-adrenoceptor stimulants.

Indications

LABAs are added to existing inhaled corticosteroid therapy to prevent asthma attacks (Fig. 10.4). They are not used for an acute asthma attack. They are also used in COPD without inhaled corticosteroids, whereas in asthma they should always be used in combination with an inhaled corticosteroid.

Preparations and dose

Salmeterol *Metered-dose inhaler: 25 μg/puff.*

Two puffs inhaled twice daily.

Accuhaler (dry powder for inhalation): 50 μg/blister.

1 blister twice daily.

Diskhaler (dry powder for inhalation): 50 μg/blister.

1 blister twice daily.

Formoterol (eformoterol) *Dry powder: 6 and 12 μg/inhalation. 6–24 μg inhaled twice daily.*

Side effects

As above.

Cautions/contraindications

As above.

Antimuscarinic bronchodilators

Mechanism of action

Ipatropium (short acting) and tiotropium (long acting) antagonize the actions of acetylcholine by competition at the type 3 muscarinic receptor (M_3) site located on airway smooth muscle. Antagonism of acetylcholine results in airway smooth muscle relaxation and bronchodilatation.

Indications

Ipatropium is used when there is a poor response to β-agonists and steroids in the emergency treatment of acute severe asthma. Antimuscarinics are not usually used as first-line bronchodilators to treat chronic asthma. Ipatropium is used for short-term relief of symptoms in COPD and tiotropium for maintenance treatment.

Preparations and dose

Ipatropium bromide *Metered-dose inhaler: 20 and 40 μg/puff.*

20–80 μg inhaled three to four times daily.

Aerocaps (dry powder for inhalation): 40 μg.

20–80 μg inhaled three to four times daily.

Nebules: 250 μg/mL.

100–500 μg inhaled up to four times daily.

    Tiotropium bromide *Dry powder for inhalation: 18 μg.*

    18 μg inhaled once daily.

Side effects

Dry mouth, nausea, constipation, tachycardia, headache, acute angle-closure glaucoma.

Cautions/contraindications

Use with caution in patients with myasthenia gravis, narrow-angle glaucoma (protect patient's eyes from nebulized drug), benign prostatic hypertrophy, bladder neck obstruction.

Theophylline

Mechanism of action

Inhibits phosphodiesterase-mediated hydrolysis and leads to an increase in intracellular concentration of cyclic nucleotides in airway smooth muscle and inflammatory cells. This in turn leads to smooth muscle relaxation and bronchodilatation. Theophylline also has anti-inflammatory/immunomodulatory and bronchoprotective effects that may be mediated by other molecular mechanisms.

Indications

It is used occasionally:

- In acute exacerbations of COPD
- In patients with chronic asthma whose asthma is not adequately controlled with inhaled corticosteroids. A single dose at night can help control nocturnal asthma and early-morning wheezing.

Preparations and dose

Aminophylline is a mixture of theophylline and ethylenediamine; the ethylene-diamine confers greater solubility in water.

    Theophylline *SR capsules: 60 mg, 125 mg, 250 mg.*

    250–500 mg every 12 hours.

SR tablets: 200 mg, 300 mg, 400 mg.

200 mg every 12 hours, increased after 1 week to 300 mg every 12 hours. Patients over 70 kg: 200–300 mg every 12 hours, increased after 1 week to 400 mg every 12 hours.

Aminophylline   *Tablets: 100 mg; SR tablets: 225 mg; Injection: 250 mg/ 10 mL.*

Oral 100–300 mg three to four times daily, or SR 225–450 mg twice daily.

IV with cardiac monitoring Loading dose 5 mg/kg (250–500 mg) over 20 minutes and then maintenance dose of 0.5 mg/kg/h (add 500 mg to 250–500 mL sodium chloride 0.9% or glucose 5%). Plasma theophylline levels are measured daily to maintain a concentration of 10–20 mg/L (55–110 µmol/L). In patients already taking oral theophylline, omit the loading dose and check plasma levels before starting the maintenance infusion.

Side effects

Tachycardia, palpitations, nausea and other gastrointestinal disturbances, headache, CNS stimulation, insomnia, arrhythmias and convulsions, especially if given rapidly by intravenous infusion. There is a narrow margin between therapeutic and toxic dose.

Cautions/contraindications

All modified-release theophylline preparations should be prescribed by brand name, as the bioavailability between different brands may vary. Plasma theophylline concentration should be monitored in patients on oral therapy (8–12 hours after the last dose) and on intravenous treatment for longer than 24 hours (stop infusion for 15 minutes before taking the blood sample). Plasma theophylline concentration for optimum response 10–20 mg/L (55–110 µmol/L).

Theophylline is metabolized in the liver; there is considerable variation in plasma theophylline concentration, particularly in smokers, in patients with hepatic impairment or heart failure, or if certain drugs are taken concurrently – check *British National Formulary* for details.

Intravenous magnesium sulphate

Mechanism of action

Relaxation of bronchial smooth muscle, leading to bronchodilatation.

Indications

A single dose of i.v. magnesium sulphate is given to patients with acute severe asthma, life-threatening or near fatal asthma (Emergency Box 11.1).

Preparations and dose

Magnesium sulphate *50% (Mg^{2+} approx. 2 mmol/mL): 2 mL (1 g), 5 mL (2.5 g), 10 mL (5 g) ampoule.*

IV (Magnesium sulphate concentration should not exceed 20%; dilute 1 part of magnesium sulphate injection 50% with at least 1.5 parts of water for injection.) 1.2–2 g i.v. infusion over 20 minutes.

Side effects

Nausea, vomiting, flushing, hypotension, arrhythmias, drowsiness and muscle weakness.

Cautions/contraindications

Profound hypotension reported with concomitant use of calcium-channel blockers.

Corticosteroids

Mechanism of action

The precise beneficial mechanism in asthma is not known. Corticosteroids induce the synthesis of inhibitory factor kappa B (IκB), a protein that traps and thereby inactivates nuclear factor kappa B. The latter protein activates cytokine genes, and thus steroids inhibit the synthesis of most cytokines. Steroids reduce airway inflammation and hence reduce oedema and secretion of mucus into the airway. Compound preparations that contain an inhaled corticosteroid and a long-acting β_2-agonist (e.g. budesonide with formoterol) are used for patients stabilized on the individual components.

Indications

Inhaled For prophylactic treatment of asthma when patients are using a β_2-agonist more than once daily. In patients with COPD who have an improvement in lung function after a trial of oral corticosteroids.

Oral Acute severe asthma and in patients with chronic asthma when the response to other anti-asthma drugs is small.

Parenteral Acute severe asthma.

Preparations and dose

Beclometasone *Metered-dose inhaler: 50, 100, 200, 250 μg/puff.*

200 μg inhaled twice daily, or for more severe cases up to 800 μg daily may be used.

Breath-activated inhaler: 50, 100, 250 μg/puff.

200 μg inhaled twice daily, or for more severe cases up to 800 μg daily may be used.

Dry powder for inhalation: 100, 200, 400 μg/puff.

400 μg inhaled twice daily.

Budesonide *Metered-dose inhaler: 50, 200 μg/puff.*

50 μg inhaled twice daily, or for more severe cases up to 400 μg twice daily.

Turbohaler (dry powder): 100, 200, 400 μg/inhalation.

100–800 μg inhaled twice daily.

Fluticasone *Metered-dose inhaler: 50, 125, 250 μg/puff.*

100–200 μg inhaled twice daily, increased up to 1 mg twice daily when necessary. Higher doses initiated by a specialist.

Dry powder for inhalation: 50, 100, 250, 500 μg/blister.

100–200 µg inhaled twice daily, increased up to 1 mg twice daily when necessary. Higher doses initiated by a specialist.

Oral See page 664.

IV See page 664.

Side effects

The adverse effects of oral corticosteroids are listed on page 665. Inhaled corticosteroids have far fewer side effects than oral corticosteroids, but adverse effects are reported. Hoarseness and oropharyngeal candidiasis are reduced by rinsing the mouth with water after inhalation of a dose and/or by using a spacer device. Higher doses of inhaled corticosteroids have the potential to induce adrenal suppression, and patients on high doses should be given a 'steroid card' and may also need corticosteroid cover during an operation or illness. High doses may also reduce bone mineral density and the dose should be reduced when asthma control is good. There is a small increased risk of glaucoma.

Cautions/contraindications

Caution with inhaled corticosteroids in active or quiescent tuberculosis. Paradoxical bronchospasm may be prevented (if mild) by inhalation of a β_2-agonist before corticosteroid treatment.

12 Intensive care medicine

Critical care medicine (or 'intensive care medicine') is concerned predominantly with the management of patients with acute life-threatening conditions ('the critically ill'). In addition to emergencies, intensive care units (ICUs) admit high-risk patients electively after major surgery. Frequently, ICU staff provide care throughout the hospital as medical emergency teams or outreach care. Teamwork and a multidisciplinary approach are central to the provision of intensive care and this functions most effectively when directed and coordinated by committed specialists.

ICUs are usually reserved for patients with established or impending organ failure. They are equipped with monitoring and technical facilities, including an adjacent laboratory (or 'near patient testing' devices) for the rapid determination of blood gases and simple biochemical data such as serum potassium, blood glucose and serum lactate levels. Technological advances have led to the development of more compact and complex mechanical ventilators that are adaptable to individual patient demands. Portable ultrasound and echocardiography equipment is commonly available. Patients receive continuous expert nursing care (in the UK a nurse/patient ratio of 1:1 in an ICU or 1:2 in a high-dependency unit [HDU]) and also the constant attention of appropriately trained medical staff.

High-dependency units offer a level of care intermediate between the general ward and that provided in an ICU. They provide monitoring and support for patients with single organ failure and for those who are at risk of developing organ failure. They can also provide a 'step-down' facility for patients being discharged from intensive care.

Patient selection – withholding and withdrawing treatment

It is essential that only patients who are likely to benefit from intensive care are admitted. For some critically ill patients, admission to ICU is inappropriate because prognosis is hopeless and this will simply prolong the process of dying, their suffering and that of their relatives as well as taking up limited resources without benefit. A decision not to admit a patient to ICU is based on their previous health and quality of life, and the prognosis of the underlying condition. These decisions should be made in conjunction with the medical and nursing staff, the patient and relatives and documented in the medical records.

Critical care outreach and early warning systems

Within an acute hospital there are patients on general wards who are 'at risk' and deteriorating who require care above the 'general level'. Prompt recognition and institution of expert treatment will often prevent progression to severe illness. Critical care outreach is an organizational approach to ensure high-quality care for these patients. Outreach services have three aims:

- Avert admissions to ICU or ensure that admissions are timely, by early identification of patients who are deteriorating
- Enable discharges from ICU by supporting the continued recovery of discharged patients, and their relatives, on wards and after discharge from hospital
- Share critical care skills with staff on the ward and in the community.

Terminal cardiovascular, neurological or respiratory collapse is often preceded by a period of abnormal basic physiological observations during which time potential life-saving therapeutic interventions may be initiated. The Modified Early Warning Score (MEWS, Table 12.1) is a cumulative score based on routine ward observations which acts as a 'tracker' to 'flag up' patients who should be given immediate priority. Hospital protocols vary but in general a MEWS score of 4 or more indicates the need for urgent medical assessment which may result in ICU admission.

ACUTE DISTURBANCES OF HAEMODYNAMIC FUNCTION (SHOCK)

The term 'shock' describes acute circulatory failure with inadequate or inappropriately distributed tissue perfusion resulting in decreased oxygen delivery to the tissues. The effects of inadequate tissue perfusion are initially reversible, but prolonged oxygen deprivation leads to critical derangement of cell processes, end-organ failure and death. Thus prompt recognition and treatment of shock is essential. The causes of shock are listed in Table 12.2. Shock is often the result of a combination of these factors: e.g. in sepsis, distributive shock is frequently complicated by hypovolaemia and myocardial depression.

Pathophysiology

The sympathoadrenal response to shock Hypotension stimulates baroreceptors and chemoreceptors, causing increased sympathetic nervous activity with 'spill-over' of noradrenaline (norepinephrine) into the circulation. Later this is augmented by the release of catecholamines (adrenaline [epinephrine]) from the adrenal medulla. The resulting vasoconstriction, together with increased myocardial contractility and heart rate, help to restore blood pressure (BP) and cardiac output.

Table 12.1 Modified Early Warning Score

Score	3	2	1	0	1	2	3
RR		≤8		9–14	15–20	21–29	>29
HR		≤40	41–50	51–100	101–110	111–129	>129
Syst BP	≤70	71–80	81–100	101–199		≥200	
Urine output	<20 mL/h for 2 h	<0.5 mL/kg/h					
Temp (°C)		≤35		35.1–37.2	37.3–37.9	≥38	
Neurological		Confused/agitated		Alert	Responds to voice	Responds to pain	Unresponsive

RR, respiratory rate, breaths/min; HR, heart rate, beats/min; syst BP, systolic blood pressure, mmHg.

Table 12.2 Causes of shock

Hypovolaemic (reduced preload)

Haemorrhage: trauma, gastrointestinal bleeding, fractures, ruptured aortic aneurysm

Fluid loss: burns, severe diarrhoea, intestinal obstruction (fluid accumulates in the intestine)

Cardiogenic (pump failure)

Myocardial infarction
Myocarditis
Atrial and ventricular arrhythmias
Bradycardias
Rupture of a valve cusp

Obstructive

Obstruction to outflow: massive pulmonary embolism, tension pneumothorax
Restricted cardiac filling: cardiac tamponade, constrictive pericarditis

Distributive (decrease in systemic vascular resistance)

Vascular dilatation: drugs, sepsis
Arteriovenous shunting
Maldistribution of flow, e.g. sepsis, anaphylaxis

Reduced perfusion of the renal cortex stimulates the juxtaglomerular apparatus to release renin. This converts angiotensinogen to angiotensin I, which is converted in the lungs and vascular endothelium to the potent vasoconstrictor angiotensin II, which also stimulates secretion of aldosterone by the adrenal cortex, causing sodium and water retention. This helps to restore the circulating volume.

Neuroendocrine response

There is *release of pituitary hormones* such as adrenocorticotrophic hormone (ACTH), vasopressin (antidiuretic hormone [ADH]) and endogenous opioid peptides. ACTH leads to *release of cortisol*, which causes fluid retention and antagonizes insulin. There is *release of glucagon*, which raises the blood sugar level. There is evidence that patients with septic shock have a blunted response to exogenous ACTH ('*relative*' *adrenocortical insufficiency*) that could be associated with an impaired vasoconstrictor response to noradrenaline and worse prognosis.

Release of mediators Severe infection, the presence of large areas of damaged tissue (e.g. following trauma or extensive surgery) or prolonged/repeated episodes of hypoperfusion can trigger a massive inflammatory response with activation of leucocytes, complement and the coagulation cascade. This is beneficial when targeted against local areas of infection or necrotic tissue but dissemination of this response can produce shock and widespread tissue damage.

- In septic shock the innate immune response and inflammatory cascade are triggered by the recognition of pathogen-associated molecular patterns (PAMPs), including bacterial and fungal DNA, cell wall components (e.g. endotoxin) and/or exotoxins (antigenic proteins produced by bacteria such as staphylococci). Cell wall components from Gram-negative and Gram-positive bacteria form a complex with specific serum proteins before attaching to a cell surface marker (CD14) and triggering a cascade of membrane-bound and intracellular signalling pathways. This in turn leads to release of reactive oxygen and nitrogen species that kill bacteria, pro-inflammatory cytokines (tumour necrosis factor, interleukin-1 [IL-1] and IL-6) which mediate inflammation and the metabolic response, and anti-inflammatory cytokines (IL-10), which if excessive can cause inappropriate immune hyporesponsiveness.
- Toxic products of tissue injury (surgery and trauma): following traumatic or surgical tissue injury, inflammatory pathways may be triggered by damage-associated molecular patterns (DAMPS) such as DNA fragments. This is why distributive shock secondary to infection can be difficult to distinguish clinically from that caused by a 'sterile' insult such as severe trauma or surgery.
- Pro-inflammatory cytokines promote adhesion of activated leucocytes to the vessel wall and subsequent extravascular migration leading to tissue damage and organ dysfunction.
- Platelet activating factor and lysosomal enzymes (by converting inactive kininogens to vasoactive kinins) cause increased vascular permeability.
- Nitric oxide produced by vascular endothelial cells under the influence of certain cytokines leads to vasodilatation, hypotension and reduced reactivity to adrenergic mediators.

Microcirculatory changes In the early stages of septic shock there is vasodilatation, increased capillary permeability with interstitial oedema and arteriovenous shunting. Vasodilatation and increased capillary permeability also occur in anaphylactic shock. In the initial stages of other forms of shock, and in the later stages of sepsis and anaphylaxis, there is capillary sequestration of blood. Fluid is forced into the extravascular space, causing interstitial oedema, haemoconcentration and an increase in plasma viscosity.

Activation of the coagulation system occurs in all forms of shock, leading to platelet aggregation, widespread intravascular thrombosis and inadequate tissue perfusion, with the development of disseminated intravascular coagulation (DIC, see p. 238).

Progressive organ failure may develop as a result of the disseminated inflammatory response and microcirculatory changes. The mortality in *multiple organ dysfunction syndrome* (MODS) is high and treatment is supportive.

Clinical features

The history will often indicate the cause of shock, e.g. a patient with major injuries will often develop hypovolaemic shock. A patient with a history of peptic ulceration may now be bleeding into the gastrointestinal tract, and rectal examination will show melaena. Anaphylactic shock develops in susceptible individuals after insect stings and after eating certain foods (Emergency Box 12.1).

✚ Emergency Box 12.1

Anaphylactic shock

Pathophysiology

Massive release of mediators from mast cells and basophils induced by cross-linking of surface IgE with trigger antigen (e.g. penicillin, latex, bee sting, radiographic contrast media, eggs, peanuts, shellfish) leads to increase in vascular permeability, vasodilatation and respiratory smooth muscle contraction.

Diagnosis

Typical symptoms and signs (p. 577) developing after exposure to an agent known to provoke anaphylaxis.

Management

- **Remove** the precipitating cause, e.g. stop administration of the offending drug.
- **Oxygen** high flow.
- **Adrenaline** 0.5 mL of a 1:1000 solution (500 μg) injected intramuscularly (i.m.) if life-threatening features (respiratory distress or shock). Repeat in 5 minutes if no clinical improvement. Intravenously (i.v.) (5 mL 1:10 000) only if cardiac arrest. Half doses of adrenaline for patients taking amitriptyline, imipramine, or β-blocker
- **Fluids** 500–1000 mL 0.9% saline i.v.
- **Chlorphenamine** (antihistamine) 10 mg i.m. or i.v. over 1–2 minutes
- **Hydrocortisone** 200 mg i.m. or i.v. over 1–2 minutes
- **Admit** patient for observation (6–8 hours) because of risk of second late reaction
- **Prevent further attacks.** Refer to an immunologist or allergist, identify responsible allergen (careful history, skin testing, serum antibody tests by RAST or ELISA). Patients who have had an attack of anaphylaxis and who are at risk of developing another should carry a preloaded syringe of adrenaline for i.m. self-administration (e.g. Epipen device) and wear an appropriate information bracelet (e.g. Medic Alert).

ELISA, enzyme-linked immunosorbent assay; IgE, immunoglobulin E; RAST, radioallergosorbent test.

Hypovolaemic shock Increased sympathetic tone causes tachycardia (pulse > 100 beats/min), sweating and peripheral vasoconstriction (blood is redirected from the periphery to vital organs), leading to inadequate tissue perfusion with cold clammy skin and slow capillary refill (>3 seconds). Capillary refill is the time for the skin of the patient's digit to turn pink again after compression for 5 seconds. The BP (particularly when supine) may be maintained initially, but later hypotension supervenes (systolic BP < 100 mmHg) with oliguria, tachypnoea, confusion and restlessness.

Cardiogenic shock Additional clinical features are those of acute heart failure, e.g. raised jugular venous pressure (JVP), pulsus alternans (alternating strong and weak pulses), a 'gallop' rhythm (additional 3rd and 4th heart sounds), basal crackles and pulmonary oedema.

Mechanical shock Muffled heart sounds, pulsus paradoxus (pulse fades on inspiration), elevated JVP and Kussmaul's sign (JVP increases on inspiration) occur in cardiac tamponade. In massive pulmonary embolism there are signs of right heart strain, with a raised JVP with prominent 'a' waves, right ventricular heave and a loud pulmonary second sound.

Anaphylactic shock Onset of symptoms is usually within 5–60 minutes of antigen exposure. Profound vasodilatation leads to warm peripheries and hypotension. Urticaria, angio-oedema, wheezing and upper airway obstruction due to laryngeal oedema may all be present.

Sepsis is an infection with evidence of a systemic inflammatory response (Table 12.3). There may be progression to severe sepsis and/or septic shock. Sepsis in elderly people or in the immunosuppressed is common without the classic clinical features of infection. The systemic inflammatory response syndrome also occurs with severe burns, trauma and acute pancreatitis, and these conditions may mimic infection.

Management

This is summarized in Emergency Box 12.2. The underlying cause must be identified and treated appropriately. Whatever the aetiology of shock, tissue blood flow and blood pressure must be restored as quickly as possible to avoid multiple organ failure.

Expansion of the circulating volume (preload) Volume replacement is necessary in hypovolaemic shock and also in anaphylactic shock. Fluid is also given to patients with severe sepsis where there is vasodilatation, sequestration of blood and loss of circulating volume secondary to capillary leakage. These patients have evidence of organ dysfunction but may not necessarily be hypotensive (Table 12.3). High filling pressures may also be needed in mechanical shock. Care must be taken to prevent volume overload, which leads to a reduction in stroke volume and a rise in left atrial pressure with a risk of pulmonary oedema. The choice of fluid depends on the clinical situation.

- Blood is given for haemorrhage as soon as it is available. Complications of massive blood transfusion are hypothermia (minimized by using a blood warmer during infusion), coagulopathy (stored blood has almost no effective

Table 12.3 Differing degrees of severity of sepsis

Sepsis – systemic inflammatory response syndrome (SIRS) associated with infection

SIRS is two or more of:
Fever >38°C or hypothermia <36°C
Tachycardia: heart rate > 90 beats/min
Tachypnoea: respiratory rate > 20 breaths/min or $P_a{CO_2} < 4.3$ kPa
Leucocytosis (white blood cell count >12 × 10⁹/L), leucopenia (white cell count <4 × 10⁹/L) or bandaemia (>10% immature forms)

Severe sepsis – sepsis with dysfunction of one or more organs:

Kidneys – creatinine > 177 µmol/L or urine output < 0.5 mL/kg/h for 2 h
Coagulation – platelets < 100, aPTT > 60 s, INR > 1.5
Respiratory – new or increased oxygen needs to keep SpO₂ > 90%
Liver – bilirubin > 34 µmol/L
Tissue hypoperfusion: systolic BP < 90 mmHg, MAP > 65 mmHg, drop in > 40 mmHg from patient's normal BP or serum lactate > 2 mmol/L

Septic shock – persisting tissue hypoperfusion after a fluid challenge:

Evidence of tissue hypoperfusion after an intravenous fluid bolus with saline 0.9% or Hartmann's solution

aPTT, activated partial thromboplastin time; BP, blood pressure; INR, international normalized ratio; MAP, mean arterial pressure over a cardiac cycle, approximated from systolic and diastolic pressures; SpO₂, peripheral capillary oxygen saturation.

✚ Emergency Box 12.2

Management of shock

Ensure adequate oxygenation and ventilation

- Maintain patent airway: use oropharyngeal airway or endotracheal tube if necessary
- Oxygen 15 L/min via face mask with reservoir bag unless oxygen restriction necessary
- Support respiratory function early: non-invasive or mechanical ventilation
- Monitor: respiratory rate, blood gases and chest X-ray

Restore cardiac output and blood pressure

- Lay patient flat or head-down
- Expand circulating volume with appropriate fluids given quickly via large-bore cannulae
- Inotropic support, vasodilators, intra-aortic balloon counterpulsation in selected cases
- Monitor in all: skin colour, pulse, blood pressure, peripheral temperature, urine output, ECG
- Monitor in selected cases: CVP monitoring, cardiac function/output

Investigations

- All cases: FBC, serum creatinine and electrolytes, blood glucose, liver biochemistry, coagulation, blood gases, ECG
- Selected cases: culture of blood, urine, sputum, pus and CSF, blood lactate, D-dimers, echocardiogram

Treat underlying cause

- Haemorrhage, sepsis, anaphylaxis

Treat complications

- Coagulopathy, acute kidney injury, etc.

CSF, cerebrospinal fluid; CVP, central venous pressure; ECG, electrocardiogram; FBC, full blood count.

platelets and is deficient in clotting factors), hypocalcaemia (citrate anticoagulation in stored blood binds calcium), hyperkalaemia (passive leakage from stored red cells) and acute lung injury due to microaggregates in stored blood. The platelet count, prothrombin time, activated partial thromboplastin time and plasma calcium and potassium should be measured after rapid transfusion of 3–5 units of blood.

- Crystalloid (0.9% saline or Hartmann's solution, p. 330) is given for acute blood loss before blood becomes available, and for volume replacement in anaphylactic shock and severe sepsis. There has been considerable debate of the merits of crystalloid versus colloid in volume resuscitation and in most situations there are no apparent clinical differences. In severe sepsis 500- to 1000-mL boluses of crystalloid are given over 30 minutes with the aim of maintaining a central venous pressure (CVP) of 8–12 mmHg, mean arterial pressure of ≥ 65 mmHg and urine output > 0.5 mL/kg/h.

Myocardial contractility and inotropic agents Myocardial contractility is impaired in cardiogenic shock and at a later stage in other forms of shock as a result of hypoxaemia, acidosis and the release of mediators. Treatment of acidosis should concentrate on correcting the cause; intravenous bicarbonate should only be administered to correct extreme (pH < 7.0) persistent metabolic acidosis. Drugs that impair cardiac performance, e.g. β-blockers, should be stopped. When the signs of shock persist despite adequate volume replacement (indicated by a CVP [see below] of 8–12 mmHg), inotropic agents are administered. Inotropic agents are administered via a large central vein and the effects must be carefully monitored. The inotropic agents used and their clinical effects are shown in Table 12.4. The particular agent used depends on the values for mean arterial pressure, cardiac output and personal preference.

Additional treatment Vasodilators, e.g. sodium nitroprusside and isosorbide dinitrate, may be useful in selected patients who remain vasoconstricted

Table 12.4 Inotropic agents used in the management of shock

Inotropic agent	Sympathomimetic and dopaminergic (D) effects and main clinical use
Adrenaline	Low dose (0.06–0.1 μg/kg/min), β-adrenergic effects predominate with increase in cardiac output and fall in systemic vascular resistance (SVR). High dose (>0.18 μg/kg/min), α_1-adrenergic effects predominate with increased SVR. This may increase renal perfusion pressure and urine output but excessive vasoconstriction leads to decreased cardiac output, oliguria and peripheral gangrene. Potent agent, used in refractory hypotension
Noradrenaline	Predominantly α-adrenergic agonist. Particularly useful in those with hypotension and a low SVR, e.g. septic shock
Dopamine	Low dose (1–3 μg/kg/min), predominantly acts on D_1 receptor, resulting in selective vasodilatation. Moderate dose – β_1 receptors also stimulated with increased heart rate, myocardial contractility and cardiac output. High dose (>10 μg/kg/min) – α-adrenergic effects predominant with an increase in SVR
Dopexamine	Dopamine analogue that activates β_2 receptors as well as D_1 and D_2 receptors. Weakly positive inotrope and powerful splanchnic vasodilator, reducing afterload and improving blood flow to vital organs. Most useful in those with low cardiac output and peripheral vasoconstriction
Dobutamine	Predominantly β_1 activity. Minimal α- and β_2-receptor activity results in vasodilatation. The net effect is increased cardiac output with decreased SVR
Milrinone and enoximone	Phosphodiesterase inhibitors with inotropic and vasodilator effects through non-adrenergic mechanisms
Vasopressin	Increases blood pressure and SVR. Used in septic shock where circulating levels of vasopressin are inappropriately low

α_1-Adrenergic receptors – located in vascular wall and heart; they increase SVR and duration of cardiac contraction.
β_1-Adrenergic receptors – located in the heart; their inotropic and chronotropic action results in increased cardiac output.
β_2-Adrenergic receptors – located in blood vessels; they mediate vasodilatation.
Postsynaptic D_1 receptors mediate vasodilatation of mesenteric, renal, coronary and cerebral circulation.
Presynaptic D_2 receptors cause vasoconstriction by inducing noradrenaline release.

and oliguric despite adequate volume replacement and a satisfactory blood pressure. Finally, in patients with a potentially reversible depression of left ventricular function (e.g. cardiogenic shock secondary to a ruptured interventricular septum), intra-aortic balloon counterpulsation (IABCP) is used as a temporary measure to maintain life until definitive surgical treatment can be carried out.

Specific treatment of the cause

- *Septic shock.* Antibiotic treatment of septicaemia is discussed on page 000. Therapy should be directed towards the probable cause. 'Blind' intravenous antibiotic therapy according to local guidelines should be started after performing an infection screen: chest X-ray and culture of blood, urine and sputum. Lumbar puncture, ultrasonography and computed tomography (CT) of the chest and abdomen are useful in selected cases. Abscesses require drainage. The administration of relatively low, 'stress' doses of hydrocortisone to selected patients with refractory vasopressor-resistant septic shock may assist shock reversal and perhaps improve outcome.
- *Anaphylactic shock* must be identified and treated immediately (Emergency Box 12.1).

Monitoring

Clinical An assessment of skin perfusion and the measurement of pulse, BP, JVP and urinary flow rate will guide treatment in a straightforward case. Additional invasive monitoring will be required in seriously ill patients who do not respond to initial treatment.

Invasive

- *Blood pressure.* A continuous recording is made with an intra-arterial cannula, usually in the radial artery.
- *CVP* is related to right ventricular end-diastolic pressure, which depends on circulating blood volume, venous tone, intrathoracic pressure and right ventricular function. CVP is measured by inserting a central venous catheter (CVC), often under ultrasound control, into the superior vena cava or right atrium via percutaneous puncture of a subclavian or internal jugular vein. The catheter is connected to a manometer system (for intermittent CVP readings) or transducer system (for continuous readings displayed on a monitor). CVP is measured in a supine patient by aligning the transducer with the mid axilla (level with the right atrium); the normal range is 5–10 cmH$_2$O (mid axilla). An isolated CVP is of limited value; a trend of readings is much more significant and should be viewed in conjunction with other parameters, e.g. blood pressure and urine output. In shock, CVP may be normal because of increased venous tone and a better guide to circulating volume is the response to a fluid challenge (Fig. 12.1). A CVC is also used to measure central venous oxyhaemoglobin saturation ($S_{cv}o_2$).
- *Pulmonary artery catheters*, also called Swan–Ganz catheters, measure cardiac output and the pulmonary artery occlusion pressure, which reflects left atrial pressure. Insertion is associated with increased complications and

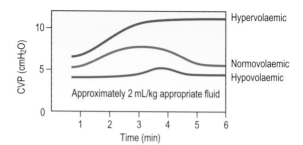

Fig. 12.1 The effect on the central venous pressure (CVP) of a rapid administration of a 'fluid challenge' to patients with a CVP within the normal range.
(From Sykes MK. Venous pressure as a clinical indication of adequacy of transfusion. Annals of the Royal College of Surgeons of England 1963; 33: 185–197.)

has not been shown to improve outcome; therefore less-invasive techniques are increasingly preferred.

- *Cardiac output* is also measured using oesophageal Doppler ultrasonography and lithium dilution.

RESPIRATORY FAILURE

Respiratory failure occurs when pulmonary gas exchange is sufficiently impaired to cause hypoxaemia with or without hypercapnia. In practical terms, respiratory failure is present when the P_aO_2 is < 8 kPa (60 mmHg) or the P_aCO_2 is >7 kPa (55 mmHg).

It can be divided into two types (Table 12.5):

- Type 1 respiratory failure in which the P_aO_2 is low and the P_aCO_2 is normal or low. It is most commonly caused by diseases that damage lung tissue. The hypoxaemia is due to ventilation–perfusion mismatch or right-to-left shunts.
- Type 2 respiratory failure in which the P_aO_2 is low and the P_aCO_2 is high is caused by alveolar hypoventilation.

Monitoring

Clinical assessment should be made of the following: tachypnoea, tachycardia, sweating, pulsus paradoxus, use of accessory muscles of respiration, intercostal recession and inability to speak. Signs of carbon dioxide retention may be present, such as asterixis (coarse tremor), bounding pulse, warm peripheries and papilloedema.

Pulse oximetry Lightweight oximeters placed on an earlobe or finger can give a continuous reading of oxygen saturation by measuring the changing amount of light transmitted through arterial blood. The normal range is 95–100%, but in general, if the saturation is greater than 90%, oxygenation can be considered to be adequate. Although simple and reliable, these

Table 12.5 Causes of respiratory failure

Type 1	Type 2
Pulmonary oedema	COPD
Pneumonia	Life-threatening acute severe asthma
Acute severe asthma	Respiratory muscle weakness, e.g. GBS
Pneumothorax	Respiratory centre depression, e.g. with sedatives
COPD	Sleep apnoea
Pulmonary embolism	Chest wall deformities
Acute respiratory distress syndrome	Inhaled foreign body
Lung fibrosis	
Right-to-left cardiac shunts	

COPD, chronic obstructive pulmonary disease; GBS, Guillain–Barré syndrome.

instruments are not very sensitive to changes in oxygenation and give no indication of carbon dioxide retention.

Forced vital capacity (FVC) In patients with acute neuromuscular problems, e.g. Guillain–Barré syndrome and myasthenia gravis, FVC is used as a guide to deterioration. ICU admission is recommended when the FVC is less than 20 mL/kg, and typically intubation and ventilation are necessary when less than 10 mL/kg.

Arterial blood gas analysis Analysis of arterial blood gives definitive measurements of P_aO_2, P_aCO_2, oxygen saturation, pH and bicarbonate. Normal values are given in Table 12.6. In type 2 respiratory failure, retention of carbon dioxide causes P_aCO_2 and $[H^+]$ to rise, resulting in respiratory acidosis. In chronic type 2 failure (e.g. chronic obstructive pulmonary disease [COPD]) the bicarbonate concentration is also raised secondary to renal retention and the pH may partially or completely normalize due to this metabolic

Table 12.6 Normal values for arterial blood gases

pH	7.35–7.45
P_aCO_2	4.3–6.0 kPa
P_aO_2	10.5–14 kPa
Base excess	±2 mmol/L
HCO_3	22–26 mmol/L
O_2 saturation	95–100%

compensation (Fig. 8.5). In type 1 respiratory failure or in hyperventilation there may be a fall in $P_a\text{co}_2$ and $[H^+]$, resulting in respiratory alkalosis. Other abnormalities of acid–base balance are discussed on page 000.

Capnography This allows the continuous breath-by-breath analysis of expired carbon dioxide concentrations and is mandatory in patients having tracheal intubation outside the ICU.

Management

This includes the administration of supplemental oxygen, control of secretions, treatment of pulmonary infection, control of airway obstruction and limiting pulmonary oedema. Correction of abnormalities which may lead to respiratory muscle weakness, e.g. hypokalaemia, hypophosphataemia and undernutrition, is also necessary. Oxygen is delivered by a face mask or by nasal cannulae. With these devices, inspired oxygen concentration varies from 35 to 55%, with flow rates between 6 and 10 L. However, in patients with chronically elevated carbon dioxide (e.g. COPD), hypoxia rather than hypercapnia maintains the respiratory drive, and thus fixed-performance masks (e.g. Venturi masks) should be used, in which the concentration of oxygen can be accurately controlled. Respiratory stimulants such as doxapram have a very limited role in treatment.

Respiratory support Respiratory support is necessary when the above measures are not sufficient. The type depends on the underlying disorder and severity. Consideration should be given to ventilating patients with severe chronic lung disease, as those who are severely incapacitated may be difficult to wean from the ventilator:

- *Continuous positive airway pressure (CPAP)* is used for acute type 1 respiratory failure. Oxygen is delivered to the spontaneously breathing patient under pressure via a tightly fitting face mask (non-invasive positive-pressure ventilation, NIPPV) or endotracheal tube. Oxygenation and vital capacity improve and the lungs become less stiff.
- *Bilevel positive airway pressure (BiPAP)* provides assistance during the inspiratory phase and prevents airway closure during the expiratory phase. The main indication for BiPAP in the emergency setting is an acute exacerbation of COPD in patients who do not require immediate intubation and ventilation. In these patients it is indicated when there is a persistent decompensated respiratory acidosis (pH < 7.35 and $P_a\text{co}_2 > 6$ kPa) following immediate maximum medical treatment on controlled oxygen for no more than 1 hour (p. 521). BiPAP reduces the need for intubation, mortality and hospital stay. It is given for as long as possible during the first 24 hours and continued until the acute exacerbation has resolved, usually 2–3 days. Contraindications are facial burns/trauma/recent facial or upper airway surgery, vomiting, fixed upper airway obstruction, undrained pneumothorax, inability to protect the airway, intestinal obstruction, confusion, agitation and patient refusal of treatment.

Table 12.7 Indications for intermittent positive-pressure ventilation (IPPV)

Indication	Comment
Acute respiratory failure	With signs of severe respiratory distress despite maximal therapy: respiratory rate > 40/min inability to speak patient exhausted, confused or agitated
	Rising $P_a\text{CO}_2$ > 8 kPa
	Extreme hypoxaemia < 8 kPa, despite oxygen therapy
Acute ventilatory failure, e.g. myasthenia gravis	Institute when vital capacity fallen to 10–15 mL/kg
Guillain–Barré syndrome	High $P_a\text{CO}_2$, particularly if rising, is an indication for urgent mechanical ventilation
Prophylactic post-operative ventilation	In poor-risk patients
Head injury	With acute brain oedema. Intracranial pressure is decreased by elective hyperventilation as this reduces cerebral blood flow
Trauma	e.g. chest injury and lung contusion
Severe left ventricular failure	
Coma with breathing difficulties	e.g. following drug overdose

- *Intermittent positive-pressure ventilation (IPPV)*. IPPV requires tracheal intubation and therefore anaesthesia if the patient is conscious. The indications for mechanical ventilation are listed in Table 12.7. The beneficial effects include improved carbon dioxide elimination, improved oxygenation and relief from exhaustion as the work of ventilation is removed. High concentrations of oxygen (up to 100%) may be administered accurately. If adequate oxygenation cannot be achieved, a positive airway pressure can be maintained at a chosen level throughout expiration by attaching a threshold resistor valve to the expiratory limb of the circuit. This is known as positive end-expiratory pressure (PEEP), and its primary effect is to re-expand underventilated lung areas, thereby reducing shunts and increasing $P_a\text{O}_2$.
- *Intermittent mandatory ventilation (IMV)*. This technique allows the ventilated patient to breathe spontaneously between mandatory tidal volumes delivered by the ventilator. These coincide with the patient's own respiratory effort. It is used as a method of weaning patients from artificial ventilation, or as an alternative to IPPV.

The major complications of intubation and assisted ventilation are:

- Trauma to the upper respiratory tract from the endotracheal tube
- Secondary pulmonary infection
- Barotrauma – overdistension of the lungs and alveolar rupture may present with tension pneumothorax (p. 561) and surgical emphysema
- Reduction in cardiac output – the increase in intrathoracic pressures during controlled ventilation impedes cardiac filling and lowers cardiac output
- Abdominal distension due to intestinal ileus – cause not known
- Increased ADH and reduced atrial natriuretic peptide secretion. Together with a fall in cardiac output and reduced renal perfusion this leads to salt and water retention.

ACUTE RESPIRATORY DISTRESS SYNDROME (ARDS)

Definition and causes The term 'acute lung injury' is no longer used. ARDS can be defined as follows:

- Respiratory distress
- Stiff lungs (reduced pulmonary compliance resulting in high inflation pressures)
- Chest radiograph: new bilateral, diffuse, patchy or homogeneous pulmonary infiltrates
- Cardiac: no apparent cardiogenic cause of pulmonary oedema (pulmonary artery occlusion pressure <18 mmHg if measured or no clinical evidence of left atrial hypertension)
- Gas exchange abnormalities: mild, P_aO_2/F_iO_2 ratio 200–300 mmHg; moderate, P_aO_2/F_iO_2 ratio 100–200 mmHg; and severe, P_aO_2/F_iO_2 ratio <100 mmHg, all with a PEEP ≥ 5 cm H_2O (Berlin) (in all cases, despite normal arterial carbon dioxide tension and with the application of PEEP)
- ARDS can occur as a non-specific reaction of the lungs to a wide variety of direct pulmonary and indirect non-pulmonary insults. By far the most common predisposing factor is sepsis, and 20–40% of patients with severe sepsis will develop ARDS.

Pathophysiology

ARDS can be viewed as an early manifestation of a generalized inflammatory response with endothelial dysfunction and is therefore frequently associated with the development of MODS. The cardinal feature is pulmonary oedema as a result of increased vascular permeability caused by the release of inflammatory mediators. Oedema may induce vascular compression resulting in pulmonary hypertension, which is later exacerbated by vasoconstriction in response to increased autonomic nervous activity. A haemorrhagic intraalveolar exudate forms, which is rich in platelets, fibrin and clotting factors. This inactivates surfactant, stimulates inflammation and promotes hyaline membrane formation. These changes may result in progressive pulmonary fibrosis.

Clinical features

Tachypnoea, increasing hypoxia and laboured breathing are the initial features. The chest X-ray shows diffuse bilateral shadowing, which may progress to a complete 'white-out'.

Management

This is based on the treatment of the underlying condition. Pulmonary oedema should be limited with fluid restriction, diuretics and haemofiltration if these measures fail. Aerosolized surfactant, inhaled nitric oxide and aerosolized prostacyclin are experimental treatments whose exact role in the management of ARDS is unclear. Repeated positional change, i.e. changing the patient from supine to prone, may allow reductions in airway pressures and the inspired oxygen fraction in those with severe hypoxaemia.

Prognosis

Mortality from ARDS has fallen over the last decade, from around 60% to between 20 and 40%, perhaps as a consequence of improved general care, lung-protective ventilator strategies, the increasing use of management protocols and attention to infection control and nutrition. Prognosis is dependent on aetiology. When ARDS occurs in association with intra-abdominal sepsis, mortality rates remain very high, whereas they are much lower in those with 'primary' ARDS (pneumonia, aspiration, lung contusion). Most of those dying with ARDS do so as a result of MODS and haemodynamic instability rather than impaired gas exchange.

DRUG PRESCRIBING

One of the most fundamental skills of being a doctor is the prescribing of medicines. Drugs should be prescribed only when necessary and in all cases the expected benefit should be considered in relation to the risk of causing adverse effects. Pregnancy and breast-feeding pose additional risks as the potential danger to the fetus or baby, as well as the mother, must be considered.

Concordance with medication

Concordance with medication aims to ensure the most effective use of drugs. This is important as it is estimated that up to one-third of medicines prescribed for chronic conditions are not used as recommended. Traditional terms such as 'non-compliance' or 'non-adherence' are no longer used, as they imply a paternalistic approach to prescribing, with little engagement by the patient in the decision-making process. A concordant consultation, however, describes an integrated approach where the views of both patient and healthcare professional are considered in reaching a consensus about management.

Simplifying a drug regimen, such as the use of once-daily administration in preference to multiple daily doses, may also help to improve concordance. Combination products also reduce the number of drugs required to be taken and, in so doing, may improve concordance, at the expense, however, of the ability to titrate individual drug doses. Finally, the use of a multi-compartment medicines system (e.g. dosette box) may be helpful in improving compliance in specific patient groups such as the elderly population.

A discussion with the patient about prescription medication should include:

- What the medicine is and how and when to take it
- The expected benefits and goals of treatment
- Possible adverse effects and what to do if they occur
- How the effect of the medicine will be monitored
- Instructions for stopping or reducing the dose of the medicine if appropriate
- Choosing between medicines and also non-pharmacological alternatives.

Adverse drug reactions

Any drug or vaccine may produce unwanted or unexpected adverse reactions. Health professionals (doctors, dentists, coroners, pharmacists and nurses) and, in some countries, patients and carers are encouraged to report suspected adverse drug reactions (even if in doubt about causality) to the relevant regulatory agency. In the UK, the reporting of adverse drug reactions is performed via the Yellow Card Scheme to the Medicines and Healthcare products Regulatory Agency (MHRA). The reporting of adverse reactions associated with new drugs or vaccines, or with established drugs where the effect has not previously been observed, acts as an early warning system for the identification of unrecognized reactions. Some patient populations such as the elderly are more susceptible to adverse drug reactions and drug interactions for a number of reasons, such as the presence of comorbidities, use of polypharmacy and differing pharmacokinetics of drugs in this population. Impairment of renal and liver function may necessitate a reduction in drug dosage or contraindicate prescribing of some medicines.

Writing a prescription

The prescribing of medicines is a complex skill requiring motor, cognitive and communicative expertise. Prescribing errors are amongst the most common medical errors and are a frequent cause of morbidity or even mortality. It is therefore essential for all prescribing healthcare professionals to become proficient in this skill in an effort to reduce the frequency of medication errors and improve patient safety. All prescriptions should be written and dated legibly in black ink with the drug name written in full. Where non-proprietary ('generic') drugs are available they should generally be used in prescribing, other than specific exceptions where stated, e.g. modified release theophylline, to avoid variable drug pharmacokinetics. The prescription should include the full name of the prescriber (and address for outpatient prescriptions), and the name, address and date of birth of the patient. Inpatient prescription drug charts should also have the patient's hospital identification number and list of drug allergies. Each prescription should be signed and printed by the prescriber. Many hospitals and local authorities provide prescribing guidelines and policies (e.g. antibiotic guidelines) which should be referred to where appropriate.

Best practice for drug prescribing

- Define the patient's problem and specify the therapeutic objective.
- Write legibly in black ink.
- Clearly document patient identifiable information and drug allergies (including the nature of the allergies) on the prescription or drug chart.
- Each drug name should be written in full, including details of the dose, frequency, route of administration and the start date. Duration of treatment for drugs such as antibiotics should also be stated.
- For prescriptions based on body weight (e.g. mg/kg), the actual total dose should be specified.

- For drugs administered via the intravenous route, the name and volume of diluent should be stated.
- A maximum dose and frequency should be clearly defined for any drug prescribed on an 'as required' basis
- Abbreviations should be avoided: e.g. the word 'microgram' should be used instead of 'μg'; 'nanogram' should be used, not 'ng'; and 'units', not 'U' or 'u'.
- Decimal points should be avoided: e.g. use 125 micrograms not 0.125 mg.
- Alterations to existing prescriptions should be avoided, and if amendments are required, the prescription should be rewritten in full.

Specific drugs

Each chapter has listed some of the drugs commonly prescribed, particularly by junior doctors. The doses given are for adults. A full list of drug interactions and dosage adjustment in renal and liver failure is beyond the scope of this book and readers should refer to the *British National Formulary*. Similarly, reference should be made for guidance during pregnancy and breast-feeding.

DRUG POISONING

Self-poisoning is one of the most common acute medical admissions to hospital in the developed world. While hospital doctors may be most familiar with acute drug poisoning, poisoning may also occur from a variety of sources such as the environment (e.g. contaminated food or water, plants, bites and stings) or occupational exposure. Poisoning may be further classified as accidental (e.g. poisoning in children, dosage error by patient or doctor) or deliberate (e.g. attempted suicide or deliberate self-harm [DSH], suicide). Other means of DSH or suicide such as hanging, shooting or drowning are less common in the UK.

The most common drugs deliberately ingested by adults in the UK include paracetamol, non-steroidal anti-inflammatory drugs (NSAIDs), benzodiazepines and antidepressants. In many cases more than one substance is taken; alcohol is frequently a secondary poison. Carbon monoxide (CO) poisoning is an important cause of non-pharmaceutical poisoning in the developed world and may be either accidental (e.g. faulty appliances using natural gas) or deliberate (e.g. inhalation of vehicle exhaust fumes). In the developing world, ingestion of pesticides and herbicides is more common than therapeutic drugs like paracetamol, reflecting patterns of habitation, work and availability of potentially toxic chemicals.

The general approach to the poisoned patient

History

On arrival at hospital the patient must be assessed urgently (**A**irway, **B**reathing, **C**irculation) and Glasgow Coma Score recorded (p. 741). In conscious patients the diagnosis of self-poisoning can be made from the history. In an unconscious patient, it may be possible to gain a history from friends or relatives, or the diagnosis may be inferred from empty tablet bottles or a suicide note. In any patient with an altered conscious level, drug overdose should be considered in the differential diagnosis.

Some drugs are associated with specific clinical signs when taken in overdose, which may aid identification (Table 13.1).

Investigations

All patients should have their vital observations recorded and an admission blood sugar checked. A 12-lead electrocardiogram (ECG) is an important initial investigation in many patients, particularly in those who have ingested a drug associated with cardiotoxicity. Routine blood sampling (full blood count, renal and liver function, coagulation screen) is required in most patients. In some cases it is possible to measure drug concentration within the plasma, and a blood sample should be taken at an appropriate time post-drug overdose if one of the following drugs are likely to have been taken: aspirin, digoxin, ethylene glycol, iron, lithium, methanol, paracetamol or theophylline. The determination of the concentration of these drugs will be valuable in management. Drug screens of blood and urine are also occasionally helpful in the seriously ill unconscious patient in whom the cause of coma is unknown. Further investigations depend on the drugs ingested and knowledge of their likely impact on metabolic and cardiorespiratory function and the clinical assessment of the patient.

Management

All patients who present with self-poisoning require good supportive care. Specific additional therapy, however, is required following ingestion of some drugs. The online poisons information database, TOXBASE (http://www.toxbase.org), provides up-to-date information about the diagnosis, management and treatment of patients suffering from exposure to a wide range of substances and products. It should be the first point of reference in all cases of poisoning. The general management of a poisoned patient is summarized in Table 13.2.

Emergency resuscitation (ABCDE, p. 742)

- Clear the airway and intubate the patient if the gag reflex is absent and airway unprotected.
- Administer high flow oxygen.

Table 13.1 Some physical signs of poisoning

Features	Likely poisons
Constricted pupils	Opioids Organophosphorus insecticides Nerve agents
Dilated pupils	Tricyclic antidepressants Amfetamines Cocaine Antimuscarinic drugs
Divergent strabismus	Tricyclic antidepressants
Nystagmus	Phenytoin Carbamazepine
Loss of vision	Methanol Quinine
Papilloedema	Carbon monoxide Methanol
Convulsions	Tricyclic antidepressants Theophylline Opioids Mefanamic acid Isoniazid Amfetamines
Dystonic reactions	Metoclopramide Phenothiazines
Delirium and hallucinations	Antimuscarinic drugs Amfetamines Cannabis Recovery from tricyclic antidepressant overdose
Hypertonia and hyperreflexia	Tricyclic antidepressants Antimuscarinic drugs
Tinnitus and deafness	Salicylates Quinine
Hyperventilation	Salicylates Phenoxyacetate herbicides Theophylline
Hyperthermia	MDMA (Ecstasy)
Blisters	Usually occur in comatose patients
Lips and skin 'cherry red'	Carbon monoxide poisoning

MDMA, 3,4-methylenedioxymethamfetamine.

Table 13.2 Principles of management of patients with self-poisoning

1. Emergency resuscitation
2. Prevent further drug absorption, if appropriate
3. Increase drug elimination, if appropriate
4. Administration of specific drug antidotes, if appropriate
5. Psychiatric assessment

- Artificial ventilation is sometimes necessary if ventilation is inadequate (p. 584).
- Treat hypotension and convulsions. Anti-arrhythmics are generally not advised in poisoned patients, but the general principles of arrhythmia management should be followed (p. 421).
- Respiratory function (arterial blood gas analysis or pulse oximetry) and ECG monitoring are often required.
- Measure temperature and treat hypothermia (p. 660).

Prevention of further drug absorption

- *Gastric lavage* is no longer recommended for routine use in the management of poisoning due to the significant risk of complications such as pulmonary aspiration and oesophageal perforation. In very rare circumstances, it may be considered within 1 hour of ingestion of a significant quantity of a potentially fatal poison. The procedure involves administration of 200–300 mL of warm water or 0.9% saline repeatedly instilled and aspirated from the stomach via a large-bore orogastric tube with the patient in the left lateral decubitus position. It is contraindicated if the airway is not protected or following an overdose of corrosives, petrol or paraffin.
- *Activated charcoal* (50 g orally) adsorbs unabsorbed drugs still present in the gut and therefore potentially reduces toxicity associated with these agents. It may be considered if the patient presents to hospital within 1 hour of ingestion of a drug that is absorbed by charcoal.
- *Whole bowel irrigation* (WBI) may be considered in cases of significant ingestion of iron, lithium, sustained-release or enteric-coated drugs and ingested drug packets where there is risk of serious toxicity. Polyethylene glycol electrolyte solution, e.g. Klean-Prep, is infused via a nasogastric tube (1–2 L/h) until the rectal effluent is clear (usually 3–6 hours). WBI is contraindicated in patients with bowel obstruction, ileus, perforation or those with a compromised airway.

Increasing drug elimination

- *Multiple-dose activated charcoal* (50 g 4-hourly until charcoal appears in the faeces or recovery occurs) interrupts the enterohepatic or enteroenteric recirculation of drugs. It is only used in patients who have ingested a life-threatening amount of carbamazepine, phenobarbital, dapsone, quinine or theophylline.

- *Urinary alkalinization* increases the urine pH by administration of intravenous sodium bicarbonate. This enhances the elimination of salicylates and may be considered in cases of severe salicylate poisoning.
- *Haemodialysis* may be used to enhance drug elimination in severe poisoning with agents such as lithium, ethanol, methanol, ethylene glycol and salicylates (see below). Haemodialysis or hemofiltration may also be used to treat acute kidney injury and acidosis which may occur as a result of poisoning.

Antagonizing the effects of specific poisons Specific antidotes are available for a small number of drugs and are discussed under the individual drug sections below.

Psychiatric assessment All patients who present to hospital with DSH should be assessed from a psychiatric perspective prior to discharge. It is important to establish the reasons behind the overdose and the degree of ongoing suicidal intent (Table 13.3).

SPECIFIC DRUG PROBLEMS

In this section, only specific treatment regimens will be discussed. The general principles of management of self-poisoning should always be applied.

Aspirin

Aspirin (salicylate), in overdose, stimulates the respiratory centre, directly increasing the depth and rate of respiration and thereby leading to respiratory alkalosis. Compensatory mechanisms include renal excretion of bicarbonate and potassium, which results in a metabolic acidosis. With this mixed metabolic picture, patients often have a normal or high arterial pH, although a fall in arterial pH indicates serious poisoning. Salicylates also interfere with carbohydrate, fat and protein metabolism, as well as with oxidative phosphorylation, giving rise to an increased lactate, pyruvate and ketone bodies, all of which contribute to the acidosis.

Clinical features

Clinical features of aspirin poisoning include tinnitus, nausea, vomiting, hyperventilation, hyperpyrexia, sweating and tachycardia.

In severe poisoning (plasma salicylate concentration >700 mg/L; 5.07 mmol/L), there may be cerebral and pulmonary oedema resulting from increased capillary permeability. Coma and respiratory depression may also be seen.

Investigations

- Plasma salicylate concentration should be measured in all patients who present with salicylate poisoning. Peak concentrations are usually reached

Table 13.3 Guidelines for the assessment of patients who harm themselves

Questions to ask: be concerned if positive answer

- Was there a clear precipitant/cause for the attempt?
- Was the act premeditated or impulsive?
- Did the patient leave a suicide note?
- Did the patient make the attempt in strange surroundings?
- Would the patient do it again?

Other relevant factors

- Has the precipitant or crisis resolved?
- Is there continuing suicide intent?
- Does the patient have any psychiatric symptoms?
- What is the patient's social support system?
- Has the patient inflicted self-harm before?
- Has anyone in the patient's family ever taken their life?
- Does the patient have a physical illness?

Indications for referral to a psychiatrist

Absolute indications include:
- Clinical depression
- Psychotic illness of any kind
- Clearly pre-planned suicide attempt which was not intended to be discovered
- Persistent suicidal intent
- A violent method used

Other common indications include:
- Alcohol and drug abuse
- Patients over 45 years, especially if male, and young adolescents
- Those with a family history of suicide in first-degree relatives
- Those with serious physical disease
- Those living alone or otherwise unsupported
- Those in whom there is a major unresolved crisis
- Persistent suicide attempts
- Any patients who give you cause for concern

2–4 hours after ingestion but can be delayed up to 24 hours. It is important to repeat the salicylate level after 2–4 hours to detect rising concentrations and ensure the peak concentration has passed.

- Serum urea and electrolytes should be checked and blood glucose monitored (hypoglycaemia may occur).
- Prothrombin time should be measured as it may be prolonged.
- Arterial blood gas should be checked to monitor acid–base disturbance.

Management

- Activated charcoal should be administered if appropriate (p. 594).
- Treat dehydration with intravenous fluids.
- Hypokalaemia should be corrected urgently, particularly if urinary alkalinisation is being considered, as sodium bicarbonate will further reduce serum potassium.
- Urinary alkalinisation may be considered to enhance urinary excretion of salicylate if plasma salicylate >500 mg/L (>3.62 mmol/L). Infuse 8.4% sodium bicarbonate intravenously to maintain urinary pH 7.5–8.5.
- Haemodialysis is the treatment of choice in severe salicylate poisoning and should be carried out if the plasma salicylate concentration is >700 mg/L (5.07 mmol/L).

Paracetamol (acetaminophen)

Paracetamol overdose is the most common form of self-poisoning in the UK. In therapeutic use, up to 90% of paracetamol ingested undergoes glucuronide and sulphate conjugation before being excreted in the urine. A small fraction (5–10%) is catalysed by the cytochrome P450 system in the liver to form a toxic metabolite, N-acetyl-p-benzoquinoneimine (NAPQI). In normal circumstances, detoxification of NAPQI occurs through conjugation with reduced glutathione to form non-toxic conjugates that are then excreted in the urine. Following paracetamol overdose, stores of glutathione are depleted, allowing a build up of NAPQI, which binds covalently with sulphydryl groups on liver cell membranes leading to hepatic necrosis.

Clinical features

Clinical features of paracetamol poisoning are often non-specific and may include nausea, vomiting and abdominal pain. Conscious level is preserved unless another drug has been co-ingested. The predominant danger of a paracetamol overdose is liver failure, which usually only becomes apparent 72–96 hours after the initial ingestion. Acute kidney injury may also occur, with or without concomitant liver failure, and is usually apparent 3–5 days after ingestion.

Management

The antidote to paracetamol poisoning is intravenous N-acetylcysteine (NAC). This acts to replenish stores of glutathione, allowing detoxification of NAPQI and so preventing hepatotoxicity. The decision as to whether or not NAC should be administered depends on the quantity of paracetamol ingested, the time interval since ingestion, and whether the overdose was a single acute ingestion (all tablets ingested in a period of less than 1 hour), or staggered ingestion (tablets ingested over a period of greater than 1 hour). Following a single acute ingestion, the need for NAC is determined by plotting the measured paracetamol concentration against the time since ingestion on the treatment nomogram (Emergency Box 13.1 and Fig. 13.1). A variety of treatment nomograms exist and have been used in both the UK and abroad. For many years, the nomogram in the UK consisted of a treatment line joining 200 mg/L at 4 hours to 30 mg/L at 15 hours (the '200' nomogram line). A lower treatment line joining 100 mg/L at 4 hours to 30 mg/L at 15 hours (the '100' nomogram line) was used when the patient was felt to be at high risk of hepatotoxicity. In 2012, the UK adopted the single '100' nomogram line for all patients. This is a lower treatment threshold than other countries, such as Australia and North America, where a '150' nomogram line (joining 150 mg/L at 4 hours to 30 mg/L at 15 hours) is used.

In the case of a staggered overdose, interpretation of the paracetamol concentration using the nomogram is more challenging and other factors should be considered. If less than 75 mg/kg in any 24-hour period has been ingested, the toxicity is unlikely to occur and treatment with NAC is usually not required. However, serious toxicity may occur in patients who have ingested more than 150 mg/kg in any 24-hour period and treatment should be administered immediately. Rarely, toxicity may occur in some patients following ingestions of between 75 and 150 mg/kg in any 24-hour period. The decision to treat such patients is complex and requires consideration of the magnitude of exposure to

---

✚ Emergency Box 13.1

Management of single acute paracetamol ingestion

- Take blood for paracetamol levels (at or after 4 hours since ingestion), full blood count, INR, ALT activity, plasma creatinine and glucose.
- Consider administration of single-dose activated charcoal if the patient has presented within an hour of ingestion (p. 594).
- Administer intravenous NAC in 5% dextrose in all patients where the measured paracetamol concentration is plotted above the treatment line on the nomogram:
  - 150 mg/kg in 200 mL over 1 hour, then
  - 50 mg/kg in 500 mL over 4 hours, then
  - 100 mg/kg in 1 L over 16 hours.
- On completion of the NAC treatment, blood tests (ALT, INR, creatinine) should be repeated. If the patient is asymptomatic and the investigations are normal, no further treatment is required. Ongoing NAC therapy is indicated in patients who are symptomatic and/or where abnormalities in ALT and INR have been detected. There is no clinical advantage in treating isolated creatinine rises with NAC and this should be managed conservatively.

ALT, alanine transaminase; INR, international normalized ratio; NAC, N-acetylcysteine.

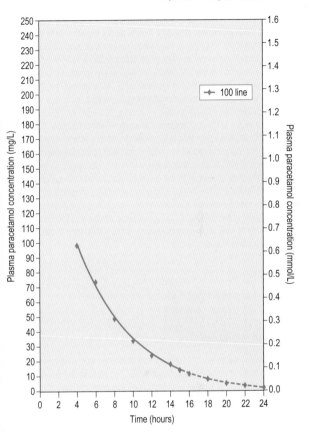

Fig. 13.1 Nomogram for treatment of paracetamol poisoning. In the UK, the single 100 nomogram treatment line is used. Note that the treatment lines are uncertain if the patient presents 15 hours or more after ingestion or has taken a modified-release preparation of paracetamol. Although these lines are often extended to 24 hours (dotted lines), the concentrations are not based on clinical trial data.

paracetamol, its duration, the reliability of the history and any other relevant factors. In cases of uncertainty, treatment with NAC should be commenced.

Adverse reactions associated with NAC are common and occur in up to 25% of patients. Clinical features may include nausea and vomiting and an anaphylactoid reaction, including urticarial rash, angio-oedema, bronchospasm and hypotension. Despite their clinical similarity to anaphylaxis, anaphylactoid reactions are not immunoglobulin E (IgE) mediated, although they are histamine mediated, and so previous exposure to NAC is not required for a reaction to occur. Additionally, if a patient has suffered a previous reaction to NAC, he/she may not suffer a further reaction on re-exposure to the antidote. Commonly, temporary cessation of the NAC infusion is all that is required. Occasionally, an antiemetic (e.g. cyclizine 50 mg intravenously), an antihistamine (e.g. chlorphenamine 10 mg intravenously) or a bronchodilator (e.g. nebulised salbutamol 2.5–5 mg) may be required.

On completion of the NAC treatment, the patient's liver function, coagulation screen and kidney function should be checked. Patients who develop liver damage with a raised international normalized ratio (INR) should remain in hospital on continuous NAC treatment until the values are returning to normal. Fresh frozen plasma or vitamin K is not normally administered to patients with a raised INR, as the trend in the INR is helpful in assessing prognosis and in determining the need for possible transplantation. The prothrombin time or the INR is the best guide to the severity of the liver damage. Advice should be sought from a specialist liver unit at an early stage as patients with severe hepatic damage may require liver transplantation.

Other drugs

Table 13.4 outlines the clinical features and management of other drugs that are commonly taken in cases of overdose.

Carbon monoxide

CO poisoning may be accidental or deliberate and is usually the result of inhalation of smoke from fires, car exhaust fumes, fumes from the use of charcoal fire grills in enclosed spaces (e.g. tents) or improperly installed domestic gas heating appliances. CO combines with haemoglobin to form carboxyhaemoglobin (COHb), thus preventing the formation of oxyhaemoglobin. Formation of COHb shifts the oxygen dissociation curve to the left, impairing liberation of oxygen to the cells. Clinical features are non-specific and include headache, mental impairment and, in severe cases, convulsions, coma and cardiac arrest. In spite of hypoxaemia, the skin is pink. A venous COHb level >3% in non-smokers and >5% in smokers confirms exposure to CO, but levels correlate poorly with symptoms. Treatment consists of removing the patient from the CO source and giving 100% oxygen via a face mask (do not use a rebreather reservoir).

RECREATIONAL DRUG USE

Drugs with a high abuse potential, drugs of addiction and other drugs with non-therapeutic psychotropic activity are categorised as controlled drugs. In the UK, The Misuse of Drugs Act categorises controlled drugs as class A, B and C and possession of a controlled drug is an offence. Class A drugs (Ecstasy, LSD,

Table 13.4 Clinical features and specific management for certain drugs taken in overdose

Drug	Clinical features	Management
TCAs	Tachycardia, hypotension, QRS prolongation on ECG, dilated pupils, convulsions, decreased conscious level, urinary retention	Intubate if airway unprotected. Treat convulsions with diazepam. Treat QRS prolongation with 8.4% sodium bicarbonate even in the absence of acidosis
Benzodiazepines	Drowsiness, ataxia, dysarthria, respiratory depression and coma. Potentiate the effects of other CNS depressants taken concomitantly	Supportive care includes intubation if necessary. Flumazenil (a benzodiazepine antagonist) may be considered in cases of isolated benzodiazepine overdose but is contraindicated in mixed ingestions where there is a risk of convulsions
NSAIDs	Often asymptomatic. Commonly transient acute kidney injury and GI irritation/haemorrhage. Rarely, convulsions, metabolic acidosis, coma	Treatment is symptomatic and supportive

CNS, central nervous system; ECG, electrocardiogram; GI, gastrointestinal; NSAIDs, non-steroidal anti-inflammatory drugs; TCAs, tricyclic antidepressants.

heroin, cocaine, crack, magic mushrooms and injected amfetamines) are those considered to be the most harmful. Three main categories of recreational drugs with specific patterns of acute toxicity can be described: stimulants, depressants and hallucinogens. While many drugs may have effects in more than one category, this distinction can be useful to predict clinical features and guide management of patients exposed to these agents.

Opioids

Opioid drugs, e.g. diamorphine (heroin), codeine and buprenorphine, are used clinically as analgesic agents for moderate to severe pain but are also frequently misused as recreational substances. They produce a well recognised toxidrome that includes depression of the respiratory and central nervous systems, constricted pupils and hypotension. Opioid drugs produce physical dependency such that an acute withdrawal syndrome (e.g. sweating, tachycardia, dilated pupils, vomiting) may develop if the drugs are stopped. Methadone, a longer-acting synthetic opiate, is used as a substitute for heroin in the treatment of heroin addiction. Drug users may inadvertently take an overdose if they consume their 'normal' dose after a period of abstinence (e.g. while in custody) or if they switch suppliers, where a more pure form may be provided. Additionally, recreational drugs are often adulterated ('cut') with other substances, which may make the clinical effects more unpredictable for the user.

The treatment of opioid toxicity is with intravenous naloxone (opiate antagonist) 0.4–2 mg, repeated at intervals of 2–3 minutes until the effect of the opioid ingested has been reversed. Naloxone has a short half-life compared to many opioid drugs and so repeated doses or a continuous infusion may be necessary, with the infusion rate titrated according to the clinical response. Intramuscular naloxone is given if intravenous access cannot be obtained. It is important to reconsider the diagnosis of opioid poisoning in patients who fail to respond to large doses of naloxone.

Cannabis

Cannabis (grass, pot, skunk, spliff, reefer) is a class B drug derived from the *Cannabis sativa* plant. This plant contains a number of chemicals known as cannabinoids, of which tetrahydrocannabinol (THC) is the predominant psychoactive toxin found in the leaves and flowering tops. Cannabis is usually smoked or ingested and rarely injected via the intravenous route. It is a mild hallucinogen and typical clinical features include initial excitement followed by calmness and euphoria. Adverse clinical features include nausea and vomiting, anxiety and paranoia. Withdrawal symptoms are uncommon. Long-term use has been associated with memory problems, apathy, manic-like psychoses and an increased risk of schizophrenia. Although cannabis use is very common, particularly among young people, cannabis itself is rarely the primary reason for hospital admission.

In recent years, use of synthetic alternatives to cannabis has increased. The synthetic cannabinoids include a large number of chemically diverse substances that act upon cannabinoid receptors with hallucinogenic and stimulant properties. Synthetic cannabinoids, however, are thought to be associated with more severe psychosis, agitation and stimulant (sympathomimetic) effects than traditional cannabis due to greater potency of cannabinoid receptors. These substances form one of the groups of recreational drugs now referred to as novel psychoactive substances (see below).

Cocaine

Cocaine (coke, charlie, bazooka, snow) is a stimulant recreational drug formerly used as a local anaesthetic. It is available either as cocaine hydrochloride, a water-soluble powder typically taken by nasal insufflation (snorting) but that may be absorbed via any mucosal surface or injected intravenously, or 'free-base' or 'crack' cocaine, where the hydrochloride moiety has been removed, leaving relatively pure cocaine crystals that are commonly smoked but also taken via other routes. Importantly, cocaine may be diluted ('cut') with a number of adulterants, including phenacetin, lidocaine, benzocaine and levamisole, which may pose an additional risk of toxicity. Cocaine toxicity produces stimulant (sympathomimetic) clinical features, including tachycardia, sweating, dilated pupils, euphoria and agitation. Cardiovascular toxicity (e.g. hypertension, acute coronary syndrome, arrhythmias, aortic or coronary dissection) and cerebrovascular toxicity (e.g. haemorrhagic stroke secondary to hypertension or ischaemia related to cerebral vasoconstriction) are important mechanisms of toxicity. Convulsions and hyperthermia may also occur in severe cases. Management of cocaine toxicity is supportive and directed by the clinical features. Intravenous benzodiazepines (e.g. diazepam) are first-line treatments for agitation, convulsions and hyperthermia. Active cooling measures (e.g. ice baths, cooled fluids) should also be instituted in patients with severe hyperthermia. Benzodiazepines, or intravenous glyceryl trinitrate, may also be considered for severe hypertension. β-adrenoceptor antagonists are contraindicated as they may lead to unopposed α-adrenoceptor agonism exacerbating hypertension. Arrhythmias and acute coronary syndromes in the context of cocaine use require specialist management and those with expertise in clinical toxicology and cardiology should be consulted.

Amfetamine-type stimulants

Amfetamine-type stimulants (ATS) are a group of substances that are similar in both pharmacological effect and chemical structure to amfetamine. These sympathomimetic drugs increase the release of, and decrease the reuptake of, sympathetic amines such as norepinephrine, serotonin and dopamine. They may be taken orally, by nasal insufflation or intravenous injection and cause a range of clinical effects, depending on the specific drug involved. Clinical features include central nervous system excitation (agitation, anxiety, hallucinations), sweating, dilated pupils, tachycardia and hypertension. More serious complications include hyperthermia, convulsions, arrhythmias, rhabdomyolysis and acute kidney injury. Management of patients with clinical features of toxicity is supportive. Patients should be managed in a quiet environment with minimal stimulation. Intravenous fluids should be administered and all patients require a 12-lead ECG and close observation of heart rate, blood pressure and temperature. Intravenous benzodiazepines (e.g. 10–20 mg diazepam) should be considered for patients with agitation, convulsions and hyperthermia. Active cooling measures (e.g. ice baths, cooled intravenous fluids) should be instituted in hyperthermic patients. Persistent hyperthermia requires discussion with a clinical toxicologist or poisons centre, as specialist treatment such as the use of a serotonin antagonist or dantrolene may be required.

Novel psychoactive substances

In recent years, many countries have experienced the rapid emergence of novel psychoactive substances (NPS), new synthetic recreational drugs designed to produce similar effects to controlled drugs. These substances, often referred to as 'legal highs', have been designed to evade drug legislation and are widely available via the Internet and retail outlets (e.g. 'head shops'), commonly branded as 'plant food', 'bath salts' or 'research chemicals' and labelled as 'not for human consumption'. Novel psychoactive substances include a wide variety of agents that can be classified according to psychotropic effects (e.g. stimulants, empathogens, hallucinogens) or chemical family (e.g. phenethylamines, amfetamines, cathinones, piperazines, tryptamines, synthetic cannabinoids). The presence of adulterants may further complicate the toxicity of these substances. Clinicians and drug users should also be aware that drugs sold under one name may on analysis contain a completely different drug, meaning that clinical features and toxicity may be unpredictable.

Body packers and stuffers

'Body packers' (also referred to as 'mules') are individuals who attempt to smuggle large amounts of well-packaged drugs internally, often heroin or cocaine, across international borders. 'Body stuffers' (also known as 'contact precipitated concealers') rapidly conceal substances internally, in poorly wrapped packages, to avoid detection by the police. Potential toxicity in these individuals is dependent upon the nature of the substance involved, the quantity, and how well wrapped the package is. Individuals may therefore present with features of toxicity following rupture of the package, gastrointestinal obstruction, perforation, or they may, in fact, be asymptomatic. All suspected body packers should undergo abdominal radiography. Unfortunately, false-negative abdominal radiographs do occur and in such cases an abdominal contrast-enhanced computed tomography (CT) scan should be performed where there is ongoing suspicion. Urine toxicological screening may also be helpful in guiding management. While a positive result cannot distinguish between perforation or previous deliberate use, an initial negative screen that subsequently becomes positive is indicative of package rupture. In the case of body stuffers, abdominal radiography is of little value in most cases and although CT may be considered, a false-negative result is possible. Urine toxicological screening should be used with caution, as most individuals will have positive results from previous use. Asymptomatic body packers and stuffers may be treated with WBI using an oral polyethylene glycol solution to speed passage of packets. Follow-up imaging should be performed to confirm clearance of packets. Packets in the vagina can be removed manually. Immediate surgery is indicated if there is evidence of intestinal obstruction, perforation or systemic toxicity, particularly if the drug involved is cocaine, for which there is no antidote.

Endocrine disease

The *endocrine* system refers to glands that release hormones (chemical messengers) directly into the bloodstream through which they travel to affect distant organs. Most hormones are secreted into the systemic circulation but hypothalamic releasing hormones are released into the pituitary portal system to reach the pituitary gland. *Exocrine* glands, in contrast, secrete their products into ducts to reach their target. The pancreas has both endocrine (glucagon, insulin and somatostatin secreted by α, β and δ cells, respectively, in the islets of Langerhans) and exocrine (digestive enzymes such as amylase secreted by acinar cells into the small intestine via the pancreatic duct) functions.

Most hormones travel in the circulation bound to proteins but it is only the free hormone that is biologically active. However, concentrations of binding proteins may be altered by disease, pregnancy or drugs and affect the amount of free hormone. Once at the target organ, hormones act by binding to specific receptors either on the target cell surface or within the cell (e.g. thyroid hormones, cortisol). The result is a cascade of intracellular reactions within the target cell which frequently amplifies the original stimulus and leads ultimately to a response by the target cell. Some hormones, e.g. growth hormone and thyroxine, act on most tissues of the body. Others act on only one tissue, e.g. thyroid-stimulating hormone (TSH) and adrenocorticotrophic hormone (ACTH), and are secreted by the anterior pituitary and have specific target tissues: namely, the thyroid gland and the adrenal cortex, respectively. Endocrine disease can involve all of the endocrine glands of the body, as illustrated in Fig. 14.1.

COMMON PRESENTING SYMPTOMS IN ENDOCRINE DISEASE

Hormones produce widespread effects upon the body and states of deficiency or excess typically present with symptoms that are generalized rather than focused on the anatomical location of the gland. Many of the presenting symptoms of endocrine disease are vague and non-specific, e.g. tiredness (which may be present in both hypo- and hyperthyroidism), weight loss or weight gain, increased thirst, anorexia and malaise, and the differential diagnosis is often wide. Precocious puberty or delayed puberty is often the result of a familial tendency, although hypothalamic–pituitary disease may present in this way, and endocrine investigations are usually undertaken.

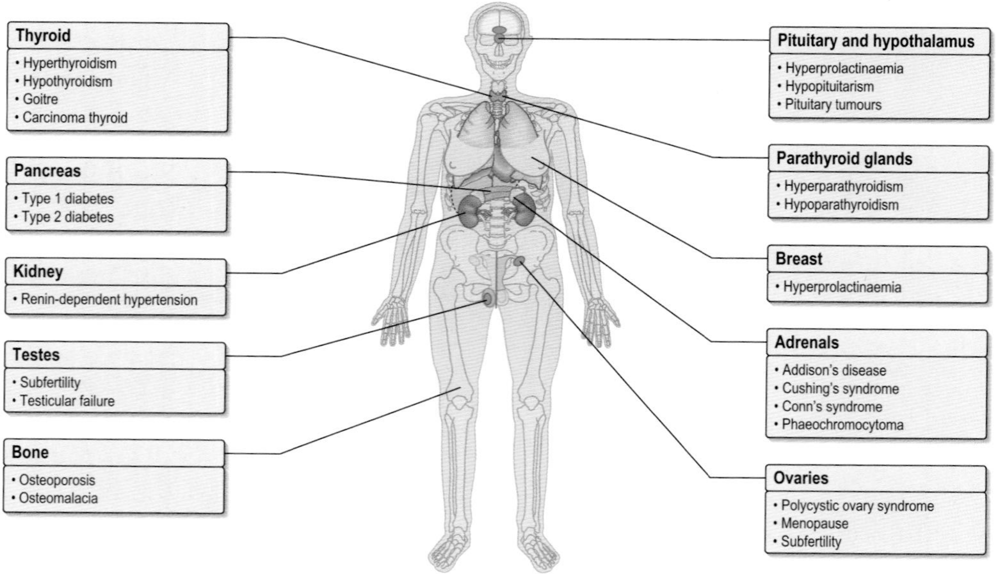

Fig. 14.1 The major endocrine organs and common endocrine problems

Pituitary and hypothalamus
• Hyperprolactinaemia
• Hypopituitarism
• Pituitary tumours

Parathyroid glands
• Hyperparathyroidism
• Hypoparathyroidism

Breast
• Hyperprolactinaemia

Adrenals
• Addison's disease
• Cushing's syndrome
• Conn's syndrome
• Phaeochromocytoma

Ovaries
• Polycystic ovary syndrome
• Menopause
• Subfertility

Thyroid
• Hyperthyroidism
• Hypothyroidism
• Goitre
• Carcinoma thyroid

Pancreas
• Type 1 diabetes
• Type 2 diabetes

Kidney
• Renin-dependent hypertension

Testes
• Subfertility
• Testicular failure

Bone
• Osteoporosis
• Osteomalacia

The hypothalamus and pituitary

The hypothalamus contains many vital centres for functions such as appetite, thirst, thermal regulation and sleep/waking. It also plays a role in circadian rhythm, the menstrual cycle, stress and mood. Releasing factors produced in the hypothalamus reach the pituitary via the portal system, which runs down the pituitary stalk. These releasing factors stimulate or inhibit the production of hormones from distinct cell types (e.g. production of growth hormone by acidophils), each of which secretes a specific hormone in response to unique hypothalamic stimulatory or inhibitory hormones. The anterior pituitary hormones, in turn, stimulate the peripheral glands and tissues. This pattern is illustrated in Fig. 14.2. The posterior pituitary acts as a storage organ for antidiuretic hormone (ADH, also called vasopressin) and oxytocin, which are synthesized in the supraoptic and paraventricular nuclei in the anterior hypothalamus and pass to the posterior pituitary along a single axon in the pituitary stalk. ADH is discussed on page 650; oxytocin produces milk ejection and uterine myometrial contractions.

Control and feedback

Most hormone systems are controlled by some form of feedback: an example is the hypothalamic–pituitary–thyroid axis (Fig. 14.3). Thyrotrophin-releasing hormone (TRH), secreted in the hypothalamus, stimulates TSH secretion from the anterior pituitary into the systemic circulation. TSH, in turn, stimulates the synthesis and release of thyroid hormones from the thyroid gland and the peripheral conversion of thyroxine (T_4) to triiodothyronine (T_3), the more active hormone. Circulating thyroid hormone feeds back on the pituitary, and possibly the hypothalamus, to suppress the production of TSH and TRH, and hence bring about a fall in thyroid hormone secretion. This is known as a 'negative feedback' system and represents the most common mechanism for regulation of circulating hormone levels. Conversely, a fall in thyroid hormone secretion (e.g. after thyroidectomy) leads to increased secretion of TSH and TRH. A patient with a hormone-producing tumour fails to show negative feedback and this is useful in diagnosis, e.g. the dexamethasone suppression test in the diagnosis of Cushing's syndrome (p. 642). In general, conditions associated with hormone excess are diagnosed by suppression tests, while conditions associated with hormone deficiency are diagnosed by stimulation tests (e.g. the short Synacthen test in Addison's disease).

Other factors influencing hormone secretion are circadian rhythms (e.g. cortisol levels are highest in the early morning), physiological stress/acute illness (producing rapid increases in cortisol, growth hormone, prolactin and adrenaline [epinephrine]) and feeding and fasting (insulin is increased and growth hormone decreased after ingestion of food).

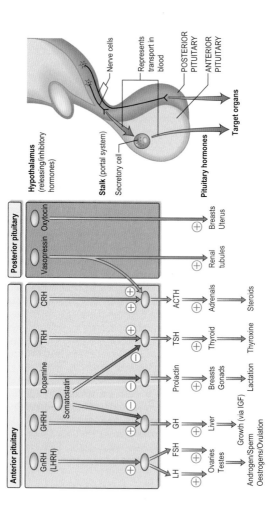

Fig. 14.2 Hypothalamic releasing hormones and the pituitary trophic hormones. ACTH, adrenocorticotrophic hormone; CRH, corticotrophin-releasing hormone; FSH, follicle-stimulating hormone; GH, growth hormone; GHRH, growth hormone releasing hormone; GnRH, gonadotrophin-releasing hormone; IGF, insulin-like growth factor; LH, luteinizing hormone; LHRH, luteinizing hormone releasing hormone; TRH, thyrotrophin-releasing hormone; TSH, thyroid-stimulating hormone.

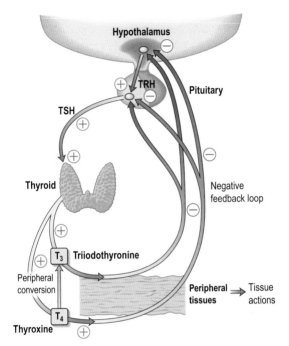

Fig. 14.3 The hypothalamic–pituitary–thyroid feedback system.
T_3, triiodothyronine; T_4, thyroxine; TRH, thyrotrophin-releasing hormone;
TSH, thyroid-stimulating hormone.

Pituitary space-occupying lesions and tumours

Benign pituitary tumours (adenomas) are the most common form of pituitary
disease. Symptoms arise as a result of inadequate hormone production, excess
hormone secretion, or from local effects of a tumour.

Underproduction

This is the result of disease at either a hypothalamic or a pituitary level, and it
results in the clinical features of hypopituitarism (p. 613).

Overproduction

There are three major conditions usually caused by secretion from pituitary
adenomas:

- Growth hormone (GH) excess – causing acromegaly in adults and
  gigantism in children

- Prolactin excess – causing galactorrhoea, amenorrhoea, erectile dysfunction or clinically silent
- Excess ACTH secretion – Cushing's disease.

Tumours producing luteinizing hormone (LH), follicle-stimulating hormone (FSH) or TSH are well described but are very rare.

Local effects

Local pressure on, or infiltration of, surrounding structures (Fig. 14.4):
- Optic chiasm, causing a bitemporal hemianopia
- Cavernous sinus, with III, IV and VI cranial nerve lesions
- Bony structures and the meninges, causing headache
- Hypothalamic centres: obesity, altered appetite and thirst, precocious puberty in children
- The ventricles, causing interruption of cerebrospinal fluid (CSF) flow and hydrocephalus.

Investigation

The purpose of investigation of a suspected pituitary mass is to confirm the diagnosis (usually by magnetic resonance imaging [MRI] of the pituitary), to determine if there is local pressure and infiltration (by clinical examination and plotting the visual fields using perimetry) and to assess for hormone

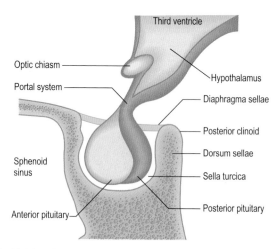

Fig. 14.4 A sagittal section of the pituitary fossa showing the anatomical relationships. The cavernous sinus lies lateral to the pituitary and is seen on a coronal view.

overproduction (discussed under the respective diseases) and/or underproduction (see hypopituitarism). Most mass lesions of the pituitary are adenomas. The history, physical examination and MRI help to exclude other rarer causes such as craniopharyngioma, secondary deposits, sarcoidosis, Wegener's granulomatosis and cystic lesions. Decisions about pituitary tumour management are made by a multidisciplinary team (including endocrinologist, pituitary surgeon and radiologist).

Hypopituitarism

Deficiency of hypothalamic-releasing hormones or pituitary hormones may be either selective or multiple. Multiple deficiencies usually result from tumour growth or other destructive lesions. There is a progressive loss of function, with GH and gonadotrophins (FSH and LH) being affected first and ACTH and TSH last. Rather than prolactin deficiency, hyperprolactinaemia occurs relatively early because of loss of tonic inhibitory control by dopamine (Fig. 14.2). Panhypopituitarism is a deficiency of all anterior pituitary hormones. ADH (vasopressin) and oxytocin secretion will only be affected if the hypothalamus is involved by either hypothalamic tumour or by extension of a pituitary lesion.

Aetiology

The most common cause of hypopituitarism is a pituitary or hypothalamic tumour, or treatment of the tumour by surgical removal or radiotherapy (Table 14.1).

Clinical features

These depend on the extent of hypothalamic–pituitary deficiencies. Gonadotrophin deficiency results in loss of libido, amenorrhoea (absent menstruation) and erectile dysfunction, whereas hyperprolactinaemia results in galactorrhoea (spontaneous flow of milk unassociated with childbirth or breast-feeding) and hypogonadism. Deficiency of GH produces short stature in children but in adults it is often clinically silent, although it may result in significant impairment in well-being and work capacity. Secondary hypothyroidism and adrenal failure lead to tiredness, slowness of thought and action, and mild hypotension. Long-standing hypopituitarism may give the classic picture of pallor with hairlessness (alabaster skin). Particular syndromes related to hypopituitarism are:

- *Congenital deficiency of gonadotrophin-releasing hormone (GnRH)* – Kallmann's syndrome, typically associated with anosmia.
- *Sheehan's syndrome* – pituitary infarction following severe post-partum haemorrhage. Rare in developed countries.
- *Pituitary apoplexy* – rapid enlargement of a pituitary tumour due to infarction or haemorrhage. There is severe headache and sudden severe

Table 14.1 Causes of hypopituitarism

Neoplastic	Traumatic
Primary tumour (pituitary or hypothalamus)	Skull fracture
Secondary deposits, especially breast	Surgery
Lymphoma	
	Infiltrations
Infective	Sarcoidosis
Basal meningitis, e.g. tuberculosis	Haemochromatosis
Encephalitis	
Syphilis	**Others**
	Radiation damage
Vascular	Chemotherapy
Pituitary apoplexy	Empty sella syndrome
Sheehan's syndrome	
Carotid artery aneurysms	**Functional**
	Anorexia
Immunological	Starvation
Pituitary antibodies	Emotional deprivation
Congenital	
Kallmann's syndrome	

visual loss, sometimes followed by acute life-threatening hypopituitarism. Ocular palsies, fever, neck stiffness or photophobia may also be seen. This is an endocrine emergency, the management of which is reviewed in Emergency Box 14.1.

- *'Empty sella' syndrome* – radiologically the sella turcica (the bony structure that surrounds the pituitary) appears devoid of pituitary tissue. In some cases, the pituitary is actually placed eccentrically and function is usually normal. In others there is pituitary atrophy (after injury, surgery or radiotherapy) and associated hypopituitarism.

Investigation

Each axis of the hypothalamic–pituitary system requires separate investigation. The presence of normal gonadal function (ovulatory menstruation or normal libido/erections) suggests that multiple defects of the anterior pituitary are unlikely. Tests range from measurement of basal hormone levels to stimulatory tests of the pituitary and tests of feedback for the hypothalamus (see under individual endocrine systems).

➕ Emergency Box 14.1

Management of pituitary apoplexy

Investigations

- Serum cortisol, IGF-1, GH, prolactin, TSH, T_4, LH, FSH, testosterone or oestradiol
- Full blood count, serum urea and electrolytes, liver function tests and clotting screen
- Bedside assessment of visual acuity and fields
- Urgent MRI to confirm diagnosis

Treatment

- Ensure haemodynamic stability with i.v. fluids
- Hydrocortisone 100 mg i.v. bolus followed by 2–4 mg/h by continuous i.v. infusion
- Liaise with regional endocrine and neurosurgical team
- Consider urgent surgery if severely reduced visual acuity/fields or deteriorating conscious level

FSH, follicle-stimulating hormone; GH, growth hormone; IGF-1, insulin-like growth factor 1; LH, luteinizing hormone; MRI, magnetic resonance imaging; T_4, thyroxine; TSH, thyroid-stimulating hormone.

Management

Steroid and thyroid hormones are essential for life and are given as oral replacement drugs (e.g. 15–25 mg hydrocortisone daily in divided doses, 100–150 µg levothyroxine daily) with the aim of restoring clinical and biochemical normality. Androgens and oestrogens are replaced for symptomatic control. If fertility is desired, LH and FSH analogues are used. GH therapy should be given to the growing child under appropriate specialist supervision and it may also produce benefits to the GH-deficient adult in terms of work capacity and psychological well-being. Two warnings are necessary:

- Thyroid replacement should not commence until normal glucocorticoid function has been demonstrated or replacement steroid therapy initiated, as an adrenal 'crisis' may otherwise be precipitated.
- Glucocorticoid deficiency masks impaired urine concentrating ability. Diabetes insipidus is apparent after steroid replacement, the steroids being necessary for excretion of a water load.

PITUITARY HYPERSECRETION SYNDROMES

Hyperprolactinaemia

Prolactin release is under tonic inhibition by dopamine from the hypothalamus and factors that increase prolactin secretion (e.g. TRH) are probably of less relevance (Fig. 14.2). There is a physiological increase in serum prolactin during pregnancy, lactation and severe stress.

Aetiology

The most common cause of pathological hyperprolactinaemia is a prolactin-secreting pituitary adenoma (prolactinoma). Other pituitary or hypothalamic tumours may also cause hyperprolactinaemia by compressing the pituitary stalk and interfering with dopamine inhibition of prolactin release ('disconnection'). Other causes are primary hypothyroidism (high TRH levels stimulate prolactin), drugs (metoclopramide, phenothiazines, oestrogens, cimetidine), polycystic ovary syndrome and acromegaly (co-secretion of prolactin with GH by the tumour). Mildly increased serum prolactin levels (400–600 mU/L) may be physiological and asymptomatic, but higher levels require investigation. Levels above 5000 mU/L always imply a prolactin-secreting pituitary tumour.

Clinical features

Hyperprolactinaemia stimulates milk production in the breast, producing galactorrhoea (spontaneous flow of milk unassociated with childbirth or breast-feeding), and inhibits GnRH, causing oligo- or amenorrhoea, decreased libido, subfertility and erectile dysfunction in men. If there is a pituitary tumour there may be headache and visual field defects.

Investigations

- Serum prolactin level. At least three measurements should be taken. Further tests are appropriate after physiological and drug causes have been excluded.
- Exclude macroprolactinaemia. Macroprolactin is a physiologically inactive higher-molecular-weight complex of prolactin bound to immunoglobulin G (IgG), which does not require treatment.
- Thyroid function tests, as hypothyroidism is a cause of hyperprolactinaemia.
- MRI of the pituitary. Tumours measuring more than 10 mm in diameter are termed macroprolactinomas while smaller tumours are microprolactinomas.
- Pituitary function and visual fields (clinical assessment and perimetry) should be checked if a prolactinoma is the cause.

Management

Causative drugs should be withdrawn if possible and hypothyroidism treated. Hyperprolactinaemia is controlled with a dopamine agonist such as cabergoline 500 μg once or twice a week judged on clinical response and prolactin levels. Bromocriptine has been longer established and is preferred if pregnancy is planned. Definitive therapy is controversial and depends on the size of the tumour, the patient's wish for fertility and the facilities available. Surgical removal of the tumour via a trans-sphenoidal approach (see acromegaly), combined with post-operative radiotherapy for large tumours, often restores normoprolactinaemia but there is a high rate of late recurrence (50% at 5 years). Small tumours (microadenomas) in asymptomatic patients may only need observation.

Acromegaly and gigantism

Pituitary GH is secreted in a pulsatile fashion under the control of two hypotha-lamic hormones: GH releasing hormone (GHRH) stimulates and somatostatin inhibits secretion. Ghrelin, which is synthesized in the stomach, also increases GH secretion. GH exerts its activity indirectly through the induction of insulin-like growth factor 1 (IGF-1), which is synthesized in the liver and other tissues, or directly on tissues such as liver, muscle, bone or fat to induce metabolic changes. Excessive GH production leads to gigantism in children (if acquired before fusion of the epiphyses of the long bones) and acromegaly in adults. Acromegaly is rare and caused by a benign pituitary GH-producing adenoma in almost all cases. Males and females are affected equally and the incidence is highest in middle age.

Clinical features

Symptoms and signs of acromegaly are shown in Fig. 14.5. The clinical man-ifestations of acromegaly can be divided into those due to local tumour expan-sion with compression of surrounding structures – headaches, visual field loss and hypopituitarism – and those due to the metabolic effects of excess GH secretion, such as sweating and soft tissue swelling. The onset is insidious, with many years between onset of symptoms and diagnosis. Inadequately trea-ted acromegaly is associated with an increased mortality rate, particularly from cardiovascular disease and cancer.

Investigations

- Plasma GH levels may exclude acromegaly if undetectable, but a detectable value is non-diagnostic.
- Serum IGF-1 levels are almost always raised in acromegaly, and fluctuate less than those of GH. A normal serum IGF-1 concentration is strong evidence that the patient does not have acromegaly.
- Glucose tolerance test is diagnostic. In a positive test there is failure of the normal suppression of serum GH below 1 mU/L.
- MRI scan of the pituitary will almost always reveal the adenoma.
- Visual field defects are common and should be plotted by perimetry.
- Pituitary function testing usually shows partial or complete hypopituitarism (p. 613).
- Serum prolactin (see hyperprolactinaemia).

Symptoms		Signs
Head and neck Change in facial appearance Headaches Visual deterioration Deep voice Goitre		**Facial** Prominent supraorbital ridge **Prognathism** **Interdental separation** **Large tongue** Visual field defects
General Tiredness Weight gain Breathlessness Excessive sweating Muscular weakness Joint pain		**General** Hirsutism Thick, greasy skin **Hands** **Spade-like hands and feet** Tight rings on fingers Carpal tunnel syndrome
Hormonal Amenorrhoea or Oligomenorrhoea in women Galactorrhoea Impotence or poor libido Increased glove or hat size		**Other** Galactorrhoea Hypertension Heart failure Oedema Arthropathy Proximal myopathy Glycosuria (plus possible signs of hypopituitarism)

Fig. 14.5 The symptoms and signs of acromegaly. Bold type indicates signs of greater discriminant value.

Management

The aim of therapy is to reduce the serum IGF-1 concentration to within the age-adjusted reference range and lower the mean GH level to below 5 mU/L (<2.5 ng/L); this has been shown to reduce mortality to normal levels. Complete cure is often slow to achieve. Hypopituitarism should be corrected and diabetes and/or hypertension treated conventionally.

Transsphenoidal surgical resection is the treatment of choice. Complications are hypopituitarism, diabetes insipidus, CSF rhinorrhoea and infection.

Medical therapy is normally used when surgery alone has failed to reduce GH and IGF-1 levels to normal. Somatostatin analogues (octreotide and lanreotide) and dopamine agonists (bromocriptine or cabergoline) inhibit GH secretion. The latter do not work as well as the somatostatin analogues, but are given orally rather than by subcutaneous or intramuscular injection.

Pegvisomant, a GH-receptor antagonist, is reserved for treatment of patients in whom IGF-1 levels cannot be reduced to safe levels with somatostatin analogues alone.

External radiotherapy is used after surgical excision is incomplete and in combination with medical treatment as the response is slow (10 years or more).

Cushing's disease

'Cushing's syndrome' is the term used to describe the clinical state of increased free circulating glucocorticoids, and it is covered on p. 642. The most common cause of Cushing's syndrome is therapeutic administration of synthetic steroids ('iatrogenic'). Spontaneous Cushing's syndrome is rare. Causes can be divided into ACTH dependent (either a pituitary adenoma – Cushing's disease – or an 'ectopic' ACTH-producing tumour elsewhere in the body) or ACTH independent, with primary excess of endogenous cortisol secretion from an adrenal tumour. Pituitary tumours account for 65% of cases of spontaneous Cushing's syndrome.

Hypersecretion of other hormones

Pituitary tumours may rarely secrete TSH or gonadotrophins.

THE THYROID AXIS

Thyroid hormones control the metabolic rate of many tissues. Disruptions of thyroid activity represent the most common endocrine problems seen in clinical practice. The thyroid gland secretes predominantly T_4 and only a small amount of the biologically active hormone T_3. Most circulating T_3 is produced by peripheral conversion of T_4. Iodine is an essential requirement for thyroid hormone synthesis. Over 99% of T_4 and T_3 circulate bound to plasma proteins, mainly thyroxine-binding globulin (TBG) but only the free hormone is available for tissue action. The feedback pathway that controls the secretion of TSH is discussed on page 609. Thyroid function is assessed by measurement of:

* Serum TSH concentration
* Serum free T_4 (or T_3) concentration.

Drugs and illness can alter the concentrations of binding proteins or interaction of the binding hormones with T_4 and T_3. Thus free and total hormone concentrations may not be concordant. For instance, oestrogens (e.g. in pregnancy and in women taking the oral contraceptive pill) increase concentrations of TBG and hence total T_4, but the physiologically important free T_4 concentrations are normal.

Table 14.2 Characteristics of thyroid function tests in thyroid disease

	TSH (0.3–3.5 mU/L)	Free T₄ (10–25 pmol/L)	Free T₃ (3.5–7.5 pmol/L)
Thyrotoxicosis	$\downarrow$ (<0.05 mU/L)	$\uparrow$	$\uparrow$
Primary hypothyroidism	$\uparrow$ (>10 mU/L)	$\downarrow$ or low-normal	$\downarrow$ or normal
TSH deficiency	$\downarrow$ or low-normal	$\downarrow$ or low-normal	$\downarrow$ or normal
T₃ toxicosis	$\downarrow$ (<0.05 mU/L)	Normal	$\uparrow$
Borderline hypothyroidism	Slightly $\uparrow$ (5–10 mU/L)	Normal	Normal

$\uparrow$, increased; $\downarrow$, suppressed; T_3, triiodothyronine; T_4, thyroxine; TSH, thyroid-stimulating hormone.

Assessment of thyroid function tests

Measurement of thyroid function is indicated in patients falling into the following categories:

- Symptoms or signs suggestive of hypo- or hyperthyroidism (Table 14.2). Thyroid function should not be assessed in patients who have coexisting acute illness such as pneumonia (unless thyroid disease is strongly suspected), since changes in binding proteins, serum thyroid hormones (low total and free T_4 and T_3) and TSH (normal) occur in severe non-thyroidal illness (the 'sick euthyroid syndrome'). Most will be euthyroid on re-testing after recovery from the acute illness.
- Receiving treatment for hypo- or hyperthyroidism.
- Treatment with drugs causing thyroid disorders, e.g. amiodarone.
- Post-irradiation – radioactive iodine therapy or external neck irradiation.
- Post-surgery – subtotal thyroidectomy.

Hypothyroidism

Underactivity of the thyroid gland may be primary, from disease of the thyroid gland, or much less commonly, secondary to hypothalamic or pituitary disease (secondary hypothyroidism).

Aetiology

Hypothyroidism affects 0.1–2% of the population. It is much more common in women, and the incidence increases with age. The most common cause of primary thyroid failure in iodine-replete areas of the world is autoimmune thyroiditis.

Autoimmune thyroiditis may be associated with a goitre (Hashimoto's thyroiditis) or thyroid atrophy. There is cell- and antibody-mediated destruction of thyroid tissue. Almost all patients have serum antibodies to thyroglobulin, thyroid peroxidase enzyme (thyroid microsomal antibodies) and antibodies that block the binding of TSH to its receptor. It is associated with other autoimmune conditions, such as pernicious anaemia and Addison's disease.

Post-partum thyroiditis is normally transient and can cause hypo- and hyperthyroidism, or both, sequentially. If conventional antibodies are present, there is a high chance of proceeding to permanent hypothyroidism.

Iatrogenic Thyroidectomy (for treatment of hyperthyroidism or goitre), radioactive iodine treatment or external neck irradiation for head and neck cancer all cause hypothyroidism.

Drug induced as a result of carbimazole, lithium, amiodarone and interferon.

Iodine deficiency still exists in some areas, particularly mountainous areas (Alps, Himalayas, South America). Goitre, occasionally massive, is common. Iodine excess can also cause hypothyroidism in patients with pre-existing thyroid disease.

Congenital hypothyroidism is related to thyroid aplasia or dysplasia or defective synthesis of thyroid hormones.

Clinical features

Symptoms and signs of hypothyroidism are illustrated in Fig. 14.6. The term 'myxoedema' refers to the accumulation of mucopolysaccharide in subcutaneous tissues. Features are often difficult to distinguish in elderly people and young women. Hypothyroidism should be excluded in all patients with oligomenorrhoea/amenorrhoea, menorrhagia, infertility and hyperprolactinaemia. Many cases are detected on routine biochemical screening.

Investigations

Measurement of serum TSH is the investigation of choice. A high TSH with a compatible clinical picture confirms primary hypothyroidism:

- Serum free T_4 levels are low.
- Thyroid antibodies and other organ-specific antibodies may be present in the serum.
- Other features include anaemia (normocytic or macrocytic), hyperlipidaemia, hyponatraemia (due to increased ADH and impaired clearance of free water) and increased serum creatine kinase levels with associated myopathy.

Management

Treatment is with lifelong levothyroxine at a daily dose of 1.6 µg/kg body weight (100–150 µg for an average-sized adult, p. 662). The adequacy of replacement is assessed clinically and by thyroid function tests after at least 6 weeks on a

Symptoms	Signs
General	**Mental slowness**
Tiredness/malaise	Psychosis/dementia
Weight gain	Ataxia
Cold intolerance	Poverty of movement
Change in appearance	Deafness
Goitre	'Peaches and cream' complexion
Depression	
Psychosis	**Dry thin hair**
Coma	Loss of eyebrows
Poor memory	Hypertension
	Hypothermia
Hair – dry, brittle, unmanageable	Heart failure
Skin – dry, coarse	**Bradycardia**
	Pericardial effusion
Arthralgia	Cold peripheries
Myalgia	Carpal tunnel syndrome
Muscle weakness/ stiffness	Oedema
Poor libido	Periorbital oedema
Puffy eyes	Deep voice
Deafness	(Goitre)
Constipation	
Anorexia	**Dry skin**
	Mild obesity
	Myotonia
	Muscular hypertrophy
	Proximal myopathy
	Slow-relaxing reflexes
	Anaemia

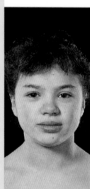

Fig. 14.6 Hypothyroidism – symptoms and signs. Bold type indicates signs of greater discriminant value. *(A history from a relative is often revealing. Symptoms of other autoimmune disease may be present.)*

steady dose. The aim of treatment is normalization of serum TSH concentrations. Annual measurement of TSH is sufficient for patients on a stable dose unless there is a change in situation, e.g. large changes in body weight or pregnancy. In older patients (>60 years) and patients with ischaemic heart disease the starting dose is 25 μg/day and then increased incrementally every 3–6 weeks until euthyroidism is achieved.

Borderline or subclinical hypothyroidism (compensated euthyroidism)

This is a slightly increased serum TSH and normal free T₄ concentration (Table 14.2). Most cases are due to early-phase chronic autoimmune thyroiditis and about 2–4% will develop overt hypothyroidism each year. The benefits of treatment, or otherwise, are controversial. Treatment with levothyroxine is normally recommended where the TSH is consistently (i.e. 3 months after the initial test) above 10 mU/L, when there are high-titre thyroid antibodies or lipid abnormalities, when pregnancy is being planned or when there are symptoms suggestive of hypothyroidism. In untreated patients, serum TSH concentrations are measured yearly to look for progression to overt hypothyroidism.

Myxoedema coma

Severe hypothyroidism may rarely present with confusion and coma, particularly in elderly people. Typical features include hypothermia (p. 660), cardiac failure, hypoventilation, hypoglycaemia and hyponatraemia. The optimal treatment is controversial and data are lacking, but a summary is given in Emergency Box 14.2. Treatment is begun on the basis of clinical suspicion, without waiting for the results of laboratory tests. Clues to the possible presence of myxoedema coma include a previous history of thyroid disease and a history from family members suggesting antecedent symptoms of thyroid dysfunction.

Myxoedema madness

Depression is common but, occasionally, with severe hypothyroidism in elderly people, the patient may become frankly demented or psychotic, sometimes with striking delusions. This may occur shortly after starting thyroxine replacement.

✚ Emergency Box 14.2

Management of myxoedema coma

Investigations

- Serum TSH, T_4 and cortisol before thyroid hormone is given
- Full blood count, serum urea and electrolytes, blood glucose and blood cultures
- ECG monitoring for cardiac arrhythmias

Treatment

- T_3 orally or intravenously 2.5–5 µg every 8 hours
- Oxygen (by mechanical ventilation if necessary)
- Gradual rewarming (Emergency Box 14.5)
- Hydrocortisone 100 mg i.v. 8-hourly (in case hypothyroidism is a manifestation of hypopituitarism)
- Glucose infusion to prevent hypoglycaemia
- Supportive management of the comatose patient

ECG, electrocardiogram; T_4, thyroxine; TSH, thyroid-stimulating hormone.

Hyperthyroidism

Hyperthyroidism (thyroid overactivity, thyrotoxicosis) is common, affecting 2–5% of all women at some time, mainly between the ages of 20 and 40 years. Three intrinsic thyroid disorders account for the majority of cases of hyperthyroidism: Graves' disease, toxic adenoma and toxic multinodular goitre. Rarer causes include viral thyroiditis (de Quervain's), thyroiditis factitia (surreptitious T_4 consumption), drugs (amiodarone), metastatic differentiated thyroid carcinoma and TSH-secreting tumours (e.g. of the pituitary).

Graves' disease is the most common cause of hyperthyroidism and is the result of IgG antibodies binding to the TSH receptor and stimulating thyroid hormone production. It is associated with characteristic clinical features (see below) and other autoimmune diseases, such as pernicious anaemia and myasthenia gravis.

Toxic multinodular goitre It commonly occurs in older women, and drug therapy is rarely successful in inducing a prolonged remission.

Solitary toxic nodule/adenoma is responsible for about 5% of cases of hyperthyroidism. Prolonged remission is again rarely induced by drug therapy.

de Quervain's thyroiditis Transient hyperthyroidism sometimes results from acute inflammation of the gland, probably as a result of viral infection. It is usually accompanied by fever, malaise and pain in the neck. Treatment is with aspirin, reserving prednisolone for severely symptomatic cases.

Post-partum thyroiditis (p. 621).

Clinical features

Typical symptoms and signs are shown in Fig. 14.7. Clinical features vary with age and the underlying aetiology. Ophthalmopathy (p. 627), pretibial myxoedema (raised, purple-red symmetrical skin lesions over anterolateral aspects of the shins) and thyroid acropachy (clubbing, swollen fingers and periosteal new bone formation) occur only in Graves' disease. Elderly patients may present with atrial fibrillation and/or heart failure, or with a clinical picture resembling hypothyroidism ('apathetic thyrotoxicosis').

Investigations

- Serum TSH is suppressed (<0.05 mU/L).
- Serum free T_4 and T_3 are elevated. Occasionally T_3 alone is elevated (T_3 toxicosis).
- TSH receptor antibodies are highly sensitive and specific for Graves' disease, although they not measured routinely in all centres.
- Thyroid ultrasound or scintigraphy can help differentiate Graves' disease from a toxic adenoma or multinodular goitre.

Symptoms

General
Weight loss
Irritability/behaviour change
Restlessness
Malaise
Itching
Sweating
Tall stature (in children)
Breathlessness
Palpitations
Heat intolerance
Stiffness
Muscle weakness

Tremor
Choreoathetosis

Thirst
Vomiting
Diarrhoea

Eye complaints*
Oligomenorrhoea
Loss of libido
Gynaecomastia
Onycholysis
Goitre

*only in Graves' disease

Tremor
Hyperkinesis
Psychosis

Tachycardia or atrial
fibrillation
Full pulse
Warm vasodilated
peripheries
Systolic hypertension
Cardiac failure

Exophthalmos*
Lid lag and 'stare'
Conjunctival oedema
Ophthalmoplegia*
Periorbital oedema
Goitre, bruit
Weight loss

Tremor
Proximal myopathy
Proximal muscle wasting
Onycholysis
Palmar erythema

Graves' dermopathy*
Thyroid acropachy
Pretibial myxoedema

*Only in Graves' disease

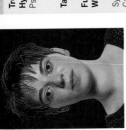
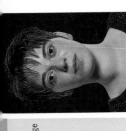

Fig. 14.7 Hyperthyroidism – symptoms and signs. Bold type indicates signs of greater discriminatory value. Additional features are hypercalcaemia and osteoporosis.

Management

Three approaches are used to decrease thyroid hormone synthesis: drugs, radioiodine ablation and surgery. Radioiodine is the first-line treatment of choice in the USA while medical treatment is first-line in the UK.

Antithyroid drugs Carbimazole (20–40 mg daily, p. 663) is most often used in the UK and its metabolite, thiamazole (methimazole), is used in the USA. They block thyroid hormone biosynthesis and also have immunosuppressive effects which will affect the Graves' disease process. As clinical benefit is not apparent for 10–20 days, β-blockers (usually propranolol) are used to provide rapid symptomatic control because many manifestations are mediated via the sympathetic system. After 4–6 weeks at full dose, carbimazole is gradually reduced over 6–24 months to 5 mg daily and discontinued when the patient is euthyroid. The aim of treatment during this time is to maintain normal free T_4 and TSH levels. At least 50% of patients with Graves' disease relapse on discontinuation of drug treatment, mostly within the following 2 years, and then need further treatment (long-term antithyroid drugs, radioactive iodine or surgery). The most severe side effect of carbimazole is agranulocytosis. All patients starting treatment must be warned to stop carbimazole and seek an urgent blood count if they develop a sore throat or unexplained fever. If toxicity occurs, propylthiouracil is used instead.

Radioactive iodine (oral sodium ^{131}I) is widely used for the treatment of hyperthyroidism but is contraindicated in pregnancy and while breast-feeding. It accumulates in the gland and results in local irradiation and tissue damage with return to normal thyroid function over 4–12 weeks. If hyperthyroidism persists, a further dose of ^{131}I can be given, although this increases the rate of subsequent hypothyroidism.

Surgery Subtotal thyroidectomy should only be performed in patients who have been rendered euthyroid. Antithyroid drugs are stopped 10–14 days before the operation and replaced with oral potassium iodide, which inhibits thyroid hormone release and reduces the vascularity of the gland. Complications of surgery include bleeding, hypocalcaemia, hypothyroidism, hypoparathyroidism, recurrent laryngeal nerve palsy and recurrent hyperthyroidism.

The choice of therapy for hyperthyroidism depends on patient preference and local expertise. Surgery is particularly indicated in patients who have a large goitre, in patients who have drug side effects or poor compliance with drug therapy but do not want radioiodine, or if there is a suspicion of malignancy in a nodule. Lifelong annual measurement of TSH to look for hypothyroidism is indicated after surgery or radioiodine treatment.

Thyroid crisis or 'thyroid storm'

This is a rare life-threatening condition in which there is a rapid deterioration of thyrotoxicosis with hyperpyrexia, tachycardia, extreme restlessness and eventually delirium, coma and death. It is usually precipitated by infection, stress and surgery or radioactive iodine therapy in an unprepared patient. With careful management it should no longer occur and most cases referred to as 'crisis' are simply severe but uncomplicated thyrotoxicosis. Treatment of thyroid storm is with large doses of carbimazole (20 mg 8-hourly orally), propranolol (80 mg 12-hourly orally), potassium iodide (15 mg 6-hourly orally, to block acutely the release of thyroid hormone from the gland) and hydrocortisone (100 mg i.v. 6-hourly, to inhibit peripheral conversion of T_4 to T_3).

Graves' orbitopathy (ophthalmopathy)

Lid retraction (white of sclera visible above the cornea as the patient looks forwards) and lid lag (delay in moving the upper eyelid as the eye moves downwards) are a result of increased catecholamine sensitivity of the levator palpebrae superioris and occur in any form of hyperthyroidism. Exophthalmos (proptosis, protruding eyeballs) and ophthalmoplegia (limitation of eye movements) only occur in patients with ophthalmic Graves' disease (or Graves' orbitopathy).

Aetiology

T lymphocytes react with one or more antigens (likely to be the TSH receptor) shared by the thyroid and orbit and trigger a cascade of events leading to retro-orbital inflammation. There is swelling and oedema of the extraocular muscles, leading to limitation of movement and proptosis. Ultimately, increased pressure on the optic nerve may cause optic atrophy. Ophthalmopathy is more common and more severe in smokers.

Clinical features

Eye involvement is usually bilateral. Symptoms are pressure or pain in the eye, a gritty sensation, decreased vision and photophobia. Exophthalmos and ophthalmoplegia are direct effects of retro-orbital inflammation, whereas conjunctival oedema (chemosis), lid lag and corneal scarring are secondary to the proptosis and lack of eye cover (Fig. 14.8). Eye manifestations do not parallel the clinical course of Graves' disease and may appear before or after the onset of hyperthyroidism.

Investigations

The diagnosis is usually made clinically by finding typical clinical features on a background of Graves' disease. MRI of the orbits will exclude other causes of proptosis, e.g. retro-orbital tumour, and show enlarged muscles and oedema. Visual acuity and visual fields should be formally assessed in all patients. TSH receptor antibodies are almost invariably positive.

Management

Thyroid dysfunction should be corrected and hypothyroidism avoided because this may exacerbate the eye problem. Smoking should be stopped. Specific

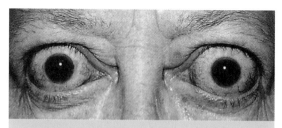

Grade 0	N: No signs or symptoms
Grade 1	O: Only signs, no symptoms
Grade 2	S: Soft tissue involvement
Grade 3	P: Proptosis (measured with exophthalmometer)
Grade 4	E: Extraocular muscle involvement
Grade 5	C: Corneal involvement
Grade 6	S: Sight loss with optic nerve involvement

Fig. 14.8 The 'NOSPECS' system of grading severity of eye involvement in Graves' orbitopathy.

treatment includes artificial tears and selenium supplements. For severe symptoms, high-dose systemic steroids (e.g. prednisolone 60 mg daily) reduce inflammation. It may be necessary to surgically decompress the orbit (particularly if sight is threatened), to perform corrective eye muscle surgery to improve diplopia or to perform corrective eyelid surgery. Occasionally, irradiation of the orbits is required.

Goitre (thyroid enlargement)

Goitre is more common in women than in men and may be physiological or pathological in origin (Table 14.3). The presence of a goitre gives no indication about the thyroid status of the patient.

Clinical features

A goitre is usually noticed as a cosmetic defect, although discomfort and pain in the neck can occur, and occasionally tracheal or oesophageal compression produces difficulty in breathing or dysphagia. The gland may be diffusely enlarged, multinodular or possess a solitary nodule. A bruit may be present in Graves' disease. Associated lymphadenopathy suggests that the goitre may be malignant.

Investigations

The purpose of assessing a goitre is to determine the patient's thyroid status, the pathological nature of the goitre and whether it is causing compressive or cosmetic problems:

Table 14.3 Goitre – causes and types

Diffuse

Physiological*: puberty, pregnancy
Autoimmune: Graves' disease, Hashimoto's disease
Acute viral thyroiditis (de Quervain's thyroiditis)*
Iodine deficiency (endemic goitre)
Dyshormonogenesis
Goitrogens, e.g. sulphonylureas

Nodular

Multinodular goitre
Solitary nodule
Fibrotic (Riedel's thyroiditis)
Cysts

Tumours

Adenoma
Carcinoma
Lymphoma

Miscellaneous

Sarcoidosis
Tuberculosis

Goitre usually resolves spontaneously.

- *Blood tests:* thyroid function tests (Table 14.2) and thyroid antibodies.
- *Imaging:* high-resolution thyroid ultrasound can delineate nodules and determine whether they are cystic or solid. Both types of nodule are usually benign, but can be malignant, and thus require fine-needle aspiration (FNA) under ultrasound control. Chest and thoracic inlet X-rays, to detect tracheal compression and large retrosternal extensions, are performed in patients with very large goitre or clinical symptoms (difficulty in breathing).
- *FNA* for cytology should be considered for solitary nodules or a dominant nodule in a multinodular goitre because there is a 5% chance of malignancy.
- *Thyroid scan* (radioiodine or technetium) distinguishes between a functioning (rarely malignant) or non-functioning (10% malignant) nodule. However, FNA has largely replaced isotope scans.

Management

Treatment is usually not required, apart from inducing euthyroidism if necessary. Surgical intervention is required for the cosmetic effects of large

Table 14.4 Characteristics of thyroid cancer

Cell type	Behaviour	Spread	Prognosis
Papillary (70%)	Young people	Local	Good
Follicular (20%)	Middle age	Lung/bone	Usually good
Anaplastic (<5%)	Aggressive	Local	Very poor
Lymphoma (2%)	Variable		Usually poor
Medullary cell (5%)	Often familial	Local and metastases	Poor

Frequency of tumour type is given as a percentage in brackets. Medullary cell carcinoma (see multiple endocrine neoplasia, p. 649).

goitres, pressure effects on the trachea or oesophagus, or confirmed (positive FNA) or possible malignancy (negative FNA but rapid growth, cervical lymphadenopathy).

Thyroid malignancy

Thyroid cancer is uncommon and most present as asymptomatic thyroid nodules. The first sign of disease is occasionally lymph node metastases or, in rare cases, lung or bone metastases. Features that suggest carcinoma in a patient presenting with a thyroid nodule are a history of progressive increase in size, a hard and irregular nodule and the presence of enlarged lymph nodes on examination. Characteristics are listed in Table 14.4. FNA cytology is the best test for distinguishing between benign and malignant thyroid nodules. Treatment of follicular and papillary cancers is total thyroidectomy with neck dissection for local nodal spread. Ablative radioiodine is subsequently given, which will be taken up by remaining thyroid tissue or metastatic lesions. External radiotherapy may produce brief respite for anaplastic carcinoma and lymphoma, but otherwise treatment is largely palliative.

MALE REPRODUCTION AND SEX

GnRH, also called luteinizing hormone-releasing hormone (LHRH), is released episodically from the hypothalamus (during and after puberty) and stimulates LH and FSH secretion from the anterior pituitary gland. LH stimulates testosterone production from Leydig cells of the testis. Testosterone circulates, bound to sex hormone-binding globulin, and acts via nuclear androgen receptors to produce male secondary sex characteristics (growth of pubic, axillary and facial hair; enlargement of the external genitalia; deepening of the voice; muscle growth; and frontal balding) and maintenance of libido. FSH stimulates the testes to produce mature sperm and the inhibins A and B; the latter feed back to the pituitary to inhibit FSH.

Male hypogonadism

Hypogonadism in a male results from disease of the testes (primary hypogonadism) or disease of the pituitary or hypothalamus (secondary hypogonadism). Occasionally there is a defect in the ability to respond to testosterone (Table 14.5). The clinical features are due to subfertility and androgen deficiency. The presentation depends on the age of onset of hypogonadism (Table 14.6). In pre-pubertal onset the patient presents with delayed puberty and eunuchoid body proportions (long legs relative to upper body and long arms relative to overall height), resulting from the continued growth of long bones, which occurs because of delayed fusion of the epiphyses.

Klinefelter's syndrome is the most common congenital abnormality and causes primary hypogonadism, with an incidence of 1 in 1000 live births. It is the result of the presence of an extra X chromosome (47, XXY). Accelerated atrophy of the testicular germ cells gives rise to sterility and small firm testes. The clinical picture varies: in the most severely affected there is complete failure of sexual maturation, eunuchoid body proportions, gynaecomastia and learning difficulties.

Table 14.5 Causes of male hypogonadism

Reduced gonadotrophins (hypothalamic–pituitary disease)

Hypopituitarism
Selective gonadotrophic deficiency (Kallmann's syndrome)
Severe systemic illness
Severe underweight

Hyperprolactinaemia

Interferes with pulsatile secretion of LH and FSH

Primary gonadal disease (congenital)

Anorchia/Leydig cell agenesis
Cryptorchidism (testicular maldescent)
Chromosome abnormality (e.g. Klinefelter's syndrome)
Enzyme defects: 5α-reductase deficiency

Primary gonadal disease (acquired)

Testicular torsion sickle cell disease
Orchidectomy
Chemotherapy/radiation toxicity
Orchitis (e.g. mumps)
Chronic kidney disease
Cirrhosis/alcohol
Sickle cell disease

Androgen-receptor deficiency/abnormality

FSH, follicle-stimulating hormone; LH, luteinizing hormone.

Table 14.6 Consequences of androgen deficiency in the male

Loss of libido
High-pitched voice (if pre-pubertal)
No temporal recession of hair
Thinning and loss of facial, axillary, pubic and limb hair
Loss of erections/ejaculations
Small soft testes
Poorly developed penis/scrotum
Subfertility
Increased height and arm span (if pre-pubertal)
Decreased muscle bulk
Osteoporosis
Gynaecomastia

Congenital deficiency of gonadotrophin-releasing hormone may occur in isolation, or be associated with anosmia (absent sense of smell), colour blindness, cleft palate and renal abnormalities, in which case it is referred to as Kallmann's syndrome.

Investigations

A low or low-normal serum testosterone confirms the clinical diagnosis of hypogonadism. Supranormal serum concentrations of FSH and LH indicate that the patient has primary hypogonadism (testicular disease), and normal or low levels of FSH/LH indicate disease of the pituitary or hypothalamus (secondary hypogonadism). Further investigations, e.g. serum prolactin, chromosomal analysis (e.g. to exclude Klinefelter's syndrome), pituitary MRI scan and pituitary function tests, will depend on the likely site of the defect.

Management

The cause can rarely be reversed and the mainstay of treatment is androgen replacement as testosterone. Patients with hypothalamic–pituitary disease are given LH and FSH or pulsatile GnRH when fertility is desired.

Loss of libido and erectile dysfunction

Erectile dysfunction is defined as failure to initiate an erection or to maintain an erection until ejaculation. Erection is the result of increased vascularity of the penis and is controlled via the sacral parasympathetic outflow; it may be impaired by vascular disease, autonomic neuropathy (most commonly from diabetes mellitus) and nerve damage after pelvic surgery. The nervous pathways for ejaculation are centred on the lumbar sympathetics, and abnormalities may occur with autonomic neuropathy and traumatic nerve damage. Psychological factors, endocrine factors (causes of hypogonadism described above), alcohol and drugs, e.g. cannabis, and diuretics may cause abnormalities of both parasympathetic and sympathetic nerves. A careful history and examination will identify the cause in many patients. The presence of nocturnal emissions and morning erections is suggestive of psychogenic erectile dysfunction.

Offending drugs should be stopped. Phosphodiesterase type-5 inhibitors (sildenafil, tadalafil, vardenafil) increase penile blood flow and are usually the first choice for therapy. Other methods of treatment include apomorphine, intracavernosal injections of alprostadil, papaverine or phentolamine, vacuum expanders and penile implants.

Many cases are the result of psychological factors, and the patient may respond to psychosexual counselling.

Gynaecomastia

Gynaecomastia is development of breast tissue in the male. It results from an increase in the oestrogen:androgen ratio (Table 14.7) and is most commonly a result of liver disease or drug side effects (e.g. spironolactone or digoxin). It may also be caused by serious diseases such as bronchial carcinoma and testicular tumours. Gynaecomastia is also seen in early puberty as a result of relative

Table 14.7 Causes of gynaecomastia

Physiological
Neonatal, resulting from the influence of maternal hormones
Pubertal
Old age
Deficient testosterone secretion
Any cause of hypogonadism (Table 14.6)
Oestrogen-producing tumours
Of the testis or adrenal gland
HCG-producing tumours
Of the testis or the lung
Drugs
Oestrogenic: oestrogens, digoxin, cannabis, diamorphine
Antiandrogens: spironolactone, cimetidine, cyproterone
Others: gonadotrophins, cytotoxics
Other
Hyperthyroidism
Carcinoma of the breast
HCG, human chorionic gonadotrophin.

oestrogen excess, and usually resolves spontaneously. Unexplained gynaecomastia may occur, especially in elderly people, and is a diagnosis of exclusion after examination and investigation. The treatment in other cases is either of the underlying cause or by removal of the drug if possible. Occasionally, surgery is needed.

FEMALE REPRODUCTION AND SEX

In the adult female, higher brain centres impose a menstrual cycle of 28 days upon the activity of hypothalamic GnRH. Pulses of GnRH stimulate the release of pituitary LH and FSH. LH stimulates ovarian androgen production and FSH stimulates follicular development and aromatase activity (an enzyme required to convert ovarian androgens to oestrogens). Oestrogens are necessary for normal pubertal development and, together with progesterone, for maintenance of the menstrual cycle; they also have effects on a variety of tissues.

The menopause

The menopause, or cessation of periods, naturally occurs about the age of 45–55 years. During the late 40s, first FSH and then LH concentrations begin to rise, probably as a result of diminishing follicle supply. Oestrogen levels fall and the cycle becomes disrupted. Menopause may also occur surgically, with radiotherapy to the ovaries and with ovarian disease (e.g. premature menopause in the 20s and 30s). Symptoms of the menopause are hot flushes, vaginal dryness and breast atrophy. There may also be vague symptoms of depression, loss of libido and weight gain. There is loss of bone density (osteoporosis) and the pre-menopausal protection against ischaemic heart disease disappears.

Oestrogen replacement is the most effective treatment available for the relief of menopausal symptoms and also reduces the risk of colorectal cancer and osteoporotic fractures. However, hormone replacement therapy (HRT) increases the risk of breast cancer, coronary heart disease (CHD), stroke and venous thromboembolism. Oestrogens, when given alone (without progestogens), increase the risk of endometrial cancer. Over 5 years of treatment, an extra 1 woman in every 100 would develop an illness that would not have occurred had she not been taking HRT. The decision about whether a woman takes HRT is an individual decision based on the severity of her symptoms and her personal risk of conditions which may be prevented or made more likely by HRT. The main indication for HRT is for control of menopausal symptoms with the lowest effective dose for the shortest time possible. It is not recommended purely for prevention of post-menopausal osteoporosis and bisphosphonates or selective oestrogen receptor modulators (SERMs), e.g. raloxifene, are the preferred treatment. SERMs have the advantage of positive oestrogen effects on bone with no effect on oestrogen receptors of breast and uterus. HRT is used in premature ovarian failure (before age 40 years) when the benefits of treatment outweigh the risks. HRT is contraindicated in women with a history of thromboembolism, stroke, CHD or breast cancer.

Female hypogonadism and amenorrhoea

Amenorrhoea is the absence of menstruation. It is often physiological, e.g. during pregnancy and lactation, and after the menopause. Primary amenorrhoea is failure to start spontaneous menstruation by the age of 16 years. Secondary amenorrhoea is the absence of menstruation for 3 months in a woman who has previously had menstrual cycles. In the female, hypogonadism almost always presents as amenorrhoea or oligomenorrhoea (fewer than nine menses per year). The other features of oestrogen deficiency include atrophy of the breasts and vagina, loss of pubic hair and osteoporosis.

Aetiology

The causes of amenorrhoea are listed in Table 14.8. Polycystic ovary syndrome (PCOS) is the most common cause of oligomenorrhoea and amenorrhoea in clinical practice, though one should always consider pregnancy as a possible cause. Severe weight loss (e.g. anorexia nervosa) has long been associated

---

Table 14.8 Pathological causes of amenorrhoea

Hypothalamic

GnRH deficiency (isolated or as part of Kallmann's syndrome)*
Weight loss, physical exercise, stress
Post oral contraceptive therapy

Pituitary

Hyperprolactinaemia
Hypopituitarism

Gonadal

Polycystic ovary syndrome
Premature ovarian failure – autoimmune basis
Defective ovarian development (dysgenesis)*
Androgen-secreting ovarian tumours
Radiotherapy

Other diseases

Thyroid dysfunction
Cushing's syndrome
Adrenal tumours
Severe illness

Uterine/vaginal abnormality

Imperforate hymen or absent uterus*

*Presents as primary amenorrhoea.
GnRH, gonadotrophin-releasing hormone.

with amenorrhoea, but less severe forms of weight loss (by dieting and exercise) are a common cause of amenorrhoea caused by abnormal secretion of GnRH.

Investigations

The cause of amenorrhoea may be apparent after a full history and examination. Basal levels of serum FSH, LH, oestrogen and prolactin will allow a distinction between primary gonadal and hypothalamic–pituitary causes. Further investigations, e.g. ultrasonography of the ovaries, laparoscopy and ovarian biopsy, pituitary MRI and measurement of serum testosterone, will depend on the probable site of the defect and the findings on clinical examination.

Management

Treatment of the cause where possible: e.g. increase weight; treat hypothyroidism and hyperprolactinaemia. In patients where the underlying defect cannot be corrected, cyclical oestrogens are given to reverse the symptoms of oestrogen deficiency and prevent early osteoporosis. Patients with isolated GnRH deficiency or hypopituitarism are treated with human FSH/LH.

Hirsutism and polycystic ovary syndrome

Hirsutism is excess hair growth in women in a male pattern (androgen dependent): beard area, abdominal wall, thigh, axilla and around the nipples. Hirsutism should be differentiated from *hypertrichosis*, which is androgen independent and refers to a general increase in body hair; this can be racial (the Mediterranean and some Asian Indian subcontinent populations), caused by drugs (e.g. ciclosporin, minoxidil, phenytoin) or anorexia nervosa, or may be familial.

Hirsutism indicates increased androgen production by the ovaries or adrenal glands, most commonly PCOS. Rarer causes are congenital adrenal hyperplasia, ovarian or adrenal androgen-secreting tumour, prolactinoma and Cushing's disease. Signs of virilization (clitoromegaly, recent-onset frontal balding, deepening of the voice and loss of female body shape) imply substantial androgen excess and usually indicate a cause other than PCOS.

PCOS is one of the most common hormonal disorders affecting women. It is characterized by multiple small cysts within the ovary (which represent arrested follicular development) and by excess androgen production from the ovaries and, to a lesser extent, from the adrenals. PCOS is frequently associated with hyperinsulinaemia and insulin resistance and there is an increased frequency of type 2 diabetes mellitus. It is also associated with hypertension, hyperlipidaemia and increased cardiovascular disease. The precise mechanisms that link this syndrome remain to be elucidated, but may play a role in the causation of macrovascular disease in women.

Clinical features

Typically, PCOS presents with amenorrhoea or oligomenorrhoea (menstrual cycles longer than 35 days or fewer than 10 periods a year), hirsutism and acne, usually beginning shortly after menarche. It is sometimes associated with marked obesity, but weight may be normal. Mild virilization occurs in severe cases.

Criteria for diagnosis

Diagnostic criteria for PCOS have been proposed by several groups. In the Rotterdam criteria the diagnosis of PCOS is made when two of the following three criteria are present and other differentials (androgen-secreting tumour, Cushing's syndrome, congenital adrenal hyperplasia) are excluded:

- Menstrual irregularity (amenorrhoea or oligomenorrhoea) due to oligo- and/or anovulation
- Clinical (hirsutism, acne, frontal balding) or biochemical evidence of hyperandrogenism
- Polycystic ovaries (multiple cysts) on ultrasound examination.

Investigations and differential diagnosis

- Sex hormones – serum total testosterone concentration may be normal in PCOS and fail to detect biochemical hyperandrogenism. This is because sex hormone-binding globulin (which affects total testosterone concentration) is suppressed, leading to high free (i.e. bioavailable) testosterone levels. Biochemical evidence of hyperandrogenism is demonstrated by a *raised free androgen index* (serum total testosterone/sex hormone-binding globulin concentration), which is a measure of bioavailable testosterone. Total testosterone concentrations more than 1.5–2 times the upper limit of normal or a history of rapid virilization are likely to be associated with an androgen-secreting tumour of the ovaries or adrenal glands.
- Serum prolactin is slightly elevated in PCOS but values more than 1.5–2 times the upper limit of normal suggest pituitary or hypothalamic disease.
- Serum 17-hydroxyprogesterone is elevated in patients with non-classic congenital adrenal hyperplasia.
- Transvaginal ultrasound gives good visualization of the ovaries.

Management

Local therapy for hirsutism Excess hair can be removed or disguised by shaving, bleaching and waxing. Eflornithine cream inhibits hair growth but is only effective in a minority of cases.

Systemic therapy for hirsutism

- Oestrogens, e.g. oral contraceptives, suppress ovarian androgen production and reduce free androgen by increasing sex hormone-binding globulin levels.

- Cyproterone acetate and flutamide are both antiandrogens. The latter is less commonly used because of a high incidence of hepatic side effects.
- Spironolactone has antiandrogen activity.
- Finasteride, a 5α-reductase inhibitor, inhibits dihydrotestosterone formation in skin.

Treatment of menstrual disturbance Cyclical oestrogen/progesterone administration regulates the menstrual cycle in addition to improving hirsutism. Metformin improves hyperinsulinaemia, regulates the menstrual cycle and helps weight loss.

Treatment for infertility Patients with PCOS who require induction of ovulation are treated with the antioestrogen, clomifene.

THE GLUCOCORTICOID AXIS

The adrenal gland consists of an outer cortex, producing steroids (cortisol, aldosterone and androgens), and an inner medulla, secreting catecholamines. Aldosterone secretion is under the control of the renin–angiotensin system (see later). Corticotrophin-releasing hormone (CRH) from the hypothalamus stimulates ACTH (from the anterior pituitary), which stimulates cortisol production by the adrenal cortex. Cortisol feeds back on the hypothalamus and pituitary to inhibit further CRH/ACTH release. CRH release, and hence cortisol release, is in response to a circadian rhythm (light–dark), stress and other factors. Random serum cortisol measurements may therefore be misleading. Suppression tests are used if excess cortisol is suspected and stimulation tests are used if cortisol deficiency is suspected. Cortisol has many effects, particularly on carbohydrate metabolism. It leads to increased protein catabolism, increased deposition of fat and glycogen, sodium retention, increased renal potassium loss and a diminished host response to infection.

Synthetic steroids are widely used in the treatment of a variety of inflammatory disorders and replacement therapy in adrenal insufficiency. They differ in their structure and potency and include cortisol, prednisolone, methylprednisolone and dexamethasone. Fludrocortisone is produced by modification of hydrocortisone. It has potent mineralocorticoid activity and is used to replace natural aldosterone in patients with primary adrenal insufficiency.

Addison's disease: primary hypoadrenalism

This is a rare condition in which there is destruction of the entire adrenal cortex.

Aetiology

Primary hypoadrenalism shows a marked female preponderance. More than 90% of cases result from destruction of the entire adrenal cortex by organ-specific autoantibodies. This is associated with other autoimmune conditions, e.g. autoimmune thyroid disease, ovarian failure, pernicious anaemia and type 1 diabetes mellitus. Rarer causes include adrenal gland tuberculosis, surgical removal, haemorrhage (in meningococcal septicaemia) and malignant infiltration. Primary hypoadrenalism must be differentiated from secondary (to pituitary disease) or tertiary (to hypothalamic disease) adrenocortical failure or after prolonged corticosteroid treatment for non-endocrine conditions (p. 641).

Clinical features

There is an insidious presentation with non-specific symptoms of lethargy, depression, anorexia and weight loss. Postural hypotension caused by salt and water loss is an early sign. Hyperpigmentation (buccal mucosa, pressure points, skin creases and recent scars) results from stimulation of melanocytes by excess ACTH in primary hypoadrenalism. There may be vitiligo and loss of body hair in women because of the dependence on adrenal androgens. Hypoadrenalism may also present as an emergency (Addisonian crisis), with vomiting, abdominal pain, profound weakness, hypoglycaemia and hypovolaemic shock.

Investigations

Investigations are three-fold: to demonstrate inappropriately low cortisol secretion; to determine if cortisol deficiency is independent or dependent on ACTH secretion, i.e. primary or secondary/tertiary hypoadrenalism; and to determine the specific cause of the adrenal failure.

- The short ACTH (tetracosactide) stimulation test is the key diagnostic investigation and demonstrates failure of exogenous ACTH to increase plasma cortisol (Table 14.9). However, it does not differentiate primary from secondary hypoadrenalism. Random cortisol measurements may be suggestive, but single values are not usually helpful.
- Plasma ACTH level – a high level (>80 ng/L at 0900 h) with low or low-normal cortisol confirms primary hypoadrenalism. Reduced ACTH and cortisol indicate secondary or tertiary hypoadrenalism.
- Plasma renin activity is high due to low serum aldosterone.
- Adrenal antibodies are detected in most cases of autoimmune adrenalitis.

Table 14.9 Short ACTH (tetracosactide) stimulation tests

1. Take blood for measurement of plasma cortisol
2. Administer tetracosactide 250 μg i.m./i.v.
3. Take blood for measurement of cortisol after 30 minutes
4. Interpretation: adrenal insufficiency is excluded if the basal plasma cortisol exceeds 170 nmol/L and exceeds 600 nmol/L at 30 minutes. Further tests (plasma ACTH and long Synacthen test) are needed to establish the cause of hypoadrenalism.

ACTH, adrenocorticotrophic hormone.

- Routine biochemical tests classically show hyponatraemia, hyperkalaemia and a raised urea. Hypoglycaemia and hypercalcaemia are occasionally seen.
- Chest and abdominal X-rays may show evidence of tuberculosis, with calcified adrenals.

Addisonian crisis is a life-threatening emergency that requires immediate treatment before full investigation (Emergency Box 14.3). Treatment should begin on the basis of clinical suspicion without waiting for the results of laboratory tests.

Management

This is with lifelong steroid replacement taken as tablets:

- *Hydrocortisone:* the usual dose is 15–25 mg in divided doses (either two or three times daily).
- *Fludrocortisone*, a synthetic mineralocorticoid, 50–300 μg daily. The dose is adequate when serum electrolytes are normal, there is no postural drop in blood pressure and plasma renin levels are suppressed to within the normal range.

✚ Emergency Box 14.3

Management of acute hypoadrenalism

Investigations

- Take blood for plasma cortisol and ACTH before administration of hydrocortisone
- Full blood count, urea and electrolytes, blood glucose, serum calcium and blood cultures

Immediate

- Hydrocortisone 100 mg intravenously
- 0.9% saline, 1 L over 30–60 minutes
- 50 mL of 50% dextrose if hypoglycaemic
- Search for precipitating cause, e.g. infection, gastroenteritis

Subsequent

- Hydrocortisone 100 mg i.m. 6-hourly until BP stable and vomiting ceased
- 0.9% saline 2–4 L i.v. in 12–24 hours; monitor by JVP or CVP
- Expect recovery, with normal BP, blood glucose and serum sodium, within 12–24 hours
- When stable, convert to oral maintenance treatment continued lifelong

ACTH, adrenocorticotrophic hormone; BP, blood pressure; CVP, central venous pressure; JVP, jugular venous pressure.

Patients should wear a Medic Alert bracelet or necklace and carry the medical information card supplied with it. Both should indicate the diagnosis, daily medications and doses. They should also keep an (up-to-date) ampoule of hydrocortisone at home in case of major illness or if they are unable to take their oral medication due to vomiting. In a normal individual, stress of any type, e.g. infection, trauma and surgery, causes an immediate and marked increase in ACTH and hence in cortisol. This is a necessary response and therefore it is essential in patients on steroid replacement that the dose is increased when they are placed in any of these situations. The usual dose is 100 mg hydrocortisone i.m. for minor surgery and, for major surgery 100 mg hydrocortisone 6-hourly until oral medication is resumed. The dose is doubled during minor illness.

Uses and problems of therapeutic steroid therapy

In addition to their use as therapeutic replacement for deficiency states, steroids are widely used for a variety of non-endocrine conditions such as inflammatory bowel disease, asthma and rheumatological conditions. Long-term steroid use is associated with side effects (Table 14.10) and also results in suppression of the adrenal axis if used continually for more than 3–4 weeks. All patients receiving steroids should carry a 'Steroid Card' and should be made aware of the following points:

- Steroid therapy must never be stopped suddenly unless treatment has been for less than 2–3 weeks. After 3 weeks, doses should be reduced very gradually.
- Doses should be doubled in times of serious intercurrent illness.
- Other physicians, anaesthetists and dentists must be told about steroid therapy.

Patients should also be informed of potential side effects and this information should be documented in the patient records. The clinical need for high-dose steroids should be continually and critically assessed. Steroid-sparing agents (e.g. azathioprine) should always be considered and screening and prophylactic therapy for osteoporosis introduced.

Secondary hypoadrenalism

This may arise from hypothalamic–pituitary disease or from long-term steroid therapy leading to hypothalamic–pituitary–adrenal suppression. The clinical features are the same as those of Addison's disease but there is no pigmentation because ACTH levels are low and, in pituitary disease, there are usually features of failure of other pituitary hormones. Treatment is with hydrocortisone; fludrocortisone is unnecessary. If adrenal failure is secondary to long-term steroid therapy, the adrenals usually recover if steroids are withdrawn very slowly.

Table 14.10 Adverse effects of corticosteroids

Physiological	
Adrenal and/or pituitary suppression	

Pathological	
Cardiovascular	*Endocrine*
Increased blood pressure	Weight gain
	Glycosuria, hyperglycaemia (diabetes mellitus)
Gastrointestinal	Impaired growth in children
Peptic ulceration exacerbation (possibly)	
Acute pancreatitis	*Bone and muscle*
	Osteoporosis
Renal	Proximal myopathy and wasting
Polyuria	Aseptic necrosis of the hip
Nocturia	Pathological fractures
Central nervous	*Skin*
Depression	Thinning
Euphoria	Easy bruising
Psychosis	
Insomnia	*Eyes*
	Cataracts
Increased susceptibility to infection	
(signs and fever are frequently masked)	
Septicaemia	
Reactivation of tuberculosis	
Skin (e.g. fungi) Oral *Candida* (including with inhaled drugs)	

Cushing's syndrome

Cushing's syndrome is caused by persistently and inappropriately elevated circulating glucocorticoid levels. Most cases result from administration of synthetic steroids or ACTH for the treatment of medical conditions, e.g. asthma. Spontaneous Cushing's syndrome is rare and two-thirds of cases result from excess ACTH secretion from the pituitary gland (Table 14.11). Cushing's

Table 14.11 Causes of Cushing's syndrome

ACTH-dependent causes

Pituitary-dependent (Cushing's disease)
Ectopic ACTH-producing tumours (small-cell lung cancer, carcinoid tumours)
ACTH administration

Non-ACTH-dependent causes

Adrenal adenomas
Adrenal carcinomas
Glucocorticoid administration

Others

Alcohol-induced pseudo-Cushing's syndrome

ACTH, adrenocorticotrophic hormone.

disease must be distinguished from Cushing's syndrome. The latter is a general term which refers to the abnormalities resulting from a chronic excess of glucocorticoids whatever the cause, whereas Cushing's disease specifically refers to excess glucocorticoids resulting from inappropriate ACTH secretion from the pituitary (usually a microadenoma, less often corticotrophin hyperplasia). Alcohol excess mimics Cushing's syndrome clinically and biochemically (pseudo-Cushing's syndrome). The pathogenesis is incompletely understood but the features resolve when alcohol is stopped.

Clinical features

Patients are obese: fat distribution is typically central, affecting the trunk, abdomen and neck (buffalo hump). They have a plethoric complexion with a moon face. Many of the features are the result of the protein-catabolic effects of cortisol: the skin is thin and bruises easily and there are purple striae on the abdomen, breasts and thighs (Fig. 14.9). Other features include proximal myopathy, hypertension, hypokalaemia and impaired glucose tolerance. Pigmentation occurs with ACTH-dependent cases. Patients with ectopic production of ACTH tend to have rapidly progressive symptoms and signs and have evidence of the primary tumour.

Investigations

In a patient with suspected spontaneous Cushing's syndrome, the purpose of investigation is firstly to confirm the presence of cortisol excess, and secondly to determine the cause.

Confirm raised cortisol

- The *48-hour low-dose dexamethasone suppression test* is the most reliable screening test. Dexamethasone 0.5 mg 6-hourly is given orally for 48 hours. Normal individuals suppress plasma cortisol to <50 nmol/L 2 hours after the last dose of dexamethasone.

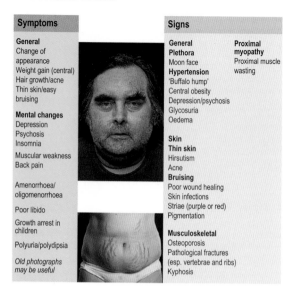

Symptoms	Signs	
General Change of appearance Weight gain (central) Hair growth/acne Thin skin/easy bruising **Mental changes** Depression Psychosis Insomnia Muscular weakness Back pain Amenorrhoea/ oligomenorrhoea Poor libido Growth arrest in children Polyuria/polydipsia *Old photographs may be useful*	**General** **Plethora** Moon face **Hypertension** 'Buffalo hump' Central obesity Depression/psychosis Glycosuria Oedema **Skin** **Thin skin** Hirsutism Acne **Bruising** Poor wound healing Skin infections Striae (purple or red) Pigmentation **Musculoskeletal** Osteoporosis Pathological fractures (esp. vertebrae and ribs) Kyphosis	**Proximal myopathy** Proximal muscle wasting

Fig. 14.9 Cushing's syndrome – symptoms and signs. Bold type indicates signs of most value in discriminating Cushing's syndrome from simple obesity and hirsutism.

- 24-hour *urinary free cortisol* is raised (normal <700 nmol/24 h) in most cases.
- *Circadian rhythm studies* show loss of the normal circadian fall of plasma cortisol at 2400 h in patients with Cushing's syndrome.
  Establishing the cause of Cushing's syndrome
- *Plasma ACTH levels* are low or undetectable in adrenal gland disease (non-ACTH dependent) and should lead to adrenal imaging. High or inappropriately normal values suggest pituitary disease or ectopic production of ACTH.
- *High-dose dexamethasone suppression test.* Dexamethasone 2 mg 6-hourly is given orally for 48 hours. Most patients with pituitary-dependent Cushing's disease suppress plasma cortisol by 48 hours. Failure of suppression suggests an ectopic source of ACTH or an adrenal tumour.
- Adrenal computed tomography (CT) or MRI will detect adrenal adenomas and carcinomas, as those which produce Cushing's syndrome are usually large.
- Pituitary MRI and CT will detect some, but not all, pituitary adenomas.
- *Corticotrophin-releasing hormone test.* An exaggerated plasma ACTH response to exogenous CRH (bolus given intravenously) suggests pituitary-dependent Cushing's disease.

- *Other tests* will depend on the probable cause of Cushing's syndrome, which has been established from the above tests. Chest X-ray, bronchoscopy and CT of the body may localize ectopic ACTH-producing tumours. Selective venous sampling for ACTH will localize pituitary tumours and an otherwise occult ectopic ACTH-producing tumour.
- *Radiolabelled octreotide* (^{111}In-octreotide) is occasionally helpful in locating ectopic ACTH sites.

Management

Surgical removal is indicated for most pituitary (usually a trans-sphenoidal approach) and adrenal tumours and may be appropriate for many cases of ectopic ACTH-producing tumours.

Drugs which inhibit cortisol synthesis (metyrapone, ketoconazole or aminoglutethimide) may be useful in cases not amenable to surgery.

External-beam irradiation of the pituitary produces a very slow response and is restricted to cases where surgery is unsuccessful, contraindicated or unacceptable to the patient.

Iatrogenic Cushing's syndrome responds to a reduction in steroid dosage when possible. Immunosuppressant drugs such as azathioprine are used in conjunction with steroids to enable lower steroid doses to be used to control the underlying disease.

Incidental adrenal tumours

With the advent of improved abdominal imaging, unsuspected adrenal masses have been discovered in about 4% of scans. Most of these masses are small non-secreting adenomas: others are secreting adenomas, carcinomas or metastases. Metastases will usually be apparent from the previous or ongoing medical history and specific imaging phenotype. If the imaging suggests an adenoma, functional tests to exclude secretory activity are indicated: dexamethasone suppression test for subclinical Cushing's syndrome; measurement of adrenal androgens; 24-hour urinary specimen for measurement of catecholamines to exclude a phaeochromocytoma; and plasma renin and aldosterone to exclude Conn's syndrome. Most authorities recommend surgical removal of large (>4–5 cm) and functional tumours but observation of smaller hormonally inactive lesions.

ENDOCRINOLOGY OF BLOOD PRESSURE CONTROL

Blood pressure is determined by cardiac output and peripheral resistance, and an increase in blood pressure may be due to an increase in one or both of these. In a few patients an underlying cause can be identified for hypertension including endocrine causes (Table 14.12). However, in 90% of cases no cause can be found and patients are said to have essential hypertension. Young patients

Table 14.12 Endocrine causes of hypertension

Excessive production of	Condition
Renin	Renal artery stenosis, renin-secreting tumours
Aldosterone	Adrenal adenoma, adrenal hyperplasia
Mineralocorticoids	Cushing's syndrome (cortisol is a weak mineralocorticoid)
Catecholamines	Phaeochromocytoma
Growth hormone	Acromegaly
Oral contraceptive pill (mechanism unclear)	

(<35 years), those with an abnormal baseline screening test or patients with malignant hypertension or hypertension resistant to conventional treatment (e.g. more than three drugs) should be screened for secondary causes.

The renin–angiotensin system

The renin–angiotensin–aldosterone system is illustrated in Fig. 14.10. *Angiotensin*, an α_2-globulin of hepatic origin, circulates in plasma. The enzyme *renin* is secreted by the kidney in response to decreased renal perfusion pressure or flow; it cleaves the decapeptide *angiotensin I* from angiotensinogen. Angiotensin I is inactive but is further cleaved by angiotensin-converting enzyme (ACE: present in lung and vascular endothelium) into the active peptide, *angiotensin II*, which has two major actions:

- It causes powerful vasoconstriction (within seconds)
- It stimulates the adrenal zona glomerulosa to increase aldosterone production.

Aldosterone causes sodium retention and urinary potassium loss (hours to days). This combination of changes leads to an increase in blood pressure, and the stimulus to renin production is reduced. Sodium deprivation or urinary loss also increases renin production, whereas dietary sodium excess will suppress production.

Primary hyperaldosteronism

Increased mineralocorticoid secretion from the adrenal cortex, termed 'primary hyperaldosteronism', is thought to account for 5–10% of all hypertension. It is caused by an adrenal adenoma secreting aldosterone (Conn's syndrome) or by bilateral adrenal hyperplasia.

Clinical features

The major function of aldosterone is to cause an exchange transport of sodium and potassium in the distal renal tubule: that is, absorption of sodium (and hence

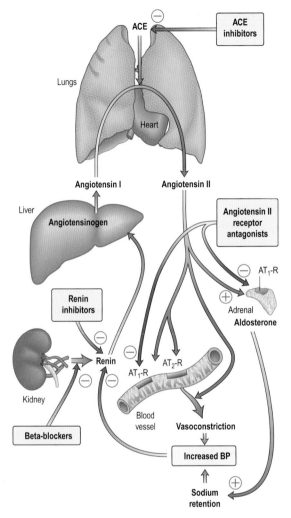

Fig. 14.10 The renin–angiotensin–aldosterone system. ACE, angiotensin-converting enzyme; BP, blood pressure. Angiotensin II antagonists act on the adrenals and blood vessels.

water) and excretion of potassium. Hyperaldosteronism causes hypertension, resulting from expansion of intravascular volume, and hypokalaemia.

Investigations

- Hypokalaemia is often but not always present.
- Plasma aldosterone:renin ratio (ARR) is the initial screening test for primary hyperaldosteronism. Spirinolactone and eplerenone should be stopped 6 weeks before the test. A raised ratio does not confirm the diagnosis, and further tests are then indicated to demonstrate inappropriate aldosterone secretion.
- The diagnosis is made by demonstrating increased plasma aldosterone levels that are not suppressed with 0.9% saline infusion (2 L over 4 hours) or fludrocortisone administration (a mineralocorticoid).
- CT or MRI of the adrenals is used to differentiate adenomas from hyperplasia.

Management

An adenoma is removed surgically. Hypertension resulting from hyperplasia is treated with the aldosterone antagonist spironolactone or eplerenone.

Phaeochromocytoma

This is a rare (0.1% of hypertension) catecholamine-producing tumour of the sympathetic nervous system; 10% are malignant and 10% occur outside the adrenal gland. Some are associated with multiple endocrine neoplasia (MEN; see below) and other genetic disorders (e.g. von Hippel–Lindau disease, neurofibromatosis type 1 and mutations in the succinate dehydrogenase gene).

Clinical features

Symptoms may be episodic and include headache, palpitations, sweating, anxiety, nausea and weight loss. The signs, which may also be intermittent, include hypertension, tachycardia and pallor. There may be hyperglycaemia.

Investigations

- A 24-hour urine collection for urinary catecholamines and metabolites (metanephrines) is a useful screening test; normal levels on three separate collections virtually exclude the diagnosis.
- Raised levels of plasma catecholamines confirm the diagnosis.
- Plasma chromogranin A (a storage vesicle protein) is raised.
- CT/MRI is useful to localize the tumour.
- Scintigraphy using meta-[^{131}I]-iodobenzylguanidine (mIBG), which is selectively taken up by adrenergic cells, is particularly useful with extra-adrenal tumours.

Management

The treatment of choice is surgical excision of the tumour under α- and β-blockade using phenoxybenzamine and propranolol, which is started before the operation. These drugs can also be used over the long term where operation is not possible.

Multiple endocrine neoplasia

The MEN syndromes are rare, but recognition is important for both treatment and evaluation of family members – inheritance is autosomal dominant. MEN is the name given to the synchronous or metachronous (i.e. occurring at different times) occurrence of tumours involving a number of endocrine glands (Table 14.13). MEN type 1 is due to a mutation in the *menin* gene on

Table 14.13 Multiple endocrine neoplasia (MEN) syndrome

Organ	Frequency	Tumours/clinical manifestations
Type 1		
Functioning adenomas in:		
Parathyroid	95%	Hypercalcaemia
Pituitary	30%	Prolactinoma, acromegaly, Cushing's disease
Enteropancreatic tumours	60%	Gastrinoma, insulinoma, glucagonoma, VIPoma
Other:		
Foregut carcinoids	10%	Thymic, bronchial gastric
Adrenal cortex adenomas	25%	Non-functional tumours
Cutaneous tumours	60%	Angiofibromas, collagenomas, lipomas
Type 2A		
Medullary thyroid carcinoma	95%	Thyroid mass, diarrhoea, raised plasma calcitonin
Adrenal medulla	40%	Phaeochromocytoma
Parathyroid hyperplasia	10%	Hypercalcaemia
Type 2B		
Like type 2A (but not parathyroid disease) with a typical phenotypic appearance: slim body habitus and neuromas of lips, tongue, and gastrointestinal tract		

VIP, vasoactive intestinal polypeptide.

chromosome 11; the normal protein product of this gene acts as a tumour suppressor. The genetic abnormality in MEN 2 lies within the *Ret* proto-oncogene on chromosome 10; the gene product plays a role in central and peripheral nerve development and function. Management involves surgical excision of the tumours if possible. Asymptomatic family members should be screened by measurement of serum calcium in MEN 1 (due to the high penetrance of hyperparathyroidism) and by genetic testing for *Ret* mutations in MEN 2 families. In a patient known to have MEN, constant surveillance is required for additional features of the syndrome, which may develop many years after the initial presentation.

THE THIRST AXIS

ADH (also called vasopressin) is synthesized in the hypothalamus and then migrates in neurosecretory granules along axonal pathways to the posterior pituitary gland. Secretion of ADH is determined principally by the plasma osmolality. The major hormonal action of ADH is on the collecting tubule of the kidney to cause water reabsorption. At high concentrations vasopressin also causes vasoconstriction. ADH secretion is suppressed at plasma osmolality below 280 mOsm/kg, thus allowing maximal water diuresis. Secretion increases to a maximum at a plasma osmolality of 295 mOsm/kg. Large falls in blood pressure or volume also stimulate vasopressin secretion.

Diabetes insipidus (DI)

Impaired vasopressin secretion (cranial diabetes insipidus [CDI]) or renal resistance to its action (nephrogenic diabetes insipidus [NDI]) leads to polyuria (dilute urine in excess of 3 L/24 h), nocturia and compensatory polydipsia. It must be distinguished from primary polydipsia, which is a psychiatric disturbance characterized by excessive intake of water, and other causes of polyuria and polydipsia, e.g. hyperglycaemia.

Aetiology

CDI is caused by disease of the hypothalamus: neurosurgery, trauma, primary or secondary tumours, infiltrative disease (sarcoidosis, histiocytosis) and idiopathic. Damage to the hypothalamo-neurohypophysial tract or the posterior pituitary with an intact hypothalamus does not lead to ADH deficiency, as the hormone can still 'leak' from the damaged end of the intact neurone. Causes of NDI are listed in Table 14.14.

Clinical features

There is polyuria (as much as 15 L in 24 hours) and polydipsia. Patients depend on a normal thirst mechanism and access to water to maintain normonatraemia.

Table 14.14 Causes of nephrogenic diabetes insipidus
Hypokalaemia
Hypercalcaemia
Drugs: lithium chloride, demeclocycline, glibenclamide
Renal tubular acidosis
Sickle cell disease
Prolonged polyuria of any cause
Familial (mutation in ADH receptor)
ADH, antidiuretic hormone.

Investigations

- Urine volume must be measured to confirm polyuria.
- Plasma biochemistry shows high or high-normal sodium concentration and osmolality. Blood glucose, serum potassium and calcium should be measured to exclude common causes of polyuria.
- Urine osmolality is inappropriately low for the high plasma osmolality.
- A water deprivation test is indicated for polyuric patients with normal blood glucose and serum electrolytes to determine if they have DI. Serum and urine osmolality, urine volume and body weight are measured hourly for up to 8 hours during fasting and without fluids. The test is abandoned if the body weight drops by >3%, as this indicates significant dehydration. Serum osmolality remaining within the normal range (275–295 mOsm/kg) and concentrated urine (>600 mOsm/kg) is a normal response. Serum osmolality >300 mOsm/kg without adequate concentration of the urine (<600 mOsm/kg) indicates DI, at which point desmopressin is given and urine osmolality is measured for a further 2–4 hours while allowing free fluids. NDI is diagnosed if urine osmolality stays the same and CDI diagnosed if urine osmolality increases by >50%.
- MRI of the hypothalamus is performed in cases of CDI.

Management

Treatment of the underlying condition seldom improves established CDI. Desmopressin, administered orally, nasally or intramuscularly, is the treatment of choice. In mild cases (3–4 L urine per day), thiazide diuretics, carbamazepine and chlorpropamide are used to sensitize the renal tubules to endogenous vasopressin. Treatment of the cause will usually improve NDI.

Syndrome of inappropriate ADH secretion

There is continued ADH secretion in spite of plasma hypotonicity and a normal or expanded plasma volume.

Table 14.15 Causes of syndrome of inappropriate ADH

Cancer	Many tumours, of which the most common is small cell cancer of the lung
Brain	Meningitis, cerebral abscess, head injury, tumour
Lung	Pneumonia, tuberculosis, lung abscess
Metabolic	Porphyria, alcohol withdrawal
Drugs	Opiates, chlorpropamide, carbamazepine, vincristine

ADH, antidiuretic hormone.

Aetiology

Syndrome of inappropriate ADH secretion (SIADH) is caused by disordered hypothalamic–pituitary secretion or ectopic production of ADH, e.g. small cell lung cancer (Table 14.15).

Clinical features

There is nausea, irritability and headache, with mild dilutional hyponatraemia (serum sodium 115–125 mmol/L). Fits and coma may occur with severe hyponatraemia (<115 mmol/L).

Investigations

SIADH must be differentiated from other causes of dilutional hyponatraemia (p. 336). Criteria for diagnosis are:

- Low serum sodium
- Low plasma osmolality with 'inappropriate' urine osmolality >100 mOsm/kg (and typically higher than plasma osmolality)
- Continued urinary sodium excretion (>30 mmol/L)
- Absence of hypokalaemia, hypotension and hypovolaemia
- Normal renal, adrenal and thyroid function.

Hyponatraemia is common during illness in frail elderly patients and it may sometimes be difficult to distinguish SIADH from salt and water depletion. Under these circumstances a trial of 1–2 L 0.9% saline is given. Sodium depletion will respond, while SIADH will not.

Management

Mild asymptomatic cases need no treatment other than that of the underlying cause. For symptomatic cases the options are:

- Water restriction: 500–1000 mL in 24 hours.
- Demeclocycline 600–1200 mg daily, inhibits the action of vasopressin on the kidney (i.e. causes nephrogenic DI) and may be useful if water restriction is poorly tolerated or ineffective.

- The specific vasopressin antagonist tolvaptan is used for treatment of hyponatraemia secondary to SIADH. It is expensive and not yet widely used.
- Hypertonic saline, with furosemide to prevent circulatory overload, is necessary in severe cases (see Emergency Box 8.1, p. 615).

DISORDERS OF CALCIUM METABOLISM

The concentration of calcium in the serum is regulated by the action of parathyroid hormone (PTH) and vitamin D on the kidneys, bones and gastrointestinal tract. PTH increases serum calcium concentration by stimulation of calcium reabsorption and activation of vitamin D in the kidney, and increasing calcium release from bone. The most active form of vitamin D (1,25-dihydroxyvitamin D) increases intestinal calcium absorption. Total plasma calcium is normally 2.2–2.6 mmol/L. Usually only 40% of total plasma calcium is ionized and physiologically relevant; the remainder is bound to albumin and thus unavailable to the tissues. Routine analytical methods measure total plasma calcium and this must be corrected for the serum albumin concentration: add or subtract 0.02 mmol/L for every 1 g/L by which the simultaneous albumin lies below or above 40 g/L. For critical measurements, samples should be taken in the fasting state without the use of an occluding cuff, which may increase the local plasma protein concentration.

Hypercalcaemia

Mild asymptomatic hypercalcaemia occurs in about 1 in 1000 of the population, especially elderly women, and is usually the result of primary hyperparathyroidism.

Aetiology

Primary hyperparathyroidism and malignancy account for >90% of cases (Table 14.16). Tumour-related hypercalcaemia is caused by the secretion of a peptide with PTH-like activity, or by direct invasion of bone and production of local factors that mobilize calcium. Ectopic PTH secretion by tumours is very rare. Severe hypercalcaemia (>3.5 mmol/L) is usually caused by malignancy.

Hyperparathyroidism

Hyperparathyroidism may be primary, secondary or tertiary.

Primary hyperparathyroidism affects about 0.1% of the population and is usually caused by a single parathyroid gland adenoma, occasionally hyperplasia, and rarely carcinoma. It may be associated with a hereditary syndrome, e.g. MEN (p. 649).

Secondary hyperparathyroidism is physiological compensatory hypertrophy of all the glands in response to prolonged hypocalcaemia (e.g. in chronic kidney disease or vitamin D deficiency). Calcium is low or low-normal.

Table 14.16 Causes of hypercalcaemia

Excess PTH

Primary hyperparathyroidism (most common cause)
Tertiary hyperparathyroidism
Ectopic PTH (very rare)

Malignant disease

Multiple myeloma
Secondary deposits in bone
Production of osteoclastic factors by tumours
PTH-related protein secretion

Excess action of vitamin D

Self-administered vitamin D
Granulomatous disease, e.g. sarcoidosis, TB
Lymphoma

Other endocrine disease (mild hypercalcaemia only)

Thyrotoxicosis
Addison's disease

Drugs

Thiazides – reduced renal tubular excretion of Ca^{2+}
Vitamin D analogues
Lithium – increased PTH secretion
Vitamin A

Miscellaneous

Long-term immobility
Familial hypocalciuric hypercalcaemia (rare)

PTH, parathyroid hormone; TB, tuberculosis.

Tertiary hyperparathyroidism is the development of apparently autonomous parathyroid hyperplasia after long-standing secondary hyperparathyroidism, most often in renal disease. Plasma calcium and PTH are both raised. Treatment is parathyroidectomy.

Clinical features

Mild hypercalcaemia (corrected serum calcium <3 mmol/L) is often asymptomatic and discovered on biochemical screening. More severe hypercalcaemia produces symptoms of general malaise and depression, bone pain, abdominal pain, nausea and constipation. Calcium deposition in the renal tubules causes polyuria and nocturia. Renal calculi and chronic kidney disease may develop. With very high levels (>3.8 mmol/L) there is dehydration, confusion, clouding of consciousness and a risk of cardiac arrest. Hypercalcaemia is rarely the presenting feature of malignancy, which is usually clinically apparent when the hypercalcaemia is first noted. Thus hypercalcaemia in an otherwise well outpatient is most likely to be due to primary hyperparathyroidism.

Investigations

- Several fasting serum calcium and phosphate samples are performed to confirm mild hypercalcaemia. The serum phosphate is low in primary hyperparathyroidism and some cases of malignancy. It is normal or high in other causes of hypercalcaemia.
- Serum PTH: normal or elevated levels during hypercalcaemia are inappropriate and imply hyperparathyroidism.
- Twenty-four-hour urinary calcium is measured in young patients and those with a family history of hypercalcaemia to exclude familial hypocalciuric hypercalcaemia in which PTH levels are also raised. Urinary calcium excretion is markedly low but normal or raised in primary hyperparathyroidism.
- An undetectable PTH in the context of hypercalcaemia excludes primary hyperparathyroidism and always requires further investigation to exclude malignancy or other pathology. The following tests may help in the diagnosis:
  - Protein electrophoresis for myeloma
  - TSH to exclude hyperthyroidism
  - Tetracosactide test to exclude Addison's disease
  - If investigations point to primary hyperparathyroidism, parathyroid imaging can be undertaken with radioisotope scanning using ^{99m}Tc-sestamibi (approximately 90% sensitive in detecting adenomas) or ultrasound.

Management

This involves lowering of the calcium levels to near normal and treatment of the underlying cause. Severe hypercalcaemia (>3.5 mmol/L) is a medical emergency which must be treated aggressively whatever the underlying cause (Emergency Box 14.4).

Treatment of primary hyperparathyroidism

The treatment of a symptomatic parathyroid adenoma is surgical removal. Conservative therapy may be indicated in asymptomatic patients older than 50 years with mildly raised serum calcium levels (2.65–3 mmol/L). In those with parathyroid hyperplasia, all four glands are removed.

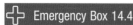

Emergency Box 14.4

Management of acute severe hypercalcaemia

- Rehydrate with intravenous fluid (0.9% saline)

    4–6 L of intravenous saline over 24 hours, then

    3–4 L for several days thereafter

    Amount and rate depend on clinical assessment and measurement of serum urea and electrolytes

- Bisphosphonate – only after rehydration, usually a minimum of 2 L

    Pamidronate disodium 60–90 mg as an i.v. infusion in 0.5 L 0.9% saline over 2–8 hours

- Measure

    Serum urea and electrolytes at least daily

    Measure serum calcium at least 48 hours after initiation of treatment, normalization may take 3–5 days, mean duration of action 28 days

- Prednisolone (30–60 mg daily)

    May be useful in some cases (myeloma, sarcoidosis and vitamin D excess) but in most cases ineffective

- Prevent recurrence

    Treat underlying cause if possible

    With untreatable malignancy, consider maintenance treatment with bisphosphonates

Hypocalcaemia and hypoparathyroidism

Aetiology

Causes of hypocalcaemia are listed in Table 14.17. Chronic kidney disease is the most common cause and results from inadequate production of active vitamin D and renal phosphate retention, leading to microprecipitation of calcium phosphate in the tissues. Mild transient hypocalcaemia often occurs after parathyroidectomy, and a few patients develop long-standing hypoparathyroidism.

Clinical features

Hypocalcaemia causes increased excitability of muscles and nerves. There is numbness around the mouth and in the extremities, followed by cramps, tetany (carpopedal spasm: opposition of the thumb, extension of the interphalangeal and flexion of the metacarpophalangeal joints), convulsions and death if untreated. Chvostek's (tapping over the facial nerve in the region of the parotid gland causes twitching of the ipsilateral facial muscles) and Trousseau's sign (carpopedal spasm induced by inflation of the sphygmomanometer cuff to a

Table 14.17 Causes of hypocalcaemia

Increased serum phosphate levels
Chronic kidney disease*
Phosphate therapy

Reduced PTH function
Post-thyroidectomy and parathyroidectomy (usually transient)*
Congenital deficiency (DiGeorge syndrome)
Idiopathic hypoparathyroidism (autoimmune)
Severe hypomagnesaemia (inhibits PTH release)
Pseudohypoparathyroidism (end-organ resistance to PTH)

Vitamin D deficiency
Reduced exposure to ultraviolet light
Malabsorption
Antiepileptic drugs (induce enzymes that increase vitamin D metabolism)
Vitamin D resistance (rare)

Drugs
Calcitonin
Bisphosphonates

Miscellaneous
Acute pancreatitis*
Citrated blood in massive transfusion

*Indicates common cause of hypocalcaemia.
PTH, parathyroid hormone.

level above systolic blood pressure) test for neuromuscular excitability. Severe hypocalcaemia may cause papilloedema and a prolonged QT interval on the electrocardiogram (ECG).

Other causes of tetany are alkalosis, potassium and magnesium deficiency and hyperventilation which decreases ionized fraction of calcium (total plasma calcium is normal) by altering the protein binding of calcium such that the ionized fraction is decreased.

Investigations

The cause of hypocalcaemia is often apparent from the history and physical examination, together with measurement of serum creatinine and estimation of the glomerular filtration rate (to look for chronic kidney disease) and magnesium. Fig. 14.11 shows an algorithm for subsequent investigation.

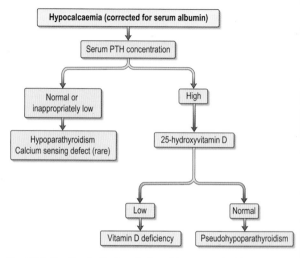

Fig. 14.11 Algorithm for the investigation of hypocalcaemia. PTH, parathyroid hormone.

Management

Acute (e.g. with tetany): 10 mL of 10% calcium gluconate (2.25 mmol) diluted in 50–100 mL 5% glucose and administered intravenously over 10 minutes with ECG monitoring. Treatment can be repeated until symptoms have resolved and continued as an infusion over 4 hours.

Persistent hypocalcaemia In vitamin D deficiency, treatment is with either ergocalciferol (vitamin D_2) or cholecalciferol (vitamin D_3) 50 000 IU orally once a week for 8 weeks. This treatment is ineffective in patients with hypoparathyroidism because PTH is needed for conversion to 1,25-dihydroxyvitamin D. Treatment is with alfacalcidol (1α-hydroxycholecalciferol) 0.25–2 µg daily to maintain serum calcium within the lower part of the normal range. Calcium levels should be checked initially weekly and 3–6 monthly once a stable dose is reached.

DISORDERS OF PHOSPHATE CONCENTRATION

Phosphate is essential for most biochemical processes in the body. The majority of body phosphate is contained within bone and regulation of plasma concentration is closely linked with calcium. Plasma phosphate concentrations are controlled in part by PTH and 1,25-dihydroxyvitamin D_3, which alter phosphate reabsorption in the proximal renal tubule. Hyperphosphataemia most commonly occurs in chronic kidney disease, and treatment is with gut phosphate binders and dialysis.

Table 14.18 Causes of hypophosphataemia

Redistribution of phosphate from extracellular fluid into the cell
Treatment of diabetic ketoacidosis
Refeeding syndrome
Acute respiratory alkalosis
Hungry bone syndrome after parathyroidectomy
Decreased intestinal absorption
Poor oral intake (rare)
Some antacids
Diarrhoea
Increased urine excretion
Hyperparathyroidism
Vitamin D deficiency
Primary renal abnormality

Hypophosphataemia

This is common and often unrecognized.

Aetiology

Hypophosphataemia is due to three major mechanisms: redistribution into cells; increased renal excretion; and decreased intake or intestinal absorption of phosphate (Table 14.18). The most common causes are treatment of patients with diabetic ketoacidosis, and carbohydrate refeeding in patients with alcohol misuse or recent weight loss and hyperparathyroidism.

Clinical features

These are due to intracellular phosphate depletion, which can impact on all organ systems. Clinical features include muscle weakness (diaphragmatic weakness leading to respiratory failure, impaired myocardial contractility and cardiac failure, and skeletal muscle weakness and rhabdomyolysis), encephalopathy (confusion, hallucinations and convulsions) and, rarely, haemolysis. More prolonged hypophosphataemia leads to osteomalacia.

Treatment

Oral phosphate supplements (e.g. effervescent tablets: four to six tablets daily if each tablet contains 16.1 mmol phosphate) and treatment of the underlying cause is generally sufficient. Tablets also contain sodium and potassium and the additional load needs to be taken into account in daily intake. Vitamin D supplementation is indicated in patients with vitamin D deficiency (p. 658).

Intravenous phosphate is potentially dangerous and may precipitate with calcium, causing hypocalcaemia and ectopic calcification in the kidneys and the heart. It is indicated for severe symptomatic hypophosphataemia (serum phosphate <0.4 mmol/L) and given as 9–18 mmol phosphate diluted in 250–500 mL glucose 5% over 6–12 hours via peripheral line. Plasma concentrations of calcium, phosphate, magnesium and potassium should be monitored during treatment.

DISORDERS OF TEMPERATURE REGULATION

Normal body temperature is 36.5–37.5°C and is controlled by temperature-sensitive cells within the hypothalamus which control heat generation and loss. Fever during an infection is due to cytokines, particularly interleukin-1, released from inflammatory cells acting in the hypothalamus affecting the thermoregulatory set-point.

Hypothermia

Hypothermia is defined as a drop in core (i.e. rectal) temperature to below 35°C. It is frequently fatal when the temperature falls below 28°C.

Aetiology

Very young and elderly individuals are particularly prone to hypothermia, the latter having a reduced ability to feel the cold. Hypothyroidism, hypnotics, alcohol or intercurrent illness may contribute. In healthy individuals, prolonged exposure to extremes of temperature or prolonged immersion in cold water is the most common underlying cause.

Clinical features

Mild hypothermia (32–35°C) causes shivering and a feeling of intense cold. More severe hypothermia leads progressively to altered consciousness and coma. This is usually associated with a fall in pulse rate and blood pressure, muscle stiffness and depressed reflexes. As coma ensues, the pupillary and other brainstem reflexes are lost. Ventricular arrhythmias or asystole is the usual cause of death.

Diagnosis

Measurement of core temperature with a low-reading thermometer makes the diagnosis. Alteration in consciousness usually indicates a core temperature of below 32°C; this is a medical emergency. With severe hypothermia there are ECG changes, including an increase in the PR interval, widening of the QRS complex and 'J' waves (prominent convex deflections at the junction of the QRS complex and ST segment, best seen in the precordial leads).

Management

The principles of treatment are to rewarm the patient gradually while correcting metabolic abnormalities (if severe) and treating cardiac arrhythmias (Emergency Box 14.5). If hypothyroidism is suspected, it should be treated with i.v. T_3.

Clues to the presence of hypothyroidism include previous radioiodine treatment or surgery for thyrotoxicosis, and preceding symptoms of hypothyroidism (p. 620). Hypothermia may protect organs from ischaemia in patients

---

 Emergency Box 14.5

Management of hypothermia

Investigations

- Arterial blood gases
- Full blood count, urea and electrolytes, blood glucose, thyroid function tests, blood cultures
- Chest X-ray, ECG

Management

- Give oxygen by face mask and attach an ECG monitor
- Search for and treat infection; pneumonia is common
- Intubate and ventilate patients who are comatose or in respiratory failure
- Warmed (37°C) i.v. fluids to achieve urine output 30–40 mL/h
- Passive external warming if core temperature >32°C
  - Place patient in a warm room (27–29°C)
  - 'Space' blankets
  - Warm bath water
- Active external rewarming if core temperature 28–32°C
  - Warm blankets, heating pads or forced warm air
  - Rewarm trunk *before* extremities to minimize peripheral vasodilatation
  - Warm bath water
- Active internal rewarming if core temperature <28°C
  - Humidified and warmed (40–46°C) oxygen
  - Lavage (gastric, peritoneal, bladder) with warm fluids (40°C)
  - Extracorporeal shunt (haemodialysis, arteriovenous or venovenous) rewarming
  - Cardiopulmonary bypass – treatment of choice for arrested hypothermic patients
- Monitor core temperature, oxygen saturation by pulse oximetry, urine output and central venous pressure

ECG, electrocardiogram.

with prolonged hypothermia-induced cardiopulmonary arrest. Therefore resuscitation should be continued (maybe for some hours) until arrest persists after rewarming or until attempts to raise the core temperature have failed. Drugs used in the usual arrest situation, e.g. adrenaline (epinephrine), have reduced efficacy at low temperatures and are withheld until the temperature is greater than 30°C.

Hyperthermia (hyperpyrexia)

Hyperpyrexia is a body temperature above 41°C. Causes include:

- Injury to the hypothalamus (trauma, surgery, infection)
- Malignant hyperpyrexia – rare autosomal dominant condition in which skeletal muscle generates heat in the presence of certain anaesthetic drugs, e.g. suxamethonium
- Ingestion of 3,4-methylenedioxy-methamfetamine (Ecstasy)
- Neuroleptic malignant syndrome: idiosyncratic reaction to therapeutic dose of neuroleptic medication, e.g. phenothiazines.

Treatment includes stopping the offending drug, cooling and the administration of dantrolene sodium.

THERAPEUTICS

Thyroid hormones

Mechanism of action
Synthetic thyroxine.

Indications
Hypothyroidism, diffuse non-toxic goitre, thyroid carcinoma.

Preparations and dose
Levothyroxine sodium (thyroxine) *Tablets: 25 μg, 50 μg, 100 μg.*

1.6 μg/kg/day body weight (100–125 μg for an average-sized adult); 25 μg/day in elderly or those with ischaemic heart disease increased in steps of 25–50 μg every 3–6 weeks until the serum TSH values return to the reference range.

Side effects
These usually occur at excessive dosage and at the start of therapy with rapid increase in metabolism: arrhythmias, palpitations, skeletal muscle cramps and weakness, vomiting, diarrhoea, tremors, restlessness, headache, flushing, sweating, fever, excessive loss of weight and, sometimes, anginal pain where there is latent myocardial ischaemia.

Cautions/contraindications

Panhypopituitarism or predisposition to adrenal insufficiency from other causes (initiate corticosteroid therapy before starting levothyroxine), lower starting dose in the elderly or cardiovascular disease, diabetes mellitus (dosage increase may be needed for antidiabetic drugs including insulin). Contraindicated in thyrotoxicosis unless with carbimazole (see below).

Antithyroid drugs

Mechanism of action

Interfere with synthesis of thyroid hormones.

Indications

Long-term management of thyrotoxicosis and to prepare patients for thyroidectomy. May be given with propranolol, 40 mg three times daily, for initial symptom control.

Preparations and dose

Carbimazole *Tablets: 5 mg, 20 mg.*

Most commonly used drug for thyrotoxicosis in the UK. Initial treatment 15–40 mg daily; higher doses required in severe disease. This dose is continued until the patient becomes euthyroid, usually after 4–8 weeks, and the dose is then gradually reduced over 6–24 months to a maintenance dose of 5–15 mg daily. A combination of carbimazole, 40–60 mg daily with levothyroxine 50–150 µg daily, is sometimes used in a *blocking–replacement regimen* (not in pregnancy).

Propylthiouracil *Tablets: 50 mg.*

Dosing schedule is as for carbimazole, but initial treatment is 200–400 mg daily and the maintenance dose is 50–150 mg daily.

Side effects

Bone marrow suppression, particularly with carbimazole; patients should be asked to report symptoms and signs suggestive of infection, especially sore throat. A white cell count should be performed if there is any clinical evidence of infection, and treatment should be stopped immediately if there is clinical or laboratory evidence of neutropenia. Nausea, gastrointestinal disturbance, headache, rashes and pruritus occur with carbimazole; cutaneous vasculitis, hepatic necrosis, nephritis and lupus-like syndrome occur with propylthiouracil.

Cautions/contraindications

Liver disorders; overtreatment can result in rapid development of hypothyroidism.

Corticosteroids

Mechanism of action

Replacement therapy The adrenal cortex normally secretes hydrocortisone (cortisol), which has glucocorticoid activity and weak mineralocorticoid activity.

It also secretes the mineralocorticoid aldosterone. In *primary adrenal insufficiency*, physiological replacement is best achieved with a combination of hydrocortisone and the mineralocorticoid fludrocortisone; hydrocortisone alone does not usually provide sufficient mineralocorticoid activity for complete replacement. In *hypopituitarism* glucocorticoids are given but aldosterone is not necessary, as production is regulated by the renin–angiotensin system.

Anti-inflammatory actions include induction of the synthesis of IκB, an inhibitory protein which binds NF-κB.

Indications

- A wide variety of inflammatory conditions of the joints, lungs, skin and bowel, acute transplant rejection, autoimmune conditions, nephritic/nephrotic syndrome (particularly in children), cerebral oedema, acute hypersensitivity reactions such as angio-oedema of the upper respiratory tract and anaphylactic shock

- For replacement therapy in adrenal insufficiency and hypopituitarism.

The type of steroid preparation used depends on the indication, e.g. dexamethasone is a very potent steroid with insignificant mineralocorticoid activity (see Table 14.19; p. 665) and this makes it particularly suitable for high-dose therapy in conditions where fluid retention (mineralocorticoid side effect) would be a disadvantage, e.g. cerebral oedema. Prednisolone has predominantly glucocorticoid activity and is the corticosteroid most commonly used by mouth for long-term disease suppression. The relatively high mineralocorticoid activity of cortisone and hydrocortisone, and the resulting fluid retention, make them unsuitable for disease suppression on a long-term basis. Hydrocortisone is used for adrenal replacement therapy and intravenously in the emergency management of some conditions, e.g. severe ulcerative colitis, anaphylactic shock. Corticosteroids are also used by inhalation in asthma, by rectal administration in inflammatory bowel disease and topically in the treatment of inflammatory conditions of the skin. These preparations are not discussed in this section.

Preparations and dose

The equivalent anti-inflammatory doses of corticosteroids and their mineralocorticoid activity are shown in Table 14.19.

Prednisolone *Tablets: 1 mg, 5 mg, 25 mg. Soluble tablets: 5 mg. Enteric-coated tablets: 2.5 mg, 5 mg.*

Oral Usual treatment dose, initially 10–40 mg daily, up to 60 mg in severe disease as a single dose after breakfast. Maintenance dose is usually 2.5–15 mg.

Hydrocortisone *Tablets: 10 mg, 20 mg. Injection: 100 mg powder for reconstitution.*

Oral Replacement therapy: 20–30 mg daily in divided doses.

IV/IM 100–500 mg, three to four times daily or as required, by a slow bolus or as an infusion in sodium chloride 0.9% or glucose 5%.

Table 14.19 Equivalent anti-inflammatory doses of corticosteroids

Corticosteroid	Mineralocorticoid activity
Prednisolone 5 mg	Slight
= Betamethasone 750 µg	Negligible
= Cortisone acetate 25 mg	High
= Deflazacort 6 mg	Slight
= Dexamethasone 750 µg	Negligible
= Hydrocortisone 20 mg	High
= Methylprednisolone 4 mg	Slight
= Triamcinolone 4 mg	Slight

Dexamethasone Tablets: 500 µg, 2 mg. Oral solution: 2 mg/5 mL. Injection: 4 mg/mL, 24 mg/5 mL.

Oral 0.5–10 mg daily in divided doses.

IV/IM Initially 0.5–20 mg daily in divided doses; i.v. injection must be given over at least 3–5 minutes or as an infusion in sodium chloride 0.9% or glucose 5%.

Methylprednisolone Tablets: 2 mg, 4 mg, 16 mg, 100 mg. Injection: 40 mg, 125 mg, 500 mg, 1 g, 2 g vial.

Oral Usual range 2–40 mg daily.

IV/IM Initially 10–500 mg daily; dose depends on condition. Slow i.v. injection or infusion.

Side effects

Glucocorticoid side effects include diabetes and osteoporosis (p. 642; Table 14.10). Precautions for patients taking prolonged therapy with corticosteroids are discussed on page 641. *Mineralocorticoid* side effects include hypertension, sodium and water retention and potassium loss.

Cautions/contraindications

Untreated systemic infection; avoid live virus vaccines in those receiving immunosuppressive doses.

15 Diabetes mellitus and other disorders of metabolism

DIABETES MELLITUS

Glucose metabolism

Blood glucose levels are closely regulated in health and rarely stray outside the range of 3.5–8.0 mmol/L (63–144 mg/dL), despite the varying demands of food, fasting and exercise. The principal organ of glucose homeostasis is the liver, which absorbs and stores glucose (as glycogen) in the post-absorptive state and releases it into the circulation between meals to match the rate of glucose utilization by peripheral tissues. The liver also combines 3-carbon molecules derived from breakdown of fat (glycerol), muscle glycogen (lactate) and protein (e.g. alanine) into the 6-carbon glucose molecule by the process of gluconeogenesis. Insulin is the key hormone involved in the storage of nutrients, in the form of glycogen in liver and muscle, and triglyceride in fat. During a meal, insulin (derived from proinsulin after splitting off C-peptide) is released from the beta (β) cells of the pancreatic islets into the portal vein and facilitates glucose uptake by fat and muscle and suppresses glucose production by the liver. In the fasting state, insulin concentrations are low and its main action is to modulate glucose production from the liver. The counter-regulatory hormones – glucagon, adrenaline (epinephrine), cortisol and growth hormone – oppose the actions of insulin and cause greater production of glucose from the liver and less utilization of glucose in fat and muscle for a given plasma level of insulin.

Classification of diabetes

Diabetes mellitus is a common group of metabolic disorders that is characterized by chronic hyperglycaemia resulting from relative insulin deficiency, insulin resistance or both. Diabetes is usually primary, but may be secondary to other conditions, which include pancreatic (e.g. total pancreatectomy, chronic pancreatitis, haemochromatosis) and endocrine diseases (e.g. acromegaly and Cushing's syndrome). It may also be drug induced, most commonly by corticosteroids and thiazide diuretics.

Primary diabetes is divided into type 1 and type 2 diabetes. In practice the two diseases are a spectrum, distinct at the two ends but overlapping in the middle (Table 15.1). At one end of the spectrum the type 1 diabetic is young, has insulin deficiency with no resistance and immunogenic markers. Type 1 diabetes is most prevalent in Northern European countries, particularly Finland, and the incidence is increasing in most populations, particularly in young

Table 15.1 The spectrum of diabetes: a comparison of type 1 and type 2 diabetes mellitus

	Type 1	Type 2
Age	Younger (usually <30 years of age)	Older (usually >30 years of age)
Weight	Usually lean	Often overweight
Higher risk ethnicity	North European	All racial groups; more common in African, Asian, Polynesian and American-Indian
Onset	Days to weeks	Months to years
Heredity	HLA-DR3 or DR4 in >90%	No HLA links
	30–50% concordance in identical twins	50% concordance in identical twins
Pathogenesis	Autoimmune disease	No immune disturbance
Clinical	Insulin deficiency	Partial insulin deficiency Insulin resistance
	May develop ketoacidosis	May develop hyperosmolar state
	Always need insulin	Sometimes need insulin
Biochemical	Eventual disappearance of C-peptide	C-peptide persists

HLA, human leucocyte antigen.

children. Type 2 diabetes is common in all populations enjoying an affluent lifestyle and is also increasing in frequency, particularly in adolescents.

Aetiology and pathogenesis

Type 1 diabetes mellitus results from an autoimmune destruction of the pancreatic β cells. This process occurs in genetically susceptible individuals and is probably triggered by one or more environmental antigens. Autoantibodies directed against insulin and islet cell antigens (e.g. glutamic acid decarboxylase) predate the onset of clinical disease by several years. There is an association with other organ-specific autoimmune diseases, e.g. autoimmune thyroid disease, Addison's disease and pernicious anaemia.

Type 2 diabetes mellitus is a polygenic disorder; the genes responsible for the majority of cases have yet to be identified. However, the genetic causes of some of the rare forms of type 2 diabetes have been identified and include mutations of the insulin receptor and structural alterations of the insulin molecule. Environmental factors, notably central obesity, trigger the disease in genetically susceptible individuals. The β-cell mass is reduced to about 50% of normal at the time of diagnosis in type 2 diabetes. Hyperglycaemia is the result of reduced insulin secretion (inappropriately low for the glucose level) and peripheral insulin resistance.

Clinical features

- *Acute presentation*. Young people present with a 2–6-week history of thirst, polyuria and weight loss. Polyuria is the result of an osmotic diuresis that occurs when blood glucose levels exceed the renal tubular reabsorptive capacity (the renal threshold). Fluid and electrolyte losses stimulate thirst. Weight loss is caused by fluid depletion and breakdown of fat and muscle secondary to insulin deficiency. Ketoacidosis (p. 677) is the presenting feature if these early symptoms are not recognized and treated.
- *Subacute presentation*. Older patients may present with the same symptoms, although less marked and extending over several months. They may also complain of lack of energy, visual problems and pruritus vulvae or balanitis due to *Candida* infection.
- *With complications,* e.g. retinopathy, noted during a visit to the optician (p. 682).
- *In asymptomatic individuals* diagnosed at routine medical examinations, e.g. for insurance purposes.

Investigations

The diagnosis of diabetes mellitus is made by demonstrating:
- Fasting (no calorie intake for at least 8 hours) plasma glucose ≥7.0 mmol/L (126 mg/dL)
- Random plasma glucose ≥11.1 mmol/L (200 mg/dL)
- One abnormal laboratory value is diagnostic in a patient with typical hyperglycaemic symptoms; two values are needed in asymptomatic people.

A glucose tolerance test (GTT, Table 15.2) is hardly ever used for clinical purposes except for screening for gestational diabetes when a random blood glucose is ≥7.0 mmol/L. It is mainly used for epidemiological studies. Glycosuria does not necessarily indicate diabetes and may be found in normoglycaemic subjects who have a low renal threshold for glucose excretion.

Glycosylated haemoglobin (HbA$_{1c}$) is an integrated measure of an individual's prevailing blood glucose concentration over several weeks. Standardization of this measure has enabled it to be proposed as an alternative diagnostic test for diabetes by the American Diabetes Association (ADA) and World Health Organization (WHO). As currently proposed, an HbA1c result of 48 mmol/mol or above would be considered diagnostic of diabetes.

Table 15.2 The oral glucose tolerance test – WHO criteria

	Fasting glucose	2 hours after glucose
Normal	≤6.0 mmol/L	<7.8 mmol/L
Diabetes mellitus	≥7.0 mmol/L	≥11.1 mmol/L
Impaired fasting glucose (IFG)	6.1–6.9 mmol/l	—
Impaired glucose tolerance (IGT)	<7.0	7.8–11.0 mmol/L

WHO, World Health Organization.
After an overnight fast, 75 g of glucose is taken in 300 mL of water. Blood samples are taken before and 2 hours after the glucose has been given. Results are for venous plasma – whole blood values are lower.

Other routine investigations at diagnosis include screening the urine for microalbuminuria (p. 683), full blood count, serum urea and electrolytes, liver biochemistry, and a fasting blood sample for cholesterol and triglyceride levels.

Impaired glucose tolerance

Impaired glucose tolerance (IGT) is not a clinical entity but a risk factor for future diabetes and cardiovascular disease. Obesity and lack of regular physical exercise make progression to frank diabetes more likely.

Management

A multidisciplinary approach – involving, among others, the hospital doctor, the general practitioner, nurse specialists, dieticians and podiatrists – is necessary in the management of this condition. It is essential that the patient understands the risks of diabetes, the potential benefits of good glycaemic control and the importance of maintaining a lean weight, stopping smoking and taking care of the feet. Education at diagnosis is the key to developing patient self-management with ongoing input from the healthcare professionals involved with care.

Management involves:

- Achieving good glycaemic control
- Advice regarding regular physical activity and reduction of body weight in the obese, both of which improve glycaemic control in type 2 diabetes
- Aggressive treatment of hypertension and hyperlipidaemia, both of which are additional risk factors for long-term complications of diabetes
- Regular checks of metabolic control and physical examination for evidence of diabetic complications (Table 15.3).

Table 15.3 Regular checks for patients with diabetes

Checked each visit

Review of monitoring results and current treatment
Review of hypoglycaemic episodes if on insulin or sulfonylurea
Talk about targets and change where necessary
Talk about any general or specific problems
Continued education

Checked at least once a year

Biochemical assessment of metabolic control (e.g. glycosylated haemoglobin test)
Measure body weight
Measure blood pressure
Measure plasma lipids (except in extreme old age)
Measure visual acuity
Examine state of retina (ophthalmoscope or retinal photo)
Test urine for proteinuria/microalbuminuria
Test blood for renal function (creatinine)
Check condition of feet, pulses and neurology
Review cardiovascular risk factors
Review self-monitoring and injection techniques
Review eating habits
Review and reinforce structured education

Discussed as needed

Driving, travel, contraception, family planning, erectile dysfunction

Principles of treatment

All patients with diabetes require diet therapy. Regular exercise is encouraged to control weight and reduce cardiovascular risk. Insulin is always indicated in a patient who presents in ketoacidosis, and is often indicated in those under 40 years of age. Insulin is also indicated in other patients who do not achieve satisfactory control with oral hypoglycaemics. Treatment of type 2 diabetes is summarized in Fig. 15.1.

Diet The diet for people with diabetes is no different from the normal healthy diet recommended for the rest of the population. Recommended food:

- Low in sugar (though not sugar-free).
- High in starchy carbohydrate (especially foods with a low glycaemic index, e.g. pasta, which is slowly absorbed and prevents rapid fluctuations in blood glucose). Carbohydrate should represent about 40–60% of total energy intake.
- Substitute artificial sweeteners instead of sugar, and limit intake of fruit juices, confectionary, cakes and biscuits.

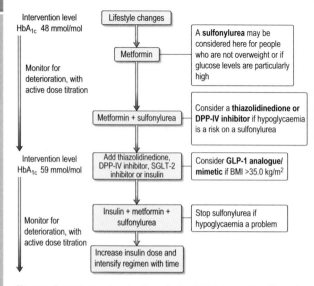

Fig. 15.1 Suggested treatment pathway for type 2 diabetes mellitus. Discussion of lifestyle changes and compliance should be undertaken at every stage. All patients require blood pressure control, statin therapy and low-dose aspirin. BMI, body mass index; HbA$_{1c}$, glycosylated haemoglobin.

- Low in fat (especially saturated fat), which should represent less than 35% of total energy intake.
- Include protein, representing about 15% of total energy intake (1 g per kg ideal body weight).

The nutrient load should be spread throughout the day (three main meals with snacks in between and at bedtime), which reduces swings in blood glucose. The overweight or obese individual should be encouraged to lose weight by a combination of changes in food intake and physical activity.

Tablet treatments for type 2 diabetes These are used in association with diet and lifestyle changes when this alone has failed to control hyperglycaemia (Fig. 15.1):

- *Biguanide.* Metformin is the only biguanide available (p. 698). It reduces glucose production by the liver and sensitizes target tissues to insulin. It is usually the first-line treatment in patients who have not achieved optimal glucose control with diet alone, particularly in overweight patients (unlike the sulfonylureas, appetite is not increased). It is the only oral agent shown to reduce cardiovascular risk in diabetes. Metformin is also used in combination treatment when single-agent use has failed to control diabetes.

Side effects include anorexia and diarrhoea. Lactic acidosis has occurred in patients with severe heart failure, liver disease or renal disease (serum creatinine > 150 µmol/L), in whom its use is contraindicated. It is not associated with either hypoglycaemia or weight gain.

- *Sulfonylureas* (p. 673) promote insulin secretion. Glibenclamide is best avoided in renal failure and in the elderly because of its relatively long duration of action (12–20 hours) and renal excretion. Gliclazide and glipizide are the most commonly used sulfonylureas in the UK. The most common side effects of the sulfonylureas are hypoglycaemia, which may be prolonged, and weight gain. Meglitinides, e.g. repaglinide and nateglinide, are also insulin secretagogues. They have a rapid onset of action and short duration of action and are administered shortly before each main meal.

- *Thiazolidinediones* ('glitazones'), e.g. pioglitazone, bind to and activate peroxisome proliferator-activated receptor-gamma (PPAR-γ), a nuclear receptor which regulates large numbers of genes including those involved in lipid metabolism and insulin action. They reduce hepatic glucose production and enhance peripheral glucose uptake. They are used alone or in combination with other agents. Side effects are weight gain, fluid retention and heart failure, anaemia and osteoporosis. They are contraindicated in patients with heart failure and there is a possible increase in the risk of bladder cancer.

- *Incretins* are agents that mimic the effect of two intestinal peptide hormones, glucose-dependent insulinotropic peptide (GIP) and glucagon-like peptide-1 (GLP-1), which are released from the intestine in response to eating. The actions of GLP-1 include promotion of insulin release, inhibition of glucagon release, prolongation of gastric emptying and a reduction in hunger mediated by receptors in the brain. These combined effects result in a decrease in body weight. Exenatide, liraglutide and lixisenatide are long-acting GLP-1 analogues given by subcutaneous injection and are used as an alternative to insulin, particularly in the overweight. The gliptins (e.g. sitagliptin, saxagliptin) inhibit dipeptidyl peptidase 4, the enzyme which inactivates GLP-1, and thus potentiates the effects of endogenous GLP-1. They have a moderate blood glucose-lowering effect and are weight neutral.

- *SGLT2 inhibitors* block the sodium/glucose transporter 2 (SGLT2), which is a sodium-dependent glucose transport protein (located in the proximal renal tubules), the function of which is to re-absorb glucose from the renal filtrate and restore it to the circulation. Its activity determines the renal threshold for glucose excretion (approximately 10 mmol/L). Specific inhibitors for this transporter increase excretion of glucose in the urine. This has the effect of removing both glucose and calories from the circulation. They are therefore associated with weight loss. Small reductions in systolic blood pressure have also been reported. Three members of this class are currently on the market: dapagliflozin, canagliflozin and empagliflozin. Side effects include an increase in genital candidiasis and urinary tract infections. This approach to therapy has the potential advantage of lowering glucose by a mechanism not mediated by insulin, but long-term safety and outcome data are not as yet available.

- *Other therapies:*
  - Acarbose inhibits intestinal α-glucosidases, impairs carbohydrate digestion and slows glucose absorption. Gastrointestinal side effects, e.g. flatulence, bloating and diarrhoea, are common and limit the dose and acceptability of this treatment.
  - Weight loss is associated with improved glycaemic control and even remission of diabetes. Orlistat is an intestinal lipase inhibitor and reduces the absorption of fat from the diet. It promotes weight loss in patients under careful dietary supervision on a low-fat diet. Gastric banding and gastric bypass surgery should be offered to those with marked obesity unresponsive to 6 months of intensive attempts at dieting and graded exercise.

Insulin treatment Almost all insulin now used in developed countries is synthetic (recombinant) human insulin. Insulin is administered by an injection into the fat below the skin (subcutaneous) on the abdomen, thighs or upper arm. The injection site should be changed frequently to prevent areas of lipohypertrophy (fatty lumps). Patients who are started on insulin have a legal duty to inform the Driver and Vehicle Licensing Agency (DVLA). In addition, those who experience complications of insulin such as frequent hypoglycaemic episodes or impaired awareness of hypoglycaemia may be unfit to drive.

There are three main types of insulin:

1. *Short-acting (soluble) insulins* start working within 30–60 minutes and last for 4–6 hours. They are given 15–30 minutes before meals in patients on multiple-dose regimens and by continuous intravenous infusion in labour, during medical emergencies, at the time of surgery and in patients using insulin pumps.

2. *Short-acting insulin analogues.* The human insulin analogues (insulin aspart, insulin lispro, insulin glulisine) have a faster onset and shorter duration of action than soluble insulin. They have a reduced carry-over effect compared to soluble insulin and are routinely used in type 1 diabetes. A *Cochrane Review* found little evidence of benefit in type 2 diabetes.

3. *Longer-acting insulins.* Insulins premixed with retarding agents (either protamine or zinc) are intermediate (12–24 hours) or long acting (more than 24 hours). The protamine insulins are also known as isophane or Neutral Protamine Hagedorn (NPH) insulins. Long-acting analogues are structurally modified. Insulin glargine precipitates in tissues and is then slowly released from the injection site. Insulin detemir binds to albumin, and its slow dissociation from the bound state prolongs its duration of action. Insulin degludec is a newer insulin analogue which is non-inferior to insulin glargine, with a small reduction in nocturnal hypoglycaemia. These insulins are much more expensive but have only a modest advantage over human

NPH, especially in the management of type 2 diabetes, although they are useful in those on intensified therapy or with troublesome hypoglycaemia.

In young patients, it is common practice to employ insulin in a basal bolus regimen, with one or two subcutaneous injections of an intermediate or long-acting insulin a day (the basal component) and a bolus of rapid-acting insulin with meals and substantial snacks. This will often involve teaching the person with diabetes to count their carbohydrate intake and administer insulin accordingly, with 1 unit for every 10 g of carbohydrate as a starting dose. In many patients who present acutely with diabetes there is some recovery of endogenous insulin secretion soon after diagnosis ('the honeymoon period') and the insulin dose may need to be reduced. Requirements rise thereafter. Target blood values should normally be 4–7 mmol/L before meals and 4–10 mmol/L after meals. An alternative to multiple injections is to use a small pump strapped to the waist, which delivers a continuous subcutaneous insulin infusion (CSII). Meal-time boluses are delivered when the patient presses a button on the pump.

In many patients with type 2 diabetes who eventually require insulin, a twice-daily regimen of premixed rapid and intermediate or long-acting insulin is suitable.

Complications of insulin therapy

- *Hypoglycaemia* is the most common complication of insulin treatment (see below)
- *At the injection site* – lipohypertrophy p. 674), local allergic reactions and rarely injection site abscesses
- *Insulin resistance* – most commonly mild and associated with obesity
- *Weight gain* – insulin makes patients feel hungry, and it is essential that they maintain a careful dietary regimen to prevent weight gain.

Hypoglycaemia This is a common complication of insulin therapy but may also occur with sulfonylurea therapy. Alcohol excess is one of the factors that can increase the risk of hypoglycaemia.

Symptoms of sympathetic overactivity usually develop when blood glucose levels fall below 3.0 mmol/L and include hunger, sweating, pallor and tachycardia. Untreated, neuroglycopenic symptoms, such as confusion, develop and later there is personality change, there are fits, occasionally hemiparesis and, finally, coma. Severe hypoglycaemia is defined by the need for external assistance, so it would include any episode where parenteral treatment is needed or where there is loss of consciousness or a seizure. However, if the person developing hypoglycaemia is too confused to either identify or self-treat the episode, it is still considered severe, even if oral treatment is used. In patients with long-standing diabetes the early 'adrenergic features' may be absent and as a result patients can develop severe hypoglycaemia without warning. Complete hypoglycaemia unawareness or more than one severe episode of severe hypoglycaemia requires the patient to inform the DVLA and stop driving.

A blood glucose confirms the diagnosis, but treatment should begin immediately (while waiting for the result) if hypoglycaemia is suspected on clinical grounds. A rapidly absorbed carbohydrate, e.g. 50–100 mL fizzy non-diet drink (e.g. lemonade or cola) or GlucoGel (40% dextrose gel) should be given orally if possible. In unconscious patients, treatment is with intravenous dextrose (50 mL of 20% dextrose into a large vein though a large-gauge needle) followed by a flush of normal saline, as concentrated dextrose is highly irritant. Intramuscular glucagon (1 mg) acts rapidly by mobilizing hepatic glycogen and is particularly useful where intravenous access is difficult. Oral glucose is given to replenish glycogen reserves once the patient revives. Hypoglycaemia may recur after treatment, particularly if it is a result of treatment with long-acting insulin preparations or sulfonylureas. These patients should be monitored with hourly (4-hourly when stable) blood glucose readings and may require a 10% dextrose infusion to prevent recurrent hypoglycaemia.

Whole pancreas and pancreatic islet transplantation

Whole pancreas transplantation is sometimes performed, usually in diabetic patients who require immunosuppression for a kidney transplant. Lasting graft function can be achieved, but the procedure adds to the risks of renal transplantation. Islet transplantation is also performed by harvesting pancreatic islets from cadavers and injecting these into the portal vein: these then seed themselves into the liver. At present, the main indication for islet cell transplants is disabling hypoglycaemia, as the majority of patients do not maintain long-term insulin independence as a result of this procedure.

Measuring the metabolic control of diabetes

Patients may feel well and be asymptomatic even if their blood glucose is consistently above the normal range. Self-monitoring at home is therefore necessary because of the immediate risks of hyper- and hypoglycaemia, and because it has been shown that persistently good control (i.e. near normoglycaemia) reduces the risk of progression to retinopathy, nephropathy and neuropathy in both type 1 and type 2 diabetes.

Home testing

- Most patients, especially those on insulin, are taught to monitor control by testing finger-prick blood samples with a glucose meter. Patients are asked to take regular profiles (e.g. four times daily samples) and to note these in a diary.
- Urine testing for glucose (using dipsticks) is a crude measure of glycaemic control because glycosuria only appears above the renal threshold for glucose (which varies between a blood glucose of 7 and 13 mmol/L).
- Urine or capillary ketones are useful if patients are unwell in order to alert them to the risk of ketoacidosis.

Hospital (clinic) testing
Single random blood glucose measurements are of limited value:

- HbA_{1c} is produced by the attachment of glucose to Hb. Measurement of this Hb fraction (expressed as millimoles per mole of haemoglobin without glucose attached) is a useful measure of the average glucose concentration over the life of the Hb molecule (8–12 weeks). The non-diabetic reference range is 20–42 mmol/mol. The target value for a diabetic patient is HbA_{1c} of 48–59 mmol/mol. Pursuing lower HbA_{1c} values risks hypoglycaemia, curtailing quality of life in the effort to achieve the target.

- Glycosylated plasma proteins (fructosamine) are less reliable than HbA_{1c} but may be useful in certain situations: e.g. thalassaemia, where haemoglobin is abnormal.

DIABETIC METABOLIC EMERGENCIES

Diabetic ketoacidosis

Diabetic ketoacidosis (DKA) results from insulin deficiency and is seen in the following circumstances:

- Previously undiagnosed diabetes
- Interruption of insulin therapy
- The stress of intercurrent illness (e.g. infection or surgery).

Most cases of DKA are preventable. The most common error is for insulin to be reduced or stopped because the patient is not eating or is vomiting. *Insulin should never be stopped in type 1 diabetes,* and most patients need a larger dose when ill.

Pathogenesis

Ketoacidosis is a state of uncontrolled catabolism associated with insulin deficiency. In the absence of insulin there is an unrestrained increase in hepatic gluconeogenesis. High circulating glucose levels result in an osmotic diuresis by the kidneys and consequent dehydration. In addition, peripheral lipolysis leads to an increase in circulating free fatty acids, which are converted within the liver to acidic ketones, leading to a metabolic acidosis. These processes are accelerated by the 'stress hormones' – catecholamines, glucagon and cortisol – which are secreted in response to dehydration and intercurrent illness.

Clinical features

There is profound dehydration secondary to water and electrolyte loss from the kidney and exacerbated by vomiting. The eyes are sunken, tissue turgor is reduced, the tongue is dry and, in severe cases, the blood pressure is low. Kussmaul's respiration (deep rapid breathing) may be present, as a sign of respiratory compensation for metabolic acidosis, and the breath smells of ketones (similar to acetone). Some disturbance of consciousness is common, but only 5% present in coma. Body temperature is often subnormal despite intercurrent infection. A few patients have abdominal pain and, rarely, this may cause confusion with a surgical acute abdomen.

Investigations

The diagnosis is based on the demonstration of hyperglycaemia in combination with acidosis and ketosis:

- Hyperglycaemia – blood glucose >11 mmol/L.
- Ketonaemia – blood ketones >3.0 mmol/L. Blood ketones are best measured using a finger-prick sample and near-patient meter which measures β-hydroxybutyrate, the major ketone in DKA. If not available, plasma ketones can be semiquantitatively measured in the supernatant of a centrifuged blood sample using a dipstick that measures ketones.
- Acidosis – blood pH <7.3 and/or bicarbonate (HCO_3) <15 mmol/L. Venous blood gives similar pH and HCO_3 to arterial. Acidosis is high anion gap (p. 348).
- Urine dipstick testing shows heavy glycosuria and ketonuria.
- Serum urea and electrolytes. Urea and creatinine are often raised as a result of dehydration. The total body potassium is low as a result of osmotic diuresis, but the serum potassium concentration is often raised because of the absence of the action of insulin, which allows potassium to shift out of cells.
- Full blood count may show an elevated white cell count even in the absence of infection.
- Further investigations are directed towards identifying a precipitating cause: blood cultures, chest radiograph and urine microscopy and culture to look for evidence of infection, and an electrocardiogram (ECG) and cardiac proteins to look for evidence of myocardial infarction (MI).

Management

Immediate emergency management (ABCDE) is necessary in all patients. Admission to the intensive care unit is recommended in the seriously ill. The aims of treatment are to replace fluid and electrolyte loss (Table 15.4), replace insulin and restore acid–base balance over a period of about 24 hours (Emergency Box 15.1). Therapy of DKA shifts potassium into cells, resulting in profound hypokalaemia and death if not treated prospectively. Cerebral oedema (presents with headache, irritability, reduced conscious level) may complicate therapy and results from rapid lowering of blood glucose and

Table 15.4 Average loss of fluid and electrolytes in an adult with ketoacidosis

Water	5–7 L
Sodium	500 mmol
Potassium	350 mmol

✚ Emergency Box 15.1

Management of diabetic ketoacidosis

Phase I management

- Fluid replacement: 0.9% sodium chloride. An average regimen would be 1 L in 30 minutes, then 1 L in 1 hour, then 1 L in 2 hours, then 1 L in 4 hours, then 1 L in 6 hours.
- Insulin: soluble insulin by intravenous infusion. A typical starting dose would be 6 units/h (or 0.1 units/kg). Aim for fall in blood glucose of approx. 5 mmol/h.
- Add KCl to 0.9% sodium chloride depending on results of blood K measurement. Temporarily delay if serum potassium >5.0 mmol/L. Add 10 mmol/L if serum potassium is 3.5–5.0 mmol/l and 20 mmol if potassium is <3.5 mmol/L. Do not routinely administer at rate of >20 mmol/h.

IF:

- Blood pressure below 80 mmHg, give plasma expander (colloid, p. 331).
- If pH below 7.0, consider 500 mL of sodium bicarbonate 1.26% plus 10 mmol KCl over 1 hour. Bicarbonate should only be given under senior supervision and some guidelines do not advocate its use.

Phase 2 management

- When blood glucose falls to <14 mmol/L, reduce NaCl and add in 10% glucose with 20 mmol KCl at 100 mL/h. Continue insulin (necessary to switch off ketogenesis) with dose adjusted according to hourly blood glucose test results (e.g. i.v. 3 units/h glucose 15 mmol/L; 2 units/h when glucose 10 mmol/L).

Phase 3 management

- Once stable and able to eat and drink normally, transfer patient to four-times-daily s.c. insulin regimen (based on previous 24 hours insulin consumption, and trend in consumption). Overlap s.c. insulin with insulin infusion by 30 minutes.

Special measures

- Broad-spectrum antibiotic if infection likely
- Bladder catheter if no urine passed in 2 hours
- Nasogastric tube if drowsy or protracted vomiting
- Consider CVP monitoring if shocked or if previous cardiac or renal impairment.
- Consider s.c. prophylactic heparin in comatose, elderly or obese patients.

Monitoring

- Vital signs, volume of fluid given and urine output hourly
- Finger-prick glucose hourly for 8 hours
- Laboratory glucose and electrolytes 2-hourly for 8 hours, then 4–6 hourly, adjust K replacement according to results.

CVP, central venous pressure.

Note: The regimen of fluid replacement set out above is a guide for patients with severe ketoacidosis. Excessive fluid can precipitate pulmonary and cerebral oedema; adequate replacement must therefore be tailored to the individual and monitored carefully throughout treatment.

osmolality. When the patient has recovered, it is necessary to determine the cause of the episode and advice and information are provided to prevent recurrence.

Hyperosmolar hyperglycaemic state

This is a life-threatening emergency characterized by marked hyperglycaemia, hyperosmolality and mild or no ketosis. It is the metabolic emergency characteristic of uncontrolled type 2 diabetes mellitus (often previously undiagnosed). Infection is the most common precipitating cause, particularly pneumonia.

Clinical features

Endogenous insulin levels are reduced but are still sufficient to inhibit hepatic ketogenesis, whereas glucose production is unrestrained. Patients present with profound dehydration (secondary to an osmotic diuresis) and a decreased level of consciousness, which is directly related to the elevation of plasma osmolality. The main biochemical differences between ketoacidosis and the hyperosmolar hyperglycaemic state are illustrated in Table 15.5.

Management

Investigations and treatment are the same as for ketoacidosis, with the exception that a lower rate of insulin infusion (3 units/h) is often sufficient, as these patients are extremely sensitive to insulin. The rate may be doubled after 2–3 hours if glucose is falling too slowly. The hyperosmolar state predisposes to stroke, MI, or arterial thrombosis, and prophylactic subcutaneous heparin is given.

Table 15.5 Typical biochemistry in diabetic ketoacidosis and the hyperosmolar hyperglycaemic state illustrating the main differences

Examples of blood values	Severe ketoacidosis	Hyperosmolar hyperglycaemic state
Na^+ (mmol/L)	140	155
K^+ (mmol/L)	5	5
Cl^- (mmol/L)	100	110
HCO_3^- (mmol/L)	15	25
Urea (mmol/L)	8	15
Glucose (mmol/L)	30	≥ 50
Serum osmolality (mOsm/kg)*	328	385
Arterial pH	7.0	7.35

*See page 327 for definition and discussion of plasma osmolality.

Prognosis

Mortality rate is approximately 20–30%, mainly because of the advanced age of the patients and the frequency of intercurrent illness. Unlike ketoacidosis, the hyperosmolar hyperglycaemic state is not an absolute indication for subsequent insulin therapy, and survivors may do well on diet and oral agents.

Lactic acidosis

This is a rare complication in patients taking metformin; the mortality is high. Patients present with severe metabolic acidosis without significant hyperglycaemia or ketosis. Treatment is by rehydration and infusion of isotonic 1.26% bicarbonate.

COMPLICATIONS OF DIABETES

Patients with diabetes have a reduced life expectancy. Cardiovascular problems (70%), followed by chronic kidney disease (10%) and infections (6%), are the most common causes of premature death in treated patients. Complications are directly related to the degree and duration of hyperglycaemia and can be reduced by improved diabetic control.

Vascular

Macrovascular complications

Diabetes is a risk factor for atherosclerosis and this is additive with other risk factors for large vessel disease, e.g. smoking, hypertension and hyperlipidaemia. Atherosclerosis results in stroke, ischaemic heart disease and peripheral vascular disease. Intensive glucose lowering has a relatively minor effect upon cardiovascular risk and it is vital to tackle all cardiovascular risk factors together in diabetes, including aggressive control of blood pressure (target <130/80 mmHg), cessation of smoking, treatment with a statin for most type 2 diabetics irrespective of serum cholesterol, and treatment with an angiotensin-converting enzyme (ACE) inhibitor (ACEI) (or angiotensin II receptor antagonist in the event of ACEI intolerance, usually a cough) for patients with one other major cardiovascular risk factor. Some patients, depending on age and other cardiovascular risk factors, are also treated with low-dose aspirin.

Microvascular complications

In contrast to macrovascular disease, microvascular disease is specific to diabetes. Small vessels throughout the body are affected, but the disease process is of particular danger in three sites: the retina, the renal glomerulus and the nerve sheath. Diabetic retinopathy, nephropathy and neuropathy tend to manifest 10–20 years after diagnosis in young patients. They present earlier in older patients, probably because they have had unrecognized diabetes for months or even years before diagnosis.

Diabetic eye disease

About one-third of young people with diabetes develop visual problems, and in the UK 5% have become blind after 30 years of diabetes. However, the prevalence is falling. Diabetes affects the eye in a variety of ways:

- Diabetic retinopathy with lesions developing in the retina and the iris.
- Cataracts develop earlier in diabetics than in the general population. Temporary blurred vision also occurs caused by reversible osmotic changes in the lens in patients with acute hyperglycaemia.
- External ocular palsies – the sixth and third nerve are most commonly affected.

Retinopathy

Diabetes is the most common cause of blindness in people under 65 years old. At diagnosis almost 30% of people with diabetes have early retinal damage (background retinopathy) which increases as the duration of diabetes increases. Diabetic retinopathy is divided into two major forms: non-proliferative and proliferative, named for the absence or presence of abnormal new blood vessels (neovascularization) arising from the retina (Table 15.6 and Fig. 15.2). Proliferative retinopathy develops as a consequence of damage to retinal blood vessels and the resultant retinal ischaemia, which occurs in non-proliferative retinopathy. Most patients are asymptomatic until the late (and often untreatable) stages. Retinal screening programmes for people with diabetes perform annual assessment of visual acuity and digital retinal photography by trained staff. Patients with background retinopathy need an annual review only to look for progression to maculopathy or proliferative retinopathy. All other forms of retinopathy require referral to an ophthalmologist, urgently in the case of proliferative and advanced retinopathy, as vision is immediately threatened. New vessel formation and maculopathy are treated by laser photocoagulation of the retina. Anti-VEGF (vascular endothelial growth factor) drugs, such as bevacizumab and ranibizumab, are also being used to control diabetic maculopathy. Recent studies have shown benefit over laser for changes affecting the central macula and leading to sight loss. The development and progression of retinopathy is accelerated by poor glycaemic control, hypertension and smoking.

The diabetic kidney

The kidney may be damaged by diabetes as a result of:

- Glomerular disease
- Ischaemic renal lesions
- Ascending urinary tract infection.

Table 15.6 Classification of diabetic retinopathy

Retinopathy grade	Retinal abnormality (cause of abnormality)
Peripheral retina	
Non-proliferative/ background	Tiny red dots (capillary microaneurysms) Larger red spots (intraretinal 'blot' haemorrhages) *Hard exudates (capillary leaks of plasma rich in lipids and protein)
Pre-proliferative	Venous beading/loops Growth of intraretinal new vessels *Multiple cotton wool spots (oedema from retinal infarcts)
Proliferative	Preretinal new (fragile) blood vessel formation Preretinal or subhyaloid haemorrhage (from above) Vitreous haemorrhage
Advanced retinopathy	Retinal fibrosis Traction retinal detachment
Central retina	
Maculopathy	Macula oedema Perimacular hard exudates

NB: *Hard exudates have a bright yellowish white colour and are often irregular in outline with a sharply defined margin. Cotton-wool spots are greyish white, have indistinct margins and a dull matt surface, unlike the glossy appearance of hard exudates.

Diabetic nephropathies Clinical nephropathy secondary to glomerular disease usually manifests 15–25 years after diagnosis and affects 25–35% of patients diagnosed under the age of 30 years. On microscopy there is thickening of the glomerular basement membrane and later glomerulosclerosis, which may be a diffuse or nodular form (Kimmelstiel–Wilson lesion). The earliest clinical evidence of glomerular damage is 'microalbuminuria' – an increase above the normal range in urinary albumin excretion but undetectable by conventional dipsticks (p. 359). This may, after some years, progress to intermittent albuminuria followed by persistent proteinuria, sometimes with a frank nephrotic syndrome. At the stage of persistent proteinuria the plasma creatinine is normal but the average patient is only some 5–10 years from end-stage kidney disease.

The urine of all patients should be checked at least once a year by dipsticks for the presence of protein. Most centres also screen for microalbuminuria, because meticulous glycaemic control and treatment with ACEIs at this stage (even in the absence of hypertension) may delay the onset of frank proteinuria. Aggressive control of blood pressure (target below 130/80 mmHg) is the most important factor to reduce disease progression in

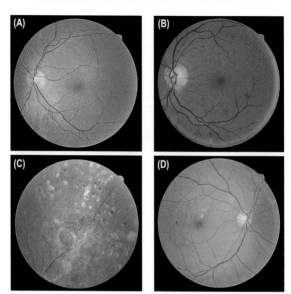

Fig. 15.2 Some features of diabetic eye disease. (A) The normal macula (centre) and optic disc. (B) Dot and blot haemorrhages (early background retinopathy). (C) Multiple frond-like new vessels, the hallmark of proliferative retinopathy. White fibrous tissue is forming near the new vessels, a feature of advanced retinopathy (this eye also illustrates multiple xenon arc laser burns superiorly). (D) Exudates appearing within a disc-width of the macula are a feature of an exudative maculopathy.

those with established proteinuria – ACEIs (or angiotensin receptor II antagonists for those intolerant) are the treatment of choice. Many patients will develop end-stage kidney disease and need dialysis and eventually renal transplantation. A segmental pancreatic graft is sometimes performed at the same time as a renal graft.

Ischaemic lesions Arteriolar lesions with hypertrophy and hyalinization of the vessels affect both afferent and efferent arterioles. The appearances are similar to those of hypertensive disease but are not necessarily related to the blood pressure in patients with diabetes.

Infective lesions Urinary tract infections are common (p. 372). A very rare complication is renal papillary necrosis, in which renal papillae are shed in the urine and may cause ureteral obstruction.

Diabetic neuropathy

The types of diabetic neuropathy are summarized in Table 15.7. Isolated mononeuropathies are thought to result from occlusion of the vasa nervorum (the

Table 15.7 Diabetic neuropathies

Progressive	Symmetrical sensory polyneuropathy
	Autonomic neuropathy
Reversible	Acute painful neuropathy

	Mononeuropathy and mononeuritis multiplex:
	   Cranial nerve lesions
	   Isolated peripheral nerve lesions

	Diabetic amyotrophy

small arteries that provide blood supply to the peripheral nerves), while the other more diffuse neuropathies may arise from accumulation of fructose and sorbitol (metabolized from glucose in peripheral nerves) that disrupts the structure and function of the nerve.

Symmetrical mainly sensory neuropathy This is the most common form of neuropathy and affects the feet first. It is often unrecognized by the patient in the early stages. Early clinical signs are loss of vibration sense, pain sensation (deep before superficial) and temperature sensation in the feet. At later stages, patients may complain of 'walking on cotton wool' and may lose their balance when walking in the dark or while washing the face due to impaired proprioception. Involvement of the hands is uncommon. Complications include unrecognized trauma, beginning as blistering caused by an ill-fitting shoe or a hot-water bottle, and leading to ulceration. Abnormal mechanical stress and repeated minor trauma, usually prevented by pain, may lead to the development of a neuropathic arthropathy (Charcot's joints) in the ankle and knee, where the joint is grossly deformed and swollen. Involvement of the motor nerves may lead to wasting of the small muscles of the hand and a distorted foot with a high arch and clawing of the toes. All patients with diabetic sensory neuropathy are at risk of insensitive foot ulceration. They should learn the principles of foot care and visit a chiropodist regularly.

Acute painful neuropathy The patient describes burning or crawling pains in the lower limbs. Symptoms are typically worse at night, and pressure from bedclothes may be intolerable. Treatment is with good diabetic control, duloxetine, tricyclic antidepressants, gabapentin or carbamazepine.

Mononeuritis and mononeuritis multiplex (multiple mononeuropathy) One or more individual nerves are affected, including involvement of a spinal root (radiculopathy). Onset may be abrupt and painful. Lesions are more likely to occur at common sites for external pressure, e.g. carpal tunnel syndrome. The most common cranial mononeuropathies are the third and sixth nerves supplying the extraocular muscles. Presentation is with unilateral pain, ptosis and diplopia, with sparing of pupillary function.

Diabetic amyotrophy presents with painful wasting, usually asymmetrical, of the quadriceps muscles. The wasting may be marked and knee reflexes are diminished or absent.

Autonomic neuropathy affects the cardiovascular system (resting tachycardia and loss of sinus arrhythmia, postural hypotension and peripheral vasodilation with a warm foot and bounding pulse), gastrointestinal tract (diarrhoea and gastroparesis leading to intractable vomiting), bladder (incomplete emptying followed by an atonic painless distended bladder) and male erectile dysfunction. There is no specific treatment, and management is based on a symptom approach.

The diabetic foot

Foot problems are a major cause of morbidity and mortality in patients with diabetes mellitus, with infection, ischaemia and neuropathy all contributing to produce tissue necrosis. On physical examination, evidence of a neuropathy is demonstrated by reduced sensation to vibration, temperature and pin-prick. There may be evidence of Charcot arthropathy. Signs of vascular disease in the lower leg include thin skin and absence of hair, bluish discoloration of the skin, reduced skin temperature and absent foot pulses. Many diabetic foot ulcers are avoidable, so patients need to learn the principles of foot care: well-fitting lace-up shoes, regular chiropody, no 'bathroom' surgery, daily inspection of feet and early advice for any damage, and finally avoiding sources of heat, such as radiators and hot bathwater. Management of foot lesions involves:

- Swabbing of ulcers for bacterial culture and early antibiotic treatment
- Good local wound care and, if necessary, surgical debridement of ulcers
- Evaluation for peripheral vascular disease by clinical examination, measurement of blood flow (by Doppler probe) and femoral angiography if clinically indicated
- Reconstructive vascular surgery for localized areas of arterial occlusion.

Infections

Poorly controlled diabetes impairs the function of polymorphonuclear leucocytes and confers an increased risk of infection, particularly of the urinary tract and skin, e.g. cellulitis, boils and abscesses. Tuberculosis and mucocutaneous candidiasis are more common in diabetic individuals. Infections may lead to loss of glycaemic control and are a common cause of ketoacidosis. Insulin-treated patients may need to increase their insulin therapy even if they feel nauseated and unable to eat. Non-insulin-treated patients may need insulin for the same reasons.

The skin

- Lipohypertrophy (fat lumps at frequently used insulin injection sites) are avoided by varying the injection site from day to day.
- Necrobiosis lipoidica diabeticorum is an unusual complication of diabetes characterized by erythematous plaques, often over the shins, which gradually develop a brown waxy discoloration.
- Vitiligo is symmetrical white patches seen in diabetes mellitus and other organ-specific autoimmune diseases.
- Granuloma annulare – flesh-coloured rings and nodules, principally over the extensor surfaces of the fingers.

SPECIAL SITUATIONS

Surgery

Diabetic patients should be screened in advance for complications (e.g. cardiovascular or renal disease, autonomic neuropathy) which increase the surgical risk. Smooth control of diabetes minimizes the risk of infection and balances the catabolic response to anaesthesia and surgery. Treatment should be intensified in poorly controlled diabetics (HbA$_{1c}$ >70 mmol/mol or random blood glucose >11 mmol/L) prior to surgery or patients admitted the night before for an insulin sliding scale if surgery is urgent, e.g. cancer. Where possible, diabetic patients should be first on the operating list and a blood glucose of 6–11 mmol/L maintained during the perioperative period. Hypoglycaemia developing perioperatively is treated as previously described (p. 675).

Major surgery (i.e. having a general anaesthetic)

- Normal subcutaneous insulin doses are given the day before surgery.
- On the day of surgery, omit morning insulin or oral hypoglycaemic (except stop metformin 24 hours before as risk of lactic acidosis). Non-insulin-treated patients with mild hyperglycaemia (fasting blood glucose below 8 mmol/L) can be treated as non-diabetic. Those with higher levels are managed in the same way as insulin-treated patients.
- Some units use a glucose/insulin/potassium infusion, starting at 08:00 with hourly glucose monitoring. A standard combination is 16 units of soluble insulin with 10 mmol of KCl in 500 mL of 10% glucose infused at 100 mL/h. Other units use a variable rate insulin infusion.
- The insulin dose is adjusted if blood sugars are persistently high or low and potassium is adjusted depending on serum measurements.

- Post-operatively, the infusion is maintained until the patient is eating and drinking normally. The normal insulin regimen is restarted with a 30-minute overlap with the infusion.

Minor surgery (e.g. endoscopy)

Insulin-treated patients On the day of surgery, omit morning insulin (unless long-acting insulin, in which case give two-thirds dose). Check blood glucose every 2 hours. Once the patient is eating and drinking after the procedure, give two-thirds of normal *morning* insulin (if twice-a-day regimen of insulin normally given) or normal dose of rapidly acting insulin (if four-times-a day regimen normally given) and teatime insulin as normal.

Tablet-controlled diabetes Omit diabetes medication on the morning of the procedure. Check blood glucose 2-hourly. Restart oral hypoglycaemics with first meal.

Pregnancy and diabetes

Poorly controlled diabetes at the time of conception and during pregnancy is associated with congenital malformations, macrosomia (large babies), hydramnios, pre-eclampsia and intrauterine death. In the neonatal period there is an increased risk of hyaline membrane disease and neonatal hypoglycaemia (unlike insulin, maternal glucose crosses the placenta and causes hypersecretion of insulin from the fetal islets, which continues when the umbilical cord is cut). Meticulous control of blood glucose levels (assessed by daily home blood testing before and 2 hours after meals) achieves results comparable to those with non-diabetic pregnancies.

Gestational diabetes is glucose intolerance that is first recognized during pregnancy; it is typically asymptomatic and usually remits following delivery. Treatment is with diet in the first instance, but patients usually require the addition of metformin or insulin during pregnancy. It is likely to recur in subsequent pregnancies, and diabetes may develop later in life.

Acutely ill hospital inpatients

Acutely ill diabetic patients are susceptible to hyperglycaemia because of increased release of counter-regulatory stress hormones (adrenaline, cortisol and growth hormone), physical inactivity and possibly an alteration in diet. Good glucose control reduces mortality in acute MI, stroke and critically ill patients on ICU. Metformin should not be given to an ill patient in hospital because of the risk of lactic acidosis. Patients who are not eating are managed with an insulin sliding scale (Table 15.8), with a target blood glucose of 4–9 mmol/L (4–7 mmol/L in stroke and MI).

Table 15.8 A sliding scale insulin regime*

Blood glucose (mmol/L)	Human Actrapid (units/hour)
<4	0.5
4.1–7	1
7.1–11	2
11.1–15	3
15.1–20	5
>20	6

*Add 50 units of human Actrapid to 49.5 mL of 0.9% sodium chloride in a syringe driver.
Give i.v. insulin as above, depending on hourly stix testing.
Fluid guide (assuming normal potassium and sodium) – if blood glucose >12 mmol/L,
give 1 L of 0.9% NaCl with 20 mmol KCL over 10 hours; if blood glucose <12 mmol/L,
give 1 L of 5% glucose with 20 mmol KCl over 10 hours. Use a separate cannula for
insulin and fluids. Patients in heart failure can be given 500 mL of 10% glucose over
10 hours.

Unstable diabetes

This is used to describe patients with recurrent ketoacidosis and/or recurrent
hypoglycaemic coma. Of these, the largest group consists of those who experience recurrent severe hypoglycaemia.

HYPOGLYCAEMIA IN THE NON-DIABETIC

The causes and mechanism of hypoglycaemia are listed in Table 15.9.

Insulinomas

These are rare pancreatic islet cell tumours (usually benign) that secrete insulin.
They may be part of the multiple endocrine neoplasia (MEN) syndrome (p. 649).

Clinical features

The classic presentation is with fasting hypoglycaemia. Hypoglycaemia produces symptoms as a result of neuroglycopenia and stimulation of the sympathetic nervous system. These include sweating, palpitations, diplopia and
weakness, progressing to confusion, abnormal behaviour, fits and coma.

Investigations

The diagnosis is made by demonstrating hypoglycaemia in association with
inappropriate or excessive insulin secretion:

Table 15.9 Causes and mechanisms of hypoglycaemia

Cause	Mechanism of hypoglycaemia
Drug induced: insulin, sulfonylureas, quinine, pentamidine, propranolol, salicylates in overdose	Variety of mechanisms
Islet cell tumour of the pancreas (insulinoma)	Inappropriately high circulating insulin levels
Non-pancreatic tumours, e.g. sarcoma, hepatoma	Secretion of IGF-1
Endocrine causes: Addison's disease	Impaired counter-regulation to the action of insulin
Fulminant liver failure	Failure of hepatic gluconeogenesis
End-stage kidney disease	Failure of renal cortical gluconeogenesis
Excess alcohol	Enhanced insulin response to carbohydrate
	Inhibition of hepatic gluconeogenesis
After gastric surgery	Rapid gastric emptying, mismatch of food and insulin
Factitious hypoglycaemia	Surreptitious self-administration of insulin or sulfonylureas, often in a non-diabetic

IGF-1, insulin-like growth factor 1: normally mainly produced by the liver, primarily a growth factor in physiological concentrations.

- Measurement of overnight fasting plasma glucose and insulin levels on three occasions
- Performing a prolonged 72-hour supervised fast if overnight testing is inconclusive and symptoms persist. Blood is taken at intervals for measurement of glucose, insulin and C-peptide.

A plasma insulin concentration of 3 μU/mL or more when the plasma glucose is below 3.0 mmol/L indicates an excess of insulin. C-peptide is co-secreted from the pancreas with insulin and is used to distinguish endogenous hyperinsulinaemia (e.g. as a result of an insulinoma or sulfonylurea overdose when C-peptide levels are detectable) from exogenous hyperinsulinaemia (e.g. due to factitious insulin administration when C-peptide levels are undetectable).

Further investigations are usually necessary to localize tumours before surgery as they are often very small. These include highly selective angiography, high-resolution computed tomography (CT) scanning, scanning with radiolabelled somatostatin (some tumours express somatostatin receptors) and endoscopic ultrasound.

Treatment

The treatment of choice is surgical excision of the tumour. Diazoxide, which inhibits insulin release from islet cells, is useful when the tumour is malignant, in patients in whom a tumour is very small and cannot be located, or in elderly patients with mild symptoms. Symptoms may also remit using a somatostatin analogue (octreotide or lanreotide).

DISORDERS OF LIPID METABOLISM

Lipids are insoluble in water, and are transported in the bloodstream as lipoprotein particles composed of lipids (principally triglycerides, cholesterol and cholesterol esters), surrounded by a coat of phospholipids. Proteins (called apoproteins) embedded into the phospholipid coating exert a stabilizing function and allow the particles to be recognized by receptors in the liver and peripheral tissues.

There are five principal types of lipoprotein particles:

- *Chylomicrons* are synthesized in the small intestine postprandially and serve to transport the digestion products of dietary fat (mainly triglycerides, small amounts of cholesterol) to the liver and peripheral tissues.
- *Very-low-density lipoproteins (VLDLs)* are synthesized and secreted by the liver and transport endogenously synthesized triglycerides (formed in the liver from plasma free fatty acids) to the periphery. In fat and muscle, triglycerides are removed from chylomicrons and VLDLs by the tissue enzyme lipoprotein lipase and the essential cofactor apoprotein C-II.
- *Intermediate-density lipoproteins (IDLs)*, derived from the peripheral breakdown of VLDLs, are transported back to the liver and metabolized to yield the cholesterol-rich particles – low-density lipoproteins (LDLs).
- *LDLs* deliver most cholesterol to the periphery and liver with subsequent binding to LDL receptors in these tissues.
- *High-density lipoproteins (HDLs)* transport cholesterol from peripheral tissues to the liver. HDL particles carry 20–30% of the total quantity of cholesterol in the blood.

The major clinical significance of hypercholesterolaemia (both total plasma and LDL concentration) is as a risk factor for atheroma and, hence, ischaemic heart disease. The risk is greatest in those with other cardiovascular risk factors, e.g. smoking and hypertension. There is a weak independent link between raised concentrations of (triglyceride-rich) VLDL particles and cardiovascular risk. More than half of all patients aged under 60 years with angiographically confirmed coronary heart disease have a lipoprotein disorder. Severe hypertriglyceridaemia (>6 mmol/L) is associated with a greatly increased risk of acute pancreatitis and retinal vein thrombosis. In contrast, HDL particles, which transport cholesterol away from the periphery, appear to protect against atheroma.

Measurement of plasma lipids

Most patients with hyperlipidaemia are asymptomatic, with no clinical signs, and they are discovered through routine screening (Table 15.10). A fasting blood sample is necessary to test for hypertriglyceridaemia; random is sufficient for cholesterol. If the total cholesterol concentration is raised, HDL cholesterol, triglyceride and LDL cholesterol should be measured on a fasting sample. Specific diagnosis of the defect (p. 693) requires the measurement of individual lipoproteins by electrophoresis, but this is not usually necessary. If a lipid disorder has been detected it is vital to carry out a clinical history, examination and simple special investigations (i.e. plasma glucose, urea and electrolytes, liver biochemistry and thyroid function tests) to detect the causes of secondary hyperlipidaemia (Table 15.11).

Table 15.10 Indications for measurement of plasma lipids

Family history of coronary heart disease (especially below 50 years of age)
First-degree relative with a lipid disorder
Prospective partner of patients with heterozygous monogenic lipid disorder (because of the risk of producing children with the disorder)
Presence of a xanthoma
Presence of xanthelasma or corneal arcus before age 40 years
Obesity
Diabetes mellitus
Hypertension
Acute pancreatitis
Patients undergoing renal replacement therapy

Table 15.11 Causes of secondary hyperlipidaemia

Hypothyroidism
Poorly controlled diabetes mellitus
Obesity
Renal impairment
Nephrotic syndrome
Dysglobulinaemia
Hepatic dysfunction
Drugs: oral contraceptives in susceptible individuals, retinoids, thiazide diuretics, corticosteroids

The primary hyperlipidaemias

Disorders of VLDL and chylomicrons – hypertriglyceridaemia alone

- Most cases of hypertriglyceridaemia are polygenic in origin i.e. many genes act together and interact with environmental factors to produce a modest elevation in serum triglyceride levels.
- Familial hypertriglyceridaemia is inherited in an autosomal dominant fashion. The exact defect is not known and the only clinical feature is a history of acute pancreatitis or retinal vein thrombosis in some individuals.
- Lipoprotein lipase deficiency and apoprotein C-II deficiency are rare diseases which usually present in childhood with severe hypertriglyceridaemia complicated by pancreatitis, retinal vein thrombosis and eruptive xanthomas – crops of small yellow lipid deposits in the skin.

Disorders of LDL – hypercholesterolaemia alone

- Familial hypercholesterolaemia is the result of underproduction of the LDL-cholesterol receptor in the liver, which results in high plasma concentrations of LDL-cholesterol. Heterozygotes may be asymptomatic or develop coronary artery disease in their 40s. Typical clinical features include tendon xanthomas (lipid nodules in the tendons, especially the extensor tendons of the fingers and the Achilles tendon) and xanthelasmas. Homozygotes have a total absence of LDL receptors in the liver. They have grossly elevated plasma cholesterol levels (>16 mmol/L) and, without treatment, die in their teens from coronary artery disease.
- Mutations in the *apoprotein B-100* gene result in a clinical picture resembling heterozygous familial hypercholesterolaemia. LDL particles normally bind to their clearance receptor in the liver through apoprotein B-100, and the mutation results in high LDL concentrations in the blood.
- Polygenic hypercholesterolaemia accounts for those patients with a raised serum cholesterol concentration, but without one of the monogenic disorders above. The precise nature of the polygenic variation in plasma cholesterol remains unknown.

Combined hyperlipidaemia (hypercholesterolaemia and hyperlipidaemia)

Polygenic combined hyperlipidaemia and familial combined hyperlipidaemia account for the vast majority of cases in this group. A small minority are the result of the rare condition, remnant hyperlipidaemia.

Management of hyperlipidaemia

Guidelines to therapy

The initial treatment in all cases of hyperlipidaemia is dietary modification, but additional measures are usually necessary. Patients with familial hypercholesterolaemia will need drug treatment. Secondary hyperlipidaemia should be managed by treatment of the underlying condition wherever possible. In all patients, other treatable cardiovascular risk factors, including smoking, hypertension and excess weight, should also be addressed in tandem with treatment of hyperlipidaemia.

Lipid-lowering diet

- Dairy products and meat are the principal sources of fat in the diet. Chicken and poultry should be substituted for red meats and the food grilled rather than fried. Low-fat cheeses and skimmed milk should be substituted for the full-fat varieties.
- Polyunsaturated fats, e.g. corn and soya oil, should be used instead of saturated fats.
- Reduction of cholesterol intake from liver, offal and fish roe.
- Increased intake of soluble fibres, e.g. pulses and legumes, which reduce circulating cholesterol.
- Avoid excess alcohol and obesity, both causes of secondary hyperlipidaemias.

Lipid-lowering drugs (Table 15.12)

- Hydroxymethylglutaryl-coenzyme A (HMG-CoA) reductase inhibitors (statins), e.g. atorvastatin, pravastatin and simvastatin, inhibit the enzyme HMG-CoA reductase, the rate-limiting enzyme in cholesterol synthesis in the liver. They are the most potent of the lipid-lowering drug classes for lowering total cholesterol and LDL cholesterol and they also raise HDL cholesterol and lower triglycerides to some extent. Side effects of statins include hepatitis, muscle injury and gastrointestinal problems (p. 701).

Table 15.12 Drugs used in the management of hyperlipidaemias (listed in the order in which they are usually selected for treatment)

Hypertriglyceridaemia	Hypercholesterolaemia	Combined
Fibrates	Statins	Fibrates
Nicotinic acid	Ezetimibe/fibrates	Nicotinic acid
Fish oil capsules	Bile acid-binding resins (ω-3 marine triglycerides)	

- Cholesterol absorption inhibitors, e.g. ezetimibe, inhibit gut absorption of cholesterol from food and also from bile. The mechanism of this inhibition is unclear. They mostly act in the gut and little is absorbed. Thus short-term safety is good. They are used when a second drug in addition to a statin is required.
- Fibrates, e.g. gemfibrozil and bezafibrate, activate peroxisome proliferator-activated nuclear receptors (especially PPAR-α) and are broad-spectrum lipid-modulating agents. They decrease serum triglycerides, raise HDL cholesterol and reduce LDL cholesterol concentrations. They are the drugs of first choice for treating isolated hypertriglyceridaemia and are used in combination with other treatments (statins, ezetimibe, fish oils) for patients with mixed dyslipidaemias. A rare but serious side effect is myositis.
- Bile acid-binding resins, e.g. cholestyramine and colestipol, bind bile acids in the intestine, preventing their reabsorption and thus lowering the cholesterol pool. They reduce LDL cholesterol and have a synergistic effect when given with a statin.
- Fish-oils, rich in ω-3 marine triglycerides, reduce plasma triglycerides.
- Nicotinic acid reduces total and LDL cholesterol levels and can reduce triglyceride levels. It is not widely used because of side effects.

Whom to treat

Primary prevention for people at risk of cardiovascular disease Lipid-lowering therapy using a statin, or alternatives as above, should be given to the following asymptomatic individuals irrespective of the total or LDL cholesterol level:

- Diabetes mellitus patients >40 years of age or irrespective of age with retinopathy or persistent microalbuminuria
- A total cardiovascular disease risk of $\geq$20% over 10 years
- Two or more of the following: positive family history of cardiovascular disease, albuminuria, hypertension and smoking
- Men with LDL cholesterol persistently >5.0 mmol/L despite dietary change. The situation for women is less clear.
- Familial hypercholesterolaemia.

Secondary prevention Statin treatment is also indicated for any patient with known macrovascular disease (coronary artery disease, transient ischaemic attack [TIA] or stroke, peripheral artery disease), irrespective of the total or LDL cholesterol level. Alternative and combination agents are ezetimibe, bile acid-binding agents or fibrates (avoid with statins due to overlapping side effects).

Aims of treatment

Statins reduce cardiovascular events and all-cause mortality. Treatment should be adjusted to achieve a target total cholesterol of less than 4 mmol/L or an LDL cholesterol concentration of less than 2.0 mmol/L.

THE PORPHYRIAS

The porphyrias form a rare heterogeneous group of inherited disorders of haem synthesis, which leads to an overproduction of intermediate compounds called porphyrins (Fig. 15.3). In porphyrias the excess production of porphyrins occurs within the liver (hepatic porphyria) or in the bone marrow (erythropoietic porphyria), but porphyrias can also be classified in terms of clinical presentation as acute or non-acute (Table 15.13). Acute porphyrias usually produce neuropsychiatric problems and are associated with excess production and urinary excretion of δ-aminolaevulinic acid (δ-ALA) and porphobilinogen. These metabolites are not increased in the non-acute porphyrias.

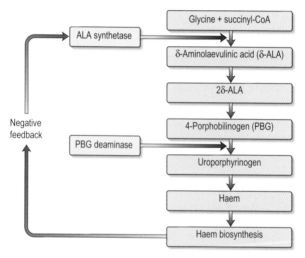

Fig. 15.3 Pathways in porphyrin metabolism.

Table 15.13 The classification of the porphyrias

	Hepatic	Erythropoietic
Acute	Acute intermittent porphyria	
	Variegate porphyria	
	Hereditary coproporphyria	
Non-acute	Porphyria cutanea tarda	Congenital porphyria
		Erythropoietic protoporphyria

Acute intermittent porphyria

This is an autosomal dominant disorder caused by a defect at the level of porphobilinogen deaminase. It is the most common of the acute porphyrias. Presentation is in early adult life, and women are affected more than men.

Clinical features

Abdominal pain, vomiting and constipation are the most common presenting features, occurring in 90% of patients (mimicking an acute abdomen, especially as there may be fever and leucocytosis). Additional features include polyneuropathy (especially motor), hypertension, tachycardia and neuropsychiatric disorder (fits, depression, anxiety and frank psychosis). The urine may turn red or brown on standing. Attacks may be precipitated by alcohol and a variety of drugs, especially those such as barbiturates, which are enzyme-inducing drugs and increase δ-ALA synthetase activity.

Investigations

During an attack there may be a neutrophil leucocytosis, abnormal liver biochemistry and a raised urea.

The diagnosis is made during an attack by demonstrating increased urinary excretion of porphobilinogen and δ-ALA. Urine turns red-brown on standing. Erythrocyte porphobilinogen deaminase is decreased and may be measured between attacks.

Management

Abdominal pain is severe and may require opiate analgesia. A high carbohydrate intake (oral or intravenous glucose) must be maintained because this depresses δ-ALA synthetase activity. Haem arginate is a stable preparation of haem and is given intravenously during an acute attack. Haem inhibits ALA synthetase (Fig. 15.3) and hence reduces levels of the intermediate precursors.

Other porphyrias

Porphyria cutanea tarda (PCT) has both sporadic and inherited forms (autosomal dominant) that are indistinguishable clinically. It presents with a bullous skin eruption on exposure to light or minor trauma. The eruption heals with scarring. Many patients with sporadic PCT have underlying chronic liver disease (particularly due to alcohol or hepatitis C infection). Diagnosis depends on demonstrating increased levels of urinary uroporphyrin.

Variegate porphyria and hereditary coproporphyria present with features similar to those of acute intermittent porphyria, together with the cutaneous features of PCT.

The erythropoietic porphyrias are very rare and present with photosensitive skin lesions.

AMYLOIDOSIS

This is a heterogeneous group of disorders characterized by extracellular deposition of an insoluble fibrillar protein called amyloid. Amyloidosis is acquired or hereditary, and may be localized or systemic. Clinical features are the result of amyloid deposits affecting the normal structure and function of the affected tissue. The diagnosis of amyloidosis is usually made with Congo red staining of a biopsy of affected tissues. In systemic amyloid a simple rectal biopsy may be used for histological diagnosis. Amyloid deposits stain red and show green fluorescence in polarized light. Scintigraphy using ^{123}I-labelled serum amyloid P component is being increasingly employed for assessment.

The features of some systemic amyloid types are shown in Table 15.14.

Localized amyloid deposits occur in the brain of patients with Alzheimer's disease and in the joints of patients on long-term dialysis.

THERAPEUTICS

Oral antidiabetic drugs

Metformin

Mechanism of action

Metformin activates adenosine monophosphate kinase, which is involved in metabolism of the membrane glucose transporter GLUT4 and fatty acid

Table 15.14 Classification of the more common types of amyloid and amyloidosis

Type	Fibril protein precursor	Clinical syndrome
AL	Monoclonal immunoglobulin light chains	Associated with myeloma, Waldenström's macroglobulinaemia and non-Hodgkin lymphoma. Presents with cardiac failure, nephrotic syndrome, carpal tunnel syndrome and macroglossia (large tongue)
ATTR (familial)	Abnormal transthyretin (plasma carrier protein)	Peripheral sensorimotor and autonomic neuropathy and cardiomyopathy
AA	Protein A, a precursor of serum amyloid A (an acute-phase reactant)	Occurs with chronic infections (e.g. TB), inflammation (e.g. rheumatoid arthritis) and malignancy (e.g. Hodgkin's disease). Presents with proteinuria and hepatosplenomegaly

TB, tuberculosis.

oxidation. It increases glucose transport into cells, decreases hepatic gluconeo-genesis and increases insulin sensitivity.

Indications

It is the drug of first choice in overweight patients in whom strict dieting has failed to control diabetes. It is also used in combination with other oral agents, injectable GLP-1 analogues or insulin if diabetes is inadequately controlled with metformin alone. It also improves fertility and weight reduction in patients with polycystic ovary syndrome.

Preparations and dose

Metformin   *Tablets: 500 mg, 850 mg.*

500 mg once daily initially, then titrate upwards in weekly increments to three times a day with meals, or 850 mg every 12 hours; maximum 3 g daily in divided doses.

Side effects

Anorexia, nausea, vomiting, diarrhoea (usually transient), abdominal pain, metallic taste, rarely type B (non-hypoxic) lactic acidosis (mortality of 30–50%), vitamin B_{12} deficiency (decreased absorption). Hypoglycaemia does not usually occur with metformin.

Cautions/contraindications

Contraindicated in severe renal impairment (estimation of the glomerular filtra-tion rate < 30 mL/min/1.73 m^2) because of increased risk of lactic acidosis. Withdraw if tissue hypoxia likely (e.g. sepsis, respiratory failure, recent MI, hepatic impairment), use of iodine-containing X-ray contrast media (do not restart until renal function returns to normal) and use of general anaesthesia (suspend metformin 2 days before surgery and restart when renal function returns to normal).

Sulfonylureas

Mechanism of action

Augment insulin secretion.

Indications

Patients with type 2 diabetes mellitus who are not overweight, or in whom met-formin is contraindicated or not tolerated.

Preparations and dose

Several sulfonylureas are available and choice is determined by side effects and the duration of action as well as the patient's age and renal function. Gliben-clamide is long acting and associated with a greater risk of hypoglycaemia and should be avoided in the elderly. Gliclazide and tolbutamide are shorter acting and are a better choice.

Gliclazide   *Tablets: 80 mg.*

Initially, 40–80 mg daily, adjusted according to response up to 160 mg as a single dose or 320 mg daily in divided doses.

Glibenclamide   *Tablets: 2.5 mg, 5 mg.*

Initially, 5 mg daily with or immediately after breakfast, adjusted according to response; maximum 15 mg daily.

Side effects

Generally mild and infrequent and include gastrointestinal disturbances such as nausea, vomiting, diarrhoea and constipation. May encourage weight gain. Sulfonylurea-induced hypoglycaemia may persist for many hours and must always be treated in hospital. Occasionally cholestatic jaundice, hepatitis, allergic skin reactions and blood disorders.

Cautions/contraindications

Use short-acting form in renal impairment. Avoid sulfonylureas in severe renal and hepatic impairment and in porphyria. Contraindicated in breast-feeding, and substitute insulin during pregnancy.

Treatment of hypoglycaemia

Initially, glucose 10–20 g (two to four teaspoons of sugar, three to six sugar lumps, 50–100 mL of fizzy drink) is given by mouth. If sugar cannot be given by mouth (e.g. unconscious patient), glucose or glucagon can be given by injection.

Mechanism of action

Glucagon mobilizes glycogen stored in the liver.

Indications

Acute hypoglycaemia, where glucose cannot be given either by mouth or intravenously.

Preparations and dose

Glucagon GlucaGen HypoKit   *1 mg vial with prefilled syringe containing water for injection.*

By subcutaneous, intramuscular, or intravenous injection 1 mg.

Side effects

Nausea, vomiting, abdominal pain, hypokalaemia, hypotension, hypersensitivity reactions.

Cautions/contraindications

Phaeochromocytoma.

Lipid-lowering drugs

Statins

Mechanism of action
Inhibition of HMG-CoA reductase, the rate-limiting enzyme involved in cholesterol synthesis. More effective at lowering LDL cholesterol than other classes of drugs but less effective than the fibrates in reducing triglycerides.

Indications
Secondary prevention of coronary and cardiovascular events in patients with history of angina or myocardial infarction, peripheral artery disease, non-haemorrhagic stroke, TIA. *Primary prevention* of coronary events in patients at increased risk of coronary heart disease such as inherited dyslipidaemias or a 10-year cardiovascular risk of 20% or more calculated using tables such as the Joint British Societies Coronary Risk Prediction Chart in the *British National Formulary.*

Preparations and dose
Atorvastatin *Lipitor tablets: 10 mg, 20 mg, 40 mg, 80 mg.*
10 mg once daily at night, increased at intervals of at least 4 weeks to 40 mg once daily. Maximum 80 mg daily.

Simvastatin *Tablets: 10 mg, 20 mg, 40 mg, 80 mg.*
10 mg at night, increased at intervals of at least 4 weeks up to 80 mg at night.

Side effects
Reversible myositis/myopathy – ask patients to report unexplained muscle pain, measure serum creatine kinase (CK) and stop statin if CK is over five times the upper limit of normal. Diagnose rhabdomyolysis if CK is over 10 times the upper limit of normal. In this case, check serum creatinine (may be acute kidney injury) and urine myoglobin. Altered liver biochemistry, which should be measured before, within 3 months of and at 12 months after starting treatment, unless indicated sooner by signs or symptoms suggestive of hepatotoxicity. Stop treatment if serum transaminase concentration is persistently raised to three times the upper limit of the reference range. Gastrointestinal effects include abdominal pain, diarrhoea, flatulence and vomiting.

Cautions/contraindications
Contraindicated in acute liver disease (acute viral hepatitis, alcoholic hepatitis), pregnancy (adequate contraception during treatment and for 1 month afterwards), breast-feeding and personal or family history of muscle disorders. Increased risk of myositis and rhabdomyolysis if statins are given with a fibrate, ezetimibe, ciclosporin, digoxin, warfarin, erythromycin and ketoconazole.

16 The special senses

Some disorders of the eye, ear, nose and throat will be discussed in this chapter. Many conditions will be managed in specialized clinics, and the purpose of this chapter is to describe common conditions or those which need an urgent referral for further specialist management.

THE EAR

The anatomy and physiology of the ear are summarized in Fig. 16.1.

Hearing loss

Hearing loss is a common problem that affects many people, at least on a temporary basis. Short-lived hearing loss occurs when flying or during an ear infection. Deafness can be conductive or sensorineural. Permanent sensorineural hearing loss often occurs with ageing and is caused by disorders of the inner ear, cochlea or cochlear nerve (Table 16.1). Conductive hearing loss is due to an abnormality of the outer or middle ear. The outer ear is examined with an auroscope, which may show wax or a foreign body in the external canal or abnormalities of the tympanic membrane such as perforation or loss of the normal light reflex.

Conductive and sensorineural deafness are differentiated at the bedside by the Rinne and the Weber tests. With normal hearing, air conduction is louder than bone conduction. The Rinne test allows comparison of sound when a vibrating tuning fork, 512 Hz, is placed on the mastoid bone behind the ear (bone conduction) versus when the tuning fork is held next to the ear (air conduction). The Rinne test is normal (positive) when the tuning fork is louder if held next to the ear. If the tuning fork is louder when placed on the mastoid (i.e. via bone conduction), then a conduction defect is present (Rinne negative). The Weber test is performed by placing the handle of the vibrating tuning fork on the bridge of the nose and asking the patient if the sound is louder in one ear or the other. The sound is heard equally in patients with normal hearing or with symmetrical hearing loss.

Vertigo

The vestibular apparatus in the inner ear comprises the semicircular canals, which indicate rotational movements, and the otoliths (utricle and saccule), which sense linear acceleration. These organs provide information to the brainstem (via the vestibular part of 8th cranial nerve) and cerebellum regarding the position and movement of the head. Vertigo is the illusion of spinning or

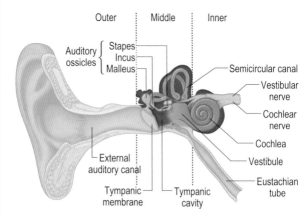

Fig. 16.1 Anatomy and physiology of the ear. Sound waves are transmitted to the fluid-filled cochlea via the external auditory canal, tympanic membrane (the ear drum) and bony ossicles (stapes, incus, malleus). Hair cells in the basilar membrane of the cochlea detect the vibrations and transduce into nerve impulses, which pass via the cochlear nerve (part of 8th cranial, vestibulocochlear, nerve) to the cochlear nucleus in the brainstem and then to the superior olivary nuclei. The vestibular nerve carries information from the semicircular canals about balance. The middle ear is normally filled with air and communicates with mastoid air cells superiorly, and nasopharynx medially via the Eustachian tube. The latter functions as a pressure-equalizing valve for the middle ear and opens for a fraction of a second periodically in response to swallowing or yawning. Anything that interferes with this periodic opening and closing or blocks the Eustachian tube may result in hearing impairment or other ear symptoms.

movement and can arise from peripheral lesions (of the vestibular apparatus or vestibular nerve) or central lesions (of the brainstem or cerebellum). Vertigo is usually rotatory when it arises from the ear. The presence of otalgia, otorrhoea, tinnitus or hearing loss suggests an otologic aetiology. Vestibular causes can be classified according to the duration of the vertigo:

- Seconds to minutes – benign paroxysmal positional vertigo
- Minutes to hours – Ménière's disease
- Hours to days – labyrinthine or central pathology.

Benign paroxysmal positional vertigo accounts for about half of cases with peripheral vestibular dysfunction. Calcium debris in one of the semicircular canals leads to recurrent episodes of vertigo lasting seconds to minutes. Episodes are provoked by specific types of head movements, e.g. turning in bed or sitting up. There is no serious underlying cause and the condition may resolve spontaneously.

Vestibular neuronitis is believed to be caused by a viral infection affecting the labyrinth. There is a sudden onset of severe vertigo, nystagmus and

Table 16.1 Causes of deafness

Conductive	Sensorineural
Rinne negative Weber – sound heard louder on affected side	Rinne positive Weber – sound heard louder in the normal ear
Congenital – atresia	**End organ**
	Advancing age
External auditory canal	Occupational acoustic trauma
Wax	Ménière's disease
Foreign body	Drugs (gentamicin, furosemide)
Otitis externa	**Eighth nerve lesions**
Chronic suppuration	Acoustic neuroma
Ear drum	Cranial trauma
Perforation/trauma Middle ear	Inflammatory lesions: tuberculous meningitis sarcoidosis, neurosyphilis, carcinomatous meningitis
Otosclerosis	
Disorder of bony ossicles	
Otitis media	**Brainstem lesions (rare)**
	Multiple sclerosis
	Infarction

vomiting, but no deafness. The attack lasts several days or weeks, and treatment is symptomatic with vestibular sedatives (e.g. prochlorperazine).

Ménière's disease is due to a build-up of endolymphatic fluid in the inner ear. It is characterized by recurrent episodes of rotatory vertigo lasting 30 minutes to a few hours. It is associated with a sensation of ear fullness, sensorineural hearing loss, tinnitus and vomiting. Treatment involves the use of vestibular sedatives, e.g. cinnarizine in the acute phase, low-salt diet, betahistine and avoidance of caffeine.

Central causes of vertigo are often vascular and may also be due to multiple sclerosis or drug-induced (e.g. anticonvulsants, alcohol or hypnotics).

Ear infections

Otitis externa is a diffuse infection (bacterial, viral or fungal) of the skin of the ear canal. There is severe pain and, on examination, debris in the ear canal sometimes with swelling. Treatment is with regular cleansing, topical antibiotics and corticosteroids. Otitis media is inflammation of the middle ear, usually due to a viral infection. There is severe pain, conductive hearing loss and a mucous discharge if the eardrum is perforated. Antibiotic treatment, amoxicillin 1 g every 8 hours for 5 days, is indicated if there are systemic features or if symptoms do not settle within 72 hours. Swelling and tenderness over the mastoid bone indicate mastoiditis and is an indication for an urgent ear, nose and throat (ENT) opinion.

THE NOSE AND NASAL CAVITY

The nasal cavity is continuous with the nose in front and the pharynx posteriorly and is divided by a midline septum formed of bone and cartilage (Fig. 16.2). The walls of the nasal cavity are formed by the maxilla (laterally), nasal bone (roof) and roof of the mouth (floor). Paranasal sinuses (frontal, ethmoidal, sphenoid, maxillary) connect to the nasal cavity via small passageways called ostia. The nasal cavity receives a rich blood supply derived from branches of the internal and external carotid arteries, which anastomose on the anterior nasal septum (Little's area).

The functions of the nose are to facilitate:

- Smell via the olfactory epithelium in the roof of the nose and the first cranial nerve
- Respiration by moistening, warming and filtering inspired air.

Common conditions of the nose are epistaxis, nasal obstruction, rhinitis (p. 513), sinusitis and nasal fracture.

Epistaxis (nose bleeds)

Local (trauma, nasal fractures, surgery, intranasal steroids, tumours of the nose, paranasal sinuses or nasopharynx) and systemic causes (anticoagulants, bleeding disorders, hypertension or familial haemorrhagic telangiectasia)

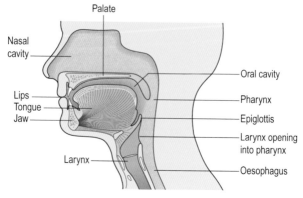

Fig. 16.2 The nasal cavity.

contribute to epistaxis. Little's area is the most common site for bleeding. Initial treatment in stable patients involves leaning the patient forward and compression of the soft nose tissues against the septum for at least 10 minutes. If this fails to control the bleeding, simple local anaesthetic cautery with a silver nitrate stick is indicated. Routine blood tests (full blood count, coagulation screen, cross-match) and an intravenous cannula with fluids are indicated in the presence of major bleeding (a minority of patients) or if a coagulopathy is suspected. If further intervention is necessary, consideration should be given to intranasal cautery of the bleeding vessel, or intranasal packing using a variety of commercially available nasal packs. If the above treatments fail, surgical ligation of the sphenopalatine artery can be undertaken endoscopically or an interventional arterial embolization can be performed for the problematic vessel.

Sinusitis

Infections of the paranasal sinuses may complicate allergic rhinitis or an upper respiratory tract infection (caused by mucosal oedema and blockage of the ostium) and are usually caused by *Streptococcus pneumoniae* or *Haemophilus influenzae*. Symptoms are frontal headache, facial pain and tenderness, fever and nasal discharge. Diagnosis is clinical and treatment is with nasal decongestants (e.g. xylometazoline), broad-spectrum antibiotics (e.g. co-amoxiclav), topical corticosteroids (e.g. fluticasone propionate nasal spray to reduce mucosal swelling) and steam inhalations. Rare complications include local and cerebral abscess formation. Indications for imaging of the sinuses with computed tomography (CT) or magnetic resonance imaging (MRI) are suspected abscess, recurrent acute (more than four episodes per year) or chronic sinusitis (symptoms >3 months).

THE THROAT

Hoarseness (dysphonia)

Most cases of a hoarse voice are due to laryngeal pathology and include inflammation of the vocal cords, nodules on the vocal cords and Reinke's oedema, which is due to a collection of tissue fluid in the subepithelial layer of the vocal cord associated with irritation of the cords due to smoking, voice abuse, acid reflux or, rarely, hypothyroidism. Acute onset of hoarseness, particularly in a smoker, is an indication for urgent referral to an ENT surgeon. It can be due to a paralysed left vocal cord secondary to mediastinal disease, e.g. bronchial carcinoma or carcinoma of the larynx.

Stridor

Stridor or noisy breathing can be divided into inspiratory (obstruction is at the level of the vocal cords or above) or expiratory (intrathoracic trachea or below) noise.

It is a medical emergency and the help of an ENT surgeon and senior anaesthetist may be needed urgently. The causes of stridor include inhalation of a foreign body (may be sudden onset of inspiratory stridor), infections (epiglottitis, diphtheria, tonsillitis), tumour of the trachea or larynx and trauma. If an infection is suspected, examination of the oropharynx should only be undertaken in an area where immediate intubation can take place. Severe stridor due to any cause may be an indication for either intubation or tracheostomy.

Sore throat

Most sore throats are viral in origin and self-limiting. Group A β-haemolytic streptococcus is the most common bacterial cause. Antibiotic treatment, phenoxymethylpenicillin 500 mg every 6 hours for 10 days, is given if there is marked systemic upset, peritonsillar cellulitis or abscess, a history of valvular heart disease or if there is an increased risk of acute infection (immunosuppressed, cystic fibrosis). Respiratory difficulty or stridor is an indication for urgent hospital admission. Infectious mononucleosis presents with a severe sore throat with exudate and anterior cervical lymphadenopathy (p. 20). Fungal infections, usually candidiasis, are uncommon and may indicate an immunocompromised patient or undiagnosed diabetes.

THE EYE

The anatomy and physiology of the eye is summarized in Fig. 16.3.

The red eye

Many patients with a red eye will have simple benign conditions (Table 16.2). However, other conditions can rapidly lead to loss of vision, which may be permanent, and these patients must be referred urgently (i.e. same-day) to a specialist (Table 16.3). Slit lamp examination and measurement of intraocular pressures will often be performed under specialist care after onward referral. The management of a patient presenting with a red eye and a history of trauma or foreign body hitting the eye is beyond the scope of this chapter and is not discussed further.

Conjunctivitis does not usually need referral for a specialist opinion unless the symptoms continue for more than 2 weeks or the eye becomes painful or vision decreases. Bacterial conjunctivitis is treated with a topical broad-spectrum antibiotic such as chloramphenicol. Conjunctival swabs for Gram stain should be taken if there is no response to treatment or in suspected gonococcal conjunctivitis (rapid onset of symptoms, copious discharge, chemosis and lid oedema). Viral conjunctivitis is usually self-limiting. The patient is highly contagious while the eye is red; strict hygiene and keeping towels separate from other family members is necessary to reduce the chance of transmission.

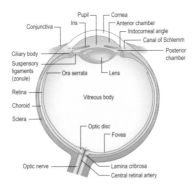

Fig. 16.3 Anatomy and physiology of the eye.

Sclera – thick protective membrane forming outer coat of eyeball (the white of the eye).

Cornea – transparent dome-shaped anterior portion of outer covering of eye, continuous with sclera. Provides most of eye's refractive power.

Conjunctiva – richly vascularized mucous membrane covering anterior surface of sclera and reflected onto undersurface of upper and lower eyelids.

Anterior chamber – contains aqueous humor (produced by ciliary body and drained via canal of Schlemm) providing nutrients and oxygen to cornea.

Iris – coloured part of eye, muscles regulate size of pupil and thus control amount of light entering eye.

Lens – transparent biconvex structure. Changes shape to alter refractive power of the eye.

Retina – contains two types of photoreceptors, rods and cones. The cones provide the eye's colour vision and are mainly confined to the central yellow spot known as the *macula*. In the centre of that region is the *fovea*.

Visual loss

Every patient with unexplained visual loss requires ophthalmic referral. The history will determine if the visual loss is transient or persistent. Temporary blurring in one or both eyes or seeing 'zig-zag' lines is most commonly due to migraine (p. 778). However, these symptoms can also occur with cerebral vascular lesions or tumours and should not automatically be attributed to migraine unless there is a history of typical migraine headache or the patient is under 50 years and has no other neurological symptoms or signs. Severe temporary visual loss (amaurosis fugax) is due to a transient lack of blood supply to the retina or visual cortex and may occur with a transient ischaemic attack (p. 746) or temporal arteritis (p. 781). Urgent assessment and treatment is necessary as amaurosis fugax is a warning sign of impending blindness or stroke. Rarely, papilloedema due to raised intracranial pressure can cause transient (lasting seconds) loss of vision in one or both eyes.

All causes of sudden severe visual loss are indications for urgent referral to an ophthalmologist (Table 16.4). Central retinal artery occlusion is an indication

Table 16.2 Causes of a red eye that do not need urgent referral

	Causes	History	Acuity/pupil/cornea	Site of redness
Conjunctivitis	Bacterial, viral, allergic, chlamydial	Often bilateral. Itchy, gritty eye. Purulent discharge with bacterial infection	Normal	Diffuse ('conjunctival') redness of ocular surface
Subconjunctival haemorrhage	Blood between sclera and conjunctiva	May occur after eye rubbing, severe coughing, rarely hypertension or blood clotting disorder	Normal	Diffuse area of bright red blood under conjunctiva of one eye
Episcleritis	Inflammation of episclera (thin membrane covering sclera)	Mild eye irritation and redness	Normal	Diffuse or localized injection of conjunctiva

Table 16.3 Causes of a red eye requiring urgent (same day) referral to an ophthalmologist

	Causes	History	Visual acuity	Site of redness	Pupil	Cornea
Keratitis (corneal inflammation)	Infections, autoimmune, exposure keratopathy, contact lens related	Pain, foreign body sensation, blurred vision, photophobia	Reduced	Ciliary injection – redness maximal around the edge of the cornea	Normal	Corneal ulceration. More easily visible with fluorescein drops and a blue light (Fig. 16.4)
Acute glaucoma	Sudden severe rise in intraocular pressure due to reduced aqueous fluid drainage	Sudden onset of severe eye pain, blurred vision, rainbow-like 'haloes' around lights ± nausea, vomiting	Reduced	Diffuse	Fixed and semi-dilated	Cloudy
Anterior uveitis (iritis)	Autoimmune diseases, sometimes infectious	Painful eye, blurred vision, photophobia	Normal or reduced	Ciliary injection	Small and fixed	Normal
Scleritis	Often underlying vasculitis	Mild to severe eye pain	Normal or decreased	Diffuse or localized	Normal	Normal
Endophthalmitis	Infection of the eyeball after eye surgery, injury or spread via the bloodstream	Blurred vision, painful eye, photophobia, 'floaters'	Decreased	Diffuse or localized	Small and fixed	Cloudy

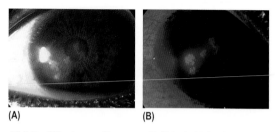

Fig. 16.4 Dendritic ulcers on the cornea. (A) Stained with fluorescein. (B) Stained with fluorescein and viewed with blue light.

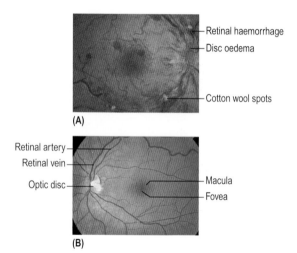

Retinal haemorrhage
Disc oedema

Cotton wool spots

(A)

Retinal artery
Retinal vein
Optic disc
Macula
Fovea

(B)

Fig. 16.5 The fundus (A) The fundus in central retinal vein occlusion compared with (B) the normal appearance of the fundus.

for very urgent referral to an ophthalmic centre (within 1 hour). Acute uveitis, acute glaucoma and keratitis present with the combination of a red eye (p. 708) and sudden or rapidly progressive visual loss. The initial history and examination of a patient presenting with sudden loss of vision is summarized in Emergency Box 16.1.

Gradual visual loss includes slowly progressive optic atrophy, chronic glaucoma, cataracts, diabetic retinopathy (p. 682), macular degeneration and chronic retinal detachment. In developing countries, trachoma due to *Chlamydia trachomatis* and onchocerciasis (river blindness) due to *Onchocerca volvulus* are also causes of visual loss.

Table 16.4 Causes of sudden or rapidly progressive visual loss

	History	Visual acuity	Pupils	Ophthalmoscopy
Acute retinal detachment	Flashing lights, floating spots (black or red), field loss (like a curtain coming in from the periphery)	Usually decreased with a visual field defect	Pupil in affected eye dilates in response to light rather than constricting (relative afferent pupillary defect, RAPD)	Abnormal red reflex. Detached retina looks grey and wrinkled. Normal examination does not exclude diagnosis
Retinal vein occlusion	Sudden loss of vision in all (central vein) or part (branch of retinal vein) of visual field	Decreased, with visual field defect	RAPD if severe	Retinal haemorrhages, tortuous dilated retinal veins, macular oedema, cotton wool spots (Fig. 16.5)
Retinal artery occlusion	Sudden painless loss of vision	Markedly reduced	RAPD	Pale retina with central macular 'cherry red spot'
Acute optic neuropathy	Rapidly progressive loss of vision; may be decreased colour vision. Symptoms of underlying disease (usually multiple sclerosis or nerve ischaemia due to atherosclerosis)	Decreased	RAPD	Normal or swollen optic disc

Continued

Table 16.4 Causes of sudden or rapidly progressive visual loss—cont'd

	History	Visual acuity	Pupils	Ophthalmoscopy
Vitreous haemorrhage	Severe visual loss if a major bleed, floating blobs or spots if mild/moderate	Normal or reduced	No RAPD	Decreased red reflex
'Wet' age-related macular degeneration	Occurs in the elderly. Sudden distortion (straight lines seem curved, central blank patch of vision) or blurring of vision	Decreased acuity with central scotoma (the macula lies in the centre of the retina and disease causes a central blank patch on field testing)	Usually no RAPD	Macular oedema (swelling) and/or subretinal haemorrhages and hard exudates -- due to abnormal new vessels under the macula leaking fluid or bleeding

✚ Emergency Box 16.1

The initial history and examination in the patient presenting with sudden loss of vision

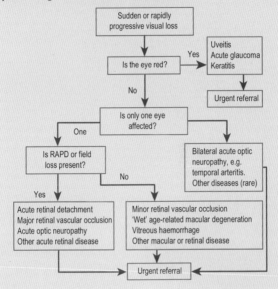

RAPD, relative afferent pupillary defect.
After Pane A, Simcock P (2005) Practical Ophthalmology. Edinburgh, Elsevier Churchill Livingstone.

COMMON NEUROLOGICAL SYMPTOMS

Pattern recognition in neurology — interpretation of history, symptoms and examination — is very reliable. There are three critical questions in formulating a diagnosis:

- What is/are the site(s) of the lesion(s)?
- What is the likely pathology?
- Does a recognizable disease fit this pattern?

Headache

Headache is a common complaint and does not usually indicate serious disease. The causes of headache can be broadly divided according to their onset and subsequent course (Table 17.1). The causes of acute or subacute headache are all potentially serious and require urgent assessment. Subarachnoid haemorrhage presents with headache which reaches maximum intensity within seconds of onset and is described as the 'worst ever' (p. 753). Neck stiffness and a positive Kernig's sign indicate meningeal irritation (e.g. caused by meningitis or subarachnoid haemorrhage).

There are often no abnormal physical signs and the history is the key to distinguishing serious from benign causes in patients with chronic or recurrent headache; most are due to tension-type headache (p. 779) and do not require further investigation. Progressively worsening headaches, or chronic headaches that change in character, may be caused by raised intracranial pressure, e.g. due to a space-occupying lesion, and require brain imaging by computed tomography (CT) scan or magnetic resonance imaging (MRI). Other features which indicate a higher risk of serious pathology and are indications for imaging are listed in Table 17.2. Headache with generalized aches and pains in the elderly suggests giant cell arteritis, which requires urgent treatment with steroids to prevent blindness (p. 781).

Difficulty walking

Change in walking pattern is a common complaint. Arthritis and muscle pain make walking painful and slow (antalgic gait). The *pattern* of gait is valuable diagnostically.

Spasticity and hemiparesis Spasticity, more pronounced in extensor muscles, causes stiff, slow walking. Pace shortens; a narrow base is maintained. In a hemiparesis when spasticity is unilateral and weakness marked, the stiff, weak leg is circumducted and drags.

Table 17.1 Causes of headache

Acute severe (onset in minutes or hours)

Intracranial haemorrhage
Cerebral venous thrombosis
Dissection of carotid/vertebrobasilar arteries
Meningitis
Head injury
Migraine
Drugs, e.g. glyceryl trinitrate
Alcohol
Infections, e.g. malaria

Subacute onset (onset in days to weeks)

Intracranial mass lesion
Encephalitis
Meningitis
Giant cell arteritis
Sinusitis
Acute glaucoma
Malignant hypertension

Recurrent/chronic

Migraine
Tension headache
Sinusitis
Cluster headaches
Paroxysmal hemicrania
Medication overuse
Intracranial mass lesion

Parkinson's disease: shuffling gait Posture is stooped and arm swing reduced. Gait becomes festinant with short rapid steps and slows to a shuffle in advanced forms. There is difficulty turning quickly. Eventually, gait initiation difficulty and freezing episodes may develop.

Cerebellar ataxia: broad-based gait In lateral cerebellar lobe disease, stance becomes broad-based and incoordinated. When walking, the person tends to veer to the side of the affected cerebellar lobe. In disease of midline structures (cerebellar vermis), truncal ataxia results in a tendency to fall backwards or sideways.

Sensory ataxia: stamping gait Peripheral sensory loss causes ataxia because of loss of *proprioception*. A broad-based, high-stepping gait develops

Table 17.2 Indications for brain imaging in patients with headache

Sudden onset

New headache in a patient over 50 years of age

Abnormal neurological signs

Headache changing with posture (may indicate raised ICP)

Headache made worse by coughing, sneezing, bending, straining (may indicate raised ICP)

Fever

History of HIV

History of cancer

HIV, human immunodeficiency virus; ICP, intracranial pressure.

as feet are placed clumsily, relying in part on vision, so balance is worse with eyes closed (positive Romberg's test).

Lower limb weakness: high-stepping and waddling gaits When weakness is distal, affecting ankle dorsiflexors – e.g. in a common peroneal nerve palsy – gait becomes high-stepping to avoid tripping. The sole returns to the ground with an audible *slap*. Weakness of proximal leg muscles (e.g. polymyositis, muscular dystrophy) causes difficulty rising from sitting. Walking becomes a *waddle*, the pelvis being poorly supported by each leg.

Gait apraxia With frontal lobe disease (e.g. normal pressure hydrocephalus), *walking skills* become disorganized despite normal motor and sensory function. The gait is shuffling with small steps *(marche à petit pas),* gait ignition failure and hesitancy. Unlike Parkinson's disease, arm swing and posture are normal. Urinary incontinence and dementia are often present.

Dizziness, faints and 'funny turns'

Episodes of transient disturbance of consciousness are common clinical problems (Table 17.3). Differentiation of seizures from other disorders often depends entirely on the medical history. An eye-witness account is invaluable. Differentiation must also be made from *narcolepsy*, a rare disorder characterized by periods of irresistible sleep in inappropriate circumstances, and *cataplexy,* a related condition in which sudden loss of tone develops in the lower limbs, with preservation of consciousness. Attacks are set off by sudden surprise or emotion.

Dizziness and syncope

Syncope describes a short duration (usually 20–30 seconds) of loss of consciousness caused by a global reduction in cerebral blood flow. There is usually

Table 17.3 Common causes of attacks of altered consciousness and falls in adults

Syncope – cardiopulmonary causes
  Underlying structural cardiopulmonary disease, e.g. aortic stenosis, PE
  Arrhythmias
Syncope – vascular causes
Reflex – vasovagal (simple faint)
  Carotid sinus hypersensitivity
  Situational: cough, micturition, postexertional
  Postural (orthostatic) hypotension: autonomic failure, volume depletion
Epilepsy
Hypoglycaemia
Psychogenic
  Panic attacks
  Hyperventilation
  Narcolepsy and cataplexy

PE, pulmonary embolism.

a rapid and complete recovery. Syncope is a symptom rather than a disease. It can be caused by several underlying conditions (Table 17.3) and is often mistaken for epilepsy.

Dizziness or faintness precedes syncope and represents an incomplete form in which cerebral perfusion has not fallen sufficiently to cause loss of consciousness. Dizziness should be differentiated from *vertigo* (p. 703), which is an illusion of rotary movement where the patient feels that the surroundings are spinning. It results from disease of the inner ear, the eighth cranial nerve, or its central connections.

The most frequent cause of dizziness is vasovagal syncope (a simple faint), which occurs as a result of reflex bradycardia and peripheral and splanchnic vasodilatation. Fear, pain and prolonged standing are the principal causes. Fainting almost never occurs in the recumbent position. A prodrome of nausea, pallor, lightheadedness and sweating usually precede a faint. Rapid recovery from the attack and the absence of jerking movements suggest a faint as opposed to a fit. Urinary incontinence may occur during syncope. Loss of consciousness due to an arrhythmia occurs without warning and may occur in the supine position. Syncope may occur after micturition in men (particularly at night), and when the venous return to the heart is obstructed by breath-holding and severe coughing. Effort syncope occurs on exercise and in patients with aortic stenosis and hypertrophic cardiomyopathy. Carotid sinus syncope is thought to be the result of excessive sensitivity of the sinus to external pressure. It occurs in elderly patients who lose consciousness following pressure on the sinus (e.g. turning the head). Postural hypotension (drop in systolic blood pressure [BP] $\geq$20 mmHg from lying to standing position after 3 minutes) occurs on standing in those with impaired autonomic reflexes, e.g. elderly people, in autonomic neuropathy and with some drugs (phenothiazines, tricyclic antidepressants).

Investigation

The history and physical examination, together with lying and standing BP and a 12-lead electrocardiogram (ECG), will provide a diagnosis in most people with transient loss of consciousness. Echocardiography is used to determine any underlying structural heart disease. Ambulatory electrography (p. 418) has a low diagnostic yield unless symptoms are frequent. Tilt table testing (p. 418) is performed to investigate patients with unexplained syncope in whom cardiac causes or epilepsy have been excluded. BP, heart rate, symptoms and ECG are recorded after head-up tilt for 10–60 minutes. Reproduction of symptoms and hypotension indicate a positive test.

Weakness

Skeletal muscle contraction is controlled by the motor axis of the central nervous system (CNS; Fig. 17.1). Muscle weakness occurs due to a defect or damage in one or more components of this system: i.e. the motor cortex, corticospinal tracts, anterior horn cells, spinal nerve roots, peripheral nerves, the neuromuscular junction and muscle fibres. It is necessary to determine whether there is true weakness rather than 'tiredness' or 'slowness', as in Parkinson's disease. The site of the lesion causing true muscle weakness is often identifiable from a detailed neurological examination. The distribution of weakness, the presence or absence of deep tendon reflexes, the plantar response (Table 17.4) and related sensory defects are all helpful in localizing the lesion in the nervous system. Lesions that affect the upper motor neurone and peripheral nerve will also often involve the sensory system because of the proximity of sensory to motor nerves in these areas.

The corticospinal (or pyramidal) tracts

The corticospinal system enables intricate, strong and organized movements. Defective function is recognized by a distinct pattern of signs – loss of skilled voluntary movement, spasticity and reflex change – seen, for example, in a hemiparesis.

The upper motor neurone The corticospinal tracts originate from neurones of the motor cortex and terminate on the motor nuclei of the cranial nerves and the anterior spinal horn cells. The pathways cross over in the medulla and pass to the contralateral cord as the crossed lateral corticospinal tracts (Fig. 17.1), which then synapse with the anterior horn cells. This is known

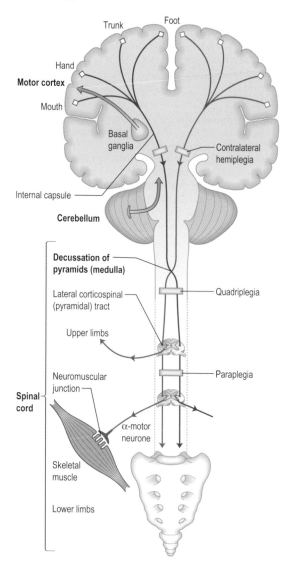

Fig. 17.1 The crossed corticospinal ('pyramidal') tracts showing cortical representation of various parts of the body.

Table 17.4 Comparison of the clinical features of upper and lower motor neurone lesions

Upper motor neurone lesion*	Lower motor neurone lesion
Signs are on the opposite side to the lesion	Signs are on the same side as the lesion
Fasciculation absent	Fasciculation present
No muscle wasting	Wasting
Spasticity ± clonus	Hypotonia
Weakness predominantly extensors in the arms, flexors in the legs	
Exaggerated tendon reflexes	Loss of tendon reflexes
Extensor plantar response	
Drift of the outstretched hand (downwards, medially with a tendency to pronate)	

Fasciculation, visible contraction of single motor units, appearing as a twitch.
*Acute injury to the upper motor neurone is, however, manifested by transient flaccid weakness and hyporeflexia.

as the pyramidal system, disease of which results in upper motor neurone (UMN) lesions with characteristic clinical features (Table 17.4).

Imaging of the CNS and spine is necessary to identify the primary disease.

Two main patterns of clinical features occur in UMN disorders: hemiparesis and paraparesis:

- Hemiparesis means weakness of the limbs of one side, and is usually caused by a lesion within the brain or brainstem, e.g. a stroke.
- Paraparesis (weak legs) indicates bilateral damage to the corticospinal tracts and is most often caused by lesions in the spinal cord below T1 (p. 782). Tetraparesis (quadriplegic, weakness of the arms and legs) indicates high cervical cord damage, most commonly resulting from trauma. Cord lesions result in UMN signs below the lesion, lower motor neurone (LMN) signs at the level of the lesion and unaffected muscles above the lesion.

The lower motor neurone The LMN is the motor pathway from the anterior horn cell or cranial nerve via a peripheral nerve to the motor endplate. Physical signs (Table 17.4) follow rapidly if the LMN is interrupted at any point in its course. Muscle disease may give a similar clinical picture, but reflexes are usually preserved.

LMN lesions are most commonly caused by the following:

- Anterior horn cell lesions, e.g. motor neurone disease, poliomyelitis
- Spinal root lesions, e.g. cervical and lumbar disc lesions
- Peripheral nerve lesions, e.g. trauma, compression or polyneuropathy.

The most common disease of the neuromuscular junction is myasthenia gravis, which characteristically produces fatiguable weakness of skeletal muscle and is rarely associated with wasting. Myopathies are discussed on page 796. Weakness of the proximal muscles, e.g. quadriceps, is typically seen with the various myopathies. Elevation of plasma muscle enzymes such as creatine kinase is highly suggestive of muscle diseases. Muscle biopsy may be necessary to determine the precise form of myopathy.

Numbness

The sensory system

The peripheral nerves carry all the modalities of sensation from nerve endings to the dorsal root ganglia and thence to the cord. These then ascend to the thalamus and cerebral cortex in two principal pathways (Fig. 17.2):

- Posterior columns, which carry sensory modalities for vibration, joint position sense (proprioception), two-point discrimination and light touch. These fibres ascend uncrossed to the gracile and cuneate nuclei in the medulla. Axons from the second-order neurones cross the midline to form the medial lemniscus and pass to the thalamus.
- Spinothalamic tracts, which carry sensations of pain and temperature. These fibres synapse in the dorsal horn of the cord, cross the midline and ascend as the spinothalamic tracts to the thalamus.

Paraesthesiae (pins and needles), numbness and pain are the principal symptoms of lesions of the sensory pathways below the level of the thalamus. The quality and distribution of the symptoms may suggest the site of the lesion.

Peripheral nerve lesions Symptoms are felt in the distribution of the affected peripheral nerve. Polyneuropathy is a subset of the peripheral nerve disorders characterized by bilateral symmetrical, distal sensory loss and burning (p. 791).

Spinal root lesions Symptoms are referred to the dermatome supplied by that root, often with a tingling discomfort in that dermatome (Fig. 17.3). This is in contrast to lesions of sensory tracts within the CNS, which characteristically present as general defects in an extremity rather than specific dermatome defects.

Spinal cord lesions Symptoms (e.g. loss of sensation) are usually evident below the level of the lesion. A lesion of the pain–temperature pathway (spinothalamic tract), whether within the brainstem or the spinal cord, will result in loss of pain–temperature sensation contralaterally, below the level of the lesion. A lesion at the spinal level of the pathway for proprioception will result in loss of these senses ipsilaterally below the level of the lesion. Dissociated sensory loss suggests a spinal cord lesion: e.g. loss of pain–temperature sensation in the right leg and loss of proprioception in the left leg.

Pontine lesions The pons lies above the decussation of the posterior columns. As the medial lemniscus and spinothalamic tracts are close together,

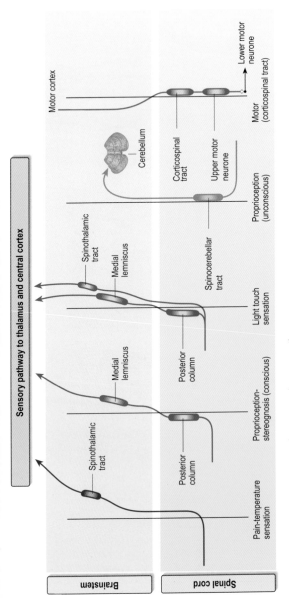

Fig. 17.2 A schematic outline of the major motor and sensory pathways.

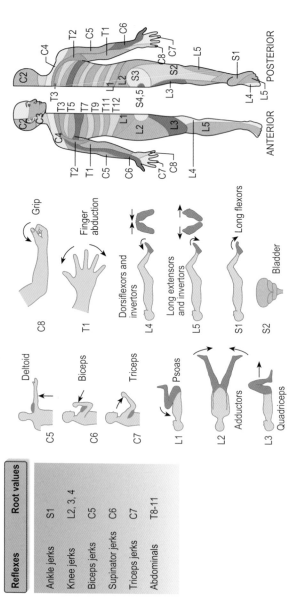

Reflexes	Root values
Ankle jerks	S1
Knee jerks	L2, 3, 4
Biceps jerks	C5
Supinator jerks	C6
Triceps jerks	C7
Abdominals	T8-11

Fig. 17.3 Simple scheme depicting motor and sensory innervation of arms and legs and root values for reflexes.

pontine lesions result in the loss of all forms of sensation on the side opposite the lesion.

Thalamic lesions A thalamic lesion is a rare cause of complete contralateral sensory loss. Spontaneous pain may also occur, most commonly as the result of a thalamic infarct.

Cortical lesions Sensory loss, neglect of one side of the body and subtle disorders of sensation may occur with lesions of the parietal cortex. Pain is not a feature of cortical lesions.

Tremor

Tremor is a rhythmic involuntary muscular contraction characterized by oscillations of a part of the body. A *resting* tremor is seen in Parkinson's disease, parkinsonism and Wilson's disease. Unlike essential tremor, Parkinsonian tremor is generally unilateral for the first few years. *Postural tremor* occurs when a patient attempts to maintain a posture such as holding the arms outstretched. Causes include physiological (due to any increase in sympathetic activity), essential tremor (p. 764), and it also occurs in some cases of Parkinson's disease and cerebellar disease. *Intention tremor* occurs during voluntary movement and gets worse when approaching the target, e.g. during finger-to-nose testing, and occurs with cerebellar disease. In many cases the cause of a tremor will be apparent from the history and examination. Investigations include thyroid function tests, testing for Wilson's disease (in anyone under 40 years) and brain imaging in selected cases.

COORDINATION OF MOVEMENT

The extrapyramidal system (p. 761) and the cerebellum coordinate movement. Disorders of these systems will not produce muscular weakness but may produce incoordination.

The cerebellum

The cerebellum and its connections have a role in coordinating movement, initiated by the pyramidal system, and in posture and balance control. Each lateral lobe of the cerebellum is responsible for coordinating movement of the ipsilateral limb. The midline vermis is concerned with maintenance of axial (midline) balance and posture. Causes of cerebellar lesions are listed in Table 17.5.

A lesion within one cerebellar lobe causes one or all of the following:

- An ataxic gait with a broad base; the patient falters to the side of the lesion.
- An 'intention tremor' (compare Parkinson's disease) with past-pointing.
- Clumsy rapid alternating movements, e.g. tapping one hand on the back of the other (dysdiadochokinesis).
- Horizontal nystagmus with the fast component towards the side of the lesion (p. 738).

Table 17.5 Some causes of cerebellar lesions

Multiple sclerosis
Space-occupying lesions
Primary tumour, e.g. medulloblastoma
Secondary tumour
Abscess
Haemorrhage
Chronic alcohol use
Antiepileptic drugs
Paraneoplastic syndrome
Spinocerebellar ataxia (rare, dominantly inherited)

- Dysarthria, usually with bilateral lesions. The speech has a halting jerking quality – 'scanning speech'.
- Titubation (rhythmic tremor of the head), hypotonia and depressed reflexes. There is no muscle weakness.
- Lesions of the cerebellar vermis cause truncal ataxia, leading to difficulty sitting up or standing.

THE CRANIAL NERVES

The 12 cranial nerves and their nuclei are distributed approximately equally between the three brainstem segments (Fig. 17.4). The exceptions are the first and second cranial nerves (nerves I and II), whose neurones project to the cerebral cortex. In addition, the sensory nucleus of nerve V extends from the midbrain to the spinal cord, and the nuclei of nerves VII and VIII lie not only in the pons but also in the medulla.

The olfactory nerve (first cranial nerve)

The olfactory nerve subserves the sense of smell. The most common cause of anosmia (loss of the sense of smell) is simply nasal congestion. Neurological causes include tumours on the floor of the anterior fossa and head injury.

The optic nerve (second cranial nerve) and the visual system

The optic nerves enter the cranial cavity through the optic foramina and unite to form the optic chiasm, beyond which they are continued as the optic tracts. Fibres of the optic tract project to the visual cortex (via the lateral geniculate body) and the third nerve nucleus for pupillary light reflexes (Figs. 17.5 and 17.6).

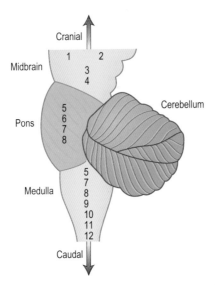

Fig. 17.4 The location of the cranial nerves and their nuclei within the midbrain, pons and medulla as seen laterally.

The assessment of optic nerve function includes measurement of visual acuity (using a Snellen test chart), colour vision (using Ishihara colour plates) and the visual fields (by confrontation and perimetry), and examination of the fundi with the ophthalmoscope. In addition, the pupillary responses, mediated by both the optic and the oculomotor nerve (third cranial nerve), must be tested.

Visual field defects

There are three main types of visual field defects (Fig. 17.5):

- Monocular, caused by damage to the eye or nerve
- Bitemporal, resulting from lesions at the chiasm
- Homonymous hemianopia, caused by lesions in the tract, radiation or a lesion in the visual cortex.

Optic nerve lesions Unilateral visual loss, starting as a central or paracentral scotoma (an area of depressed vision within the visual field), is characteristic of optic nerve lesions. Complete destruction of one optic nerve results in blindness in that eye and loss of the pupillary light reflex (direct and consensual). Optic nerve lesions result from demyelination (e.g. multiple sclerosis), nerve compression and occlusion of the retinal artery (e.g. in giant cell arteritis). Other causes include trauma, papilloedema, severe anaemia and drugs or toxins (e.g. ethambutol, quinine, tobacco and methyl alcohol).

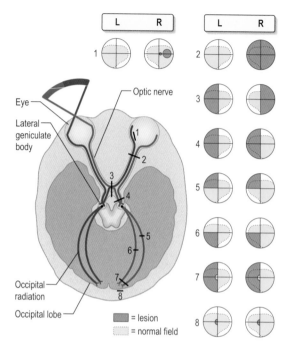

1, Paracentral scotoma – retinal lesion.
2, Mononuclear field loss – optic nerve lesion.
3, Bitemporal hemianopia – chiasmal lesion.
4, Homonymous hemianopia – optic tract lesion.
5, Homonymous quadrantanopia – temporal lesion.
6, Homonymous quadrantanopia – parietal lesion.
7, Homonymous hemianopia – occipital cortex or optic radiation.
8, Homonymous hemianopia – occipital pole lesion.

Fig. 17.5 Diagram of the visual pathways demonstrating the main field defects. At the optic chiasm (3), fibres derived from the nasal half of the retina (the temporal visual field) decussate, whereas the fibres from the temporal half of the retina remain uncrossed. Thus the right optic tract (4) is composed of fibres from the right half of each retina which 'see' the left half of both visual fields. Lesions of the retina (1) produce scotoma (small areas of visual loss) or quadrantanopia. Lesion at 2 produces blindness in the right eye with loss of direct light reflex. Lesion at 3 produces bitemporal hemianopia. Lesions at 4, 5 and 6 produce homonymous hemianopia with macular involvement. Lesions at 7 and 8 produce homonymous hemianopia with macular sparing at 7.

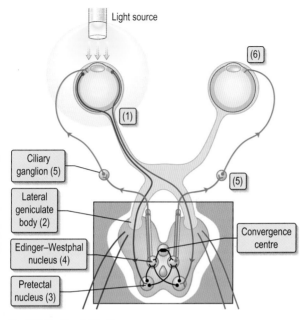

Fig. 17.6 Pupillary light reflex.

Afferent pathway

(1) A retinal image generates action potentials in the optic nerve.

(2) These travel via axons, some of which decussate at the chiasm and pass through the lateral geniculate bodies.

(3) Synapse at each pretectal nucleus.

Efferent pathway

(4) Action potentials then pass to each Edinger–Westphal nucleus of III,

(5) then, to the ciliary ganglion via the third nerve,

(6) leading to constriction of the pupil being illuminated (direct reflex) and, by the consensual reflex, the contralateral pupil.

Defects of the optic chiasm The most common cause of bitemporal hemianopia (i.e. blindness in the outer half of each visual field) is a pituitary adenoma, which compresses the decussating fibres from the nasal half of each eye. Other causes are craniopharyngioma and secondary neoplasm.

Defects of the optic tract and radiation Damage to the tracts or radiation, usually by tumour or a vascular accident, produces a homonymous hemianopia (blindness affecting either the right or the left half of each visual field) in one half of the visual field contralateral to the lesion.

Defects of the occipital cortex Homonymous hemianopic defects are caused by unilateral posterior cerebral artery infarction. The macular region may be spared in ischaemic lesions as a result of the dual blood supply to this area from the middle and posterior cerebral arteries. In contrast, injury to one occipital pole produces a bilateral macular (central) field defect.

Optic disc oedema (papilloedema) and optic atrophy

The principal pathological appearances of the visible part of the nerve, the disc, are:

- Swelling (papilloedema)
- Pallor (optic atrophy).

Papilloedema Papilloedema produces few visual symptoms in the early stages. As disc oedema develops, there is enlargement of the blind spot and blurring of vision. The exception is optic neuritis, in which there is early and severe visual loss. The common causes of papilloedema are:

- Raised intracranial pressure, e.g. from a tumour, an abscess or meningitis
- Retinal vein obstruction (thrombosis or compression)
- Optic neuritis (inflammation of the optic nerve, often caused by demyelination)
- Accelerated hypertension.

Optic atrophy Optic atrophy is the end result of many processes that damage the nerve (see Optic nerve lesions, p. 729). The degree of visual loss depends upon the underlying cause.

The pupils

The pupils constrict in response to bright light and convergence (when the centre of focus shifts from a distant to a near object). The parasympathetic efferents that control the constrictor muscle of the pupil arise in the Edinger—Westphal nucleus in the midbrain, and run with the oculomotor (third) nerve to the eye. The Edinger—Westphal nucleus receives afferents from the optic nerve (for the light reflex) and from the convergence centre in the midbrain (Fig. 17.6).

Sympathetic fibres which arise in the hypothalamus produce pupillary dilatation. They run from the hypothalamus through the brainstem and cervical cord and emerge from the spinal cord at T1. They then ascend in the neck as the cervical sympathetic chain, and travel with the carotid artery into the head.

The main causes of persistent pupillary dilatation are:

- A third cranial nerve palsy (p. 733)
- Antimuscarinic eye drops (instilled to facilitate examination of the fundus)
- The myotonic pupil (Holmes—Adie pupil): this is a dilated pupil seen most commonly in young women. There is absent (or much delayed) reaction to light and convergence. It is of no pathological significance and may be associated with absent tendon reflexes.

The main causes of persistent pupillary constriction are:

- Parasympathomimetic eye drops used in the treatment of glaucoma.
- Horner's syndrome, resulting from the interruption of sympathetic fibres to one eye. There is unilateral pupillary constriction, slight ptosis (sympathetic fibres innervate the levator palpebrae superioris), enophthalmos (backward displacement of the eyeball in the orbit) and loss of sweating on the ipsilateral side of the face. A lesion affecting any part of the sympathetic pathway to the eye results in a Horner's syndrome. Causes include diseases of the cervical cord, e.g. syringomyelia, involvement of the T1 root by apical lung cancer (Pancoast's tumour) and lesions in the neck, such as trauma, surgical resection or malignant lymph nodes.
- Argyll Robertson pupil: this is the pupillary abnormality seen in neurosyphilis and occasionally in diabetes mellitus. There is a small irregular pupil which is fixed to light but which constricts on convergence.
- Opiate addiction.

Cranial nerves III–XII

The cranial nerves III–XII may be damaged by lesions in the brainstem or during their intracranial and extracranial course. The site of a lesion may be suggested if clinical examination shows the involvement of other cranial nerves at that site.

- A seventh-nerve palsy, together with cerebellar signs and involvement of the fifth, sixth and eighth cranial nerves, suggests a lesion of the cerebellopontine angle, commonly a meningioma or acoustic neuroma.
- An isolated seventh-nerve palsy in a patient with a parotid tumour suggests involvement during its extracranial course in the parotid.
- Cavernous sinus lesions (thrombosis, tumours, internal carotid artery aneurysm) involve the oculomotor nerves and the ophthalmic and sometimes maxillary division of the fifth cranial nerve during their intracranial course.
- Conditions which can affect any cranial nerve are diabetes mellitus, sarcoidosis, vasculitis, syphilis and brainstem tumours, multiple sclerosis and infarction.

The ocular movements and the third, fourth and sixth cranial nerves

These three cranial nerves supply the six external ocular muscles, which move the eye in the orbit (Fig. 17.7). The abducens nerve (sixth cranial nerve) supplies the lateral rectus muscle and the trochlear (fourth cranial nerve) supplies the superior oblique muscle. All the other extraocular muscles, the sphincter pupillae (parasympathetic fibres) and the levator palpebrae superioris are supplied by the oculomotor nerve (third cranial nerve). Normally the brainstem (with input from the cortex, cerebellum and vestibular nucleus) coordinates the

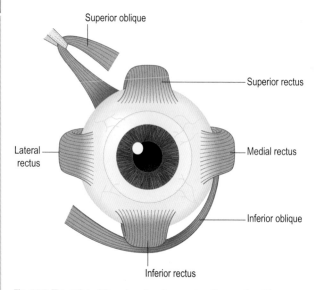

Fig. 17.7 The action of the external ocular muscles. The muscles of the eye move the eyeball in various directions. The lateral rectus muscle moves the eyeball to the temple, away from the midline of the face. The medial rectus muscle moves the eyeball to the nose, toward the midline of the face. The superior rectus muscle moves the eyeball upward, and the inferior rectus muscle moves the eyeball downward. The superior oblique muscle moves the eyeball downward and outward. The inferior oblique muscle moves the eyeball upward and outward.

functions of these three cranial nerves, so that eye movement is symmetrical (conjugate gaze). Thus *infranuclear (lower motor neurone)* lesions of the third, fourth and sixth cranial nerves lead to paralysis of individual muscles or muscle groups. *Supranuclear (upper motor neurone)* lesions, e.g. brainstem involvement by multiple sclerosis, lead to paralysis of conjugate movements of the eyes.

- Oculomotor (third) nerve lesions cause unilateral complete ptosis, the eye faces 'down and out', and the pupil is dilated and fixed to light and convergence. This is the picture of a complete third-nerve palsy, of which the most common cause is a 'berry' aneurysm arising in the posterior communicating artery, which runs alongside the nerve. Frequently the lesion is partial, particularly in diabetes mellitus, when parasympathetic fibres are spared and the pupil reacts normally.

- In lesions on the abducens (sixth) nerve the eye cannot be abducted beyond the midline. The unopposed pull of the medial rectus muscle causes the eye to turn inward, thereby producing a squint (squint, or *strabismus*, is the appearance of the eyes when the visual axes do not meet at the point of fixation). Patients complain of diplopia or double vision, which worsens when they attempt to gaze to the side of the lesion.

- Trochlear nerve lesions in isolation are rare. The patient complains of torsional diplopia (two objects at an angle) when attempting to look down (e.g. descending stairs); the head is tilted away from that side.

Disordered ocular movements may also result from disease of the ocular muscles (e.g. muscular dystrophy, dystrophia myotonica) or of the neuromuscular junction (e.g. myasthenia gravis). In these conditions all the muscles tend to be affected equally, presenting a generalized restriction of eye movements.

The trigeminal nerve (fifth cranial nerve)

The trigeminal nerve has both motor and sensory functions and enters the brainstem at the level of the pons. The neurones for pain and temperature descend to the upper cervical spine before they synapse with neurones of the descending tract of the fifth nerve. Second-order neurones then cross over and ascend to the thalamus. The sensory portion of this nerve supplies sensation to the face and scalp as far back as the vertex through its three divisions (Fig. 17.8). It also supplies the mucous membranes of the sinuses, the nose, mouth, tongue and teeth. The motor root travels with the mandibular division and supplies the muscles of mastication.

Diminution of the corneal reflex is often the first sign of a fifth-nerve lesion. A complete fifth-nerve lesion on one side causes unilateral sensory loss on the face, tongue and buccal mucosa. The jaw deviates to the side of the lesion

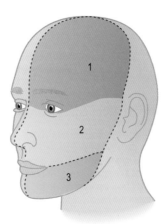

Fig. 17.8 Cutaneous distribution of the trigeminal nerve. (1) Ophthalmic or first division; (2) maxillary or second division; (3) mandibular or third division.

when the mouth is opened. A brisk jaw jerk is seen with UMN lesions, i.e. above the motor nucleus in the pons.

A fifth-nerve lesion is due to pathology within the brainstem (tumour, multiple sclerosis, infarction, syringobulbia), at the cerebellopontine angle (acoustic neuroma, other tumour), within the petrous temporal bone (spreading middle ear infection) or within the cavernous sinus (aneurysm of the internal carotid artery, tumour, thrombosis of the cavernous sinus).

Trigeminal neuralgia

Trigeminal neuralgia *(tic douloureux)* is of unknown cause, seen most commonly in old age, and is almost always unilateral.

Clinical features

Severe paroxysms of knife-like pain occur in one or more sensory divisions of the trigeminal nerve (Fig. 17.8), although rarely in the ophthalmic division. Each paroxysm is stereotyped, brought on by stimulation of a specific 'trigger zone' in the face. The stimuli may be minimal, and include washing, shaving and eating. There are no objective physical signs and the diagnosis is based on the history.

Management

The anticonvulsant carbamazepine suppresses attacks in most patients. Phenytoin and gabapentin are also used but are less effective. If this fails, thermocoagulation of the trigeminal ganglion or section of the sensory division may be necessary.

Differential diagnosis

Similar pain may occur with structural lesions involving the trigeminal nerve. These lesions are often accompanied by physical signs, e.g. a depressed corneal reflex.

The facial nerve (seventh cranial nerve)

The facial nerve is largely motor in function, supplying the muscles of facial expression. It has, in addition, two major branches: the chorda tympani, which carries taste from the anterior two-thirds of the tongue, and the nerve to the stapedius muscle (this has a damping effect to protect the ear from loud noise). These two branches arise from the facial nerve during its intracranial course through the facial canal of the petrous temporal bone. Therefore damage to the facial nerve in the temporal bone (e.g. Bell's palsy, trauma, herpes zoster, middle-ear infection) may be associated with undue sensitivity to sounds (hyperacusis) and loss of taste to the anterior two-thirds of the tongue.

Lower motor neurone lesions

A unilateral LMN lesion causes weakness of all the muscles of facial expression (cf. UMN, p. 738) on the same side as the lesion. The face, especially the angle of the mouth, falls and dribbling occurs from the corner of the mouth. There is weakness of frontalis, the eye will not close and the exposed cornea is at risk of ulceration. LMN facial palsy is caused by a lesion in the pons/medulla (and involving the seventh cranial nerve nuclei) or by a lesion in the course of the facial nerve outside of the brainstem (posterior fossa, facial canal in the temporal bone, middle ear, parotid gland). The nerve may also be affected in polyneuritis (e.g. Guillain–Barré syndrome [GBS], Lyme disease), when there may be bilateral involvement. The most common cause of LMN facial palsy is Bell's palsy.

Bell's palsy This is a common, acute, isolated unilateral facial nerve palsy that is probably the result of a viral infection (often herpes simplex) that causes swelling of the nerve within the petrous temporal bone. Peak incidence is between the ages of 65 and 74 years and it is more common in pregnancy.

Clinical features

There is LMN weakness of the facial muscles, sometimes with loss of taste on the anterior two-thirds of the tongue. There may be hyperacusis and decreased production of tears.

Investigations

The diagnosis is clinical. The differential diagnosis of LMN facial weakness includes the Ramsay Hunt syndrome and parotid gland tumour. In addition, the facial nerve is the most common cranial nerve lesion in meningitis associated with Lyme disease (erythema migrans on the limbs and trunk in a patient with a history of tick bite) and in sarcoidosis (p. 546), in which bilateral involvement may occur. Bilateral Bell's palsy is rare. A prolonged steadily progressive weakness suggests a tumour.

Management

The eyelid must be closed to protect the cornea from ulceration (either adhesive tape or, in prolonged cases surgical tarsorrhaphy). Oral prednisolone (60 mg/day for 10 days) given within 72 hours of onset increases the chance of a full recovery. Antivirals (e.g. valaciclovir) are used in addition in severe cases.

Prognosis

Most patients recover completely, although 30% are left with a permanent weakness.

Ramsay Hunt syndrome This is herpes zoster (shingles) of the geniculate ganglion (the sensory ganglion for taste fibres) situated in the facial canal. There is an LMN facial palsy, with herpetic vesicles in the external auditory meatus and sometimes in the soft palate. Deafness may occur as a result of involvement of the eighth nerve in the facial canal. Treatment is with aciclovir.

Upper motor neurone lesions

A UMN lesion causes weakness of the lower part of the face on the side oppo-site the lesion. Upper facial muscles are spared because of the bilateral cortical innervation of neurones supplying the upper face. Wrinkling of the forehead (frontalis muscle) and eye closure are normal. The most common cause is a stroke, when there is an associated hemiparesis.

The vestibulocochlear nerve (eighth cranial nerve)

The eighth cranial nerve has two components – cochlear and vestibular – subserving hearing and equilibrium, respectively (see Fig. 16.1). The clinical features of a cochlear nerve lesion are sensorineural deafness and tinnitus. Causes of a cochlear nerve lesion are within the brainstem (tumour, multiple sclerosis, infarction), cerebellopontine angle (acoustic neuroma and other tumours) and petrous temporal bone (trauma, middle-ear infection, tumour). Sensorineural deafness may also be the result of disease of the cochlea itself: Ménière's disease (p. 705), drugs (e.g. gentamicin) and presbycusis (deafness of old age).

The main symptom of a vestibular nerve lesion is vertigo, which may be accompanied by vomiting. Nystagmus is the principal physical sign, often with ataxia (loss of balance).

Vertigo

Vertigo is the definite illusion of movement – a sensation as if the external world were revolving around the patient. It results from disease of the inner ear, the eighth nerve or its central connections (p. 703).

Nystagmus

Nystagmus is a rhythmic oscillation of the eyes, which must be sustained for more than a few beats to be significant. It is a sign of disease of either the ocular or the vestibular system and its connections. Nystagmus is described as either pendular or jerk.

Pendular nystagmus A pendular movement of the eye occurs; there is no rapid phase. It occurs where there is poor visual fixation (i.e. long-standing severe visual impairment) or a congenital lesion.

Jerk nystagmus Jerk nystagmus has a fast and a slow component to the rhythmic movement:

- Horizontal or rotary nystagmus may be either peripheral (middle ear) or central (brainstem and cerebellum) in origin. In peripheral lesions it is usually transient (minutes or hours); in central lesions it is long lasting (weeks, months or more).
- Vertical nystagmus is caused only by central lesions.

Glossopharyngeal, vagus, accessory and hypoglossal nerves (ninth to twelfth cranial nerves)

The lower four cranial nerves (ninth to twelfth) which lie in the medulla (the 'bulb') are usually affected together; isolated lesions are rare. A *bulbar palsy* is a weakness of the LMN type, of the muscles supplied by these cranial nerves. There is dysarthria, dysphagia and nasal regurgitation. The tongue is weak, wasted and fasciculating. The most common causes of a bulbar palsy are motor neurone disease (p. 787), syringobulbia (p. 785) and GBS (p. 793). Poliomyelitis is now rare. *Pseudobulbar palsy* is caused by bilateral UMN lesions causing weakness of the same muscle groups. There is also dysarthria, dysphagia and nasal regurgitation, but the tongue is small and spastic and there is no fasciculation. The jaw jerk is exaggerated, the gag and palatal reflexes are preserved and the patient is emotionally labile. In many patients there is a partial palsy with only some of these features. The most common cause of pseudobulbar palsy is a cerebrovascular disease, typically after multiple infarcts, but it may also occur in motor neurone disease and multiple sclerosis.

COMMON INVESTIGATIONS IN NEUROLOGICAL DISEASE

Blood tests

An elevated erythrocyte sedimentation rate (ESR) or C-reactive protein (CRP) may point to inflammatory conditions such as vasculitis. Comatose patients may be hypoglycaemic or hyponatraemic, and hypocalcaemia may lead to spasms and tetany.

Imaging

Skull and spinal X-rays are used to identify fractures, metastases, destructive lesions, osteomyelitis and degenerative osteomyelitis.

Computed tomography CT is of value in identifying cerebral tumours, intracerebral haemorrhage and infarction, subdural and extradural haematoma, midline shift of intracranial structures and cerebral atrophy. However, small lesions (<1 cm) or lesions with the same attenuation as bone or brain (e.g. plaques of multiple sclerosis, isodense subdural haematoma) are poorly seen. In addition, lesions in the posterior fossa are sometimes missed. CT scans can be performed much more rapidly than MRI scans (seconds) and are better than MRI for detailed evaluation of bone. They are also safe with implanted devices.

Magnetic resonance imaging MRI is of particular value in imaging tumours, infarction, haemorrhage, clot, multiple sclerosis plaques, the posterior fossa, the foramen magnum and the spinal cord. Patients with pacemakers or metallic fragments in the brain cannot be imaged and claustrophobia is an issue for some patients. The lack of ionizing radiation is an advantage over CT scanning.

Positron emission tomography PET is principally used in the detection of occult neoplasms.

Doppler studies B-mode and colour ultrasound are valuable in the detection of stenosis of the carotid arteries.

Electroencephalography The electroencephalogram (EEG) measures brain electrical activity and is recorded from scalp electrodes on 20 channels simultaneously. Its main value is to characterize epilepsy syndromes and it is a sensitive test for encephalopathies; different patterns are seen with different encephalopathies. Patients with epilepsy often have a normal EEG between seizures. Evoked potentials record brain responses to sound (auditory evoked potentials), touch (somatosensory) and visual stimuli (visual evoked potentials).

Lumbar puncture and cerebrospinal fluid examination Lumbar puncture (LP) is central to the diagnosis of meningitis and encephalitis, but it is also helpful in the diagnosis of other conditions, such as subarachnoid haemorrhage, multiple sclerosis, sarcoidosis and Behçet's disease. It is used therapeutically for intrathecal injection of drugs or for removal of cerebrospinal fluid (CSF) in idiopathic intracranial hypertension. Brain imaging (CT or MRI) should be performed before LP in patients who have clinical features that increase the likelihood of having intracranial mass lesions or increase in CSF pressure which would preclude LP: immunosuppression, bleeding tendency, focal neurological signs, papilloedema, loss of consciousness or seizure. CSF pressure (normally 80–180 mm H_2O with small visible excursions related to pulse and respiration) is measured with a manometer and CSF fluid is collected into at least three separate numbered bottles. It should normally be clear and colourless. A decreasing concentration of red blood cells from bottles one to three indicates a traumatic tap, rather than blood in the CSF (indicating subarachnoid haemorrhage). Fluid should be sent for microscopy and culture, protein, and glucose concentration with a simultaneous plasma glucose sample. Additional investigations depend on the suspected diagnosis. Complications of LP are post-procedure headache, infection and herniation of the brainstem through the foramen magnum ('coning').

Electromyography The electromyogram (EMG) records the electrical activity of muscles at rest and during voluntary contraction. Recordings are made by placing a small electrode needle into the muscle. Electromyography is usually performed in conjunction with *nerve conduction studies*, which measure the speed of conduction of impulses through a nerve. They will differentiate between axonal and demyelination neuropathy and determine whether pathology is focal or diffuse. These tests are used to investigate disease of the muscles, nerves or neuromuscular junction.

Investigation of suspected muscle disease

Measurement of serum creatine phosphokinase (CK) and aldose, EMG and muscle biopsy for histology and immunohistochemical staining are the three main investigations used in the diagnosis of muscle disease. Muscle biopsy is performed under local anaesthetic with a small skin incision and muscle biopsy needle. MRI demonstrates areas of muscle inflammation, oedema and fibrosis. It can image a large bulk of muscle and avoids the sampling error associated with muscle biopsy. Serial images can be used to assess the response to treatment. Currently it is used as well as and not in place of biopsy.

UNCONSCIOUSNESS AND COMA

The central reticular formation, which extends from the brainstem to the thalamus, influences the state of arousal. It consists of clusters of interconnected neurones throughout the brainstem, with projections to the spinal cord, the hypothalamus, the cerebellum and the cerebral cortex.

Coma is a state of unconsciousness from which the patient cannot be roused. A *stuporous* patient is sleepy but will respond to vigorous stimulation. The Glasgow Coma Scale (GCS; Table 17.6) is a simple grading system used to

Table 17.6 Glasgow Coma Scale

Category	Score
Eye opening (E)	
Spontaneous	4
To speech	3
To pain	2
None	1
Best verbal response (V)	
Orientated	5
Confused	4
Inappropriate	3
Incomprehensible	2
None	1
Best motor response (M)	
Obeying commands	6
Localizing – use limb to resist a painful stimulus	5
Limb withdrawing	4
Limb flexing	3
Limb extending	2
None	1

The scores in each category are added up to give an overall score, which may vary from 3 (in the deeply comatose patient) to 15.

assess the level of consciousness. It is easy to perform and provides an objective assessment of the patient. Serial measurements are used to detect a deterioration which may indicate the need for further investigation or treatment. A very rapid assessment in an unstable patient is obtained using the AVPU score: Alert, responds to Voice, responds to Pain, Unresponsive. A patient responding to pain only, broadly corresponds to a GCS of less than 8.

Coma must be differentiated from persistent vegetative state (PVS, a state of wakefulness in which sleep–wake cycles persist but without detectable awareness), brain death (p. 745) in which there is no possibility of recovery and the locked-in syndrome (p. 749). Patients in coma may progress to a PVS.

Aetiology

Altered consciousness is produced by four types of processes:

- Diffuse brain dysfunction due to severe metabolic, toxic or neurological disorders
- Brainstem lesions which damage the reticular formation
- Pressure effect on the brainstem such as a cortical or cerebellar lesion which compresses the brainstem, inhibiting the ascending reticular activating system
- Extensive damage of the cerebral cortex and cortical connections can cause coma, e.g. meningitis or hypoxic-ischaemic damage after cardiac arrest.

The principal causes of coma are shown in Table 17.7. The most common causes of coma are metabolic disorders, drugs and toxins and mass lesions.

Assessment

In all patients presenting in coma, a history should be obtained from any witnesses and relatives (e.g. speed of onset of coma, diabetes, drug or alcohol abuse, past medical history and medication).

Immediate assessment takes only seconds, but is essential:

- **A**irway. Clear the airway of vomit, secretions and foreign bodies. A patient not protecting his airway may need intubating.
- **B**reathing. Assess for cyanosis, respiratory rate (normal 12–20 breaths/min), use of accessory muscles of respiration (p. 505), chest auscultation, oxygen saturation by pulse oximetry. Consider intubation and ventilation.
- **C**irculation. Assess pulse, BP and capillary refill (p. 577).
- **D**isability. Conscious level using the Glasgow Coma Score.
- **E**xposure. Full examination of the patient, e.g. head injury, rash.

Further assessment A full general examination should be carried out. Clues to the cause of coma should be looked for: e.g. the smell of alcohol or ketones (in diabetic ketoacidosis) on the breath; needle-track marks in a

Table 17.7 Principal causes of coma

Diffuse brain dysfunction

Drug overdose, alcohol excess
CO poisoning, anaesthetic gases
Hypo- or hyperglycaemia
Hypo- or hypercalcaemia – if severe
Hypo- or hypernatraemia – if severe
Hypoadrenalism
Severe uraemia
Hepatocellular failure
Metabolic acidosis
Respiratory failure with CO_2 retention
Hypoxic/ischaemic brain injury
Subarachnoid haemorrhage
Hypertensive encephalopathy
Encephalitis, cerebral malaria, septicaemia

Direct effect within the brainstem

Haemorrhage/infarction
Tumour
Demyelination, e.g. multiple sclerosis
Wernicke–Korsakoff syndrome
Trauma

Pressure effect on brainstem

Tumour
Haemorrhage/infarction
Abscess
Encephalitis

drug abuser; or a Medic-Alert bracelet, as carried by some people with diabetes and patients on steroid-replacement therapy. Immediate assessment of capillary glucose is essential if the patient has diabetes.

The neurological examination must include:

- Head and neck. Look for evidence of trauma, bruits and neck stiffness (indicating meningitis or subarachnoid haemorrhage).
- Pupils. Record size and reaction to light:
  - *A unilateral fixed dilated pupil* indicates herniation of the temporal lobe ('coning') through the tentorial hiatus and compression of the third cranial nerve (p. 733). This indicates the need for urgent neurosurgical intervention.

- *Bilateral fixed dilated pupils* are a cardinal sign of brain death. They also occur in deep coma of any cause, but particularly coma caused by barbiturate intoxication or hypothermia.
- *Pinpoint pupils* are seen with opiate overdose or with pontine lesions that interrupt the sympathetic pathways to the dilator muscle of the pupil.
- *Midpoint pupils* that react to light are characteristic in coma of metabolic origin and coma caused by most CNS depressant drugs.
- Fundi. Look for papilloedema, which indicates raised intracranial pressure.
- Eye movements. *Conjugate lateral deviation of the eyes* indicates ipsilateral cerebral haemorrhage or infarction (the eyes look away from the paralysed limbs), or a contralateral pontine lesion (towards the paralysed limbs). Passive head rotation normally causes conjugate ocular deviation in the direction opposite to the induced head movement (doll's head reflex). This reflex is lost in very deep coma and is absent in brainstem lesions. Dysconjugate eyes (divergent ocular axes) indicate a brainstem lesion.
- Motor responses. Asymmetry of spontaneous limb movements, tone and reflexes indicates a unilateral cerebral hemisphere or brainstem lesion. The plantar responses are often both extensor in coma of any cause.

Investigations

In many cases the cause of coma will be evident from the history and examination, and appropriate investigations should then be carried out. However, if the cause is still unclear, further investigations will be necessary.

Blood and urine tests

- Blood glucose by immediate Stix testing and then formal laboratory testing
- Serum for urea and electrolytes, liver biochemistry and calcium
- Arterial blood gases
- Blood cultures
- Serum and urine for drug analysis, e.g. salicylates
- Thyroid function tests and serum cortisol.

Radiology

CT of the head may indicate an otherwise unsuspected mass lesion or intracranial haemorrhage.

CSF examination

If a mass lesion is excluded on CT, lumbar puncture (p. 740) is performed if subarachnoid haemorrhage or meningoencephalitis is suspected.

Management

The immediate management consists of treatment of the cause, careful nursing, meticulous attention to the airway and frequent observation to detect any change in vital function. Naloxone (400 µg i.v.) is given if opiate poisoning (pinpoint pupils, hypoventilation, drug addict) is suspected. Flumazenil is given if coma is a complication of benzodiazepines. Give thiamine 100 mg i.v. to alcohol dependents or malnourished patients.

Prognosis

The outlook depends upon the cause of coma. A cause must be established before decisions are made about withdrawing supportive care.

Brain death

Brain death means the irreversible loss of the capacity for consciousness, combined with the irreversible loss of the capacity to breathe. Two independent senior medical opinions are required for the diagnosis to be made. The three main criteria for diagnosis are as follows:

- Irremediable structural brain damage. A disorder that can cause brainstem death, e.g. intracranial haemorrhage, must have been diagnosed with certainty. Patients with hypothermia, significant electrolyte imbalance or drug overdose are excluded, but may be reassessed when these are corrected.
- Absent motor responses to any stimulus. Spinal reflexes may be present.
- Absent brainstem function, demonstrated by:
  - Pupils fixed and unresponsive to light
  - Absent corneal, gag and cough reflexes
  - Absent doll's head reflex (p. 744)
  - Absent caloric responses: ice-cold water run into the external auditory meatus causes nystagmus when brainstem function is normal
  - Lack of spontaneous respiration.

In suitable cases, and provided the patient was carrying a donor card and/or the consent of relatives has been obtained, the organs of those in whom brainstem death has been established may be used for transplantation.

STROKE AND CEREBROVASCULAR DISEASE

Stroke is the third most common cause of death and a major cause of disability world-wide. The death rate following stroke is 20–25%. The incidence rises steeply with age; it is uncommon in those under 40 years and is slightly more common in men. A FAST (Face, Arm, Speech, Time) approach is used outside of hospital by paramedics or relatives to facilitate early recognition of the symptoms of stroke and allow early action to be taken.

Definitions

Stroke is defined as rapid onset of neurological deficit (usually focal), lasting >24 hours, which is the result of a vascular lesion and associated with infarction of central nervous tissue. A completed stroke is when the neurological deficit has reached its maximum (usually within 6 hours).

Stroke in evolution is when the symptoms and signs are getting worse (usually within 24 hours of onset).

A minor stroke is one in which the patient recovers without a significant neurological deficit, usually within 1 week.

Transient ischaemic attack A TIA is a transient episode of neurological dysfunction caused by focal brain, spinal cord or retinal ischaemia without acute infarction. TIAs have a tendency to recur and may herald thromboembolic stroke.

Pathophysiology

Different pathological events cause similar clinical events in cerebrovascular disease.

Completed stroke Most strokes (85%) are caused by cerebral infarction due to arterial embolism or thrombosis. Thrombosis occurs at the site of an atheromatous plaque in carotid, vertebral or cerebral arteries. Emboli arise from atheromatous plaques in the carotid/vertebrobasilar arteries, or from cardiac mural thrombi (e.g. following myocardial infarction), or from the left atrium in atrial fibrillation. In about 15% of cases, stroke is caused by intracranial or subarachnoid haemorrhage.

Less commonly, the clinical picture of stroke may be caused by intracranial venous thrombosis, multiple sclerosis relapse and a space-occupying lesion in the brain, e.g. a tumour or abscess. With an abscess, the onset of symptoms and signs is usually much slower than in a stroke. In young adults, one-fifth of strokes are caused by carotid or vertebral artery dissection allowing blood to track within the wall of the artery and occlude the lumen. It should be considered in those with recent neck pain, trauma or manipulation of the neck. Diagnosis is by magnetic resonance (MR) angiography.

Transient ischaemic attacks TIAs are usually the result of passage of microemboli (which subsequently lyse) arising from atheromatous plaques or from cardiac mural thrombi. The risk factors and causes of TIAs are the same as those for thromboembolic stroke. A TIA may also be caused by a temporary drop in cerebral perfusion (e.g. cardiac dysrhythmia, severe hyper- or hypoperfusion) and, rarely, tumours and subdural haematomas may produce a similar clinical picture.

Risk factors

The major risk factors for thromboembolic stroke are those for atheroma: i.e. hypertension, diabetes mellitus, cigarette smoking and hyperlipidaemia. Hypertension is the most modifiable risk factor: others are obesity, oestrogen-containing oral contraceptives, excessive alcohol consumption and polycythaemia (hyperviscosity syndromes). Atrial fibrillation is a major risk factor for embolic stroke (rate 1–5% per year depending on age). Rarer causes of stroke are migraine, vasculitis, cocaine (by causing vasoconstriction), antiphospholipid syndrome (p. 305) and the thrombophilias (predispose to cerebral venous thrombosis).

Transient ischaemic attacks

There is a sudden onset of focal neurological deficit (usually hemiparesis and dysphasia) with symptoms maximal at the onset and usually lasting 5–15 minutes. The classical definition of resolution within 24 hours is not used now. Gradual progression of symptoms suggests a different pathology such as demyelination, tumour or migraine. Symptoms and signs depend on the site of the brain involved (Table 17.8). Amaurosis fugax is painless transient monocular blindness as a result of the passage of emboli through the retinal arteries. Dizziness, loss of consciousness and temporary memory loss (transient global amnesia) occurring on their own are not due to TIAs. The history and physical examination must include a search for risk factors and possible sources of emboli (atrial fibrillation, valve lesion, carotid bruits in the neck).

Investigations

The diagnosis of TIA is clinical.

Blood is taken for measurement of glucose, full blood count (to identify polycythaemia), ESR (raised in the few cases of vasculitis), creatinine and electrolytes, cholesterol and international normalized ratio (INR; if taking warfarin).

Brain imaging by diffusion-weighted MRI, together with specialist review, should be performed within 24 hours in patients with an ABCD2 score ≥ 4 (Table 17.9) or if they have crescendo TIAs (defined as two or more in a week); these patients are at highest risk of stroke. CT is used where MRI is contra-indicated or unavailable. Brain imaging should be performed within 1 week in lower-risk patients.

Table 17.8 Features of transient ischaemic attacks in different arterial territories

Carotid territory symptoms	Vertebrobasilar territory symptoms
Amaurosis fugax	Diplopia, vertigo, vomiting
Aphasia	Choking and dysarthria
Hemiparesis	Ataxia
Hemisensory loss	Hemisensory loss
Hemianopic visual loss	Hemianopic or bilateral visual loss
	Tetraparesis
	Loss of consciousness (rare)

Table 17.9 ABCD2 risk of stroke after a transient ischaemic attack (TIA)

	Score
Age ≥ 60 years	1 point
Blood pressure ≥ 140 mmHg systolic or 90 mmHg diastolic	1 point
Clinical features	
Unilateral weakness	2 points
Speech disturbance without weakness	1 point
Other	0 point
Duration of TIA	
≥ 60 minutes	2 points
10–59 minutes	1 point
< 10 minutes	0 point
Presence of diabetes mellitus	1 point

Two-day risk of stroke is 4.1% with a score 4–5 and 8.1% with a score 6–7.

Carotid artery imaging Carotid Doppler and duplex ultrasound scanning are performed (ideally within 1 week of onset of symptoms) to look for carotid atheroma and stenosis. MR angiography or CT angiography are performed if ultrasound suggests carotid stenosis to determine the degree of carotid artery stenosis.

Other investigations include ECG to confirm sinus rhythm and cardiac echo.

Treatment

Antithrombotic treatment Aspirin 300 mg should be given immediately and continued long term (75 mg once daily). Clopidogrel (75 mg daily) is given for those patients intolerant of aspirin. Long-term anticoagulation with warfarin (after brain imaging) is given to patients in atrial fibrillation, with some valvular lesions (uninfected) or dilated cardiomyopathy.

Other secondary prevention This involves advice and treatment to reverse risk factors (p. 746). Control of hypertension (p. 484) is the single most important factor in the prevention of stroke. Treatment with a statin (e.g. simvastatin 40 mg daily) should be given to patients with a total cholesterol >3.5 mmol/L or low-density lipoprotein cholesterol >2.5 mmol/L.

Carotid endarterectomy is recommended in patients with internal carotid artery stenosis >70%. Successful surgery reduces the risk of further TIA/stroke by about 75%. Endarterectomy is associated with a mortality of approximately 3% and a similar risk of stroke.

Patients should not drive for a month after TIA.

Cerebral infarction

Most thromboembolic cerebral infarctions cause an obvious stroke. Following vessel occlusion brain ischaemia occurs, followed by infarction. The infarcted area is surrounded by a swollen area which can regain function with neurological recovery.

Clinical features

The neurological deficit produced by the occlusion of a vessel may be predicted by a knowledge of neuroanatomy and vascular supply (Fig. 17.1 and Fig. 17.9). In practice it is less clear-cut because of collateral supply to brain areas.

Cerebral hemisphere infarcts The most common stroke is the hemiplegia caused by infarction of the internal capsule (the narrow zone of motor and sensory fibres that converges on the brainstem from the cerebral cortex; Fig. 17.1) following occlusion of a branch of the middle cerebral artery. The signs are contralateral to the lesion: hemiplegia (arm > leg), hemisensory loss, upper motor neurone facial weakness and hemianopia. Initially the patient has a hypotonic hemiplegia with decreased reflexes; within days this develops into a spastic hemiplegia with increased reflexes and an extensor plantar response, i.e. an upper motor neurone lesion (Table 17.4). Weakness may recover gradually over days or months. Lacunar infarcts are small infarcts that produce localized deficits, e.g. pure motor stroke, pure sensory stroke.

Brainstem infarction Brainstem infarction causes complex patterns of dysfunction depending on the sites involved:

- *The lateral medullary syndrome*, the most common of the brainstem vascular syndromes, is caused by occlusion of the posterior inferior cerebellar artery. It presents with sudden vomiting and vertigo, ipsilateral Horner's syndrome, facial numbness, cerebellar signs and palatal paralysis with a diminished gag reflex. On the side opposite the lesion there is loss of pain and temperature sensation.
- *Coma* as a result of involvement of the reticular activating system.
- *The locked-in syndrome* in which all voluntary muscles are paralysed except for those that control eye movement is caused by upper brainstem infarction.
- *Pseudobulbar palsy* (p. 739) is caused by lower brainstem infarction.

Multi-infarct dementia (vascular dementia) is a syndrome caused by multiple small cortical infarcts, resulting in generalized intellectual loss; there is a stepwise progression with each infarct. The final picture is of dementia, pseudobulbar palsy and a shuffling gait resembling Parkinson's disease.

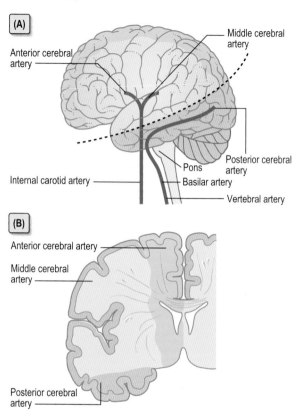

Fig. 17.9 The arterial supply to the brain. (A) The area above the dotted line is supplied by the internal carotid artery and the area below the line is supplied by the vertebral artery. **(B)** A coronal section through the brain. The anterior cerebral artery supplies the medial surface of the hemisphere and the middle cerebral artery supplies the lateral surface of the hemisphere, including the internal capsule.

Management

Stroke is a medical emergency – 'time lost is brain lost'. Immediate management is summarized in Emergency Box 17.1. Patients with a cerebellar infarct causing hydrocephalus or a large cerebral infarct with brain oedema and a risk of brain herniation should be referred for immediate neurosurgical evaluation.

Detailed clotting studies and autoantibody screen to look for evidence of conditions associated with thrombophilia are indicated in younger patients with unexplained stroke. Echocardiography (in suspected cardioembolic stroke) and

✚ Emergency Box 17.1

Immediate management of acute stroke

Investigations

- *Brain CT (or MRI)*. Demonstrates the site of the lesion; distinguishes between ischaemic/haemorrhagic stroke; identifies conditions mimicking stroke, e.g. cerebral tumour or abscess. Imaging is performed immediately (at the next scanning slot) in the following circumstances:
  - patient presents within the time frame for thrombolysis
  - early anticoagulation is indicated
  - recent history of head injury
  - severe headache at onset of stroke symptoms
  - patient is taking anticoagulant treatment or has a known bleeding tendency
  - depressed level of consciousness (Glasgow Coma Score <13).
- Otherwise brain imaging is performed within 24 hours of onset of symptoms. MRI is indicated if the underlying pathology is uncertain, the diagnosis is in doubt (CT may not show an infarct in the first few hours), or imaging is delayed for more than 10 days after stroke.
- *Blood tests* are similar to a transient ischaemic attack (TIA; p. 747).
- *ECG:* to look for atrial fibrillation, myocardial infarction.

Treatment

- *Aspirin*. Aspirin 300 mg daily (orally, via nasogastric tube or rectally) should be given as soon as possible after the onset of stroke symptoms once a diagnosis of primary intracerebral haemorrhage has been excluded by brain imaging.
- *Thrombolysis*. Intravenous alteplase (tPA, p. 251) improves functional outcome if given within 4.5 hours of the onset of symptoms in *acute ischaemic stroke*. It is given immediately if haemorrhage has been excluded in the emergency department provided that patients can be managed in an acute stroke service with appropriate support from a stroke physician. Contraindications are listed on page 252.
- *Hypertension*. Blood pressure should only be lowered in the acute phase where there are likely to be complications of hypertension such as hypertensive encephalopathy, heart failure or aortic dissection.
- Endovascular thrombectomy is of benefit for patients with stroke caused by occlusion of the proximal anterior circulation.

Supportive care

- *Stroke unit*. Dedicated stroke units improve outcome compared to management on a general ward.
- *Swallowing and feeding*. Dysphagia is common and may cause aspiration pneumonia and nutritional deficit. Formal assessment of swallowing by trained staff is performed on admission and, if the admission screen

indicates swallowing problems, specialist assessment (Speech and Language Therapy, SALT) is made within 24–72 hours. Feeding by fine-bore nasogastric tube or percutaneous gastrostomy may be necessary.

- *Unconscious patient.* Maintenance of hydration, frequent turning to avoid pressure sores and other supportive measures.
- *Prevention of deep venous thrombosis* by anti-embolism (T.E.D.) stockings. Heparin is not given.

syphilis serology are performed in selected patients. High-dose aspirin (300 mg daily) is continued for 2 weeks before converting to clopidogrel. Anticoagulation is initiated immediately for cerebral venous thrombosis or arterial dissection, but delayed for 14 days after the onset of ischaemic stroke in atrial fibrillation due to the risk of bleeding into the infarcted area. Carotid artery imaging, anti-thrombotic treatment and secondary prevention is similar to TIA (p. 748). Internal carotid endarterectomy or stenting reduces the risk of recurrent stroke (by 75%) in patients who have had an infarct and who have internal carotid artery stenosis which narrows the arterial lumen by more than 70%. It is considered in patients with a non-disabling stroke who are likely to have some recoverable function.

Further management of the stroke patient centres on identification and treatment of risk factors (p. 746) and rehabilitation to restore function. BP should not be lowered within the first 72 hours after an ischaemic stroke and any sudden falls in perfusion should be avoided. Statins should be offered to all patients unless there is a contraindication. Optimal care is on a stroke rehabilitation unit that provides multidisciplinary services, coordinates disability-related medical care and trains caregivers. Physiotherapy is particularly useful in the first few months in reducing spasticity, relieving contractures and teaching patients to use walking aids. Following recovery, the occupational therapist plays a valuable role in assessing the requirement for and arranging the provision of various aids and modifications in the home, such as stair rails, hoists, or wheelchairs. Patients and relatives may gain useful information and support from a Stroke Association (e.g. http://www.stroke.org.uk).

Prognosis

About one-quarter of patients will die in the first 2 years following a stroke; the prognosis is worse for bleeds than for infarction. Gradual improvement usually follows stroke, with a plateau reached 3–4 months after stroke onset, although one-third of long-term survivors are permanently dependent on the help of others. Only 25% of patients return to a level of everyday participation and physical functioning of community-matched persons who have not had a stroke. About 10% of all patients will suffer a recurrent stroke within 1 year.

Primary intracranial haemorrhage

Intracerebral haemorrhage

Intracerebral haemorrhage causes approximately 10% of strokes. It is associated with a higher mortality than ischaemic stroke (up to 50%). Major risk factors for intracerebral haemorrhage are hypertension, excess alcohol consumption, increasing age and smoking. These risk factors lead to secondary vascular changes such as small vessel disease and arterial aneurysms which may eventually rupture and bleed. Presentation is with sudden loss of consciousness and stroke (p. 745) often accompanied by a severe headache. Diagnosis is made on brain imaging by CT or MRI. Anticoagulants should be stopped in patients with intracerebral haemorrhage and the effects reversed by prothrombin complex concentrate. A decision to restart anticoagulants (usually stopped for 7–10 days after an intracerebral haemorrhage) is made on a case-by-case basis. Control of hypertension is vital – with intravenous drugs in an intensive care unit setting for systolic BP > 160–180 mmHg. Measures to reduce intracranial pressure may be required, including mechanical ventilation and mannitol. Patients with a large intracerebral haematoma causing deepening coma or brainstem compression or patients with a cerebellar bleed causing hydrocephalus as a result of obstruction of the drainage pathways for CSF fluid should be referred for immediate neurosurgical evaluation.

Subarachnoid haemorrhage

Subarachnoid haemorrhage (SAH) means spontaneous rather than traumatic arterial bleeding into the subarachnoid space.

Incidence

SAH accounts for 5% of strokes and has an annual incidence of 6 per 100 000. The mean age of patients at presentation is 50 years.

Aetiology

SAH is caused by rupture of:

- Saccular ('berry') aneurysms in 70% of cases. These are acquired lesions that are most commonly located at the branching points (Fig. 17.10) of the major arteries coursing through the subarachnoid space at the base of the brain (the circle of Willis).
- Congenital arteriovenous malformations (AVMs) in 10%. The risk of a first haemorrhage in unruptured AVMs (20% fatal and 30% resulting in permanent disability) is approximately 2–3% per year. Once an AVM has ruptured, the risk of re-bleeds is approximately 10% per year. In 20% of cases, no lesion can be found.

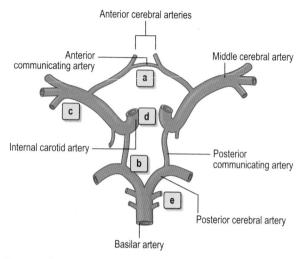

Fig. 17.10 The main cerebral arteries showing the circle of Willis and the most common sites for berry aneurysms. Frequency of occurrence, a–e (decreasing order): a, anterior communicating artery; b, origin of the posterior communicating artery; c, trifurcation of the middle cerebral artery; d, termination of the internal carotid artery; e, basilar artery.

Clinical features

Most intracranial aneurysms remain asymptomatic until they rupture and cause an SAH. Some, however, become symptomatic because of a mass effect, and the most common symptom is a painful third-nerve palsy. The typical presentation of SAH is the sudden onset of severe headache, often occipital, that reaches maximum intensity immediately or within minutes. The headache is typically described as the 'worst ever' and there is absence of similar headaches in the past. It is often accompanied by nausea and vomiting, and sometimes loss of consciousness. On examination there may be signs of meningeal irritation (neck stiffness and a positive Kernig's sign), focal neurological signs and subhyaloid haemorrhages (between the retina and vitreous membrane) with or without papilloedema. Some patients have experienced small warning headaches a few days before the major bleed.

Investigation

- CT scan is the investigation of choice and should be undertaken as soon as possible. It shows subarachnoid or intraventricular blood in 95% of cases undergoing scanning within 24 hours of the haemorrhage; the sensitivity decreases after that time.
- LP (p. 740) is indicated if there is a strong clinical suspicion of an SAH but the CT scan is normal. An increase in pigments (bilirubin and/or

oxyhaemoglobin released from lysis and phagocytosis of red blood cells) is the key finding which supports the diagnosis of SAH. LP must be performed at least 12 hours after symptom onset to allow sufficient time for haemoglobin to degrade into oxyhaemoglobin and bilirubin. Detection of oxyhaemoglobin without bilirubin makes SAH less likely. Pigments in the CSF are detected by spectrophotometry of the supernatant after centrifugation of the last fraction of CSF taken at lumbar puncture. The specimen should be protected from light. Bilirubin can be detected in the CSF for up to 2 weeks after SAH.

- MR angiography is usually performed to establish the source of bleeding in all patients potentially fit for surgery.

Management

Immediate management consists of bed rest and supportive measures with cautious control of hypertension. Nimodipine, a calcium-channel blocker, is given by mouth (60 mg 4-hourly) or by intravenous infusion (1–2 mg per hour via a central line) to reduce cerebral artery spasm, a cause of ischaemia and further neurological deterioration. Hyponatraemia (which contributes to delayed cerebral ischaemia) occurs due to urinary salt loss and patients may require large volumes of intravenous 0.9% saline to maintain normal sodium concentrations. All patients should be discussed with a neurosurgeon. Obliteration of the aneurysm by surgical clipping or endovascular coiling under radiological guidance prevents re-bleeding. Surviving patients should be advised on secondary prevention, especially on treatment of hypertension and the need to stop smoking.

Prognosis

Approximately 50% of patients die suddenly or soon after the haemorrhage. A further 10–20% die in the early weeks in hospital from further bleeding. The outcome is variable in the survivors; some patients are left with major neurological deficits. Glasgow Coma Score on admission has the most prognostic significance; patients with a score >12 usually have a good outcome.

Subdural haematoma

Subdural haematoma (SDH) means accumulation of blood in the subdural space following the rupture of a vein running from the hemisphere to the sagittal sinus. It is almost always the result of head injury, often minor, and the latent interval between injury and symptoms may be weeks or months. Elderly patients and alcoholics are particularly susceptible because they are accident prone and their atrophic brains make the connecting veins more susceptible to rupture. The main clinical symptoms are headache, drowsiness and confusion, which may fluctuate. The diagnosis is usually made on CT, and treatment is by surgical removal of the haematoma.

Extradural haemorrhage

Extradural haematomas are caused by injuries that fracture the temporal bone and rupture the underlying middle meningeal artery. Clinically there is the picture of a head injury with a brief period of unconsciousness followed by a lucid interval of recovery. This is then followed by rapid deterioration with focal neurological signs and deterioration in conscious level if surgical drainage is not immediately carried out.

EPILEPSY AND LOSS OF CONSCIOUSNESS

Epilepsy

A seizure is a convulsion or transient abnormal event caused by a paroxysmal discharge of cerebral neurones. Epilepsy is the continuing tendency to have such seizures. Epilepsy is common, with 2% of the UK population having two or more seizures during their lives, and in 0.5% epilepsy is an active problem.

Classification

Seizures are classified clinically as partial or generalized (Table 17.10). Partial seizures involve only a portion of the brain at their onset (e.g. temporal lobe),

Table 17.10 The more common types of seizure

Generalized seizure types

Bilateral abnormal electrical activity with bilateral motor manifestations and impaired consciousness
Absence seizures (petit mal)
Generalized tonic–clonic seizures (grand mal)
Myoclonic seizures
Tonic seizures
Akinetic seizures

Partial seizure types

Electrical activity starts in one area of the brain
Simple partial seizures (without impaired awareness, e.g. Jacksonian seizures)
Complex partial seizures (with impaired awareness, e.g. temporal lobe seizure)
Partial seizures evolving to tonic–clonic seizures
Apparent generalized tonic–clonic seizures, with ECG but not clinical evidence of focal onset

Unclassifiable seizures

Seizures that do not fit a category above

although these may later become generalized (secondarily generalized tonic–clonic seizures):

- *Generalized tonic–clonic seizures (grand mal seizures).* There is a sudden onset of a rigid tonic phase followed by a convulsion (clonic phase) in which the muscles jerk rhythmically and the eyes remain open. The episode lasts typically for seconds to minutes, may be associated with tongue biting and incontinence of urine, and is followed by a period of (post-ictal) flaccid unresponsiveness followed by confusion or drowsiness lasting several hours. Headache is common after a tonic–conic seizure.

- *Typical absence seizures (petit mal).* This is usually a disorder of childhood in which the child ceases activity, stares and pales for a few seconds only. It is characterized by 3-Hz spike and wave activity on the EEG. Children with petit mal tend to develop generalized tonic–clonic seizures in adult life.

- *Myoclonic, tonic and akinetic seizures.* There is isolated muscle jerking (myoclonic), intense stiffening of the body (tonic) or cessation of movement, falling and loss of consciousness (akinetic).

- *Partial seizures* involve epileptic activity in a part of the brain and are simple (not affecting consciousness or memory) or complex (affecting awareness or memory before, during or immediately after the seizure). Patients with focal seizures have symptoms depending on the area of the brain where the seizure starts, often the temporal lobe. The seizures may become generalized to affect the whole brain (secondary generalization). Jacksonian (motor) seizures originate in the motor cortex. They typically result in jerking movements, typically beginning in the corner of the mouth or thumb and index finger, and spreading to involve the limbs on the opposite side of the epileptic focus. Paralysis of the involved limbs may follow for several hours (Todd's paralysis). Temporal lobe seizures are associated with olfactory and visual hallucinations, blank staring, feelings of unreality (jamais-vu) or undue familiarity (déjà-vu) with the surroundings.

Aetiology and precipitants

Flashing lights or a flickering television screen may provoke an attack in susceptible patients. A cause for epilepsy is found in less than one-third of cases in UK surveys. Known causes include cerebrovascular disease (15%), cerebral tumours (6%), alcohol-related seizures (6%) and post-traumatic epilepsy (2%). Hippocampal sclerosis is the main pathological cause of temporal lobe epilepsy. Childhood febrile convulsions are the main risk factor. It is usually visible on MRI and is one of the more common causes of refractory epilepsy, in which case it may be amenable to surgical resection of the damaged temporal lobe.

Occasionally, metabolic disturbances such as hypoglycaemia, acute hypoxia, hypocalcaemia, hyponatraemia, uraemia and hepatocellular failure present with convulsions.

About 30% of patients have a first-degree relative with epilepsy, although the exact mode of inheritance is unknown. Primary epilepsies are due to complex developmental abnormalities of neuronal control; there are abnormalities in synaptic connections and distribution and release of neurotransmitters.

Evaluation and investigation

There are three steps in the evaluation of a patient with possible epilepsy:

1. Confirm if the patient has epilepsy. The diagnosis is made clinically and a detailed description of the attack from an eye-witness is invaluable. Disorders causing attacks of altered consciousness must be differentiated from epilepsy (Table 17.3).
2. Determine the patient's seizure type (see classification).
3. Identify any underlying cause for epilepsy:
   - The EEG is used to assist in the classification of epilepsy and to confirm the clinical suspicion. It is frequently normal between attacks and false-positive 'non-specific' abnormalities may be present in non-epileptics. During a seizure the EEG is almost always abnormal and is shown typically by a cortical spike focus (e.g. in a temporal lobe) or by generalized spike and wave activity. Video-EEG recording is used where the diagnosis of epilepsy is in doubt.
   - Brain imaging is indicated in all new cases to exclude an underlying lesion. CT is used in the emergency setting to look for a space-occupying lesion, e.g. tumour. MRI with imaging of the hippocampi is used routinely to study epilepsy.

Management

Emergency measures

The emergency treatment is to ensure that patients harm themselves as little as possible and that the airway remains patent. Most seizures stop spontaneously. A prolonged seizure (longer than 3 minutes) or repeated seizures are treated with rectal (10 mg) or i.v. diazepam or lorazepam. Repeated seizures with brief periods of recovery may lead to status epilepticus.

Status epilepticus This is a medical emergency. There are continuous seizures for 30 minutes or longer (or two or more seizures without recovery of consciousness between them over a similar period). When grand mal seizures follow one another, there is a risk of death from cardiorespiratory failure. Precipitating factors in a known epileptic include abruptly stopping antiepileptic treatment, intercurrent illness, alcohol abuse and poor compliance with therapy; over 50% of all episodes occur in patients without any history of epilepsy. Rectal diazepam or buccal midazolam (10 mg) is given out of hospital. Management in hospital is summarized in Emergency Box 17.2. EEG monitoring should be considered in refractory status or if the diagnosis is in doubt (consider pseudostatus – non-epileptic attacks with a psychological basis).

✚ **Emergency Box 17.2**

Management and investigation of status epilepticus

General measures

- Administer oxygen.
- Secure venous access via a large vein; many anticonvulsants cause phlebitis.
- Blood glucose, FBC, U/E, calcium, magnesium, drug screen, anticonvulsant levels.
- Cardiorespiratory monitoring and pulse oximetry.
- Thiamine, 250 mg i.v. over 10 minutes, if nutrition poor or alcohol abuse suspected. In the UK give Vitamin B and C, high-potency ampoules, one pair i.v. over 10 minutes.

Control of seizures

- *First line.* Lorazepam 4 mg i.v. at 2 mg/min, repeated after 10 minutes if no response. Give rectal diazepam (10–20 mg) if no i.v. access. Lorazepam may cause respiratory depression and hypotension, and facilities for resuscitation should be available.

- *Second line.* If seizures continue, give phenytoin 15 mg/kg i.v. 50 mg/min or fosphenytoin (p. 806). Both may cause cardiac dysrhythmias, and ECG monitoring is necessary.

- *Third line.* Phenobarbital 10 mg/kg at a rate not exceeding 100 mg/min and repeated at intervals of 6–8 hours if necessary. Valproate i.v. (>25 mg/kg) is an alternative. For refractory seizures (>90 min) intubation, ventilation and anaesthesia in an intensive care setting may be needed.

Investigations

- Consider brain CT scan, lumbar puncture and blood cultures, depending on clinical circumstances.

CT, computed tomography; ECG, electrocardiogram; FBC, full blood count; U/E, urea and electrolytes.

Once status is controlled, regular anticonvulsant therapy is continued to prevent subsequent fits. Intravenous treatment is withdrawn when anticonvulsant therapy is established.

Antiepileptic drugs

Antiepileptic drugs (AEDs) are indicated when there is a firm clinical diagnosis of recurrent seizures or after a first seizure with features associated with a high risk of seizure recurrence (abnormal EEG and/or structural brain abnormality on imaging). Treatment is started with a single first-line antiepileptic drug (Table 17.11). Monotherapy is the aim and the dose is increased until seizure control is achieved or tolerance exceeded. Routine measurement of serum drug levels is necessary only for phenytoin and phenobarbital. Levels should also be

Table 17.11 First-line treatment depending on seizure type

Seizure type	Drug	Major side effects of drug treatment
Generalized tonic–clonic	Sodium valproate†	Weight gain, hair loss, liver damage, blood dyscrasias
	Levetiracetam	Headaches, drowsiness
	Lamotrigine	TEN
	Carbamazepine	Rashes, leucopenia, TEN
	Topiramate	Weight loss, renal stones, glaucoma
Petit mal	Sodium valproate†	
	Ethosuximide	Rashes, blood dyscrasias, night terrors
Partial seizures	Lamotrigine Carbamazepine	
	Levetiracetam	
	Sodium valproate	
	Phenytoin*	Rashes, blood dyscrasias, lymphadenopathy, SLE, TEN, gum hypertrophy, hirsutism, osteomalacia, folate deficiency

TEN, toxic epidermal necrolysis. SLE, systemic lupus erythematosus.
*In developing countries.
†Avoid in women of child-bearing age; associated with highest risk of major congenital malformation in fetuses exposed to drug during pregnancy.

measured if non-compliance is suspected or if there are signs of toxicity. Idiosyncratic side effects (i.e. non-dose related), which tend to be more common than dose-related effects, are listed in Table 17.11. Intoxication with all anticonvulsants causes a syndrome of ataxia, nystagmus and dysarthria. Side effects of chronic administration of phenytoin as listed in Table 17.11 are reduced by maintaining serum levels within the therapeutic range. Phenytoin is a potent hepatic enzyme inducer and will reduce the efficacy of the contraceptive pill. Many new drugs have been developed and there remain different views about the most appropriate drugs for each seizure type. Epilepsy is one of the few disorders where non-generic ('brand name') prescribing is justified to ensure consistent drug levels.

Drug withdrawal Gradual withdrawal of drugs should only be undertaken when the patient has been seizure-free for at least 2 years, and is only achieved successfully in less than 50%. Many patients will have further fits, resulting in a threat to employment and driving (p. 761).

Neurosurgical treatment

Surgical treatment, e.g. amputation of the anterior temporal lobe, cures epilepsy in 50% of patients with poorly controlled epilepsy and a clearly defined focus of abnormal electrical activity (<1% of all patients with epilepsy).

Advice to patients

Patients should restrict their lives as little as possible but follow simple advice: for example, avoid swimming alone; avoid dangerous sports, such as rock climbing; and leave the door open when taking a bath. In European Union member states, patients with epilepsy (whether on or off treatment) may drive a motor vehicle (cars, vans, motorcycles) provided that they have been seizure-free for a year. Patients who wish to drive heavy goods vehicles (buses, lorries, etc.) must have been seizure-free and off all AEDs for 10 years or more.

MOVEMENT DISORDERS

The extrapyramidal system is a general term for the basal ganglia and their connections with other brain areas. The overall function of this system is the initiation and modulation of movement. Defective function produces slowness (bradykinesia), stiffness (rigidity) and/or disorders of movement (rest tremor, chorea and other dyskinesias). Table 17.12 outlines the clinical varieties: Parkinson's disease and essential tremor are the most common.

Table 17.12 Movement disorders
Akinetic–rigid syndromes
Idiopathic Parkinson's disease
Drug-induced parkinsonism, e.g. phenothiazines
MPTP-induced parkinsonism
Postencephalitic parkinsonism
'Parkinsonism plus'
Wilson's disease
Childhood akinetic–rigid syndromes
Dyskinesias
Essential tremor
Chorea
Hemiballismus
Myoclonus
Tics
Dystonias
Paroxysmal dyskinesias
MPTP, methylphenyltetrahydropyridine.

Akinetic–rigid syndromes

Idiopathic Parkinson's disease

Parkinson's disease (PD) is a common neurodegenerative disease developing predominantly in older people. The clinical features principally result from the progressive depletion of dopamine-secreting cells in the substantia nigra. These neurones project to the striatum and their loss leads to alteration of activity of the neural circuits within the basal ganglia that regulate movement. Disruption of dopamine along the non-striatal pathways accounts for the neuropsychiatric pathology associated with PD. Cell loss in PD is thought to be due to abnormal accumulation of α-synuclein bound to ubiquitin which forms cytoplasmic inclusions called Lewy bodies.

Aetiology

The cause of the disease is unknown. Factors possibly involved are:

- MPTP (methylphenyltetrahydropyridine), an impurity produced during illegal synthesis of opiates produces severe parkinsonism.
- Survivors of an epidemic of encephalitis lethargica in the early 20th century developed parkinsonism. However, there is no evidence that idiopathic PD is caused by an environmental toxin or an infective agent.
- Parkinson's disease is less prevalent in tobacco smokers than in lifelong abstainers.
- Genetic factors. There is clustering of early-onset PD in some families. Mutations in the parkin gene, α-synuclein gene and ubiquitin carboxyl-terminal hydrolase L1 gene have been found in some of these families. Relevance to the common sporadic older PD cases is unclear.

Clinical features

The combination of rest tremor, rigidity and bradykinesia (slow movements) develops over months or several years together with changes in posture. These features are initially more prominent on one side:

- *Tremor*. This is a characteristic 4–7 Hz resting tremor (cf. cerebellar disease), usually most obvious in the hands ('pill-rolling' of the thumb and fingers), improved by voluntary movement and made worse by anxiety.
- *Rigidity* refers to the increase in tone in the limbs and trunk. The limbs resist passive extension throughout movement (lead pipe rigidity, or cogwheel when combined with tremor), in contrast to the hypertonia of an upper motor neurone lesion (p. 721), where resistance falls away as the movement continues (clasp-knife).
- *Akinesia ('poverty of movement')*. There is difficulty in initiating movement (starting to walk, or rising from a chair). The face is expressionless and unblinking. Speech is slow and monotonous. The writing becomes small (micrographia) and tends to tail off at the end of a line. There is a progressive fatiguing and decrement in the amplitude of repetitive movements.

- *Postural changes.* A stoop is characteristic. The gait is shuffling, festinant (hurrying) and with poor arm swinging. The posture is sometimes called 'simian', to describe the forward flexion, immobility of the arms and lack of facial expression. Balance is poor, with a tendency to fall.

Non-motor features may predate motor features and consist of neuropsychiatric symptoms (depression, hallucinations, dementia, impulsive behaviours), sleep disorders (insomnia, sleep fragmentation, vivid dreams), gastrointestinal and autonomic disorders (drooling of saliva, excess sweating, dysphagia, constipation) and fatigue and weight loss. Anosmia is present in 90% of patients, as the olfactory bulb is one of the first structures to be affected. There is gradual progression of the disease over 10–15 years, with death resulting most commonly from bronchopneumonia.

Investigations

The diagnosis is clinical. Other brain diseases (e.g. multi-infarct dementia, repeated head injury) can cause features of *parkinsonism,* i.e. slowing, rigidity and tremor, which can usually be differentiated from idiopathic PD on clinical grounds. MRI is normal and not necessary in typical cases. Dopamine transporter (DaT) imaging makes use of a radiolabelled ligand binding to dopaminergic terminals to assess the extent of nigrostriatal cell loss. It may occasionally be needed to distinguish PD from other causes of tremor, or drug-induced parkinsonism, but it cannot discriminate between PD and other akinetic-rigid syndromes.

Management

The decision to start treatment is determined by the degree to which the patient is functionally impaired. Treatment does not alter the natural history. Dopamine replacement improves motor symptoms and is the basis of pharmacological therapy. Initial therapy is with one of the following medicines:

Levodopa (L-dopa, a dopamine precursor) is combined with a peripheral dopa-decarboxylase inhibitor – benserazide (co-beneldopa) or carbidopa (co-careldopa) – to reduce peripheral side effects (e.g. nausea, hypotension). A typical starting dose would be 50 mg of L-dopa (e.g. co-careldopa 62.5 mg) three times daily, increasing after 1 week to 100 mg three times daily. Therapy may become less effective with time. Patients may also switch between periods of dopamine-induced dyskinesias (choreas and dystonic movements) and periods of immobility ('on–off' syndrome).

Dopamine agonists are non-ergot dopamine agonists (ropinirole, pramipexole, rotigotine). Possible side effects are impulse control disorders (pathological gambling, compulsive shopping, hypersexuality) and excessive daytime sleepiness.

Monoamine oxidase B inhibitors (e.g. selegiline, rasagiline) inhibit the catabolism of dopamine in the brain.

The options for managing disease progression and the loss of smooth motor control associated with levodopa-based drugs are shortening the interval between drug dosing and increasing the dose, adding or swapping to other antiparkinsonian drugs using catechol-*O*-methyl transferase inhibitors (entacapone, tolcapone) to prevent peripheral breakdown of L-dopa or using apomorphine by subcutaneous pump or by subcutaneous injection as an intermittent 'rescue' for off periods.

Additional treatment Physiotherapy can improve gait and help to prevent falls. Selective serotonin reuptake inhibitors are the treatment of choice for depression. Deep brain stimulation (DBS) using stereotactic insertion of electrodes into the brain has proved to be a major therapeutic advance in selected patients (usually under age 70 years) with disabling dyskinesias and motor fluctuations not adequately controlled with medical therapy. Dopaminergic drugs can be reduced (but not withdrawn) after DBS. There is a trend towards earlier use of DBS before motor complications become severe. Information and support for patients and relatives is provided by the Parkinson's Disease Society (http://www.parkinsons.org.uk).

Other akinetic-rigid syndromes

Drug-induced parkinsonism

Reserpine, phenothiazines and butyrophenones block dopamine receptors and may induce a parkinsonian syndrome with slowness and rigidity, but usually with little tremor. These syndromes tend not to progress, they respond poorly to L-dopa, and the correct management is to stop the offending drug.

'Parkinsonism plus'

This describes rare disorders in which there is parkinsonism and evidence of a separate pathology. *Progressive supranuclear palsy* is the most common disorder and consists of axial rigidity, dementia and signs of parkinsonism, together with gaze paresis. Other examples are *multiple system atrophy* (early severe autonomic neuropathy), such as olivo-ponto-cerebellar degeneration and primary autonomic failure (Shy–Drager syndrome). Unlike idiopathic PD, there is a poor response to L-dopa in these conditions.

Dyskinesias

Benign essential tremor

This is usually a familial (autosomal dominant) tremor of the arms and head (titubation) which occurs most frequently in elderly people. Unlike the tremor of Parkinson's disease it is not usually present at rest, but is most obvious when the hands adopt a posture such as holding a glass or a spoon (p. 762). It is made worse by anxiety and improved by alcohol, propranolol, primidone (an anticonvulsant) and mirtazapine (an antidepressant).

Table 17.13 Causes of chorea

Huntington's disease
Dentatorubropallidoluysian atrophy
Sydenham's chorea
Benign hereditary chorea
Drug-induced: phenytoin, levodopa, alcohol
Thyrotoxicosis
Pregnancy and the oral contraceptive pill
Hypoparathyroidism
Systemic lupus erythematosus
Polycythaemia vera
Stroke (basal ganglia)
Other CNS disease: tumour, traumatic subdural haematoma, following carbon
monoxide poisoning, Wilson's disease

Chorea

Chorea is a continuous flow of jerky, quasi-purposive movements, flitting from one part of the body to another. They may interfere with voluntary movements but cease during sleep. The causes of chorea are listed in Table 17.13.

Huntington's disease

This is a rare autosomal dominant condition with full penetrance. There is a relentlessly progressive course, with chorea and personality change preceding dementia and death. Symptoms usually begin in middle age. Expansion of CAG repeats in the Huntington's disease gene on chromosome 4 leads to production of mutant *huntingtin* protein. It is not known how the mutant protein causes disease. There is loss of neurones within the basal ganglia, leading to depletion of GABA (γ-aminobutyric acid) and acetylcholine but sparing dopamine. No treatment arrests the disease, and the management is symptomatic treatment of chorea and genetic counselling of family members.

Hemiballismus

Hemiballismus (also called hemiballism) describes violent swinging movements of one side of the body, usually caused by infarction or haemorrhage in the contralateral subthalamic nucleus.

Myoclonus

Myoclonus is the sudden, involuntary jerking of a single muscle or group of muscles. The most common example is benign essential myoclonus, which is the sudden jerking of a limb or the body on falling asleep. Myoclonus also occurs with epilepsy and some encephalopathies.

Tics

Tics are brief, repeated stereotypical movements, usually involving the face and shoulders. Unlike other involuntary movements, it is usually possible for the patient to control tics.

Dystonias

Dystonias are prolonged spasms of muscle contraction. They occur as a symptom of neurological disease, e.g. Wilson's disease, but are usually focal, of unknown cause and occur without other neurological problems, e.g. blepharospasm (spasms of forced blinking) or spasmodic torticollis (the head is turned and held to one side or drawn backwards or forwards). Targeted injection of minute amounts of botulinum toxin (which inhibits the release of acetylcholine from nerve endings) into the muscle provides temporary relief. Acute dystonic reactions are seen with phenothiazines, butyrophenones and metoclopramide, and can occur after a single dose of the drug. Spasmodic torticollis, trismus and oculogyric crises (i.e. episodes of sustained upward gaze) may occur. Acute dystonias respond promptly to an anticholinergic drug administered by intravenous or intramuscular injection, e.g. benztropine (1–2 mg) or procyclidine (5 mg).

Multiple sclerosis

Multiple sclerosis (MS) is a chronic debilitating autoimmune disorder of the central nervous system in which there are multiple plaques of demyelination within the brain and spinal cord. These plaques are disseminated both in time and place: hence the old name 'disseminated sclerosis'.

Epidemiology

MS typically begins in early adulthood and the disease is twice as common in women as in men. The prevalence varies widely (12 per 10 000 in the UK) and rises with increasing distance from the equator. People moving from a low- to a high-risk area (e.g. from southern to northern UK) acquire the level of risk of the population they migrated to, indicating that environmental influences are a factor in pathogenesis.

Aetiology

Although the precise mechanism is unknown, there is an inflammatory process in the white matter of the brain and spinal cord mediated by B cells and CD4 T cells. It is thought that exposure to a specific infectious agent (Epstein–Barr virus [EBV]) in childhood may predispose to the later development of MS in a genetically susceptible host. Antibodies produced by B cells and T cells directed against EBV nuclear antigens may be redirected to attack CNS myelin because of molecular mimicry. The increased frequency of other autoimmune disorders in people with MS and their relatives indicates a genetic predisposition to autoimmunity.

Pathology

Inflammation, demyelination and axonal loss are the major feature of the MS plaque and cause the clinical manifestations. Plaques are perivenular and have a predilection for distinct CNS sites: optic nerves, periventricular white matter, brainstem and its cerebellar connections and the cervical spinal cord (corticospinal tracts and posterior columns). The peripheral nerves are never affected.

Clinical features

The typical patient presents as a young adult (onset of MS is rare before puberty or after 60 years) with two or more clinically distinct episodes of CNS dysfunction followed by a remission during which symptoms and signs resolve to some extent within weeks. The regression of symptoms is attributed to the resolution of inflammatory oedema and to partial remyelination. Three characteristic common presentations of relapsing and remitting MS are optic neuropathy, brainstem demyelination and spinal cord lesions.

Optic neuropathy Inflammation of the optic nerve produces blurred vision and unilateral eye pain. A lesion in the optic nerve head produces disc swelling (optic neuritis) and pallor (optic atrophy) following the attack. When inflammation occurs in the optic nerve further away from the eye (retrobulbar neuritis) examination of the fundus is normal.

Brainstem demyelination produces diplopia, vertigo, dysphagia, dysarthria, facial weakness/numbness and nystagmus. A typical picture is sudden diplopia and vertigo with nystagmus, but without tinnitus or deafness. Bilateral internuclear ophthalmoplegia is pathognomonic of MS.

Spinal cord lesions Sensory symptoms, including numbness and pins and needles, are common in MS and reflect spinothalamic and posterior column lesions. Spastic paraparesis is the result of plaques of demyelination in the cervical or thoracic cord.

There are four main clinical patterns:

- Relapsing-remitting MS (RRMS) (85–90%), the most common pattern of MS: symptoms occur in attacks (relapses) with onset over days and typically recovery, either partial or complete, over weeks. Patients may accumulate disability over time if relapses do not recover fully.
- Secondary progressive MS: this late stage of MS consists of gradually worsening disability progressing slowly over years; 75% of patients with RRMS will eventually evolve into a secondary progressive phase.

- Primary progressive MS (PPMS) (10–15%) is characterized by gradually worsening disability without relapses or remissions and typically presents later and is associated with fewer inflammatory changes on MRI.
- Relapsing-progressive MS (<5%) is the least common form of MS and is similar to PPMS but with occasional supra-added relapses on a background of progressive disability from the outset.

Late MS causes severe disability with spastic tetraparesis, ataxia, optic atrophy, nystagmus, brainstem signs, pseudobulbar palsy and urinary incontinence. Cognitive impairment, often with frontal lobe features, may also occur.

Differential diagnosis

Initially, individual plaques (in the optic nerve, brainstem or cord) may cause diagnostic difficulty and must be distinguished from inflammatory (Behçet's disease, systemic lupus erythematosus [SLE], sarcoid), mass or vascular lesions. A single lesion in the cord may produce paraparesis and a sensory level and mechanical cord compression (p. 782) must be excluded by MRI. In young patients with a relapsing and remitting course, the diagnosis is straightforward, as few other diseases produce this clinical picture.

Investigations

- MRI of brain and spinal cord is the definitive investigation and shows plaques particularly in the periventricular area and brainstem. Lesions are rarely visible on CT.
- Electrophysiological tests. Visual, auditory and somatosensory evoked potentials may be prolonged, even in the absence of any past or present visual symptoms.
- CSF examination is usually unnecessary as the diagnosis is made with MRI or evoked potentials and a compatible clinical picture. Protein concentration and cell count (5–60 mononuclear cells/mm^3) are raised. CSF electrophoresis shows oligoclonal immunoglobulin G (IgG) bands in 90% cases but these are not specific.

Management

- Short courses of steroids, e.g. i.v. methylprednisolone 1000 mg/day for 3 days, are used in relapses and may reduce severity. However, they do not influence long-term outlook.
- Subcutaneous administration of β-interferon reduces the relapse rate by one-third in relapsing/remitting disease and may delay the time to severe debility. Treatment is prolonged, expensive and associated with side effects, such as 'flu-like symptoms'.
- Glatiramer acetate is antigenically similar to myelin basic protein and competes with various myelin antigens for their presentation to T cells. It has similar efficacy to interferons and is given by subcutaneous injection.

- Natalizumab and mitoxantrone are reserved as second-line therapy due to side effects (progressive multifocal leucoencephalopathy and cardiac toxicity, respectively).
- Newer oral agents include fingolimod, teriflunomide and dimethyl fumarate. They all reduce relapse rate significantly.
- Physiotherapy and occupational therapy maintain the mobility of joints, and muscle relaxants (e.g. baclofen, dantrolene and benzodiazepines) reduce the discomfort and pain of spasticity. Multidisciplinary team liaison between patient, carers, medical practitioners and therapists is essential for any patient with chronic disabling disease. Urinary catheterization is eventually needed for those with bladder involvement. The Multiple Sclerosis Society provides information and support for patients and relatives (http://www.mssociety.org.uk).

NERVOUS SYSTEM INFECTION AND INFLAMMATION

Meningitis

Meningitis (inflammation of the meninges) can be caused by infection, intrathecal drug, malignant cells and blood (following subarachnoid haemorrhage). The term is, however, usually reserved for inflammation caused by infective agents (Table 17.14). Microorganisms reach the meninges either by direct extension from the ears, nasopharynx, cranial injury or congenital meningeal defect, or by bloodstream spread. Immunocompromised patients (human immunodeficiency virus [HIV], cytotoxic drug therapy) are at risk of infection by unusual organisms.

Clinical features

Acute bacterial meningitis Headache, neck stiffness and fever develop over minutes to hours. Photophobia (intolerance of light) and vomiting are often present. Kernig's sign (inability to allow full extension of the knee when the hip is flexed 90°) is usually present. Consciousness is usually not impaired, although the patient may be delirious with a high fever. Papilloedema may occur. Progressive drowsiness, lateralizing signs and cranial nerve lesions indicates the existence of a complication, e.g. venous sinus thrombosis, severe cerebral oedema or cerebral abscess. In meningococcal septicaemia there is a non-blanching petechial and purpuric skin rash and signs of shock.

Viral meningitis is usually a benign self-limiting condition lasting for about 4–10 days. There are no serious sequelae.

Chronic meningitis presents with a long history and vague symptoms of headache, lassitude, anorexia and vomiting. Signs of meningism may be absent or appear late in the course of the disease.

Differential diagnosis

Subarachnoid haemorrhage, migraine, viral encephalitis and cerebral malaria can mimic meningitis.

Table 17.14 Infective causes of meningitis in the UK

Bacteria

*Neisseria meningitidis**
*Streptococcus pneumoniae**
Staphylococcus aureus
Streptococcus group B
Listeria monocytogenes
Gram-negative bacilli, e.g. *E. coli*
Mycobacterium tuberculosis[†]
Treponema pallidum[†]

Viruses

Enterovirus (ECHO, Coxsackie)
Poliomyelitis
Mumps
Herpes simplex virus
HIV
Epstein–Barr virus

Fungi[†]

Cryptococcus neoformans
Candida albicans
Coccidioides immitis
Histoplasma capsulatum

*Account for most cases of acute bacterial meningitis outside of the neonatal period.
[†]May cause chronic meningitis with signs and symptoms for longer than 4 weeks.

Management

Suspected bacterial meningitis is a medical emergency with a high mortality rate and requires urgent investigation and treatment (Emergency Box 17.3).

Notification

All cases of meningitis must (by law in the UK) be notified to the local public health authority; this allows contact tracing and provides data for epidemiological studies.

Meningococcal prophylaxis

Oral rifampicin or ciprofloxacin is given to eradicate nasopharyngeal carriage of the organism. It is given to patients and those who have had prolonged close contact in a household setting during the 7 days before onset of the illness.

⊹ Emergency Box 17.3

Investigation and treatment of suspected bacterial meningitis

Note: A non-blanching petechial or purpuric skin rash is indicative of meningococcal infection. It is an indication for immediate treatment with third-generation cephalosporin, e.g. ceftriaxone 2 g every 12 hours. If the patient is aged >50 years, pregnant, immunocompromised or on steroids, add amoxicillin 2 g every 6 hours i.v. to provide *Listeria* cover. Give dexamethasone 0.6 mg/kg i.v. with first dose of antibiotic.

Investigations

- *Head CT scan* should be performed if there is any suspicion of an intracranial mass lesion such as focal neurological signs, papilloedema, loss of consciousness or seizure.
- *Lumbar puncture (LP)* should not be performed if meningococcal sepsis is suspected because coning of the cerebellar tonsils may follow – the organism is confirmed by blood culture. In other cases, urgent CSF microscopy, white cell count and differential, and analysis for protein and glucose concentration (Table 17.15). Auramine stain (tuberculous) and Indian ink stain (cryptococcal infection) in immunocompromised or other at-risk individual.
- *Other.* Blood cultures, blood glucose, chest X-ray, viral and syphilis serology.

Treatment

Note: Antimicrobial therapy should not be delayed if there is a contraindication or inability to perform immediate LP.

- Close liaison between clinician and microbiologist is essential
- After initial treatment with third-generation cephalosporin +/− amoxicillin, subsequent treatment will depend on results of Gram stain and culture, and antibiotic sensitivities of the organism
- Intravenous fluids and inotropes are given if there is also septicaemia (p. 577)
- Tuberculous meningitis is treated for 12 months (p. 544).

A vaccine for meningococcal group C and *Haemophilus influenzae* is part of routine childhood UK immunization.

Encephalitis

Encephalitis is inflammation of the brain parenchyma. Unlike meningitis, cerebral function is usually abnormal, with altered mental status, motor and sensory deficits. It is caused by a wide variety of viruses and may also occur in bacterial and other infections. In certain groups (e.g. men who have sex with men,

Table 17.15 Typical changes in the CSF in viral, bacterial and TB meningitis

	Normal	Bacterial	Viral	Tuberculous
Appearance	Clear	Turbid/purulent	Clear/turbid	Turbid/viscous
Mononuclear cells/mm^3	<5	<50	10–100	100–300
Polymorphs/mm^3	Nil	200–3000	Nil	0–200
Protein (g/L)	0.2–0.4	0.5–2.00	0.4–0.8	0.5–3.0
Glucose (% blood glucose)	>50	<50	>50	<50

Note: Malignant meningitis, e.g. with lymphoma, may give similar changes to TB.

intravenous drug users), HIV infection and opportunistic organisms (e.g. *Toxoplasma gondii* in patients with full-blown acquired immune deficiency syndrome [AIDS]) are causes.

Acute viral encephalitis

A viral aetiology is often presumed, although not confirmed serologically or by culture. In the UK the common organisms are herpes simplex viruses, varicella-zoster virus (VZV), ECHO, Coxsackie and mumps. Epidemic and endemic viral encephalitides occur world-wide, e.g. Japanese encephalitis (arbovirus) in South-East Asia, West Nile encephalitis in Egypt and Sudan. Tick-borne encephalitis (TBE) is caused by the TBE virus, and exists in two major forms: Central European and Far Eastern. An inactivated vaccine is available for travellers spending time in endemic areas.

Clinical features

Many of these infections cause a mild self-limiting illness with fever, headache and drowsiness. Less commonly, the illness is severe, with focal signs (e.g. hemiparesis, dysphasia), seizures and coma. Death or brain injury follows; herpes simplex virus (HSV-1) accounts for many of these in the UK.

Investigations

- CT and MR imaging shows areas of oedema often in the temporal lobes
- CSF analysis shows an elevated lymphocyte count (5–500 cells/mm^3). Protein may also be increased
- Viral serology of blood and CSF may identify the causative virus
- EEG often shows non-specific slow-wave activity.

Treatment

Suspected herpes simplex and VZV encephalitis is immediately treated with intravenous aciclovir (10 mg/kg every 8 hours for 14–21 days). If the patient is in a coma, the prognosis is poor, whether or not treatment is given.

Brain and spinal abscesses

An intracranial abscess may develop in the epidural, subdural or intracerebral sites. Epidural abscesses are uncommon; subdural abscess presents similarly to intracerebral abscess.

Cerebral abscess

Infection follows the direct spread of organisms from a parameningeal infective focus (e.g. paranasal sinuses, middle ear or skull fracture) or a distant source of infection via the bloodstream (lung, heart, abdomen). Frequently no cause is found. The most common organisms are *Streptococci anginosus*, *Bacteroides* spp. and staphylococci. Infection with tubercle bacilli may result in chronic caseating granulomata (tuberculomas) presenting as intracranial mass lesions.

Clinical features

These include headache, focal neurological signs, seizures and sometimes evidence of raised intracranial pressure (p. 776) developing over days to weeks. Fever is usual but not invariable.

Investigations

Contrast-enhanced CT scan will show the abscess. Lumbar puncture is not performed because of the danger of coning in the presence of raised intracranial pressure (p. 776). Aspiration with stereotactic guidance allows the organism to be identified.

Management

Treatment is with a combination of intravenous antibiotics and sometimes surgical decompression.

Spinal epidural abscess

Back pain and fever are followed by paraparesis and/or root lesions. The abscess is shown on MR imaging and treatment is with antibiotics (organism is usually *Staphylococcus aureus*) and surgical decompression.

Neurosyphilis

Syphilis is described on page 47. Neurosyphilis occurs late in the course of untreated infection and is now rarely seen in the UK because of treatment at

Table 17.16 The clinical syndromes of neurosyphilis

Asymptomatic neurosyphilis	Positive CSF serology without symptoms or signs
Meningovascular syphilis (3–4 years)	Subacute meningitis with cranial nerve palsies and papilloedema Gumma (an expanding intracranial mass) causes raised intracranial pressure and focal deficits Paraparesis caused by spinal meningovasculitis
General paralysis of the insane (10–15 years)	Progressive dementia Brisk reflexes Extensor plantar responses Tremor
Tabes dorsalis (10–35 years)	Demyelination in the dorsal roots causes lightning pains (short, sharp, stabbing) in the legs Ataxia, loss of reflexes and sensory loss Neuropathic joints (Charcot's joints) Argyll Robertson pupils (p. 733), ptosis and optic atrophy

The numbers in brackets are the years after the primary infection.

an earlier stage. The different clinical syndromes (Table 17.16) occur alone or in combination.

Management

Treatment is with benzylpenicillin 1 g daily i.m. for 10 days, which may arrest (but not reverse) the neurological disease.

Transmissible spongiform encephalopathy (Creutzfeldt–Jakob disease)

In Creutzfeldt–Jakob disease (CJD) there is progressive dementia, usually developing after 50 years of age, characterized pathologically by spongiform changes in the brain. It is caused by prions (a proteinaceous infectious particle) and the pathology is similar to bovine spongiform encephalopathy (BSE) of cattle. Prions are resistant to many of the usual processes that destroy proteins. CJD occurs as a sporadic form or an iatrogenic form as a result of contaminated material such as corneal grafts or human growth hormone. There is no treatment and death usually occurs within 6 months of onset.

Variant CJD (vCJD) presents with neuropsychiatric symptoms, followed by ataxia and dementia, and affects a younger age group. Diagnosis can be confirmed by tonsillar biopsy and CSF gel electrophoresis. vCJD and BSE are caused by the same prion strain, suggesting transmission from BSE-infected cattle to the human food chain.

HIV and neurology

HIV-infected individuals frequently present with or develop neurological conditions. The HIV virus itself is directly neuroinvasive and neurovirulent. Immunosuppression leads to indolent, atypical clinical patterns. HIV patients also have a high incidence of stroke. The pattern of disease is changing where antiretroviral therapy (ART) is available.

CNS and peripheral nerve disease in HIV

HIV seroconversion can cause meningitis, encephalitis, GBS and Bell's palsy (the most common cause of Bell's palsy in South Africa).

Chronic meningitis occurs with fungi (e.g. *Cryptococcus neoformans* or *Aspergillus*), tuberculosis (TB), *Listeria*, coliforms or other organisms. Raised CSF pressure is common in cryptococcal meningitis.

AIDS-dementia complex (ADC) is a progressive, HIV-related dementia, sometimes with cerebellar signs, that is still seen where antiretroviral therapy is unavailable.

Encephalitis and brain abscess *Toxoplasma*, cytomegalovirus, herpes simplex and other organisms cause severe encephalitis. Multiple brain abscesses develop in HIV infection, usually due to toxoplasmosis.

CNS lymphoma is typically fatal.

Progressive multifocal leucoencephalopathy (PML) is due to JC virus and occurs with very low CD4 counts.

Spinal vacuolar myelopathy occurs in advanced disease.

Peripheral nerve disease HIV-related peripheral neuropathy is common (70%) and can be difficult to distinguish from the effects of ART, which is also toxic to peripheral nerves.

BRAIN TUMOURS

Primary intracranial tumours account for 10% of all neoplasms, and in the UK about half of all intracranial tumours are metastatic. Primary intracranial tumours are derived from the skull itself, or from any of the structures lying within it, or from their tissue precursors. They may be malignant on histological investigation but rarely metastasize outside the brain. The most common intracranial tumours occurring in adults are listed in Table 17.17. Pituitary tumours are discussed separately on page 611.

Clinical features

The clinical features of a cerebral tumour are the result of the following:

- Progressive focal neurological deficit
- Raised intracranial pressure
- Focal or generalized epilepsy.

Table 17.17 Common brain tumours

Tumour	Relative frequency (%)
Primary malignant	35
Glioma	
Embryonal tumours, e.g. medulloblastoma	
Lymphoma	
Benign	15
Meningioma	
Neurofibroma	
Metastases	50
Bronchus	
Breast	
Stomach	
Prostate	
Thyroid	
Kidney	

Gliomas, meningiomas and embryonal tumours account for 95% of primary brain tumours.

Neurological deficit is the result of a mass effect of the tumour and surrounding cerebral oedema. The deficit depends on the site of the tumour, e.g. a frontal lobe tumour will initially cause personality change, apathy and intellectual deterioration. Subsequent involvement of the frontal speech area and motor cortex produces expressive aphasia and hemiparesis. Parietal lobe tumours cause a homonymous field defect, cortical sensory loss, hemiparesis and partial seizures on the side contralateral to the tumour. Rapidly growing tumours destroy cerebral tissue and loss of function is an early feature.

Raised intracranial pressure produces headache, vomiting and papilloedema. The headache typically changes with posture and is made worse by coughing, sneezing, bending and straining.

As the tumour grows there is downward displacement of the brain and pressure on the brainstem, causing drowsiness, which progresses eventually to respiratory depression, bradycardia, coma and death. Distortion of normal structures at a distance from the growing tumour leads to focal neurological signs (false localizing signs). The most common are a third and sixth cranial nerve palsy (p. 733), resulting from stretching of the nerves by downward displacement of the temporal lobes.

Epilepsy Fits may be generalized or partial in nature. The site of origin of a partial seizure is frequently of value in localization.

Differential diagnosis

The main differential is from other intracranial mass lesions (cerebral abscess, tuberculoma, subdural haematoma and intracranial haematoma) and a stroke, which may have an identical clinical presentation. Benign (idiopathic) intracranial hypertension presents with headache and papilloedema in young obese females. Neuroimaging is normal but at lumbar puncture there is raised CSF pressure.

Investigations

- *Imaging.* CT and MRI are useful in detecting brain tumours. MRI is of particular value in investigation of tumours of the posterior fossa and brainstem. MR angiography is sometimes necessary to define the site or blood supply of a mass, particularly if surgery is planned. PET is sometimes helpful to locate an occult primary tumour with metastasis. Plain skull X-rays have no value in brain tumour diagnosis.

- *Other investigations.* These include routine tests, e.g. chest X-ray if metastatic disease is suspected. Lumbar puncture and examination of the CSF is contraindicated with the possibility of an intracranial mass lesion because of danger of immediate herniation of the cerebellar tonsils, impaction within the foramen magnum and compression of the brainstem ('coning').

Management

- *Surgery.* Surgical exploration, and either biopsy or removal of the mass, is usually carried out to ascertain its nature. Some benign tumours, e.g. meningiomas, can be removed in their entirety without unacceptable damage to surrounding structures.

- *Radiotherapy* is given for gliomas and radiosensitive metastases and improves survival slightly. Selected centres offer stereotactic (gamma knife) radiotherapy to deliver high doses of radiation to small targets with precision.

- *Medical treatment.* Cerebral oedema surrounding a tumour is rapidly reduced by corticosteroids – intravenous or oral dexamethasone. Epilepsy is treated with anticonvulsants. Chemotherapy has little real value in the majority of primary or secondary brain tumours. The prognosis is very poor in patients with malignant tumours, with only 50% survival at 2 years for high-grade gliomas.

HYDROCEPHALUS

Hydrocephalus is characterized by an excessive amount of CSF within the cranium. CSF is produced in the cerebral ventricles and normally flows downwards into the central canal of the spinal cord and then out into the subarachnoid space, from where it is reabsorbed. Hydrocephalus occurs when there is obstruction to the outflow of CSF; rarely is it the result of increased production of CSF.

Aetiology

In children, hydrocephalus may be caused by a congenital malformation of the brain (e.g. Arnold–Chiari malformation, where the cerebellar tonsils descend into the cervical canal), meningitis or haemorrhage causing obstruction to the flow of CSF. In adults, hydrocephalus is caused by:

- A late presentation of a congenital malformation
- Cerebral tumours in the posterior fossa or brainstem which obstruct the aqueduct or fourth-ventricle outflow
- Subarachnoid haemorrhage, head injury and meningitis
- A third ventricle colloid cyst causing intermittent hydrocephalus – recurrent prostrating headaches with episodes of lower limb weakness
- Normal-pressure hydrocephalus, in which there is dilatation of the cerebral ventricles without signs of raised intracranial pressure. It presents in elderly people with dementia, urinary incontinence and ataxia.

Clinical features

There is headache, vomiting and papilloedema caused by raised intracranial pressure. There may be ataxia and bilateral pyramidal signs.

Management

Treatment is by the surgical insertion of a shunt between the ventricles and the right atrium or peritoneum (ventriculoatrial or ventriculoperitoneal).

HEADACHE, MIGRAINE AND FACIAL PAIN

Headache is common and the history and examination is the key to diagnosis. Neuroimaging is not indicated in patients who have a clear history of migraine and have no 'red flag' symptoms or signs (Table 17.2). When taking a headache history, ask about:

- Location (e.g. hemicranial), severity and character (e.g. throbbing vs non-throbbing)
- Associated symptoms, e.g. nausea, photophonia, phonophobia and motion sensitivity
- Presence of autonomic symptoms, e.g. tearing or ptosis
- Triggers; relieving or exacerbating features, e.g. effect of posture
- Is headache episodic and part of a pattern? Age at onset and frequency
- Duration of headache episodes
- Pattern of analgesic use

- Family history of headache
- 'Red flag' symptoms – fever (meningitis, sinusitis)
- Sudden onset in less than 1 minute (SAH)
- Features of raised intracranial pressure
- Jaw claudication (giant cell arteritis).

Tension headache

Most chronic daily and recurrent headaches are tension headaches. They are thought to be generated by neurovascular irritation and referred to scalp muscles and soft tissues. There is a feeling of pressure or tightness all around the head and there are no associated features of classic migraine (aura, nausea, photophobia). Treatment consists of explanation and reassurance, analgesic withdrawal (to avoid analgesic overuse headache) and tricyclic antidepressants in some cases.

Migraine

Migraine is recurrent headache associated with visual and gastrointestinal disturbance. It is a common condition, occurs more frequently in women and onset is usually before 40 years of age. The diagnosis is clinical.

Pathogenesis

Genetic and environmental factors play a role. Changes in brainstem blood flow lead to an unstable trigeminal nerve nucleus and nuclei in the basal thalamus. This results in release of vasoactive neuropeptides including calcitonin generelated peptide (CGRP) and substance P; this then results in the process of neurogenic inflammation, of which the two components are vasodilatation and plasma protein extravasation. Cortical spreading depression is a self-propagating wave of neuronal and glial depolarization that spreads across the cerebral cortex. It is proposed to cause the aura of migraine and lead to release of inflammatory mediators which impact on the trigeminal nerve nucleus. Precipitating factors include stress, too much or too little sleep, noise and irritating lights, hormonal factors (e.g. premenstrual migraine or worsening migraine with the combined oral contraceptive pill [OCP]), alcohol and skipping meals (contrary to popular belief, individual foods are rarely a trigger).

Clinical features

Migraine is classified into three types:
- Migraine with aura (classic migraine)
- Migraine without aura (common migraine)
- Migraine variants (unilateral motor or sensory symptoms resembling a stroke).

The headache is characteristically unilateral, throbbing and builds up over minutes to hours. It may be associated with nausea, vomiting and photophobia. It may last for some days and is made worse by physical exertion. The patient is irritable and prefers the dark. Premonitory symptoms of fatigue, nausea, changes in mood and appetite may occur in the hours or days before the headache. Auras are related to depression of visual cortical function or retinal function and persist for minutes to hours before the headache. There may be scotomata, unilateral blindness, hemianopic field loss, flashes and fortification spectra. Other aura include aphasia, tingling, numbness and weakness of one side of the body. The most common way in which a migraine attack resolves is through sleep.

Differential diagnosis

A sudden migraine headache may resemble meningitis or subarachnoid hae-morrhage. The hemiplegic, visual and hemisensory symptoms must be distin-guished from thromboembolic TIAs. In TIAs the maximum deficit is present immediately, visual symptoms are negative (i.e. visual loss rather than visual distortion) and headache is unusual (p. 746).

Management

General measures Avoidance of dietary precipitating factors is rarely helpful. Women taking the OCP may be helped by stopping the drug or changing the brand. Hormonal contraceptives are contraindicated in migraine with focal aura.

Treatment of the acute attack

- *Mild attacks.* Simple analgesics such as paracetamol (p. 320), high-dose soluble aspirin (900 mg) or non-steroidal anti-inflammatory drugs (NSAIDs) are given at the start of the headache and combined with an antiemetic such as metoclopramide (p. 136).
- *Moderate/severe attacks.* Triptans, (e.g. sumatriptan, almotriptan, eletriptan, or rizatriptan) are serotonin (5-hydroxytryptamine; 5-HT) 1B/1D agonists. They inhibit the release of vasoactive peptides, promote vasoconstriction and block pain pathways in the brainstem. They vary in their onset of action, recurrence rate and route of administration, e.g. tablets, subcutaneous injection, nasal spray. They are contraindicated when there is vascular disease and in migraine variants. Frequent use of medication for acute attacks may lead to analgesia overuse headache. CGRP antagonists, e.g. telcagepant, are effective for acute treatment of migraine.

Prophylaxis

Prophylaxis is indicated in patients with frequent attacks (more than two per month) or who respond poorly to treatment for acute attacks.
Options are:

- Anticonvulsants. Valproate (800 mg) used off licence or topiramate (100–200 mg daily) are generally the most effective options.

- β-Blockers, e.g. propranolol 10 mg three times daily increased to 40–80 mg three times daily.
- Amitriptyline 10 mg (or more) at night.
- Botulinum toxin was recently recommended as a treatment for chronic migraine. The technique involves 31 injections over the scalp and neck repeated every 3 months.
- Pizotifen is rarely used. Flunarizine (a calcium antagonist) and methysergide are used in refractory patients.

Facial pain

The face is richly supplied with pain-sensitive structures – the teeth, gums, sinuses, temporomandibular joints, jaws and eyes – disease of which causes facial pain. Trigeminal (fifth) nerve lesions (p. 735) and trigeminal neuralgia (p. 736) also present with facial pain.

Trigeminal autonomic cephalgias

These headaches are characterized by unilateral trigeminal distribution of pain in association with ipsilateral cranial autonomic features. The group comprises cluster headache, paroxysmal hemicrania, hemicrania continua, and short-lasting unilateral neuralgiform headache attacks with conjunctival injection and tearing (SUNCT syndrome). They are rare, other than cluster headache.

Cluster headaches (migrainous neuralgia)

These are rapid-onset, severe, short-lived (1–2 hours) unilateral headaches with a clustering of painful attacks over weeks or months followed by periods of remission. Men are affected more commonly than women, with a peak age of onset of 20–50 years. The pain often begins around the eye or temple. Autonomic features are lacrimation and redness of the eye, rhinorrhoea and Horner's syndrome. Treatment of an acute attack is with subcutaneous or nasal triptans or inhalation of 100% oxygen. Verapamil, topiramate, lithium carbonate and/or a short course of steroids helps to bring about an end to a bout of clusters.

Giant cell arteritis (cranial or temporal arteritis)

This is a granulomatous arteritis of unknown aetiology occurring chiefly in those over the age of 60 years and affecting, in particular, the extradural arteries. Giant cell arteritis is closely related to polymyalgia rheumatica (p. 310) and this can occur in the same patient.

Clinical features

There is headache, scalp tenderness (e.g. on combing the hair) and, occasionally, pain in the jaw and mouth which is characteristically worse on eating (jaw claudication). The superficial temporal artery may become tender, firm and pulseless. Blindness, caused by inflammation and occlusion of the ciliary and/ or central retinal artery, occurs in 25% of untreated cases. Systemic features include weight loss, malaise and a low-grade fever.

Investigations

- ESR is always elevated >50 mm/h. Liver enzymes are usually also elevated.
- Full blood count may show a normochromic, normocytic anaemia.
- Histology. A temporal artery biopsy, which can be performed under local anaesthetic, usually confirms the diagnosis. However, the granulomatous changes may be patchy and therefore missed.

Management

High doses of steroids (oral prednisolone, initially 60–100 mg daily) should be started *immediately* in a patient with typical features, and a temporal artery biopsy obtained as soon as possible (the histological changes remain for up to a week after starting treatment). The steroid dose is gradually reduced, guided by symptoms and the ESR. Long-term steroids may be needed because the risk of visual loss persists.

SPINAL CORD DISEASE

The cord extends from C1 (its junction with the medulla) to the vertebral body of L1. The spinal canal below L1 is occupied by lumbar and sacral nerve roots, which group together to form the cauda equina and ultimately extend into the pelvis and thigh (Fig. 17.11). Paraplegia (weakness of both legs) is almost always caused by a spinal cord lesion, as opposed to hemiplegia (weakness of one side of the body), which is usually the result of a lesion in the brain.

Spinal cord compression

This is a medical emergency.

Clinical features

There is progressive weakness of the legs with upper motor neurone pattern (Table 17.4) and eventual paralysis. The onset may be acute (hours to days) or chronic (weeks to months), depending on the cause. The arms are affected if the lesion is above the thoracic spine. There is a *sensory level*, with sensation abruptly diminishing one to two spinal cord segments below the anatomical level of spinal cord compression. Sometimes there is loss of sphincter control with urinary incontinence. There may be painless urinary retention and constipation in the later stages.

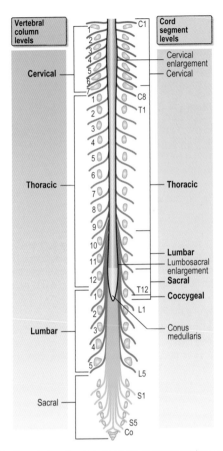

Fig. 17.11 The spinal cord and cauda equina. The bony vertebrae are indicated on the left-hand side (7 cervical, 12 thoracic, 5 lumbar and 5 sacral). The spinal cord extends from C1 (its junction with the medulla) to the vertebral body of L1. The spinal cord segments indicated on the right are not necessarily situated at the same vertebral levels as the bony vertebra. For instance, the lumbar cord is situated between T9 and T11 vertebrae. A T8 vertebral injury will result in a T12 cord or neurological level (i.e. sensation is diminished below the T12 dermatome, and motor function is reduced in muscles innervated by T12 and below). The cord segmental levels are indicated for cervical (blue), thoracic (red), lumbar (green) and sacral (yellow). The spray of spinal roots below the conus is called the cauda equina and is damaged by lesions below the L2 vertebra.

Aetiology

The most common cause of acute spinal cord compression is a vertebral tumour (metastases from lung, breast, kidney, prostate or multiple myeloma [Table 17.18]). Spinal tuberculosis is a frequent cause in endemic areas (p. 540). Chronic compression due to cervical spondylotic myelopathy is the most common cause of a spastic paraparesis in an elderly person.

Investigations

Urgent investigation is essential in a patient with suspected cord compression, especially with acute or subacute onset, because irreversible paraplegia may follow if the cord is not decompressed.

- MRI identifies the cause and site of cord compression
- X-ray of the spine may show degenerative bone disease and destruction of vertebrae by infection or neoplasm.

Management

The treatment depends on the cause, but in most cases the initial treatment involves surgical decompression of the cord and stabilization of the spine. Dexamethasone (16 mg/day, p. 664) reduces oedema around the lesion and improves outcome in patients with cord compression due to malignancy.

Differential diagnosis

The differential diagnosis is from intrinsic lesions of the cord causing paraparesis. Transverse myelitis (acute inflammation of the cord resulting from viral infection, syphilis or radiation therapy), anterior spinal artery occlusion and

Table 17.18 Causes of spinal cord compression

Vertebral body neoplasms	Metastases, e.g. from lung, breast, prostate
	Myeloma
	Lymphoma
Disc and vertebral lesions	Trauma
	Chronic degenerative disease
Inflammatory	Epidural abscess
	Tuberculosis (Pott's paraplegia)
Spinal cord neoplasms	Primary cord neoplasm, e.g. glioma, neurofibroma
	Metastases
Rarities	Paget's disease, bone cysts, osteoporotic vertebral collapse
	Epidural haemorrhage, e.g. patients on warfarin

multiple sclerosis may present with a rapid onset of paraparesis. A more insidious onset of weakness occurs with motor neurone disease (in which there is no sensory deficit), subacute combined degeneration of the cord, and as a non-metastatic manifestation of malignancy. MRI should always be performed in a patient with a sensory or motor level. Rarely, a parasagittal cortical lesion, e.g. meningioma, may cause paraplegia.

Cauda equina lesion

Spinal damage at or distal to L1 (a common cause is lumbar disc prolapse at the L4/L5 and L5/S1 level) injures the cauda equina (p. 783). Cauda equina syndrome can present acutely or with a more insidious onset of typical signs and symptoms. Involvement of multiple sacral and lumbar nerve roots in the lumbar vertebral canal causes bladder (reduced desire to void progressing to painless urinary retention) and bowel dysfunction and perianal and perineal ('saddle') numbness. There may also be back pain, numbness and weakness in the legs with reduced reflexes. MRI is the imaging method of choice in patients with suspected cauda equina syndrome and surgical decompression if a potentially reversible cause is shown.

Syringomyelia and syringobulbia

Fluid-filled cavities within the spinal cord (myelia) and brainstem (bulbia) are the essential features of these conditions.

Aetiology

The most frequent cause is blockage of CSF flow from the fourth ventricle in association with an Arnold–Chiari malformation (congenital herniation of the cerebellar tonsils through the foramen magnum). The normal pulsatile CSF pressure waves are transmitted to the delicate tissues of the cervical cord and brainstem, with secondary cavity formation. Hydrocephalus may also occur as a result of disturbed CSF flow.

Clinical features

Patients usually present in the third or fourth decade with pain and sensory loss (pain and temperature) in the upper limbs. The clinical features are demonstrated in Fig. 17.12.

Investigation

MRI is the investigation of choice and demonstrates the intrinsic cavities.

Treatment

Surgical decompression of the foramen magnum sometimes slows deterioration.

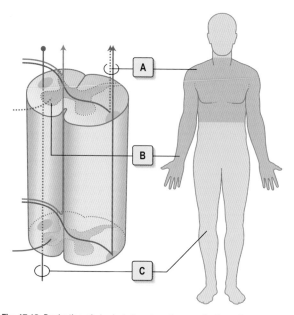

Fig. 17.12 Production of physical signs in syringomyelia. Expanding cavities distend the cord. Pain and temperature (A) fibres crossing at that level are destroyed, but sensory fibres in the posterior columns (other sensory modalities) and those that enter the spinothalamic tract at a lower level are spared. Sensory loss is therefore 'dissociated' and confined to the upper trunk and limbs. Further extension damages the anterior horn cells (B), the pyramidal tracts (C) and the medulla, causing wasting in the hands, a spastic paraplegia, nystagmus and a bulbar palsy.
(From Parsons M [1993] A Colour Atlas of Clinical Neurology. London, Mosby-Wolfe.)

Friedreich's ataxia

This autosomal recessive disorder is the most common of the hereditary spinocerebellar degenerations. There is a progressive degeneration of the spinocerebellar tracts and cerebellum, causing cerebellar ataxia, dysarthria and nystagmus. Degeneration of the corticospinal tracts causes weakness and an extensor plantar response. The tendon reflexes are absent as a result of peripheral nerve damage. Loss of the dorsal columns causes absent joint position and vibration sense. Other features are pes cavus, optic atrophy, cardiomyopathy and death by middle age.

Management of the paraplegic patient

The paraplegic patient requires skilled and prolonged nursing care. A pressure-relieving mattress and turning the patient every 2 hours helps to prevent pressure sores. Bladder catheterization (sometimes intermittent self-catheterization) prevents urinary stasis and infection. Patients may need manual evacuation of faeces. This may become unnecessary as reflex emptying of the bladder and rectum develops. Passive physiotherapy helps to prevent contractures in paralysed limbs. Severe spasticity may be helped by dantrolene sodium, baclofen or diazepam. Many patients graduate to a wheelchair and maintain some degree of independence.

DEGENERATIVE NEURONAL DISEASES

Motor neurone disease

There is relentless and unexplained destruction of upper motor neurones and anterior horn cells in the brain and spinal cord. Most patients die within 3 years from respiratory failure as a result of bulbar palsy and pneumonia. It presents in middle age and is more common in men. Most cases are sporadic with no family history but the rare familial cases may give clues to the pathophysiology. Mutations in the free radical scavenging enzyme, copper/zinc superoxide dismutase (SOD-1), are responsible for one familial form, suggesting that oxidative stress and free radicals are implicated in the destruction of motor neurones.

Clinical features

Four clinical patterns are seen at diagnosis. However, as the disease progresses most patients develop a mixed picture. There is no involvement of the sensory system or motor nerves to the eyes and sphincters in any of the clinical types:

- *Progressive muscular atrophy* is a predominantly lower motor neurone lesion of the cord, causing weakness, wasting and fasciculation (spontaneous, irregular and brief contractions of part of a muscle) in the hands and arms.
- *Amyotrophic lateral sclerosis* is a combination of disease of the lateral corticospinal tracts and anterior horn cells, producing a progressive spastic tetraparesis or paraparesis with added lower motor neurone signs (wasting and fasciculation).
- *Progressive bulbar and pseudobulbar palsy* results from destruction of upper (pseudobulbar palsy) and lower (bulbar palsy) motor neurones in the lower

cranial nerves. There is dysarthria, dysphagia with wasting, and
fasciculation of the tongue.

- *Primary lateral sclerosis* is rare. There is progressive tetraparesis.

Investigations

The diagnosis is clinical; fasciculation is characteristic. An EMG shows muscle
denervation, but this is not a specific finding.

Differential diagnosis

The differential diagnosis is a cervical spine lesion, which may present with
upper and lower motor neurone signs in the arms and legs. It is often distinguished by the presence of sensory signs. Idiopathic multifocal motor neuropathy (Table 17.21) presents with weakness predominantly in the hands and
profuse fasciculation.

Management

Riluzole, a sodium-channel blocker that inhibits glutamate release, slows
progression slightly. Ventilatory support and feeding via a percutaneous endoscopic gastrostomy (PEG) tube helps prolong survival for some months. Survival
for more than 3 years is unusual.

Spinal muscular atrophies

This is a group of rare disorders which destroy the anterior horn cells of the
spinal cord. There is a slowly progressive, usually symmetrical wasting and
weakness of the limbs.

Dementia

Dementia is a clinical syndrome with multiple causes defined by a progressive
acquired loss of higher mental function of sufficient severity to cause social or occupational impairment. It occurs in clear consciousness and is therefore distinct from
delirium. Dementia affects about 10% of those aged 65 years and over, and 20% of
those over 80 years. The most common causes are Alzheimer's disease, frontotemporal dementia, vascular dementia and dementia with Lewy bodies (Table 17.19).

Alzheimer's disease

Alzheimer's disease is a primary degenerative cerebral disease of unknown
aetiology that accounts for over 65% of dementia in any age group. There
are characteristic pathological features, which include neuronal reduction
in several areas of the brain, neurofibrillary tangles, argentophile plaques, consisting largely of amyloid protein, and granulovacuolar bodies.

Table 17.19 Causes of dementia

Alzheimer's disease
Dementia with Lewy bodies
Frontotemporal dementia
Vascular dementia
Vitamin deficiency: B_{12}, thiamin
Hypothyroidism
Intracranial mass: subdural haematoma, hydrocephalus, tumour
Chronic traumatic encephalopathy, e.g. punch drunkenness
Infections: neurosyphilis, Creutzfeldt–Jakob disease, HIV
Huntington's disease
Parkinson's disease

Clinical features

There is an insidious onset, with steady progression over years. Short-term memory loss is usually the most prominent early symptom, but, subsequently, there is slow disintegration of the personality and intellect, eventually affecting all aspects of cortical function. There is decline in language (difficulty in naming and in understanding what is being said), visuospacial skills, apraxia (impaired ability to carry out skilled motor tasks) and agnosia (failure to recognize objects, e.g. clothing, people, places).

Investigations

There is no single test that will make a diagnosis of dementia. Memory problems are not always due to dementia, and alternative diagnoses which mimic dementia should be considered: delirium, depression, drugs, normal age-associated memory problems. The Mini Mental State Examination (MMSE) is commonly used to screen for cognitive function: a score of 25 or above out of 30 is considered normal; a score of 18–24 indicates mild to moderate impairment; and a score of 17 or below indicates serious impairment. The MMSE is relatively insensitive to milder cognitive impairment and to frontal lobe dysfunction. The Addenbrooke's Cognitive Examination is a tool developed to address the deficiencies of the MMSE. The Abbreviated Mental Test Score is a quick and simple assessment of the mental state (Table 17.20). Exclusion of rare treatable causes of dementia (Table 17.19) should also be considered and blood taken for a full blood count, liver biochemistry, thyroid function tests and measurement of vitamin B_{12} and folate. A brain CT scan should be performed in younger patients or those with an atypical presentation. MRI typically shows characteristic atrophy of mesial temporal lobe structures, including hippocampi, progressing eventually to generalized cerebral atrophy. Characteristic MRI and psychometric testing abnormalities are sufficient to make a diagnosis if the clinical picture is suggestive (a progressive amnestic cognitive disorder in an older person). Amyloid imaging is now beginning to enter clinical practice in

Table 17.20 Abbreviated Mental Test Score

1. Age
2. Time to nearest hour
3. Address for recall at the end of the test (house number and street name)
4. Year
5. Place – name of hospital
6. Recognition of two people (e.g. doctor, nurse)
7. Date of birth
8. Year of First World War
9. Name of present monarch
10. Count backwards 20 to 1
11. Address recall correct?
12. Each correct answer scores one mark.

At the 7/8 cut off, sensitivity is 70–80% and specificity is 70–90% for diagnosis of dementia.

some specialist centres. A social and family history will help to assess how vulnerable the person is in the community and what plans for support will need to be made.

Management

In most cases there is no specific therapy, although the associated anxiety and depression often need treatment. Attempts to therapeutically augment cholinergic activity have been based on the observations that there is impaired cortical cholinergic function as a result of reduced cerebral production of choline acetyl transferase and a decrease in acetylcholine synthesis. Acetylcholinesterase inhibitors (donepezil, rivastigmine and galantamine) increase cholinergic transmission by inhibiting cholinesterase at the synaptic cleft. They have a modest symptomatic benefit in mild to moderate Alzheimer's disease, equivalent to an increase in 1–2 points on the MMSE. They are not disease modifying, so do not slow progression. Memantine (an N-methyl-D-aspartate [NMDA] receptor antagonist) is used in moderate or severe Alzheimer's or where cholinesterase inhibitors are not tolerated. There is some evidence that the combination of memantine and cholinesterase inhibitors is better than either used alone. Patients should be managed in the community as much as possible. Home care, day care, respite care and sitter services are all needed at various points during the progression of the disease. At some point, long-term institutional care in a residential or nursing home may be required.

Prognosis

The typical course is one of progressive decline. The average survival is 8–10 years.

Vascular (multi-infarct) dementia

This is the second most common cause of dementia, with a stepwise deterioration and declines followed by short periods of stability. There is usually a history of TIAs, although the dementia may follow a succession of acute cerebrovascular accidents or, less commonly, a single major stroke. There may be other evidence of arteriopathy.

Dementia with Lewy bodies

This is characterized by fluctuating cognition with pronounced variation in attention and alertness. Prominent or persistent memory loss may not occur in the early stages. Impairment in attention, frontal, subcortical and visuospatial ability is often prominent. Depression and sleep disorders occur. Recurrent formed visual hallucinations (e.g. strange faces, frightening creatures) are a feature. Parkinsonism (e.g. slowing, rigidity) is common, with repeated falls. Delusions and transient loss of consciousness occur. Cortical Lewy bodies are prominent at autopsy. These inclusions were first described in idiopathic Parkinson's disease, but are a hallmark of this clinical pattern of dementia. Neuroleptic drugs should not be used.

DISEASES OF THE PERIPHERAL NERVES

Six principal mechanisms cause nerve malfunction: demyelination; axonal degeneration, e.g. due to a toxin; Wallerian degeneration following nerve section; compression; infarction (in arteritis); and infiltration by inflammatory cells, e.g. sarcoid.

Mononeuropathies

Mononeuropathy is a process affecting a single nerve, and multiple mononeuropathy (or mononeuritis multiplex) is a process affecting several or multiple nerves. Mononeuropathy may be the result of acute compression, particularly where the nerves are exposed anatomically (e.g. the common peroneal nerve at the head of the fibula), or entrapment, where the nerve passes through a relatively tight anatomical passage (e.g. the carpal tunnel). It may also be caused by direct damage, e.g. major trauma, surgery or penetrating injuries.

Carpal tunnel syndrome

Carpal tunnel syndrome is the most common entrapment neuropathy. It results from pressure on the median nerve as it passes through the carpal tunnel.

Aetiology It is usually idiopathic but may be associated with hypothyroidism, diabetes mellitus, pregnancy, obesity, rheumatoid arthritis, acromegaly and amyloid (including renal dialysis patients).

Clinical features The history is of pain and paraesthesiae in the hand, typically worse at night, when it may wake the patient. On examination there may be no physical signs; there may be weakness and wasting of the thenar muscles and sensory loss of the palm and palmar aspects of the radial three and a half fingers. Tapping on the carpal tunnel may reproduce the pain (Tinel's sign). In Phalen's test, symptoms are reproduced on passive maximal wrist flexion.

Management Treatment with nocturnal splints or local steroid injections gives temporary relief. Surgical decompression is the definitive treatment unless the condition is likely to resolve (e.g. with pregnancy, obesity).

Compression neuropathies may also affect the ulnar nerve (at the elbow), the radial nerve (caused by pressure against the humerus) and the common peroneal nerve (resulting from pressure at the head of the fibula).

Mononeuritis multiplex

Mononeuritis multiplex often indicates a systemic disorder (Table 17.21); treatment is that of the underlying disease. Acute presentation is most commonly due to vasculitis when prompt treatment with steroids may prevent irreversible nerve damage.

Polyneuropathy

Polyneuropathy is an acute or chronic, diffuse, usually symmetrical, disease process and may involve motor, sensory and autonomic nerves, either alone or in combination. Sensory symptoms include numbness, tingling, 'pins and needles', pain in the extremities and unsteadiness on the feet. Numbness typically affects the distal arms and legs in a 'glove and stocking' distribution. Motor symptoms are usually those of weakness. Autonomic neuropathy causes postural hypotension, urinary retention, erectile dysfunction, diarrhoea (or occasionally constipation), diminished sweating, impaired pupillary responses and cardiac arrhythmias. Many varieties of neuropathy affect autonomic function to some

Table 17.21 Causes of mononeuritis multiplex

Diabetes mellitus
Leprosy (the most common cause world-wide)
Vasculitis
Sarcoidosis
Amyloidosis
Malignancy
Neurofibromatosis
HIV and hepatitis C infection
Guillain–Barré syndrome
Idiopathic multifocal motor neuropathy (distal motor, unknown cause)

Table 17.22 Varieties of polyneuropathy

Guillain–Barré syndrome
Chronic inflammatory demyelinating polyradiculoneuropathy
Diphtheritic polyneuropathy
Idiopathic sensorimotor neuropathy
Drugs: e.g. isoniazid, metronidazole, cisplatin, phenytoin
Toxins: alcohol, lead, arsenic, thallium
Metabolic: diabetes mellitus, uraemia, thyroid disease, porphyria, amyloidosis
Vitamin deficiency: B_1 (thiamin), B_6 (pyridoxine), nicotinic acid, B_{12}
Hereditary sensorimotor neuropathy
Neuropathy in cancer: paraneoplastic manifestation, myeloma
Autonomic neuropathy
HIV-associated neuropathy
Neuropathy in systemic disease: SLE, PAN, Churg–Strauss, RA, sarcoidosis, GCA
Critical illness neuropathy – ICU patients with multiorgan failure

GCA, giant cell arteritis; PAN, polyarteritis nodosa; RA, rheumatoid arthritis; SLE, systemic lupus erythematosus.

degree, but occasionally autonomic features predominate. This occurs in diabetes mellitus, amyloidosis and the GBS.

A classification is given in Table 17.22. In Europe, diabetes mellitus is the most common cause. First-line investigations in a patient presenting with polyneuropathy include full blood count and erythrocyte sedimentation rate, serum vitamin B_{12}, blood glucose, urea and electrolytes, liver biochemistry and sometimes nerve conduction studies (p. 740).

Guillain–Barré syndrome

GBS is the most common acute neuropathy and is usually an inflammatory demyelinating, but occasionally axonal, polyneuropathy. It can lead to life-threatening respiratory failure.

Pathogenesis

GBS is usually triggered by an infection: *Campylobacter jejuni,* Epstein–Barr virus and cytomegalovirus have all been associated. It is thought that the infectious organism shares epitopes with an antigen in peripheral nerve tissue (ganglioside GM_1 and GQ1b), leading to autoantibody-mediated nerve cell damage formation.

Clinical features

There is progressive onset of distal limb weakness and/or numbness (usually symmetrical) that reaches its nadir within 4 weeks. Reflexes are lost early in the illness and low back pain is a frequent early feature. There are often sensory symptoms, e.g. paraesthesias, but few sensory signs on examination. Disability ranges from mild to very severe, with involvement of the respiratory and facial muscles. Autonomic features, such as postural hypotension, cardiac arrhythmias, ileus and bladder atony, are sometimes seen. The Miller Fisher syndrome is a rare variant that affects the cranial nerves to the eye muscles and is characterized by ophthalmoplegia and ataxia.

Investigations

The diagnosis is established on clinical grounds and confirmed by nerve conduction studies showing slowing of motor conduction, prolonged distal motor latency and/or conduction block. CSF protein is non-specifically elevated, with a normal sugar and cell count. In the Miller Fisher syndrome antibodies against GQ1b have a sensitivity of 90%.

Differential diagnosis

Other causes of neuromuscular paralysis (hypokalaemia, polymyositis, myasthenia, botulism, poliomyelitis) can usually be excluded on clinical grounds and investigation. MRI of the spine may be needed to exclude transverse myelitis or cord compression.

Management

Vital capacity is monitored 4-hourly to recognize respiratory muscle weakness. A fall below 80% of predicted or 20 mL/kg is an indication for transfer to ICU and possible mechanical ventilation. There is ECG monitoring to document cardiac dysrhythmias associated with autonomic dysfunction.

Intravenous immunoglobulin (0.4 g/kg body weight daily for 5 consecutive days) is the standard treatment. It reduces duration and severity of paralysis and has fewer side effects that plasma exchange. Immunoglobulin is contraindicated in patients with IgA deficiency (measure serum levels before treatment) in whom it causes severe allergic reactions. Plasma exchange is an alternative. Supportive treatment includes heparin to prevent thrombosis, physiotherapy to prevent contractures and nasogastric or PEG feeding for patients with swallowing problems. Visiting and counselling services are offered by past patients through the Guillain–Barré Syndrome Support Group (http://www.gbs.org.uk).

Recovery begins between several days and 6 weeks from the outset. Prolonged ventilation may be necessary. Improvement towards independent mobility is gradual over many months but may be incomplete. About 10% of patients die (respiratory failure, pulmonary emboli or infection) and 20% have permanent neurological damage.

Vitamin deficiency neuropathies

Vitamin deficiencies cause nervous system damage that is potentially reversible if treated early, and progressive if not. Deficiencies, often of multiple vitamins, develop in malnutrition.

Thiamin (vitamin B_1)

Thiamin deficiency occurs in chronic alcohol-dependent patients (where little food is consumed), in starvation from any cause, and in beriberi (poorest areas of South East Asia where only polished rice is consumed). Presentation is with the Wernicke–Korsakoff syndrome, polyneuropathy and cardiac failure (rarely seen in Western countries). Treatment is with thiamin (250 mg daily i.m. or i.v.) for 3 days. Anaphylaxis can occur with parenteral thiamin. Thiamin must always be given before intravenous glucose in these high-risk patients.

Pyridoxine (vitamin B_6)

Deficiency causes mainly a sensory neuropathy. It may be precipitated during isoniazid therapy (which complexes with pyridoxal phosphate) for tuberculosis in those who acetylate the drug slowly. Prophylactic pyridoxine (10 mg daily) is given with isoniazid.

Vitamin B_{12}

Deficiency causes a polyneuropathy and the syndrome of *subacute combined degeneration of the cord*. This comprises distal sensory loss (particularly the posterior column), absent ankle jerks (as a result of the neuropathy) and evidence of cord disease (exaggerated knee jerk reflexes, extensor plantar responses). Treatment is with intramuscular vitamin B_{12} (p. 244), which reverses the peripheral nerve damage but has little effect on the CNS (cord and brain signs).

Hereditary sensorimotor neuropathy

This is a large and complex group with variable genetic mutations. Charcot–Marie–Tooth disease, also called peroneal muscular atrophy, is the most common with autosomal dominant inheritance in most cases. There is distal limb wasting and weakness that progress over many years, mostly in the legs, with variable loss of sensation and reflexes. In advanced cases the distal wasting below the knees is so marked that the legs resemble 'inverted champagne bottles'.

MUSCLE DISEASES

Weakness is the predominant feature of muscle disease. In contrast to weakness secondary to a neuropathy, reflexes and sensation are normal in muscle

Table 17.23 Muscle disease: classification

Acquired	Genetic
Inflammatory	**Dystrophic**
Polymyositis/dermatomyositis	Duchenne
Inclusion body myositis	Facioscapulohumeral
Viral, bacterial, parasitic infection	Limb girdle and others
Sarcoidosis	
Endocrine	**Myotonic**
Corticosteroids/Cushing's syndrome	Myotonic dystrophy
Thyroid disease	Myotonia congenital
Hypocalcaemia	**Channelopathies**
Osteomalacia	Hypokalaemic periodic paralysis
Hypokalaemia	Hyperkalaemic periodic paralysis
Alcohol excess	Normokalaemic periodic paralysis
Drugs (diamorphine, amfetamine, statin)	
Myasthenic	**Metabolic (all rare)**
Myasthenia gravis	Myophosphorylase deficiency
Lambert–Eaton myasthenic syndrome (LEMS)	(McArdle's disease)
	Other defects of glycogen and fatty acid metabolism
	Mitochondrial disease
	Malignant hyperpyrexia (p. 662)

disease and wasting of muscle occurs late. Muscle disease is acquired or congenital (Table 17.23). Investigation of suspected muscle disease is discussed on page 740.

Acquired muscle disease

Polymyositis and dermatomyositis are discussed on page 308. Inclusion body myositis is a rare idiopathic inflammatory myopathy occurring in men over 50 years. There is pharyngeal muscle weakness and slowly progressive weakness of the distal muscles. There is no specific treatment. Muscle disease associated with drugs, toxins and endocrine disease usually produces weakness of the limb girdles (proximal myopathy). Typically, the patient is unable to rise from a seated position without the use of their arms.

Myasthenia gravis

Myasthenia gravis (MG) is an autoimmune disorder of neuromuscular junction transmission characterized by weakness and fatiguability of ocular, bulbar and proximal limb muscles. It can present at any age but peaks occur in the third and sixth decade. It is twice as common in women as in men.

Aetiology

In most cases, autoantibodies to acetylcholine receptors (anti-AChR antibodies) at the postsynaptic membrane of the neuromuscular junction cause receptor loss. MG is associated with thymic hyperplasia in about 70% of patients under 40 years of age, and in about 10% a thymic tumour is found. There is an association with other autoimmune disorders such as thyroid disease, rheumatoid disease and pernicious anaemia.

Clinical features

Presentation is usually with fatiguability of muscle on sustained or repeated activity that improves after rest. The ocular muscles are the first to be involved in about 65% of patients, resulting in ptosis that is often partial or unilateral and improves after sleep or with the application of an ice pack on the lid (specific to MG). There is extraocular progression of weakness, usually from top down, leading to difficulty in talking, chewing, swallowing and respiratory difficulties. Fatigue can be demonstrated by ptosis on sustained upward gaze or asking the patient to sit with the arms outstretched and looking for a slow downward drift.

Investigations

- Anti-AChR antibodies are specific for MG and are found in the serum in 90% of cases of generalized MG but in less than 30% of pure ocular disease. Antibodies against a muscle-specific receptor tyrosine kinase (anti-MuSK antibodies) are found in Anti-AChR negative disease.
- Nerve stimulation tests show a characteristic decrement in evoked potential following stimulation of the motor nerve.
- Mediastinal imaging with CT or MRI to look for a thymoma.
- The Tensilon test (positive if intravenous injection of edrophonium, an anticholinesterase, results in rapid temporary improvement in weakness) is seldom required.

Differential diagnosis

Thyroid ophthalmopathy, myotonic dystrophy and brainstem cranial nerve lesions present with ocular and/or bulbar symptoms. Botulism causes rapid onset of muscle weakness, often with pupillary paralysis and there is a history of ingestion of contaminated food. Generalized muscle weakness occurs in motor neurone disease (differs in involvement of upper and lower motor neurones). Lambert–Eaton myasthenic syndrome (LEMS) is due to a presynaptic defect on the neuromuscular junction in patients with small cell lung cancer. Limb muscle weakness is the usual presenting symptom; exercise improves symptoms and reflexes are decreased or absent.

Management

Anticholinesterases (e.g. oral pyridostigmine: starting dose 60 mg three times a day and then titrated according to the response) increase availability of acetylcholine at the receptor and are the mainstay of treatment. Excessive treatment may cause a 'cholinergic crisis' with worsening weakness, hypersalivation, abdominal pain and diarrhoea. However, weakness is more often due to myasthenia unless high doses of pyridostigmine are used (>360 mg per day).

Immunosuppressant drugs are used in patients who do not respond to pyridostigmine or who relapse on treatment. Corticosteroids produce an improvement in 70% of cases. Azathioprine, mycophenolate and other immunosuppressants are also used.

Plasmapheresis and intravenous immunoglobulin have rapid onset and transient benefit and are used occasionally in myasthenic crisis (life-threatening condition with weakness of respiratory and bulbar muscles and may be drug induced, e.g. aminoglycosides, β-blockers) or as a bridge to other therapies (thymectomy or immunosuppressants).

Thymectomy is performed in patients with a thymoma (because of the potential for malignancy) and in selected patients without a thymoma who are most likely to benefit (<50 years, + ve anti-AChR antibodies) and enter a remission without medication.

Muscular dystrophies

This is an inherited group of progressive myopathic disorders resulting from defects in a number of genes needed for normal muscle function (though one-third of cases are spontaneous mutations). The Duchenne and Becker muscular dystrophies are inherited as X-linked recessive traits caused by a mutation in the dystrophin gene on chromosome 21. Patients with Duchenne muscular dystrophy present in early childhood with weakness in the proximal muscles of the leg. CK is grossly elevated ($100–200 \times$ normal). There is progression to other muscle groups with severe disability and death in the late teens. There is no curative treatment but new gene-editing therapies are in development. Steroids may delay progression. Patients with Becker muscle dystrophy present later and the degree of clinical involvement is milder. Other dystrophies present later in life and are summarized in Table 17.24.

MYOTONIAS

These conditions are characterized by myotonia (delayed muscle relaxation after contraction), which can be demonstrated by difficulty releasing the grasp after shaking hands. Patients tolerate general anaesthetics poorly. Dystrophia myotonica and myotonia congenita are the most common and both are autosomal dominant conditions.

Table 17.24 Limb girdle and facioscapulohumeral dystrophies

	Limb girdle	Facioscapulohumeral
Inheritance	Autosomal, various	Dominant, usually
Onset	10–20 years	10–40 years
Muscles affected	Shoulders, pelvic girdle	Face, shoulders, pelvic girdle
Progress	Severe disability in 20–25 years	Normal life expectancy
Pseudohypertrophy	Rare	Very rare

Dystrophia myotonica

This autosomal dominant condition causes progressive distal muscle weakness with myotonia, ptosis, facial muscle weakness and wasting. Other features commonly present are cataracts, frontal baldness, cardiomyopathy, mild mental handicap, glucose intolerance and hypogonadism. Phenytoin or procainamide sometimes helps the myotonia.

Myotonia congenita

There is mild isolated myotonia often accentuated by rest and cold. This autosomal dominant condition becomes evident in childhood.

DELIRIUM

Delirium (toxic confusional state)

Delirium is an acute or subacute condition in which impairment of consciousness is accompanied by abnormalities of perception and mood. Impairment of consciousness can vary in severity and often fluctuates (compare with dementia). Confusion is usually worse at night and may be accompanied by hallucinations, delusions, restlessness and aggression. Many diseases (Table 17.25) can be accompanied by delirium, particularly in the elderly. Infection and drugs are the most common causes.

Management

Investigation and treatment of the underlying disease should be undertaken. General measures include withdrawing all drugs where possible, rehydration, and adequate pain relief and sedation. The patient should be nursed in a quiet area of the ward. Sedation should only be used if the patient is at risk of self-injury or aggressive behaviour interferes with management. Benzodiazepines

Table 17.25 Causes of delirium

Systemic infection	
Drugs	Tricyclic antidepressants
	Benzodiazepines
	Opiates
	Anticonvulsants
Drug/alcohol withdrawal	
Metabolic disturbance	Hepatic failure
	Renal failure
	Disorders of electrolyte balance
	Hypoxia
	Hypoglycaemia
Vitamin deficiency	Vitamin B_{12}
	Vitamin B_1 (Wernicke–Korsakoff syndrome)
Brain damage	Trauma
	Tumour
	Abscess
	Subarachnoid haemorrhage

are usually the drugs of choice, although in severe delirium intramuscular haloperidol (2.5–5 mg) may be preferred. Management of alcohol withdrawal is summarized on page 163.

THERAPEUTICS

Hypnotics

Hypnotics should be reserved for short courses (because dependence and tolerance may occur with long-term use) to alleviate acute conditions after causal factors have been established. Benzodiazepines are the most commonly used hypnotics.

Mechanism of action

Benzodiazepines bind to specific receptor sites that are closely linked to the $GABA_A$ receptor, inducing a conformational change that enhances the action of the inhibitory neurotransmitter γ-aminobutyric acid (GABA). Zopiclone is not a benzodiazepine but binds to the same receptor.

Indications

Transient or short-term insomnia due to extraneous factors such as shift work or an emotional problem or serious medical illness. Short-term use only – up to 4 weeks.

Preparations and dose

Temazepam

Tablets: 10 mg, 20 mg. Oral solution: 10 mg/5 mL.
   Oral 10–20 mg at bedtime.

Zopiclone

Tablets: 3.75 mg, 7.5 mg.
   Oral 7.5 mg at bedtime; elderly, initially 3.75 mg.

Side effects

Drowsiness and lightheadedness, confusion and ataxia, especially in the elderly (avoid if possible). Hangover effects of a night-time dose may impair driving the following day. Paradoxical increase in anxiety and aggression; adjustment of the dose up or down usually improves the problem. Tolerance may develop within 3–14 days.

Cautions/contraindications

Contraindicated in respiratory depression, acute breathlessness, severe liver disease, myasthenia gravis and sleep apnoea syndrome. Withdrawal symptoms (may be delayed for 3 weeks with long-acting preparation) if drug stopped abruptly after long-term use, consisting of anxiety, insomnia, depression, psychosis and convulsions.

Anxiolytics

Anxiolytics, as with hypnotics, should only be prescribed in short courses (danger of dependence and tolerance following long-term use) to alleviate acute conditions after establishing the causal factors. Benzodiazepines are again the most commonly used anxiolytics.

Mechanism of action

As above.

Indications

- Short-term relief in severe anxiety
- In panic disorders resistant to antidepressant treatment

- Intravenously for short-term sedation with medical procedures, e.g. colonoscopy
- Prevention of the alcohol withdrawal syndrome
- Benzodiazepines also used in the acute management of status epilepticus.

Preparations and dose

Diazepam

Tablets: 2 mg, 5 mg, 10 mg. Oral solution: 2 mg/5 mL, 5 mg/5 mL. Emulsion injection: 10 mg/2 mL. Rectal solution: 2.5 mg/1.25 mL, 5 mg/2.5 mL, 10 mg/ 2.5 mL.

Oral Anxiety: 2 mg three times daily, increasing if necessary to 15–30 mg daily in divided doses. Elderly: half adult dose. Insomnia associated with anxiety: 5–15 mg at bedtime.

IM/IV for severe acute anxiety and control of panic attacks: 10 mg repeated if necessary after not less than 4 hours (into a large vein at a rate not more than 5 mg/min). In status epilepticus: 10–20 mg i.v. repeated if necessary after 30–60 minutes; may be followed by infusion to maximum 3 mg/kg over 24 hours.

By rectum 500 μg/kg up to maximum 30 mg (elderly, half dose) repeated after 12 hours if necessary.

Lorazepam

Tablets: 1 mg, 2.5 mg. Injection: 4 mg/mL.

Oral Anxiety: 1–4 mg daily in divided doses (elderly, half dose). Insomnia associated with anxiety: 1–2 mg at bedtime.

IM/IV for severe acute anxiety and control of panic attacks: 25–30 μg/kg, repeated if necessary every 6 hours (into a large vein by slow injection). In status epilepticus: 4 mg, by intravenous injection into a large vein.

Chlordiazepoxide

Capsules: 5 mg, 10 mg. Tablets: 5 mg, 10 mg.

Oral Anxiety: 10 mg three times daily in anxiety, increased if necessary to 60–100 mg daily. In alcohol withdrawal: 10–50 mg four times daily (under supervision) and reduced gradually over 7–14 days.

Oxazepam

Tablets: 10 mg, 15 mg, 30 mg.

Oral Anxiety: 15–30 mg three to four times daily (half dose in elderly). Insomnia associated with anxiety: 15–25 mg (max. 50 mg) at bedtime.

Short acting and used as an alternative to chlordiazepoxide in alcohol withdrawal for patients with severe liver dysfunction, 15–30 mg four times daily (under supervision) and reduced gradually over 7–14 days.

Antipsychotics ('neuroleptics')

Mechanism of action

Blockade of CNS dopamine (D_2) receptors.

Indications

In the short term to quieten disturbed patients whatever the underlying psychopathology: e.g. schizophrenia, mania or toxic delirium. Used in the long-term management of schizophrenia. Also used in intractable hiccup and nausea and vomiting.

Preparations and dose

Chlorpromazine

Tablets: 10 mg, 25 mg, 50 mg, 100 mg. Oral solution: 25 mg/5 mL, 100 mg/5 mL. Suppositories: 100 mg.

Initially 25–50 mg three times daily or 75 mg at night; adjust according to response.

Haloperidol

Capsules: 500 μg. Tablets: 500 μg, 1.5 mg, 5 mg, 10 mg, 20 mg. Oral liquid: 5 mg/5 mL, 10 mg/5 mL. Injection: 5 mg/mL, 20 mg/mL.

Oral Psychoses: initially 1.5–3 mg (3–5 mg in severe cases) two to three times daily, which may be increased to a maximum 30 mg daily in divided doses and then reduced to maintenance dose when control has been achieved. Hiccup and vomiting: 1–1.5 mg three times daily.

IM/IV 2–10 mg repeated every 4–8 hours according to response, to a maximum of 18 mg daily.

Side effects

Acute drowsiness, hypotension, tachycardia, convulsions, antimuscarinic symptoms (dry mouth, constipation, difficulty with micturition, blurred vision), neuroleptic malignant syndrome (hyperthermia, fluctuating conscious level, muscular rigidity, autonomic dysfunction). Extrapyramidal, haematological and endocrine side effects with longer-term use (check with *British National Formulary*).

Cautions/contraindications

Use with caution in liver disease, renal impairment, cardiovascular disease, Parkinson's disease, epilepsy, myasthenia gravis, glaucoma. Contraindicated in coma and phaeochromocytoma. Many drug interactions (check with *British National Formulary*).

Antiepileptics

Drug of choice for seizure type in adults. The newer antiepileptic drugs are not described here and should be initiated by a specialist.

Carbamazepine

Mechanism of action

Inhibition of repetitive neuronal firing is produced by reduction of transmembrane Na^+ influx, by blockade of Na^+ channels.

Indications

Drug of choice for simple and complex partial seizures, and for tonic–clonic seizures secondary to a focal discharge.

Preparations and dose

Tablets: 100 mg, 200 mg, 400 mg. Liquid: 100 mg/5 mL. Suppositories: 100 mg. Modified-release tablets: 200 mg, 400 mg.

Initially 100 mg once or twice daily, increased slowly to usual dose of 0.8–1.2 g daily (epilepsy) or 200 mg three to four times daily (trigeminal neuralgia). Total daily doses are the same for modified-release preparations but given twice daily (may provide better steady-state levels).

Side effects

Nausea and vomiting, especially early in treatment. CNS toxicity leads to double vision, dizziness, drowsiness and ataxia. Transient leucopenia is common, especially early in treatment – severe bone marrow depression is rare. Hyponatraemia caused by potentiation of antidiuretic hormone.

Cautions/contraindications

Contraindicated in AV conduction abnormalities (unless paced), history of bone marrow depression, porphyria. Hepatic enzyme induction leads to accelerated metabolism of the oral contraceptive pill (dose of oestrogen should be increased to avoid failure of contraception), warfarin (reduced anticoagulant effect), ciclosporin and others (check with *British National Formulary*). Interactions also with other antiepileptic drugs.

Valproate

Mechanism of action

Blockade of transmembrane Na^+ channels, thus stabilizing neuronal membranes.

Indications

Effective for all forms of epilepsy.

Preparations and dose

Tablets: 100 mg, 200 mg. Solution: 200 mg/5 mL. Injection powder for reconstitution: 400 mg.

600 mg/day in two divided doses, increasing by 200 mg/day at 3-day intervals to usual dose of 1–2 g/day in divided doses.

Side effects

Gastrointestinal upset (nausea, vomiting, anorexia, abdominal pain, acute pancreatitis), increased appetite and weight gain, transient hair loss, dose-related tremor, thrombocytopenia, rarely severe hepatotoxicity. Drug concentration in plasma does not correlate with therapeutic effect and monitoring is only necessary to assess complications of suspected toxicity.

Cautions/contraindications

Acute liver disease, porphyria. Monitor liver biochemistry 6-monthly in those most at risk of severe liver damage (check with *British National Formulary*). Many drug interactions with antiepileptics and other drugs (check with *British National Formulary*).

Phenytoin

Mechanism of action

Inhibits sodium influx across the cell membrane, reduces cell excitability.

Indications

All forms of epilepsy except absence seizures, but used much less in developed countries. Also used in management of status epilepticus and in trigeminal neuralgia.

Preparations and dose

Capsules: 25 mg, 50 mg, 100 mg, 300 mg. Suspension: 30 mg/5 mL. Injection: 50 mg/mL.

Oral 150–300 mg daily (single dose or two divided doses) increased gradually as necessary (with plasma phenytoin concentration monitoring); usual dose 200–500 mg. Reference range for concentration 40–80 μmol/L (10–20 mg/L) immediately before the next dose.

IV Give with BP and ECG monitoring. 18 mg/kg diluted to 10 mg/mL in 0.9% sodium chloride at a rate not exceeding 50 mg/min (average-sized adult 1000 mg over 20 min) as a loading dose. Maintenance dose 100 mg i.v. at intervals of 6–8 hours monitored by measurement of plasma concentration.

Side effects

Intravenous injection may cause CNS, cardiovascular (hypotension, heart block, arrhythmias) and respiratory depression. If hypotension occurs, reduce infusion rate or discontinue. Other side effects are dose related and include impaired brainstem and cerebellar function (nystagmus, double vision, vertigo, ataxia, dysarthria), chronic connective tissue effects (gum hyperplasia, coarsening of facial features, hirsutism), skin rashes (withdraw treatment), folate deficiency, increased vitamin D metabolism and deficiency, blood dyscrasias, lymphadenopathy and teratogenic effects.

Cautions/contraindications

Contraindicated in sinus bradycardia, heart block and porphyria. Many drug interactions (check with *British National Formulary*). Highly protein bound and can be displaced by valproate and salicylates, which therefore enhance the effect. Induction of hepatic drug-metabolizing enzymes and metabolism of warfarin and ciclosporin increased (see *British National Formulary* for full list).

Fosphenytoin

Mechanism of action

As for phenytoin.

Indications

As for phenytoin.

Preparations and dose

Injection: 75 mg/mL.

Pro-drug of phenytoin which can be given more rapidly and causes fewer infusion site reactions. Dose expressed as phenytoin sodium equivalent (PE) (fosphenytoin 1.5 mg = phenytoin sodium 1 mg).

Status epilepticus: initially 15 mg PE/kg by i.v. infusion (with BP, ECG and respiratory rate monitoring during and for at least 30 minutes after infusion) at a rate of 100–150 mg PE/min. Maintenance 4–5 mg PE/kg daily (in one to four divided doses) by i.v. infusion at a rate of 50–100 mg PE/min.

Side effects

As for phenytoin.

Cautions/contraindications

As for phenytoin.

18 Dermatology

INTRODUCTION

Skin diseases are extremely common, although their exact prevalence is unknown. There are over 1000 different entities described, but two-thirds of all cases are the result of fewer than 10 conditions. In developing countries, infectious diseases such as tuberculosis, leprosy and onchocerciasis are common, whereas in developed countries, inflammatory disorders such as acne and eczema are common. Some conditions may be part of normal development, e.g. acne; others may be inherited, e.g. Ehlers–Danlos syndrome; still others are part of a systemic disease, e.g. the rash of systemic lupus erythematosus (SLE). The most common skin conditions and those which can be fatal (e.g. malignant melanoma, pemphigus), will be described in this chapter. The structure and functions of the skin are summarized in Fig. 18.1.

SKIN AND SOFT TISSUE INFECTIONS

Infections of the skin and soft tissues beneath are common. The majority are caused by the Gram-positive cocci *Staphylococcus aureus* (part of the normal microflora of the skin) and *Streptococcus pyogenes*. Sometimes infection is introduced by an animal bite or a penetrating foreign body and in these cases more unusual organisms can be found.

Cellulitis is a spreading infection involving the deep subcutaneous layer and is the most common skin infection leading to hospitalization. It falls into a continuum of skin infections that includes impetigo (superficial vesiculopustular infection in children), folliculitis (multiple erythematous lesions with a central pustule localized to the hair follicles) and carbuncles (abscesses in the subcutaneous tissue that drain via hair follicles). The last three infections are usually caused by *S. aureus*.

CELLULITIS AND ERYSIPELAS

Cellulitis and erysipelas are caused by superficial and deeper infection of the dermis and subcutaneous tissues, respectively. Cellulitis preferentially involves the lower extremities, while erysipelas tends to affect the face. Risk factors include lymphoedema, site of entry (leg ulcer, trauma, presence of tinea pedis – 'athlete's foot'), venous insufficiency, leg oedema and obesity. It is usually caused by a streptococcus, rarely a staphylococcus, and sometimes community acquired methicillin-resistant *S. aureus* (MRSA).

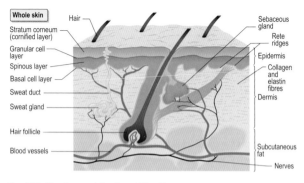

Fig. 18.1 Structure and function of the skin.

- Physical barrier against friction and shearing forces
- Protection against infection, chemicals, ultraviolet radiation
- Prevention of excessive water loss or absorption
- Ultraviolet-induced synthesis of vitamin D
- Temperature regulation
- Sensation (pain, touch, temperature)
- Antigen presentation/immunological reactions/wound healing.

Clinical features

Cellulitis presents as erythema in the involved area, with poorly demarcated margins, swelling, warmth and tenderness. There may be a low-grade fever. In erysipelas the area is raised and erythematous and sharply demarcated from normal skin.

Diagnosis

The diagnosis is clinical. Patients should also be evaluated for risk factors for cellulitis (p. 808) which may prevent recurrence if treated. In the majority of cases, culturing blood or skin aspirates does not reveal a pathogen. Deep venous thrombosis is the main differential diagnosis.

Treatment

Treatment is with flucloxacillin (or erythromycin if penicillin allergic). If disease is widespread, treatment is given intravenously for 3–5 days followed by at least 2 weeks of oral therapy. Approximately 25% of patients suffer from recurrent episodes of cellulitis and it is not clear whether prophylactic treatment with low-dose antibiotics (e.g. phenoxymethylpenicillin) is beneficial.

Necrotizing fasciitis

This is a deep-seated infection of the subcutaneous tissue that results in a fulminant and spreading destruction of fascia and fat but may initially spare the skin. There is a high mortality rate. Spreading erythema and underlying crepitus with pain and systemic toxicity (that are both out of proportion to the skin findings) are typical. Type 1 is caused by a mixture of aerobic and anaerobic bacteria and is usually seen following abdominal surgery or in people with diabetes. Type 2, caused by group A streptococci, occurs in previously healthy patients. The treatment is urgent surgical debridement and aggressive broad-spectrum antibiotic treatment with benzylpenicillin and clindamycin (plus metronidazole in type 1).

Gas gangrene

This is a deep-tissue infection with *Clostridium* spp., especially *C. perfringens*, and follows contaminated penetrating wounds. Toxins produced by the organism cause muscle necrosis with severe pain and tissue swelling, gas production and sepsis with rapid progression to shock. The treatment is urgent surgical debridement and intravenous antibiotics. Clostridial species are sensitive to a combination of benzylpenicillin and clindamycin. However, it may be difficult to differentiate gas gangrene from necrotizing fasciitis and treatment is initially with broad-spectrum antibiotics, as for necrotizing fasciitis above.

Fungal infections

Dermatophytes is the common label for the three types of fungus that cause infections of the outer layer of skin, hair and nails. The main genera responsible are *Trichophyton*, *Microsporum* and *Epidermophyton*. They tend to form expanding annular lesions due to lateral growth: hence, the name 'ringworm'. All are spread by direct contact from infected humans or animals or indirect contact with exfoliated skin or hair; communal showers, swimming baths and the sharing of towels or sportswear aids transmission. Types of dermatophyte infections are:

- Tinea corporis – ringworm of the body usually presents with slightly itchy, asymmetrical, scaly patches which show central clearing and an advancing, scaly, raised edge.
- Tinea faciei – ringworm of the face often arises after the use of topical steroids. It tends to be more erythematous and less scaly than trunk lesions.
- Tinea cruris – is more common in men than women and presents with an intensely itchy rash in the groin with a scaly border that extends onto the thighs.
- Tinea pedis – athlete's foot is confined to the toe clefts where the skin is white, macerated and fissured or is more diffuse causing a scaly erythema of the soles spreading on to the sides of the foot.

- Tinea manuum – ringworm of the hands presents with a diffuse erythematous scaling of the palms with variable skin peeling and skin thickening.
- Tinea capitis – scalp ringworm is more common in children. There is a spectrum from mild diffuse scaling with no hair loss to circular scaly patches with associated alopecia and broken hairs.
- Tinea unguium – ringworm of the nails presents as asymmetrical whitening or yellowish black discoloration of one or more nails with nail plate thickening and crumbly white material under the nail.

A host immune response in these infections is associated with the appearance of vesicles and pustules and sometimes an exudate.

Diagnosis is clinical and by microscopy of scrapings from skin, hair or nail. Fungal culture medium is used to identify the species. Localized ringworm is treated with topical antifungal cream (clotrimazole, miconazole or terbinafine applied three times daily for 1–2 weeks). Oral antifungal therapy (itraconazole 100 mg daily, terbinafine 250 mg daily for 1–2 months) is used to treat more widespread infection.

Candida albicans

This is a yeast that is sometimes found as part of the body's flora, especially in the gastrointestinal tract. It takes hold in the skin where there is a suitable warm, moist environment, such as in the groin, interdigital clefts of the toes and around the nails. Infection can mimic ringworm but in the groin there are small circular areas of erythema in front of the advancing edge (satellite lesions). Treatment of localized infection is with topical antifungal cream or systemic antifungal therapy (itraconazole 100 mg daily for 3–6 months) for nail infection. *Candida* can also infect mucosal surfaces of the mouth or genital tract particularly in patients taking antibiotics (due to suppression of protective bacterial flora) or in immunosuppressed patients where infection can also be widespread and life-threatening. Screening for diabetes should be considered.

COMMON SKIN CONDITIONS

Acne vulgaris

This is a common condition occurring in adolescence and frequently continuing into early and middle adult life.

Clinical features

Increased sebum production by sebaceous glands, blockage of pilosebaceous units, follicular epidermal hyperproliferation and infection with *Propionibacterium acnes* all contribute to produce the clinical features of open comedones (blackheads) or closed comedones (whiteheads), inflammatory papules and pustules. Other features that may be present include hypertrophic or keloidal scarring, and hyperpigmentation, which occurs predominantly in patients with darker complexions. There is a tendency for spontaneous improvement over a number of years.

Management

Acne should be actively treated to avoid unnecessary scarring and psychological distress. The aims of treatment are to decrease sebum production, reduce bacteria, normalize duct keratinization and decrease inflammation. There are a variety of approaches, the choice of which depends on the severity of the disease. Regular washing with acne soaps to remove excess grease is helpful (normal soaps can be comedogenic). 'Picking' should be discouraged.

First-line therapy Topical agents such as keratolytics (benzoyl peroxide), topical retinoids (tretinoin or isotretinoin), retinoid-like agents (adapalene) and antibiotics for inflammatory acne (erythromycin, clindamycin) are used in mild disease.

Second-line therapy Low-dose oral antibiotics (e.g. oxytetracycline, minocycline, erythromycin, trimethoprim) often help but must be given for 3–4 months. Hormonal treatment with cyproterone acetate 2 mg/ethinylestradiol 35 µg (co-cyprindiol) is useful in women if there is no contraindication to oral contraception.

Third-line therapy with an oral retinoid (isotretinoin or acitretin) is given if the above measures fail, there is nodulocystic acne with scarring or there is severe psychological disturbance. Retinoids are synthetic vitamin A analogues that affect cell growth and differentiation. Although effective, they are highly teratogenic and are absolutely contraindicated during pregnancy. All women of child-bearing age should have a pregnancy test and contraceptive advice prior to treatment and pregnancy testing repeated monthly during the 4-month course. Over 90% of individuals will respond to therapy and 65% of people will obtain a long-term 'cure'.

Psoriasis

Psoriasis is a common chronic hyperproliferative disorder characterized by the presence of well-demarcated red scaly plaques over extensor surfaces such as the elbows and knees, and in the scalp. There is an equal sex incidence, with age of onset occurring in two peaks: 16–22 years and 55–60 years.

Aetiology

The condition is polygenic (nine genetic psoriasis susceptibility loci have been identified) but is dependent on certain environmental triggers (infection with group A streptococcus, drugs such as lithium, ultraviolet light, high alcohol use and stress). It is thought that psoriasis is a T-lymphocyte driven disorder to an unidentified antigen(s). T-cell activation results in upregulation of

Th1-type T-cell cytokines, e.g. interferon-γ, interleukins (IL-1, -2, -8), tumour growth factors (TGF-α, TNF-α) and adhesion molecules (ICAM-1).

Clinical features

- *Chronic plaque psoriasis* is the most common. Well-demarcated, salmon-pink silvery scaling lesions occur on the extensor surfaces of the limbs, particularly the elbows and knees (Fig. 18.2). Scalp involvement is common and is most often seen at the hair margin or over the occiput. New plaques of psoriasis occur at sites of skin trauma ('Koebner phenomenon').
- *Flexural psoriasis* – red glazed non-scaly plaques confined to flexures such as the groin, natal cleft and submammary areas. The rash is sometimes misdiagnosed as *Candida* intertrigo, but the latter will normally show satellite lesions.
- *Guttate* ('raindrop-like') psoriasis occurs most commonly in children and young adults. An explosive eruption of very small circular or oval plaques appears over the trunk about 2 weeks after a streptococcal sore throat.
- *Erythrodermic* and *pustular* psoriasis are the most severe forms and may be life-threatening. There is widespread intense inflammation of the skin which may be associated with malaise, pyrexia and circulatory disturbances.

Associated features

Nail involvement occurs in 50% of patients with psoriasis and is manifest as pitting of the nail plate, onycholysis (separation of the nail from the underlying vascular bed), yellow–brown discoloration, subungual hyperkeratosis and,

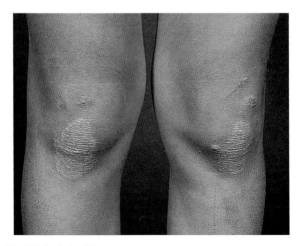

Fig. 18.2 Psoriasis of the knees.

rarely, a damaged nail matrix and lost nail plate. Arthritis occurs in 5–10% of patients (p. 295).

Management

Topical treatment For mild disease, reassurance and treatment with an emollient may be all that is necessary. Emollients (e.g. aqueous cream, emulsifying ointment, white soft paraffin) hydrate the skin and may have an antiproliferative effect. More specific topical treatments for chronic plaque psoriasis on the extensor surfaces of the trunk and limbs include vitamin D_3 analogues (e.g. calcipotriol, calcitriol, tacalcitol) that affect cell division and differentiation, coal tar (antiscaling and anti-inflammatory properties), tazarotene (a vitamin A antagonist, i.e. a retinoid) and corticosteroids in combination with other treatments. Topical dithranol (inhibits DNA synthesis) can also be helpful but it causes staining of the skin and clothing and it may prove difficult to use at home on a regular basis. Salicylic acid acts as a keratolytic and is particularly useful for scalp psoriasis.

Phototherapy Ultraviolet A radiation (UVA) in conjunction with a photosensitizing agent, oral or topical psoralen (PUVA), is usually highly effective for treating extensive psoriasis. Repeated treatments exaggerate skin ageing and carry the risk of UV-induced skin cancer.

Systemic therapy is with oral retinoic acid derivatives (acitretin or etretinate), immunosuppression (methotrexate, ciclosporin) or biological agents (TNF-α blockers and efalizumab, an anti-CD11a monoclonal antibody). They are used in resistant disease or for severe erythrodermic or pustular psoriasis. The retinoic acid derivatives are teratogenic and in women of child-bearing age the possibility of pregnancy must be excluded before treatment and effective contraception must be used during treatment and for 3 years afterwards.

Urticaria/angio-oedema

These are inflammatory, predominantly dermal processes in which degranulation of mast cells is the final common pathway. The involved skin in urticaria (hives, 'nettle rash') is red and swollen due to vasodilatation and increased vascular permeability. The predominant symptom is itch. Similar processes operate in angio-oedema, but involvement is predominantly below the dermis and the swelling is less red and not itchy.

Aetiology

Viral or parasitic infection, drug reactions (non-steroidal anti-inflammatory drugs [NSAIDs], penicillin, angiotensin-converting enzyme inhibitors [ACEIs], opiates), food allergy (strawberries, food colourings, seafood) or, rarely, SLE are all causes but in most cases the underlying cause is unknown. Physical urticarias can be caused by cold, deep pressure, stress, heat, sunlight or water. *Hereditary angio-oedema* is a rare autosomal dominant condition. A mutation in the C1-esterase inhibitor leads to unchecked activation of the complement system. There are recurrent episodes of non-pruritic, non-pitting subcutaneous or submucosal oedema typically involving the arms, legs, hands, feet, abdomen (nausea, vomiting, pain) and sometimes larynx (respiratory difficulty and sudden death).

Management

Urticaria is managed by avoiding precipitating factors (including opiates and salicylates which degranulate mast cells) and oral non-sedating antihistamines (H$_1$ blocker), e.g. cetirizine 10 mg daily. Sedating antihistamines, H$_2$ blockers and dapsone are added if necessary. Intramuscular adrenaline and intravenous hydrocortisone are used in angio-oedema involving the mouth or throat. Hereditary angio-oedema is treated with C1 esterase inhibitor concentrates and fresh frozen plasma in the acute setting. Maintenance treatment is with the anabolic steroid stanozolol or danazol, which stimulates an increase in synthesis of C1 esterase inhibitor.

Eczema

Eczema (dermatitis) is characterized by superficial skin inflammation with vesicles (when acute), redness, oedema, oozing, scaling and usually pruritus. The most common type of eczema is atopic eczema.

Atopic eczema

Aetiology

There is a significant hereditary predisposition. The primary defect is thought to be an abnormal epithelial barrier function allowing antigenic and irritant agents to penetrate the barrier and come into contact with immune cells. Loss-of-function mutations in the epidermal barrier protein filaggrin predispose to atopic eczema in Caucasian individuals. An initial selective activation of Th2–type CD4 lymphocytes drives the inflammatory process with Th0 and Th1 cells predominating in the chronic phase. There are high levels of serum immunoglobulin E (IgE) antibodies, although their significance in contributing to the pathogenesis is unclear. Exacerbating factors include strong detergents and chemicals, cat and dog fur and some dietary antigens.

Clinical features

There are itchy, erythematous scaly patches, especially in the flexures such as in front of the elbows and ankles, behind the knees and around the neck (Fig. 18.3). Scratching can produce excoriations and repeated rubbing produces skin thickening (lichenification) with exaggerated skin markings. Pigmented skin may become hyper- or hypopigmented and extensor surfaces are often involved (reverse pattern). Broken skin may become secondarily infected by *S. aureus* (appearing as crusted weeping impetigo-like lesions) or herpes simplex virus causing multiple small blisters or punched-out lesions (eczema herpeticum) which can occasionally be fatal.

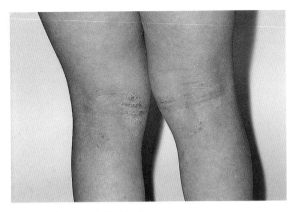

Fig. 18.3 Atopic eczema behind the knees.

Management

Known irritants should be avoided. Regular use of emollients, such as aqueous cream or emulsifying ointments, is useful in hydrating the skin. Topical corticosteroids form the mainstay of treatment. Mild steroids (e.g. 1% hydrocortisone) are used for the face and more potent steroids (e.g. betamethasone, fluocinolone) are used on the body and soles. Topical immunomodulators such as tacrolimus and pimecrolimus are particularly helpful for treatment in sensitive areas such as the face and eyelids. Antibiotics are indicated for bacterial superinfection and bandaging helps absorption of treatment and acts as a barrier to prevent scratching. Sedating antihistamines can be useful at nighttime.

Second-line treatments in severe non-responsive cases include ultra-violet phototherapy, azathioprine, ciclosporin and short courses of oral prednisolone.

Exogenous eczema (contact dermatitis)

In this condition there is acute or chronic skin inflammation, often sharply demarcated, produced by substances in contact with the skin. It may be caused by a primary chemical irritant, or may be the result of a type IV hypersensitivity reaction. Common chemical irritants are industrial solvents used in the workplace, or cleaning and detergent solutions used in the home. With allergic dermatitis there is sensitization of T lymphocytes over a period of time, which results in itching and dermatitis upon re-exposure to the antigen.

Clinical features

An unusual pattern of rash with clear-cut demarcation or odd-shaped areas of erythema and scaling should arouse suspicion and, in combination with a careful history, should indicate a cause. Patch testing, where the suspected allergen is placed in contact with the skin, is often useful in identifying a suspected allergen.

Management

Causative agents should be removed where possible. Steroid creams are useful for short periods in severe disease. Antipruritic agents are used for symptomatic relief of itching.

CUTANEOUS SIGNS OF SYSTEMIC DISEASE

Erythema nodosum

Erythema nodosum is an acute and sometimes recurrent paniculitis which produces painful dusky blue–red nodules over the shins or lower limbs, with occasional spread to the thighs or arms. Causes are listed in Table 18.1.

Clinical features

Painful nodules or plaques up to 5 cm in diameter appear in crops over 2 weeks and slowly fade to leave bruising and staining of the skin. Systemic upset is common, with malaise, fever and arthralgia.

Management

Symptoms should be treated with NSAIDs, light compression bandaging and bed rest. Recovery may take weeks, and recurrent attacks can occur. Dapsone, colchicine or oral prednisolone is used in resistant cases.

Table 18.1 Common causes of erythema nodosum

Streptococcal infection*
Drugs (e.g. sulphonamides, oral contraceptive pill)
Sarcoidosis*
Idiopathic*
Bacterial gastroenteritis, e.g. *Salmonella, Shigella, Yersinia*
Fungal infection (histoplasmosis, blastomycosis) diseases
Tuberculosis
Leprosy
Inflammatory bowel disease*
Chlamydia infection

Indicates most common causes.

Erythema multiforme

Erythema multiforme is an acute self-limiting symmetrical rash characterized by target lesions on the distal limbs, palms and soles. A cell-mediated cutaneous lymphocytotoxic response is present. Children and young adults are most commonly affected. The cause is unknown in 50% of cases, but the following should be considered:

- Infections: herpes simplex virus (HSV) and *Mycoplasma* are the most common causes. Others are Epstein–Barr virus (EBV), orf and human immunodeficiency virus (HIV)
- Drugs (e.g. sulfonamides, anticonvulsants)
- Autoimmune rheumatic conditions, e.g. SLE
- Wegener's granulomatosis
- Carcinoma, lymphoma.

Clinical features

Symmetrically distributed erythematous papules occur most commonly on the back of the hands, the palms and the forearms. There may be a central lesion surrounded by pale red rings ('target lesions'). Eye changes include conjunctivitis, corneal ulceration and uveitis. Occasionally there is severe mucosal involvement leading to necrotic ulcers of the mouth and genitalia.

Management

The diagnosis is based on the appearance of the skin lesion and a history of risk factors or related disease. The disease usually resolves in 2–4 weeks. Treatment is symptomatic and involves treating the underlying cause. Rarely, recurrent erythema multiforme can occur. This is triggered by herpes simplex infection in 80% of cases, and oral aciclovir can be helpful. In resistant cases, azathioprine (1–2 mg/kg daily) is used.

Differential diagnosis

Erythema multiforme falls within a spectrum of drug-induced skin reactions that includes toxic epidermal necrolysis (widespread separation of the epidermis from the dermis) and the variant, Stevens–Johnson syndrome (damage is restricted to the mucosal surfaces with <10% bullous involvement of the skin).

Pyoderma gangrenosum

This condition presents with erythematous nodules or pustules which frequently ulcerate. The ulcers, which are often large, have a classic bluish-black undermined edge and a purulent surface. The main causes are inflammatory bowel disease, rheumatoid arthritis, haematological malignancy (myeloma, lymphoma, leukaemia) and primary biliary cirrhosis. In 20% of cases no cause is identified.

Management

The underlying condition should be treated. High-dose topical and/or oral steroids are used to prevent progressive ulceration. Other immunosuppressants such as ciclosporin are sometimes used. Debridement is contraindicated as it worsens the condition.

Acanthosis nigricans

There is thickened, hyperpigmented skin predominantly of the flexures which can appear warty. It is associated with obesity, insulin resistance, underlying malignancy (especially gastrointestinal) and hyperandrogenism in females.

Neurofibromatosis

Type 1 (von Recklinghausen's disease) neurofibromatosis is an autosomal dominant disease caused by mutations in the *NF1* gene (encoding for a protein, neurofibromin) on chromosome 17. Clinical features include multiple fleshy skin tags and deeper soft tissue tumours (neurofibromas), 'café-au-lait' spots (light-brown macules of varying size), axillary freckling, scoliosis and an increased incidence of a variety of neural tumours, e.g. meningioma, eighth-nerve tumours and gliomas. Type 2 is caused by a mutation in the gene encoding for the protein merlin or schwannomin (chromosome 22) and presents with bilateral acoustic neuromas, other neural tumours and cutaneous neurofibromas.

Tuberous sclerosis

Tuberous sclerosis is an autosomal dominant condition which in most cases is due to a mutation in either the tuberous sclerosis complex 1 *(TSC1)* gene (encodes hamartin) or the tuberous sclerosis complex 2 *(TSC2)* gene (encodes tuberin). There is mental retardation, epilepsy and cutaneous abnormalities. The skin signs include adenoma sebaceum (reddish papules around the nose), periungual fibroma (nodules arising from the nail bed), shagreen patches (flesh-coloured plaques on the trunk), ash-leaf hypopigmentation and café-au-lait patches. There may be pitting of dental enamel.

Other diseases

Chronic kidney disease, liver disease and endocrine diseases all may have skin manifestations which are discussed in the relevant chapters.

OTHER DISEASES AFFECTING THE SKIN

Marfan's syndrome

Marfan's syndrome is an autosomal dominant disorder associated with mutations in the fibrillin 1 gene on chromosome 15. Abnormalities of collagen synthesis cause fragility of the skin and bruising. The most obvious abnormalities are skeletal: tall stature, arm span greater than height, arachnodactyly (long spidery fingers), sternal depression, hypermobile joints and a high arched palate. There is often upward dislocation of the lens as a result of weakness of the suspensory ligament. Cardiovascular complications (ascending aortic aneurysm formation, aortic dissection and aortic valve incompetence) are responsible for a greatly reduced life span.

Ehlers–Danlos syndrome

Inherited defects of collagen lead to fragility and hyperelasticity of the skin, with easy bruising, 'paper-thin' scars and hypermobility of the joints. The walls of the aorta and gut are weak and may rarely rupture with catastrophic results.

BULLOUS DISEASE

Primary blistering diseases of the skin are rare. Skin biopsy for light and electron microscopy together with immunofluorescence is necessary for diagnosis. Much more common causes of skin blistering are chickenpox, herpes, impetigo, pompholyx eczema and inset bite reactions.

Autoimmune bullous diseases

Pemphigus vulgaris Autoantibodies against desmoglein 3, an adhesion protein of the keratinocyte membrane, disrupt intraepithelial junctions and result in formation of cutaneous and mucosal blisters (particularly oral mucosa) which evolve into erosions. Blisters can be extended with gentle sliding pressure (Nikolsky's sign). Blistering and erosions disrupt the skin's main functions (Fig. 18.1) and the disease can be fatal. Treatment is with high-dose oral prednisolone (60–100 mg/day) or pulsed methylprednisolone. Immunosuppressants (azathioprine, mycophenolate mofetil, cyclophosphamide, ciclosporin) are used long term as steroid-sparing agents. Intravenous immunoglobulin infusions and rituximab (p. 256) have also been used.

Bullous pemphigoid Autoantibodies against hemidesmosomal proteins (BP230 and BP180) disrupt the dermal–epidermal junction, leading to formation of large tense bullae, especially on the limbs and torso. It most commonly affects those over the age of 60 years. Treatment is with high-dose oral prednisolone (30–60 mg daily) and immunosuppressants as for pemphigus vulgaris.

Mechanobullous disease (epidermolysis bullosa)

This is a group of inherited disorders with blisters in the skin and mucous membranes after minor trauma. Epidermolysis bullosa (EB) simplex is due to mutations of cytoskeletal proteins (keratin 5, keratin 14) within the basal layer of the epidermis and is generally a mild disease. EB dystrophica is a more severe disease and results from a mutation in the *COL-7A1* gene that causes a loss of collagen V11 in the basement membrane. There is blistering with scarring, joint contractures, and involvement of the nails, mucosae and larynx. Squamous cell carcinoma is a complication and results in death in early adult life. The most severe form, junctional EB, causes death in infancy or early childhood.

MALIGNANT SKIN TUMOURS

All of these are related to sun exposure.

Basal cell carcinomas (rodent ulcer)

Basal cell carcinomas (BCCs) are the most common malignant skin tumours. They are common later in life and occur on sun-exposed areas, although rarely on the ear. Most present as a shiny pearly nodule which may go on to ulcerate (Fig. 18.4). They rarely metastasize but can invade surrounding local structures. Treatment is by surgical excision. Radiotherapy, photodynamic therapy, cryotherapy or 5% imiquimod cream are used for the flat, diffuse superficial forms.

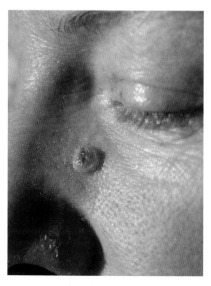

Fig. 18.4 Ulcerating basal cell carcinoma.

Squamous cell carcinoma

Squamous cell carcinoma (SCC) is a more aggressive tumour than BCC and it can metastasize. It presents as rather ill-defined nodules that ulcerate and grow rapidly. Solar keratoses (erythematous silver-scaly papules with a red base) and Bowen's disease (isolated scaly red plaques resembling psoriasis) are pre-malignant. Multiple tumours may occur in patients who have had prolonged periods of immunosuppression. Treatment of SCC is with wide local excision or, occasionally, radiotherapy.

Malignant melanoma

This is the most serious form of skin cancer, as metastasis can occur early; it causes a number of deaths, even in young people. The clinical signs listed in Table 18.2 help distinguish malignant from benign moles. Four clinical types exist:

- *Lentigo maligna melanoma* – a patch of lentigo maligna (slow-growing macular area of pigmentation, often on the face, occurring in the elderly) that develops a nodule, signalling invasive malignancy.
- *Superficial spreading malignant melanoma* – a large flat irregularly pigmented lesion that grows laterally before vertical invasion develops.
- *Nodule malignant melanoma* – a rapidly growing pigmented (rarely non-pigmented) nodule that bleeds or ulcerates.
- *Acral lentiginous malignant melanomas* – pigmented lesions on the palm, sole or under the nail.

Table 18.2 Clinical criteria for the diagnosis of malignant melanoma

ABCDE criteria (USA)	
Asymmetry of mole	
Border irregularity	
Colour variation	
Diameter	
Elevation	
The Glasgow 7-point checklist	
Major criteria	Change in size
	Change in shape
	Change in colour
Minor criteria	Diameter >6 mm
	Inflammation
	Oozing or bleeding
	Mild itch or altered sensation

Treatment

Treatment is by wide surgical excision: 1-cm margin for thin melanomas (<1 mm) and 3-cm margin for thicker melanomas (>2 mm). Staging (by tumour thickness, metastasis and lymph node status) helps predict prognosis and 5-year survival. Metastatic disease responds poorly to treatment of all modalities.

Cutaneous T-cell lymphoma (mycosis fungoides)

This is a rare type of skin tumour with a benign course. Scaly patches, resembling eczema or psoriasis, often on the buttocks, come and go or persist for many years. In elderly males, the disease may progress and be accompanied by lymphadenopathy and blood involvement (Sézary's syndrome). Early cutaneous disease can be left untreated or treated with topical steroids or PUVA (p. 813). More advanced disease may require radiotherapy, chemotherapy, immunotherapy or electron beam therapy.

Kaposi's sarcoma

This is a tumour of vascular and lymphatic endothelium that presents as purplish nodules and plaques in elderly males (especially Jewish people from Eastern Europe), as an endemic form in males from central Africa, and in patients with HIV infection. Infection with human herpesvirus 8 has an aetiological role. Treatment is with radiotherapy, immunotherapy or chemotherapy.

Normal values

Haemoglobin
    Male   135–175 g/L
    Female   115–160 g/L

Haemoglobin	
Male	135–175 g/L
Female	115–160 g/L
Mean corpuscular haemoglobin (MCH)	27–32 pg
Mean corpuscular haemoglobin concentration (MCHC)	32–36 g/dL
Mean corpuscular volume (MCV)	80–96 fL
Packed cell volume (PCV)	
Male	0.40–0.54 L/L
Female	0.37–0.47 L/L
White blood count (WBC)	$4–11 \times 10^9$/L
Basophil granulocytes	$<0.01–0.1 \times 10^9$/L
Eosinophil granulocytes	$0.04–0.4 \times 10^9$/L
Lymphocytes	$1.5–4.0 \times 10^9$/L
Monocytes	$0.2–0.8 \times 10^9$/L
Neutrophil granulocytes	$2.0–7.5 \times 10^9$/L
Platelet count	$150–400 \times 10^9$/L
Serum vitamin B_{12}	160–925 ng/L (150–675 pmol/L)
Serum folate	2.9–18 µg/L (3.6–63 nmol/L)
Red cell folate	149–640 µg/L
Red cell mass	
Male	25–35 mL/kg
Female	20–30 mL/kg
Reticulocyte count	0.5–2.5% of red cells ($50–100 \times 10^9$/L)
Erythrocyte sedimentation rate (ESR)	<20 mm in 1 hour

Bleeding time (Ivy method)	3–10 min
Activated partial thromboplastin time (APTT)	30–50 s
Prothrombin time	12–16 s
International normalized ratio (INR)	1.0–1.3
D-dimer	<500 ng/mL

Cholesterol	3.5–6.5 mmol/L (ideal <5.2 mmol/L)

High-density lipoprotein (HDL) cholesterol

Male	0.8–1.8 mmol/L
Female	1.0–2.3 mmol/L

Low-density lipoprotein (LDL) cholesterol <4.0 mmol/L

Triglycerides

Male	0.70–2.1 mmol/L
Female	0.50–1.70 mmol/L

BIOCHEMISTRY (SERUM/PLASMA)

Alanine aminotransferase (ALT)	5–40 U/L
Albumin	35–50 g/L
Alkaline phosphatase	39–117 U/L
Amylase	25–125 U/L
Aspartate aminotransferase (AST)	12–40 U/L
Bicarbonate	22–30 mmol/L
Bilirubin	<17 µmol/L (0.3–1.5 mg/dL)
Calcium	2.20–2.67 mmol/L (8.5–10.5 mg/dL)
Chloride	98–106 mmol/L
C-reactive protein (CRP)	<10 mg/L
Creatinine	79–118 µmol/L (0.6–1.5 mg/dL)
Creatine kinase (CPK)	
Female	24–170 U/L
Male	24–195 U/L
CK-MB fraction	<25 U/L (<60% of total activity)
Ferritin	
Female	6–110 µg/L
Male	20–260 µg/L
α-Fetoprotein	<10 kU/L
Glucose (fasting)	4.5–5.6 mmol/L (70–110 mg/dL)
γ-Glutamyl transpeptidase (γ-GT)	
Male	11–58 U/L
Female	7–32 U/L
Glycosylated (glycated) haemoglobin (HbA$_{1c}$)	3.7–5.1%
Iron	13–32 µmol/L (50–150 µg/dL)
Iron-binding capacity (total) (TIBC)	42–80 µmol/L (250–410 µg/dL)
Lactate	0.6–2.4 mmol/L
Magnesium	0.7–1.1 mmol/L

Osmolality	275–295 mOsm/kg
Phosphate	0.8–1.5 mmol/L
Potassium	3.5–5.0 mmol/L
Prostate-specific antigen (PSA)	$\leq$4.0 µg/L
Protein (total)	62–77 g/L
Sodium	135–146 mmol/L
Urate	0.18–0.42 mmol/L
	(3.0–7.0 mg/dL)
Urea	2.5–6.7 mmol/L
	(8–25 mg/dL)

BLOOD GASES (ARTERIAL)

$P_{a}CO_2$	4.8–6.1 kPa
	(36–46 mmHg)
$P_{a}O_2$	10.6–13.3 kPa
	(80–100 mmHg)
[H$^+$]	35–45 nmol/L
pH	7.35–7.45
Bicarbonate	22–26 mmol/L

Dictionary of terms

There are excellent on-line medical dictionaries with definitions for thousands of medical words and conditions. Sites for two of them are:

http://www.medterms.com

http://cancerweb.ncl.ac.uk/omd/

Adenoma A benign epithelial neoplasm in which the cells form recognizable glandular structures or in which they are clearly derived from glandular epithelium.

Adjuvant Term applied to chemotherapy or hormone therapy given after local treatment, in tumours where dissemination is undetectable but can be assumed to have occurred. If effective, it should lead to an increase in cure rate or overall disease-free survival.

Aerobic In microbiology refers to growing, living or occurring in the presence of molecular oxygen. Bacteria that require oxygen to survive (aerobic bacteria).

Afterload The load against which the cardiac muscle exerts its contractile force, i.e. the peripheral vascular tree.

Agonist A drug that has affinity for and in some way activates a receptor when it occupies it.

Alkaptonuria Inborn error of amino acid metabolism caused by a defect in the enzyme homogentisic acid oxidase. There is ochronosis (accumulation of a blue–black pigment in connective tissues) and arthritis. The slate blue–black pigmentation is most apparent in the sclera of the eyes, the external ears, and the tympanic membranes.

Allogeneic transplantation When another individual acts as the donor.

Alopecia Hair loss from areas where it is normally present.

Alport's syndrome Hereditary disorder characterized by progressive sensorineural hearing loss, nephritis and renal failure, and, occasionally, ocular defects; transmitted as an autosomal dominant or X-linked trait.

Ambulant (ambulatory) Able to walk; may be used to describe patients who do not require a wheelchair or are not confined to bed.

Anaerobic Lacking molecular oxygen. Growing, living or occurring in the absence of molecular oxygen, pertaining to an anaerobe.

Angiography A radiographic technique where a radio-opaque contrast material is injected into a blood vessel for the purpose of identifying its anatomy on X-ray.

Anisocytosis Increased variation in the size of the red blood cells.

Annular lesions Lesions occurring in rings.

Antagonist A drug that binds to a cell receptor and does not activate it.

Antibody An immunoglobulin molecule that has a specific amino acid sequence by virtue of which it interacts only with the antigen that induced its synthesis in cells of the lymphoid series (especially plasma cells), or with an antigen closely related to it.

Antigen Any substance, organism or foreign material recognized by the immune system as being 'non-self', which will provoke the production of a specific antibody, disease and rheumatological disease which is not associated with a vasculitis.

Antioxidant An enzyme or other organic substance that has the ability to counteract the damaging effects of oxygen in tissues. It has been suggested that antioxidant vitamins such as vitamin E may provide protection against certain diseases, including atherosclerosis.

Aphasia (dysphasia) A disturbance of the ability to use language, whether in speaking, writing or comprehending. It is caused by left frontoparietal lesions, often a stroke:

- Broca's aphasia (expressive aphasia) is due to a lesion in the left frontal lobe. There is reduced fluency of speech, with comprehension relatively preserved. The patient knows what he/she wants to say but cannot get the words out.
- Wernicke's aphasia (receptive aphasia) is due to a left temporoparietal lesion. The patient speaks fluently but words are put together in the wrong order, and in the most severe forms the patient speaks complete rubbish with the insertion of non-existent words. Comprehension is severely impaired.
- Global aphasia is due to widespread damage to the areas concerned with speech. The patient shows combined expressive and receptive dysphasia.

Apoptosis Programmed cell death, as signalled by the nuclei in normally functioning cells when age or state of cell health dictates.

Apraxia Loss of the ability to carry out familiar purposeful movements in the absence of paralysis or other motor or sensory impairment.

Ataxia Is due to failure of coordination of complex muscular movements despite intact individual movements and sensation.

Atrophy Thinning (e.g. of the skin).

Autoantibody An antibody that reacts with an antigen, which is a normal component of the body.

Autocrine Autocrine signalling is where a cell secretes a chemical messenger that binds to receptors on the same cell, leading to changes in the cell (see also Paracrine or Endocrine signalling).

Autologous The patient acts as his or her own source of cells.

Autosomal dominant Only one affected parent is required to have the trait to pass it on to offspring.

Autosomal recessive Mutation carried on an autosome (i.e. a chromosome not involved in sex determination) that is deleterious only in homozygotes (identical alleles of the gene are carried). Both affected parents must have the trait to pass it on to their offspring.

Bone marrow   Is obtained for examination by aspiration from the anterior iliac crest or sternum. In many cases a trephine biopsy (removal of a core of bone marrow tissue) is also necessary.

Bulla   A large vesicle.

Bursa   A closed fluid-filled sac lined with synovium that functions to facilitate movement and reduce friction between tissues of the body. Bursitis is inflammation of a bursa.

Carcinoma   A malignant neoplasm arising from epithelium.

Caseating   Developing a necrotic centre.

CD (cluster differentiation) antigens   Antigens on the cell surface that can be detected by immune reagents and which are associated with the differentiation of a particular cell type or types. Many cells can be identified by their possession of a unique set of differentiation antigens, e.g. CD4, CD8.

Chagas disease   caused by the parasite *Trypanosoma cruzi*. Transmitted to animals and people by blood-sucking triatomine bugs present only in the Americas. Acute symptoms are mild and non-specific but persist to chronic disease (cardiomyopathy, megaoesophagus, megacolon) if untreated. Treatment is with benznidazole and nifurtimox.

Cheyne–Stokes respiration   An abnormal breathing pattern in which there are periods of rapid breathing alternating with periods of no breathing or slow breathing.

Choledochal cyst   A congenital anatomical malformation of a bile duct, including cystic dilatation of the extrahepatic bile duct or the large intrahepatic bile duct. Classification is based on the site and type of dilatation. Type I is most common.

Chronic granulomatous disease   A recessive X-linked defect of leucocyte function in which phagocytic cells ingest but fail to digest bacteria, resulting in recurring bacterial infections with granuloma formation.

Chronotropic   Positively chronotropic means to increase the rate of contraction of the heart; negatively chronotropic is the opposite.

Clone   A population of identical cells or organisms that are derived from a single cell or ancestor and contain identical DNA molecules.

Clubbing   Broadening or thickening of the tips of the fingers and toes with increased lengthwise curvature of the nail and a decrease in the angle normally seen between cuticle and fingernail. Causes include congenital, respiratory (lung cancer, tuberculosis, bronchiectasis, lung abscess or empyema, lung fibrosis), cardiac (bacterial endocarditis, cyanotic congenital heart disease) and, rarely, gastrointestinal (Crohn's disease, cirrhosis).

Clubfoot (talipes equinovarus)   A deformed foot in which the foot is plantar flexed, inverted and adducted.

Congenital   Something that is present at birth. It may or may not be genetic (inherited).

Constructional apraxia   Inability to copy simple drawings: often seen in hepatic encephalopathy when the patient is unable to copy a five-pointed star.

Contraindication Any condition, especially a disease or current treatment, which renders some particular line of treatment undesirable.

C-reactive protein (CRP) Synthesized in the liver and produced during the acute-phase response, it is quick and easy to measure and is replacing measurement of the erythrocyte sedimentation rate (ESR) in some centres.

Crust Dried exudate on the skin.

Cryoglobulins Immunoglobulins that precipitate when cold or during exercise. They may be monoclonal or polyclonal, e.g. mixed essential cryoglobulinaemia, and result in a cutaneous vasculitis or occasionally a multisystem disorder.

Cryptogenic A disease of obscure or unknown origin.

CT scan (computed axial tomography) CT combines the use of X-rays with computed analysis of the images to assimilate multiple X-ray images into two-dimensional cross-sectional images ('slices'). With helical or spiral CT scanning, computer interpolation allows reconstruction of standard transverse scans to make three-dimensional images. Often a contrast agent is given by mouth or intravenously to highlight specific areas. Risks of CT scanning are exposure to radiation, and allergies and renal impairment after intravenous contrast agents.

Cytokines Soluble messenger molecules which enable the immune system to communicate through its different compartments. Cytokines are made by many cells, such as lymphocytes (lymphokines) and other white cells (interleukins). Examples of cytokines, other than interleukins, include tumour necrosis factor (TNF), interferons and granulocyte colony-stimulating factor (G-CSF).

Dextrocardia The heart is in the right hemithorax, with the apex directed to the right.

DIDMOAD syndrome (Wolfram's syndrome) Hereditary association of diabetes insipidus, diabetes mellitus, optic atrophy and deafness.

Distal A term of comparison meaning farther from a point of reference; it is the opposite of proximal.

Doppler ultrasound A form of ultrasound that can detect and measure blood flow. Doppler ultrasound depends on the Doppler effect, a change in the frequency of a wave resulting from the motion of a reflector, i.e. the red blood cell in the case of Doppler ultrasound.

Down's syndrome Chromosome disorder associated either with a triplication or translocation of chromosome 21. Clinical manifestations include mental retardation, short stature, flat hypoplastic face with short nose, prominent epicanthic skinfolds, small low-set ears with prominent antihelix, fissured and thickened tongue, laxness of joint ligaments, pelvic dysplasia, broad hands and feet, stubby fingers, transverse palmar crease, lenticular opacities and heart disease. Patients with Down's syndrome have an increased risk for leukaemia, thyroid disorders, coeliac disease and early-onset Alzheimer's disease.

Dupytren's disease   Collagen cords form in the palm and eventually thicken and shorten, causing flexion contractures of the hand. Ring and little fingers are most commonly affected. It is associated with increasing age, alcoholism, diabetes and epilepsy. Treatment for those with severely impaired hand function is fasciotomy.

Dysarthria   Disordered articulation. Any lesion that produces paralysis, slowing or incoordination of the muscles of articulation, or local discomfort, will cause dysarthria. Examples are upper and lower motor lesions of the lower cranial nerves, cerebellar lesions, Parkinson's disease and local lesions in the mouth, larynx, pharynx and tongue.

Dysplasia   Abnormal cell growth or maturation of cells.

Ecchymoses   Bruises >3 mm in diameter.

Ectopic   Located away from its normal position, such as an ectopic pregnancy.

Empirical   Based on experience. Empirical treatment refers to treatment given to an individual that is based on the experience of the physician in treating previous patients with a similar presentation. It is not completely 'scientific' treatment.

End-diastolic volume   The volume of blood in the ventricle at the end of diastole.

Endemic   Present in a community at all times.

Endocrine   Endocrine signalling refers to cells secreting hormones into the bloodstream to exert their action on cells distant to the cell of origin (see also Autocrine and Paracrine signaling).

Endogenous   Related to or produced by the body.

Enzyme-linked immunosorbent (ELISA) assay   A serologic test used for the detection of particular antibodies or antigens in the blood. ELISA technology links a measurable enzyme to either an antigen or antibody. In this way it can then measure the presence of an antibody or an antigen in the bloodstream.

Epidemic   An outbreak of a disease affecting a large number of individuals in a community at the same time. The number of people affected is in excess of the expected.

Epidemiology   The study of the distribution and determinants of health-related states and events in populations.

Epitope   That part of an antigenic molecule to which an antibody or T-cell receptor responds.

Erythema   Redness.

Erythrocyte sedimentation rate   The rate of fall of red cells in a column of blood: a measure of the acute-phase response. The speed is mainly determined by the concentration of large proteins, e.g. fibrinogen. The ESR is higher in women and rises with age. It is raised in a wide variety of systemic inflammatory and neoplastic diseases. The highest values (>100 mm/h) are found in chronic infections (e.g. tuberculosis [TB]), myeloma, connective tissue disorders and cancer.

Erythroderma   Widespread redness of the skin, with scaling.

Euthanasia   The illegal act of killing someone painlessly, especially to relieve suffering from an incurable disease.

Excoriation   Linear marks caused by scratching.

Exogenous   Developed or originated outside of the body.

Exudate   Fluid rich in protein and cells, which has leaked from blood vessels and has been deposited in tissues.

Factitious   Artificial, self-induced.

Familial Mediterranean fever   Inherited disorder more common in those of Mediterranean descent. Recurrent episodes of abdominal pain (due to peritoneal inflammation), fever and arthritis.

Fissure   A cleft, groove or slit: e.g. an anal fissure is an ulcer in the anal canal.

Fistula   A tunnel or abnormal passage connecting two epithelial surfaces, frequently designated according to the organs or parts with which it communicates: e.g. a vesico–colic fistula connects the bladder to the colon.

Fitz-Hugh–Curtis syndrome   Inflammation of the liver capsule associated with genital tract infection – occurs in about 25% of patients with pelvic inflammatory disease. *Neisseria gonorrhoeae* and *Chlamydia trachomatis* are the main causes. Women present with sharp right upper quadrant pain with or without signs of salpingitis. Diagnosis is often clinical and treatment is with appropriate antibiotics.

Gaucher's disease   Inherited (autosomal recessive) disorder of lipid metabolism caused by a deficiency of the enzyme β-glucocerebrosidase. Clinical features include hepatosplenomegaly and sometimes neurological dysfunction.

Generic drugs   Non-proprietary drugs. They should usually be used when prescribing in preference to proprietary titles.

Hallucinations   Perceptions that occur in the absence of external stimuli and while an individual is awake. They may involve any of the senses, including hearing (auditory hallucinations), vision (visual hallucinations), smell (olfactory hallucinations), taste (gustatory hallucinations) and touch (tactile hallucinations). Hallucinations may be drug induced or caused by chronic alcohol excess, temporal lobe epilepsy, psychotic illnesses, or certain organic disorders, such as Huntington's disease.

Histocompatibility antigens   Genetically determined isoantigens present on the membranes of nucleated cells. They incite an immune response when grafted on to genetically disparate individuals, and thus determine the compatibility of cells in transplantation.

Howell–Jolly bodies   DNA remnants in peripheral RBCs seen post-splenectomy and in leukaemia and megaloblastic anaemia.

Human leucocyte antigens (HLA)   Human histocompatibility antigens determined by a region on chromosome 6. There are several genetic loci, each having multiple alleles, designated HLA-A, HLA-B, HLA-C, HLA-DP, -DQ and -DR. The susceptibility to some diseases is associated with certain HLA alleles (e.g. HLA-B27 in 95% of patients with ankylosing spondylitis), although their exact role in aetiology is unclear.

Hyperplasia   The abnormal multiplication or increase in the number of normal cells in normal arrangement in a tissue.

Hypertrophy   The enlargement or overgrowth of an organ or part due to an increase in size of its constituent cells.

Iatrogenic   Induced inadvertently by medical treatment or procedures, or activity of attending physician.

Idiopathic   Of unknown cause.

Idiosyncratic   Relates to idiosyncrasy – an abnormal susceptibility to a drug or other agent which is peculiar to the individual.

Incidence   An expression of the rate at which a certain event occurs, as in the number of new cases of a specific disease occurring during a certain period.

Incubation period   Period between transmission of the infecting organism and the start of symptoms.

Inotropic   Positively inotropic means increasing the force of cardiac muscle contraction.

Insidious   Subtle, gradual, or imperceptible development. It may be used to refer to the onset of symptoms or signs before the diagnosis of a disorder.

In vitro   Outside of the body in an artificial environment such as a test tube.

In vivo   Within the body.

Kawasaki's disease   An acute febrile illness (lasting more than 5 days) of unknown aetiology that occurs mainly in children. Features include damage to the coronary arteries, which is reduced by treatment with aspirin and intravenous γ-globulin.

Macule   A flat circumscribed area of discoloration.

Maculopapule   A raised and discolored circumscribed lesion.

Magnetic resonance imaging (MRI)   Uses the body's natural magnetic properties to produce detailed images from any part of the body. It does not involve radiation. Gadolinium is used as an intravenous contrast medium – rarely causes nephrogenic systemic fibrosis (p. 000) in patients with renal impairment. MRI scanning is potentially life-threatening for patients who have had medical or surgical (or accidental) metal implants (e.g. pacemakers, metallic clips, metal valves and joints) because of potential movement within a magnetic field. A metal check (including foreign bodies in the eye) should be done before requesting an MRI. Some implants are MRI safe and some are not. Most MRI departments will have a comprehensive safety check list of such devices and implants.

Marfan's syndrome   Autosomal dominant connective tissue disorder associated with mutations in the fibrillin 1 gene on chromosome 15. Up to one-third are new mutations. Clinical features include tall stature, long thin digits (arachnodactyly), high-arched palate, hypermobile joints, lens subluxation, incompetence of aortic and mitral valves, aortic dissection and spontaneous pneumothorax.

Ménétrier's disease (giant hypertrophic gastritis)   Gastritis with hypertrophy of the gastric mucosa. Characterized by giant gastric folds, diminished acid secretion, excessive secretion of mucus and hypoproteinaemia. Symptoms include vomiting, diarrhoea and weight loss.

Metaplasia   A change in the type of cells in a tissue to a form which is not normal for that tissue.

Methaemoglobinaemia   A condition in which the iron within haemoglobin is oxidized from the ferrous (Fe^{2+}) state to the ferric (Fe^{3}) state, resulting in the inability to transport oxygen and carbon dioxide. Clinically, there is cyanosis. May be congenital or acquired (after exposure to certain drugs and toxins).

Mirizzi's syndrome   Obstructive jaundice caused by compression of the common hepatic duct by a stone in the cystic duct or the neck of the gall bladder.

Multidisciplinary team (MDT)   A group of healthcare professionals working in a team with clear protocols and management pathways leading to more tailored and efficient patient care. For instance the core elements of a lung cancer MDT would be respiratory physicians, thoracic surgeons, specialist nurses, radiologists, oncologists and palliative care physicians. The specialist nurse usually acts as the key source of support and information for the patient, bridging the gap to the clinical team.

Mutation   A change in a gene, such as loss, gain or substitution of genetic material, which alters its function or expression. This change is passed along with subsequent divisions of the affected cell. Gene mutations may occur randomly for unknown reasons or may be inherited.

National Institute for Health and Care Excellence (NICE)   This is part of the National Health Service (NHS) in the UK and its role is to provide patients, health professionals and the public with authoritative, robust and reliable guidance on current 'best practice'.

nd   Notifiable disease.

Necrosis   Morphological changes indicative of cell death that are caused by the progressive degradative action of enzymes; necrosis may affect groups of cells or part of a structure or an organ.

Nephrogenic systemic fibrosis (see MRI)   Formation of connective tissue in the skin which becomes thickened, coarse and hard and may lead to contractures and joint immobility. Systemic involvement – e.g. of lung, liver, muscles and heart – can occur.

Nodule   A circumscribed large palpable mass >1 cm in diameter.

Objective Structured Clinical Examination (OSCE)   Examination based on planned clinical encounters in which the candidate (student, doctor or nurse) interviews, examines, informs, or otherwise interacts with a standardized patient (SP). SPs are individuals who are scripted and rehearsed to portray an actual patient with a specific set of symptoms or clinical findings. SPs may be able-bodied individuals or actual patients with stable findings.

Oligoarticular   Affecting a limited number of joints.

Oncogene   Gene coding for proteins which are either growth factors, growth factor receptors, secondary messengers or DNA-binding proteins. Mutation of the gene promotes abnormal cell growth.

Osmolality   The concentration of osmotically active particles in solution expressed in terms of osmoles of solute per kilogram of solvent.

Osmolarity   The concentration of osmotically active particles expressed in terms of osmoles of solute per litre of solution.

Papule   A circumscribed raised palpable area.

Paracrine   Paracrine signalling is where a cell secretes a chemical messenger that binds to receptors on cells nearby (see also Autocrine and Endocrine signalling).

Pathognomonic   A symptom or sign that, when present, points unmistakably to the presence of a certain definite disease.

Persistent vegetative state   A condition of life without consciousness or will as a result of brain damage.

Petechiae   Bruises <3 mm in diameter.

Phenotype   The appearance and function of an organism as a result of its genotype and its environment.

Plaque   A disc-shaped lesion that can result from coalescence of papules.

Poikilocytosis   Increased variation in the shape of the red blood cell.

Polychromasia   Blue tinge to red blood cells in the blood film caused by the presence of young red cells.

Polymerase chain reaction (PCR)   Technique for rapid detection and analysis of DNA and, by a modification of the method, RNA. Using oligonucleotide primers and DNA polymerase, minute amounts of genomic DNA can be amplified over a million times into measurable quantities.

Positron emission tomography (PET) scanning   PET facilitates the imaging of structures by virtue of their ability to concentrate specific molecules that have been labelled with a positron-emitting isotope, e.g. a glucose analogue (that is not metabolized by the cell) tagged with fluorine (fluorodeoxyglucose [FDG]). Metabolically active cells, including malignant cells, utilize and import more glucose than other tissues and thus take up FDG more avidly. False positives occur with active infections or inflammatory processes.

Prevalence   Total number of cases of a disease in existence at a certain time in a designated area.

Prognosis   A forecast as to the probable outcome of an attack or disease.

Promyelocytes, myelocytes and metamyelocytes   Immature white cells seen in the peripheral blood in leucoerythroblastic anaemia.

Prophylaxis   Prevention of disease.

Proximal   A term of comparison meaning nearer or closer to a point of reference; for example, proximal myopathy is weakness of muscles nearest to the trunk, e.g. quadriceps.

Purpura   Extravasation of blood into the skin; does not blanch on pressure.

Pustule   A pus-filled blister.

Radioimmunoassay (RIA)   Any system for testing antigen–antibody reactions in which use is made of radioactive labelling of antigen or antibody to detect the extent of the reaction.

Refractory   Resistant to or not responding readily to treatment.

Rhabdomyolysis   The destruction of skeletal muscle cells that may be due to electrical injury, alcoholism, injury, drug side effects or toxins.

Scales   Dried flakes of dead skin.

Serum   The cell-free portion of blood from which fibrinogen has been separated in the process of clotting. Serum is the supernatant obtained by high-speed centrifugation of whole blood collected in a plain tube.

Sinus   A blind track opening onto the skin or a mucous surface.

Stomatocyte   A red blood cell with a central slit (stoma).

Syndrome   A set of signs or a series of events occurring together that point to a single condition as the cause.

Target cells ('Mexican hat cells')   Red blood cells with central staining surrounded by a ring of pallor and an outer ring of staining. They occur in thalassaemia, sickle cell disease and liver disease.

Telangiectasia   A visible, dilated blood vessel creating small focal red lesions in skin, mucous membranes or gut.

Teratogenic   Possessing the ability to disrupt normal fetal development and cause fetal abnormalities.

TNM classification (tumour, node, metastasis)   Staging system for many cancers. T is the extent of primary tumour, N is the involvement of lymph nodes and M indicates the presence or absence of metastases. For instance T0–T4 indicates increasing local tumour spread.

Transudate   A plasma-derived fluid that accumulates in tissues/cavities as a result of venous and capillary pressure.

Tumour suppressor genes   Genes, the protein products of which induce the repair or self-destruction (apoptosis) of cells containing damaged DNA. Unlike oncogenes, they restrict undue cell proliferation.

Turner's syndrome   Females with chromosomes 45X instead of the normal female chromosomes, 46XX. They experience growth failure, gonadal dysgenesis, widely spaced nipples, webbed neck and cardiac abnormalities but their intelligence is usually normal.

Vesicle   A small, visible, fluid-filled blister.

Von Hippel–Lindau syndrome   Autosomal dominant disorder characterized by cerebellar and retinal neoplasms, clear cell renal carcinoma, phaeochromocytoma, pancreatic tumours and inner ear tumours. Associated with germline mutations of the VHL tumour suppressor gene.

Weal   A transiently raised reddened area associated with scratching.

Xenotransplantation   Transplantation of organs or tissues between different species.

Zoonosis   Transmission of a disease from an animal or non-human species to humans. The reservoir for the disease is not human.

Index

Note: Page numbers followed by *f* indicate figures, *t* indicate tables and *b* indicate boxes.

W

X

Y

Z